Health Care from Patients' Perspective

Health Care from Patients' Perspective

Editor

Andrea Glässel

MDPI • Basel • Beijing • Wuhan • Barcelona • Belgrade • Manchester • Tokyo • Cluj • Tianjin

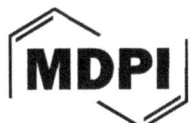

Editor
Andrea Glässel
University of Zurich
Zürich, Switzerland

Editorial Office
MDPI
St. Alban-Anlage 66
4052 Basel, Switzerland

This is a reprint of articles from the Special Issue published online in the open access journal *International Journal of Environmental Research and Public Health* (ISSN 1660-4601) (available at: https://www.mdpi.com/journal/ijerph/special_issues/health_care_patients_perspective).

For citation purposes, cite each article independently as indicated on the article page online and as indicated below:

LastName, A.A.; LastName, B.B.; LastName, C.C. Article Title. *Journal Name* **Year**, *Volume Number*, Page Range.

ISBN 978-3-0365-7286-4 (Hbk)
ISBN 978-3-0365-7287-1 (PDF)

© 2023 by the authors. Articles in this book are Open Access and distributed under the Creative Commons Attribution (CC BY) license, which allows users to download, copy and build upon published articles, as long as the author and publisher are properly credited, which ensures maximum dissemination and a wider impact of our publications.
The book as a whole is distributed by MDPI under the terms and conditions of the Creative Commons license CC BY-NC-ND.

Contents

About the Editor . . . . **vii**

Preface to "Health Care from Patients' Perspective" . . . . **ix**

Yolanda María Chacón Gámez, Florian Brugger and Nikola Biller-Andorno
Parkinson's Disease and Deep Brain Stimulation Have an Impact on My Life: A Multimodal Study on the Experiences of Patients and Family Caregivers
Reprinted from: *Int. J. Environ. Res. Public Health* **2021**, *18*, 9516, doi:10.3390/ijerph18189516 . . . **1**

Joelle Ott, Nikola Biller-Andorno and Andrea Glässel
First Insights into Barriers and Facilitators from the Perspective of Persons with Multiple Sclerosis: A Multiple Case Study
Reprinted from: *Int. J. Environ. Res. Public Health* **2022**, *19*, 10733, doi:10.3390/ijerph191710733 . **39**

Fabienne Schmid, Slavko Rogan and Andrea Glässel
A Swiss Health Care Professionals' Perspective on the Meaning of Interprofessional Collaboration in Health Care of People with MS—A Focus Group Study
Reprinted from: *Int. J. Environ. Res. Public Health* **2021**, *18*, 6537, doi:10.3390/ijerph18126537 . . . **61**

Laura Lorenz, Franziska Krebs, Farah Nawabi, Adrienne Alayli and Stephanie Stock
Preventive Counseling in Routine Prenatal Care—A Qualitative Study of Pregnant Women's Perspectives on a Lifestyle Intervention, Contrasted with the Experiences of Healthcare Providers
Reprinted from: *Int. J. Environ. Res. Public Health* **2022**, *19*, 6122, doi:10.3390/ijerph19106122 . . . **77**

Doris Arnold, Andrea Glässel, Tabea Böttger, Navina Sarma, Andreas Bethmann and Petra Narimani
"What Do You Need? What Are You Experiencing?" Relationship Building and Power Dynamics in Participatory Research Projects: Critical Self-Reflections of Researchers
Reprinted from: *Int. J. Environ. Res. Public Health* **2022**, *19*, 9336, doi:10.3390/ijerph19159336 . . . **101**

Tabea Böttger, Silke Dennhardt, Julia Knape and Ulrike Marotzki
"Back into Life—With a Power Wheelchair": Learning from People with Severe Stroke through a Participatory Photovoice Study in a Metropolitan Area in Germany
Reprinted from: *Int. J. Environ. Res. Public Health* **2022**, *19*, 10465, doi:10.3390/ijerph191710465 . **127**

Shan Jiang, Udday Datta and Christine Jones
Promoting Health and Behavior Change through Evidence-Based Landscape Interventions in Rural Communities: A Pilot Protocol
Reprinted from: *Int. J. Environ. Res. Public Health* **2022**, *19*, 12833, doi:10.3390/ijerph191912833 . **153**

Eun-Jeong Kim, Inn-Chul Nam and Yoo-Ri Koo
Reframing Patient Experience Approaches and Methods to Achieve Patient-Centeredness in Healthcare: Scoping Review
Reprinted from: *Int. J. Environ. Res. Public Health* **2022**, *19*, 9163, doi:10.3390/ijerph19159163 . . . **167**

Seth Ayisi Addo, Reidar Johan Mykletun and Espen Olsen
Validation and Adjustment of the Patient Experience Questionnaire (PEQ): A Regional Hospital Study in Norway
Reprinted from: *Int. J. Environ. Res. Public Health* **2021**, *18*, 7141, doi:10.3390/ijerph18137141 . . . **187**

Faten Amer, Sahar Hammoud, David Onchonga, Abdulsalam Alkaiyat, Abdulnaser Nour, Dóra Endrei and Imre Boncz
Assessing Patient Experience and Attitude: BSC-PATIENT Development, Translation, and Psychometric Evaluation—A Cross-Sectional Study
Reprinted from: *Int. J. Environ. Res. Public Health* **2022**, *19*, 7149, doi:10.3390/ijerph19127149 . . . 207

Anna Maria Hage, Pimrapat Gebert, Friedrich Kühn, Therese Pross, Ulrike Grittner and Maria Margarete Karsten
Examining the Feasibility of an Application-Based Patient-Reported Outcome Monitoring for Breast Cancer Patients: A Pretest for the PRO B Study
Reprinted from: *Int. J. Environ. Res. Public Health* **2022**, *19*, 8284, doi:10.3390/ijerph19148284 . . . 237

Sarah H. Al-Mazidi and Laila Y. Al-Ayadhi
National Profile of Caregivers' Perspectives on Autism Spectrum Disorder Screening and Care in Primary Health Care: The Need for Autism Medical Home
Reprinted from: *Int. J. Environ. Res. Public Health* **2021**, *18*, 13043, doi:10.3390/ijerph182413043 . 245

Susanne Schnitzer, Raphael Kohl, Hella Fügemann, Kathrin Gödde, Judith Stumm, Fabian Engelmann, et al.
Patient Navigation—Who Needs What? Awareness of Patient Navigators and Ranking of Their Tasks in the General Population in Germany
Reprinted from: *Int. J. Environ. Res. Public Health* **2022**, *19*, 2846, doi:10.3390/ijerph19052846 . . . 259

Charity Ngoatle and Tebogo Maria Mothiba
How Is It to Live with Diabetes Mellitus? The Voices of the Diabetes Mellitus Clients
Reprinted from: *Int. J. Environ. Res. Public Health* **2022**, *19*, 9638, doi:10.3390/ijerph19159638 . . . 273

Maya Maor, Moflah Ataika, Pesach Shvartzman and Maya Lavie Ajayi
"I Had to Rediscover Our Healthy Food": An Indigenous Perspective on Coping with Type 2 Diabetes Mellitus
Reprinted from: *Int. J. Environ. Res. Public Health* **2022**, *19*, 159, doi:10.3390/ijerph19010159 . . . 283

Gregory A. Thompson, Jonathan Segura, Dianne Cruz, Cassie Arnita and Leeann H. Whiffen
Cultural Differences in Patients' Preferences for Paternalism: Comparing Mexican and American Patients' Preferences for and Experiences with Physician Paternalism and Patient Autonomy
Reprinted from: *Int. J. Environ. Res. Public Health* **2022**, *19*, 10663, doi:10.3390/ijerph191710663 . 299

Barbara Groot, Annyk Haveman, Mireille Buree, Ruud van Zuijlen, Juliette van Zuijlen and Tineke Abma
What Patients Prioritize for Research to Improve Their Lives and How Their Priorities Get Dismissed again
Reprinted from: *Int. J. Environ. Res. Public Health* **2022**, *19*, 1927, doi:10.3390/ijerph19041927 . . . 323

Sean A. Aspinall, Kelly A. Mackintosh, Denise M. Hill, Bethany Cope and Melitta A. McNarry
Evaluating the Effect of Kaftrio on Perspectives of Health and Wellbeing in Individuals with Cystic Fibrosis
Reprinted from: *Int. J. Environ. Res. Public Health* **2022**, *19*, 6114, doi:10.3390/ijerph19106114 . . . 339

Isabel Baumann, Frank Wieber, Thomas Volken, Peter Rüesch and Andrea Glässel
Interprofessional Collaboration in Fall Prevention: Insights from a Qualitative Study
Reprinted from: *Int. J. Environ. Res. Public Health* **2022**, *19*, 10477, doi:10.3390/ijerph191710477 . 353

About the Editor

Andrea Glässel

Since July 2017, Andrea Glässel has been a research associate at the Institute for Biomedical Ethics and History of Medicine (IBME). She is working in the group of DIPEx Swiss (Database of Individual Patient Experiences). In 2017, she received her DIPEx certificate from the Nuffield Department of Primary Care Health Sciences of the University of Oxford, focusing on qualitative research into people's experiences of health and illness. In addition to her research at IBME, Andrea has been a lecturer and researcher in qualitative research methods and interprofessional teachings at the Department of Health Sciences, Institute of Public Health (IPH), Zurich Applied University of Sciences (ZHAW) since 2015. In 2017 she was appointed Professor of Interprofessional Collaboration and Communication at ZHAW.

Andrea has been a qualified physiotherapist for 32 years. She has worked for ten years in outpatient and inpatient settings, including five years as director of an interprofessional motor neurorehabilitation unit. 2001 Andrea completed her Bachelor's in physical therapy at the University of Applied Sciences and Arts in Hildesheim, Germany. She also completed a semester at the Faculty of Health at Linköping University, Sweden. Andrea also holds a Master's in Neurorehabilitation from the Danube University in Krems, Austria, a master's in public health from the University of Bielefeld, Germany, and received a master's in applied Ethics with a focus on Biomedical Ethics in 2022. 2012 she completed her Ph.D. in Human Biology at the Ludwig-Maximilians-University, Munich, Germany. Her topic was "Functioning and Disability after Stroke: The Perspective of Patients and Healthcare Professionals".

Her research interests are:

Health experiences from patient and health professional perspective

Illness Narratives and Qualitative Research

Interprofessional Collaboration in the rehabilitation and health care settings

International Classification of Functioning, Disability, and Health (ICF)

Preface to "Health Care from Patients' Perspective"

We have initiated this Special Issue, entitled "Health Care from the Patient's Perspective", in the *International Journal of Environmental Research and Public Health*, a peer-reviewed journal that publishes articles and communications in the interdisciplinary field of environmental health sciences and public health. Detailed information about the journal can be found at https://www.mdpi.com/journal/ijerph.

This *IJERPH* Special Issue—"Health Care from the Patient's Perspective"—focuses on the perspective of patients as experts, on their challenges and experiences with health care, embedded in a biopsychosocial framework. In doing so, the Special Issue offers contributions across the entire health and disease continuum, ranging from health promotion to rehabilitation and the outpatient setting. These issues are described from different perspectives on disease-related situations such as Parkinson's disease, stroke, or multiple sclerosis, diabetes mellitus, and others. These works highlight methodological innovations, with a focus on qualitative, but also participatory research as well as quantitative approaches. Experiential research forms the core of this issue. The articles within will not only provide insights into complex health care situations and ethical issues, but also highlight patient-centered problems as a possible starting point for health system and/or policy improvement. Additionally, this Special Issue will take an interprofessional perspective on patients' care providers, family members, and caregivers.

This Special Issue includes high-quality articles on health and illness stories, focusing particularly on health-related topics based on qualitative research. This includes participatory research methods from across the spectrum of health care, such as health promotion, prevention, chronic disease, or rehabilitation. Also, contributions to reviews, especially to a scoping review, is part of this issue.

We would like to thank all the authors who published their contributions in the Special Issue and who are instrumental in shaping every issue with us. We received 19 impressive and important contributions to healthcare that we encourage all to read. We further thank all reviewers for their time in assisting us with a comprehensive peer review.

We would be pleased if this Special Issue serves as a trigger for the provision insightful data on the design of teaching-relevant studies, based on narratives used in study programs for health professionals such as therapists, nurses, midwives, physicians, and other professions. We hope you enjoy reading the issue.

Andrea Glässel
Editor

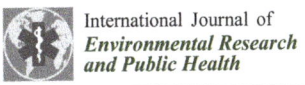

Article

Parkinson's Disease and Deep Brain Stimulation Have an Impact on My Life: A Multimodal Study on the Experiences of Patients and Family Caregivers

Yolanda María Chacón Gámez [1,*], Florian Brugger [2] and Nikola Biller-Andorno [1]

1 Institute of Medical Bioethics and History of Medicine, University of Zurich, Wintherthurerstrasse 30, 8006 Zurich, Switzerland; biller-andorno@ibme.uzh.ch
2 Kantonsspital St. Gallen, Klinik für Neurologie, Haus 04 Rorsacher Strasse 95, 9007 St. Gallen, Switzerland; florian.brugger@kssg.ch
* Correspondence: Yolanda.chacon@ibme.uzh.ch

Abstract: Parkinson's disease (PD) has a large impact on patients' physical and mental health, which also greatly affects their family caregivers. Deep brain stimulation (DBS) has emerged as an effective treatment for PD, but different authors have expressed their concerns about the potential impact of DBS on personality and identity. Our study aims at better understanding how patients and family caregivers experience life with PD and DBS, the impact of both on their personal and social lives, and their perception of the changes that have occurred as a result of the disease and the treatment. Our study applies a multimodal approach by means of narrative semi-structured interviews and drawings. Seven principal themes have been identified: "everyone's Parkinson's is different", "changing as a person during the disease", "going through Parkinson's together", "DBS improved my life", "I am treated with DBS but I have Parkinson's still", "DBS is not perfect", and "being different after DBS". PD is perceived as an unpredictable and heterogeneous disease that changes from person to person, as does the effect of DBS. While DBS side-effects may have an impact on patients' personality, behavior, and self-perception, PD symptoms and drug side-effects also have a great impact on these aspects.

Keywords: deep brain stimulation; drawings; Parkinson's disease; qualitative methods; patients' and family caregivers' narratives; personality; post-operative changes

Citation: Chacón Gámez, Y.M.; Brugger, F.; Biller-Andorno, N. Parkinson's Disease and Deep Brain Stimulation Have an Impact on My Life: A Multimodal Study on the Experiences of Patients and Family Caregivers. *Int. J. Environ. Res. Public Health* **2021**, *18*, 9516. https://doi.org/10.3390/ijerph18189516

Academic Editor: Andrea Glässel

Received: 6 May 2021
Accepted: 21 July 2021
Published: 9 September 2021

Publisher's Note: MDPI stays neutral with regard to jurisdictional claims in published maps and institutional affiliations.

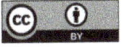

Copyright: © 2021 by the authors. Licensee MDPI, Basel, Switzerland. This article is an open access article distributed under the terms and conditions of the Creative Commons Attribution (CC BY) license (https://creativecommons.org/licenses/by/4.0/).

1. Introduction

Parkinson's disease (PD) is one of the most common neurodegenerative disorders [1]. From 1990 to 2015, the number of people with PD doubled to over 6 million, and it is estimated to double to over 12 million by 2040 [2]. Although the incidence of PD increases with age, rising sharply around the age of 65, it does not affect only older individuals because cases of people with PD under 50 are not uncommon [2–4]. PD has become over the past two centuries one of the best-investigated disorders in neurology. It was first described in 1817 by James Parkinson when reporting six cases of 'shaking palsy', which was the term used at the time to refer to the phenomenology of disease [5]. In his monograph, he provided an already detailed description of this disorder including non-motor symptoms. A century later, Charcot provided a detailed description of this disorder including a description of non-motor symptoms associated with PD, which facilitated the diagnosis of PD worldwide [6]. Although PD is widely known for its motor and axial symptoms (e.g., tremor, slow movement, muscular rigidity, or postural instability) caused by the loss of striatal dopaminergic neurons, nonmotor symptoms are also very characteristic of PD and are due to the loss of non-dopaminergic neurons [7,8]. The non-motor manifestations of PD are very heterogeneous and can appear several years before the first motor symptoms [3,6]. They include fatigue, autonomic dysfunction (e.g., constipation, sexual dysfunction, or urinary retention), neuropsychiatric symptoms (e.g., anxiety, depression, dementia, or hallucinations), sensory symptoms (e.g., pain), and sleep disturbances (e.g., insomnia, REM-sleep behavior disorder or restless legs syndrome) [9,10]. Communication impairment is also common in PD and is associated with both motor and cognitive dysfunction [11,12]. All these symptoms have a large impact on PD patients' physical and mental health, which can alter their individual and social identities and lead to a loss of autonomy and self-esteem, altered relationships, and social isolation [13]. Furthermore, it is a disease with a significant economic burden on society, payers, patients, and caregivers [14,15].

Motor and non-motor symptoms are managed through a variety of pharmacological treatments that include dopamine-based therapies for PD motor symptoms (e.g., levodopa, dopamine agonists) and nondopaminergic approaches (e.g., cholinesterase inhibitors, selective serotonin reuptake inhibitors) for nonmotor manifestations of PD. However, it has been known for a long time that under long-term levodopa therapy, patients often develop fluctuations in their motor performance ("wearing-off effect") and dyskinesia [16]. Strategies to manage these complications include adding a dopamine agonist or inhibitors of levodopa-degrading enzymes such as catechol-O-methyltransferase or monoamine oxidase B inhibitors as adjuncts. However, these agents may also cause adverse side effects including a worsening of non-motor symptoms such as hallucinations, impulse control disorders, or gastrointestinal discomfort [17].

Device-aided therapies such as deep brain stimulation (DBS) can manage motor symptoms and improve the quality of life of patients with refractory tremor [18] or who suffer from intolerable side effects from oral treatment (e.g., dyskinesias from levodopa [19] or impulse control disorders from dopamine agonists [20]). Deep brain stimulation (DBS) emerged in the late 1960s as a possible therapeutic alternative for patients with chronic pain. In 1987, it was introduced as a therapy for PD by the French neurosurgeon Alim Benabid [21]. In 1997, the US Food and Drug Administration (FDA) approved the first DBS implant to treat tremor in PD and essential tremor [22]. In 2003, this approval was extended to treat other symptoms of PD. To date, this intervention is approved as a standard treatment by the European Union CE mark for PD, essential tremor, dystonia, obsessive compulsive disorder, and epilepsy [23], and several clinical studies are underway worldwide to extend the use of DBS to the treatment of other neurological and psychiatric diseases such as Tourette's Syndrome [24] or treatment-resistant depression [25]. Although DBS has emerged over the past two decades as a treatment for both neurological and neuropsychiatric disorders, the main medical indication for DBS use is still represented by patients with PD [26].

DBS requires an invasive neurosurgical intervention that involves the insertion of electrodes deep into the brain, which are connected to a pulse generator placed in the chest region [27]. The device generates electrical pulses that stimulate a defined area of the brain. The most common stimulation targets for PD are the subthalamic nucleus (STN) or the globus pallidus internus (GPi) [28]. Therefore, this procedure works similarly to a pacemaker but for the brain [29]. In the bioethics literature, there is controversy about whether DBS has an impact on personality or identity. While different authors have expressed their concerns about the potential impact of DBS on personality and identity [30–32], others argue that there is not enough scientific evidence supporting this claim [33]. However, some quantitative studies show significant changes in personality and mood after applying DBS in PD [34,35]. We agree with other authors that pre-determined scales or standardized questionnaires may not capture the magnitude of all the changes in personality, identity, or self-perception that patients may face while being treated with DBS [36,37]. These changes could be due not only to DBS side effects but also to its interaction with PD progression and oral medication, as many patients continue to require medication, although usually in lower doses than before DBS intervention [7]. Furthermore, the changes that the patient undergoes are not only due to the disease or the treatment directly but also due to the process of adaptation that the patient goes through to become used to them [38]. Therefore, both from a clinical and from an ethics point of view, we consider it necessary to better understand qualitatively the experience of both having PD and being treated for it with DBS not only quantitatively but also qualitatively [39].

Although healthcare research is very much dominated by evidence based on quantitative research methods, qualitative approaches complement the medical doctors' work in clinical routine because the approach applied by health professionals when seeing patient in day-to-day medical practice (e.g., when taking medical history) resembles methods used in qualitative research (e.g., interviews). Therefore, the results of qualitative studies are of great interest for neurologists and other clinicians as they serve to better understand the patients' needs and tailor individualized treatment (e.g., choosing between DBS or medical pumps to treat motor fluctuations and dyskinesias). The available qualitative studies in the field have typically focused either on specific aspects of PD [40–42], the perception of DBS [38,43], or some side effects of DBS affecting patients' personality or identity [44–46]. However, there are few studies with a comprehensive approach encompassing the patients' experiences with both PD and DBS and deepening their perception of both [37,47]. To our knowledge, no qualitative studies have yet been carried out applying a multimodal approach [48].

Our study aims at collecting and analyzing a wide range of experiences of PD patients treated with DBS and their family caregivers. We applied a multimodal approach by means of narrative semi-structured interviews and drawings to better understand how they experience life with PD and DBS and the impact of both on their personal and social lives. We decided to include the point of view of family caregivers (FCs) because their experiences are a highly valuable source of knowledge for two reasons [49,50]. First, FCs are sometimes more sensitive to changes in the patients caused by either disease or therapy than patients themselves, and hence their experiences are of great value to complement the patient's account [51]. Second, FCs provide daily care at home with PD and the different treatments for it, which modifies their personal routine and social life. Therefore, it is also worth to explore the impact of the disease and the treatment on the FCs' personal lives.

This paper will present the experiences of nineteen patients and seventeen FCs with PD and DBS. We will first present our methodology and after the following themes will be covered: "everyone's Parkinson's is different", "changing as a person during the disease", "going through Parkinson's together", "DBS improved my life", "I am treated with DBS but I still have Parkinson's", "DBS is not perfect", and "being different after DBS". Next, we will discuss our results and the strengths, limitations, and relevance for future research of our study. Finally, we will present our conclusions.

2. Materials and Methods

The set of data presented in this study is part of a bigger qualitative study conducted in Switzerland between 2018 and 2020, which explores a wide range of experiences of 44 patients and family caregivers with PD and two device-aided treatments: DBS and intrajejunal infusion of levodopa (known commercially as Duodopa® pump). It applies a multimodal approach including narrative semi-structured interviews and drawings. This approach allowed a better exploration of the participants' perception of PD and device-aided treatments incorporating both language-based and nonverbal communication. This study identified four groups of experiences reported by the patients and their family caregivers that can be classified in the following way: daily life and perception of PD and the effects of device-aided treatments, self-perception, social interaction and partnership/family dynamics, and experiences with different healthcare professionals including the receipt of PD diagnosis and the specific health needs of PD patients [52]. Due to the enormous amount of data obtained with this study and the different research questions we had, we decided to divide the results into three articles answering different questions [52,53]. Therefore, this article will focus on the first three categories mentioned above that are related to the experiences of PD patients treated with DBS and their FCs.

2.1. Researcher Characteristics and Reflexivity

The interviews have been conducted and analyzed by Researcher 1 (the first author) and Researcher 2. Researcher 1 (R1) is a PhD candidate working full time on the study from which this paper is derived. Researcher 2 (R2) is a postdoctoral researcher with extensive experience in qualitative methods. Both researchers are female and have been trained in DIPEx methodology [54]. There was no previous relationship between the researchers and the study participants. The participants did not know the professional characteristics of the researchers until the end of the interview.

2.2. Recruitment and Collaborations

The study has been conducted in collaboration with the Department of Neurology of different Swiss hospitals (Kantonspital St Gallen, Luzerner Kantonspital, and the University Hospital of Lausanne). We chose maximum variation purposeful sampling for the selection of participants to identify the individuals whose experiences were especially informative and would vary from each other as much as possible [55]. We therefore include participants from different parts of Switzerland with different symptoms and disease progression, different length of time with the disease and treatment, and different family environments and lifestyles. The participants were recruited through a combination of neurologists, PD nurses, and patients' support groups belonging to the Swiss Parkinson's association (Parkinson Schweiz).

For better dissemination of these results, they are part of the International Database of Patients Experiences research initiative (DIPEx International). This platform applies an established narrative method developed by the Health Experiences Research Group at the Nuffield Department of Primary Care at the University of Oxford [54]. The international DIPEx network comprises fourteen countries implementing their own national DIPEx platforms, which are based on qualitative studies. The aim of DIPEx is to present to a wide public (patients, family caregivers, health professionals, and students) a wide spectrum of diverse perspectives about different illnesses and health conditions [56,57]. Therefore, the Selected Material of the presented data in this paper will be uploaded to the Swiss DIPEx website in 2022 (www.dipex.ch, accessed on 4 May 2021) [53].

2.3. Study Population and Inclusion Criteria

A total of thirty-six Swiss people, including nineteen patients and seventeen FCs, participated in the study. In Table 1, the description of the patients (e.g., average age at interview, average age at diagnosis) can be found. One of the patients was treated simultaneously with DBS and the Duodopa® pump (DP). Fourteen of the interviewed FCs were spouses of the patients, two of them were children (one son and one daughter), and one was the mother in law of one of the patients. Three participants participated alone. For two of them, the reason was that neither their spouses nor their children wanted to participate, and the other participant had no family in Switzerland. One of the FCs also participated alone because her husband was physically unable to participate in an interview. However, the patient was aware that his wife would participate in the study and agreed that she should share their story.

Table 1. Description of DBS patients and FCs. [a] Averages are given in the order range, mean, and median.

Group	Average Age at Diagnosis [a]	Number	Average Age at Interview [a]	Gender (F, M)	Average Years with DBS [a]
Patients	37–71, 50.4, 50	19	54–75, 67.2, 71	6, 13	1–10, 4.7, 2
FCs	21–65, 48.7, 48	17	30–88, 64.2, 64	13, 4	-

The inclusion criteria were as follows: (i) patients diagnosed with PD or relatives providing care to a PD patient and (ii) patients treated with DBS for at least six months or family caregivers providing care to PD patients treated with DBS for at least six months. The following exclusion criteria were applied: (i) lack of legal competency, (ii) people experiencing moderate or severe dementia or experiencing substance addiction at the moment of the interview, (iii) and lack of physical and psychological resilience to participate in an interview or difficulties interacting with an interviewer [53]. The inclusion and exclusion criteria were first evaluated and applied by the healthcare professionals that helped us to recruit our participants. They conducted a previous assessment of the participants who, according to their medical judgement, qualified for the study. Hereafter, R1 received a list of participants from the healthcare professionals and contacted the participants by telephone to make the appointment and ensure that the participants were able to maintain a rich conversation for a long time. To this aim, they were asked some questions about the disease and the treatment over the phone to ensure that they could share their experiences over different time frames (pre-disease, post-disease, and post DBS treatment).

2.4. Informed Consent Process

The participants were informed in great detail about the study before participating. On the day of the interview, they signed the informed consent form that allowed us to proceed with the interview and its subsequent analysis for our qualitative research. In this form, they also expressed their preference between being video- or audiotaped. After the interview, the participants received the interview transcripts for verification and the second informed consent form, through which they could accept or reject the use of the interview—either in video, audio, or text format—for the DIPEx website [54,56]. As a result, the number of participants in the DIPEx platform will be less than the number of participants in the study ($n = 26/36$ patients).

2.5. Data Collection

We applied a multimodal approach that includes the conduction of narrative semi-structured interviews and the collection of drawings. This multimodal methodology allows the collection of data about the experience with the disease and the treatment, incorporating both language-based and nonverbal communication to express their individual experiences and give them meaning [48,53,58]. We collected the data of the presented dataset, collecting drawings and conducting thirty-six interviews, of which thirty were conducted in 2019 and six took place in 2020. The German interviews were conducted by the first author (Researcher 1) and the French interviews by one of the members of our team (Researcher 2). The average duration of the interviews was 66 min for the patients and 53 min for the FCs. The duration of the interviews ranged from 27 min to 150 min. This duration does not include the time devoted to drawings. We conducted thirty interviews in German (with some parts in Swiss German) and six in French.

Thirty-two interviews were conducted at the participants' homes, one was carried out in the nursing home where the patient lived, and three took place in our institute. They were conducted alone with the participant or in the company of the spouse, depending on the participant's desire. Given that this study is part of the DIPEx databank, the narrative DIPEx method developed by the research group of the department of Public Health of the University of Oxford was applied to conduct the interviews [54,56]. Therefore, all interviews started with a narrative part to learn about the participants' individual experiences, which was introduced with the following question: "Could you explain your experience with PD and DBS since the beginning?". This question gave the participants great freedom to put their personal narrative into words [53].

This narrative part was further explored and complemented by semi-structured questions in the second part of the interview, which were structured in two sections. The first one was focused on the impact of PD on the participants' lives (either as a patient or FC), including aspects such as the perception of PD, coping strategies, the experience with previous treatments (normally oral medication), and changes in self-perception, social life, and/or partnership/family dynamics due to PD. The second section comprehended questions focused on the participants' perception of the DBS effects, their daily life with the treatment (either as patient or FC), the reasons to choose DBS as treatment, and the aspects that have improved or worsened with therapy. It also included changes in self-perception, social life, and/or partnership/family dynamics due to DBS. An extract of the interview guide for patients translated into English can be found in Appendix A Figure A1.

To offer additional insights to the researcher into the patients' and FCs' experiences with PD and DBS, we employed the drawings as a complementary qualitative method to the semi-structured interviews [53]. We collected drawings from 23 participants (14 patients and 9 FCs), and each of them made two drawings (one about their perception of the disease and another about the perception of DBS). One person only made the drawing about the perception of DBS. Therefore, we collected a total of 45 drawings. Thirteen participants opted not to draw due to physical incapability or the lack of a visual image of the disease or therapy. Although other authors asked their participants to draw after the interview [59], we decided to ask our participants to draw before conducting the interview to provide our participants with the opportunity to reflect on their own story before recounting it. We considered that this preliminary reflection would contribute to enriching the results obtained from the study [53]. Both patients and FCs were invited to draw and received a sketching pencil, a set of twelve color pencils, an eraser, and two pieces of paper. It was not required that the participants would know how to draw, as the only important thing was that what they drew had a meaning for them that they could explain. During the interview, the participants who drew were asked different questions about the drawings they made [53].

2.6. Data Analysis

We performed data analysis, applying a hybrid process of inductive and deductive thematic analysis, which required a continuous back and forth between data collection and data analysis [52,60,61]. To proceed with the analysis, the interviews were transcribed verbatim by our team of trained transcribers based on established rules [54]. After the participants' verification, we fed the transcripts and the drawings into the qualitative data analysis software MAXQDA, which allowed us to perform multimodal analysis. After a first reading of each interview to familiarize with our data, we read every transcript several times while thematically coding the data using a coding scheme (coding tree). This coding tree was primarily created based on the interview guide, which served as a template [62]. For this reason, twelve initial codes were created from the questions included in the interview guide. These initial codes were the following: the meaning of drawings, getting the diagnosis, life with PD, the decision to undergo DBS, the DBS intervention, life with DBS, technical issues of DBS, relationships, wishes for the future, experiences with the medical team or in healthcare settings, suggestions or recommendations, and the reasons to participate in the study. This deductive approach was adopted in order to answer our research questions that sought to assess whether our findings were in line with the concerns expressed in the bioethics literature, which will be addressed in the discussion.

As we analyzed the interviews, we added more sub-codes within the initial codes created from the interview guide. In this way, the coding tree was continuously enriched with sub-codes that emerged from the interview transcripts and drawings (mix coding). Every time that we created a new sub-code, we reviewed all coded segments to ensure homogeneity within the entire data set [63]. This way, the concepts that we used to develop the final coding tree stemmed from the participants' life experiences collected through semi-structured interviews and drawings, which were subsequently systematized, categorized, and analyzed following the coding tree [53,56]. Therefore, the analysis required a continuous back and forth between data collection and analysis to allow a constant comparison of the participants' experiences and perspectives [64]. An extract of the final coding treatment can be found in Appendix A Figure A2.

Once we had analyzed all interviews and completed our coding tree, we sorted our codes into the descriptive themes presented in Table 2. We reviewed all themes to ensure that all extracts supported the theme and to avoid contradictions. We are aware that our themes allowed further abstraction, but we decided to stay with the descriptive themes that we present in this paper because they allowed us to more easily perform the next stage of the analysis in order to select the material for the Swiss DIPEx website. However, we do not rule out the possibility of a secondary study in the future to further develop themes that will allow us to further differentiate between the different nuances of our results.

Table 2. Descriptive themes.

1. Everyone's Parkinson is different	1.1. Different symptoms and disease duration 1.2. Different perception of the disease 1.3. Different reaction to drugs 1.4. Different difficulties and changes that led to different daily routines 1.5. Different impact on the family and couple relationships and on social life 1.6. Different coping strategies
2. Changing through PD together	
3. Changing as a person during the disease	
4. DBS improved my life	
5. I am treated with DBS, but I still have PD	
6. DBS is not perfect	
7. Being different after DBS	

The method for selection of relevant material for the DIPEx platforms is called the "one sheet of paper" (OSOP) method. It involves reading through each section of coded data for each topic and summarizing on a single sheet of paper the key points of all interviews in relation to the same topic [56,57]. The resulting text will constitute the summary of the different topics for the website. The website will be organized into the categories derived from the coding tree (e.g., PD symptoms, patients' or caregivers' difficulties with PD, work life with PD). All texts and video or audio clips on the website will be classified into these categories [53,54].

2.7. Quality Assurance of Data

Two interview guides were created, one for patients and one for FCs, which were tested before conducting the first interview to ensure that interview questions align with research questions. A total of 16% of the interviews were coded and analyzed by R1 and R2. They were first coded and analyzed by R2, and then by R1. Finally, both researchers reviewed both analyses, and after a thorough discussion, they decided on the final coding and analysis of this set of interviews. The rest of the interviews were coded and analyzed only by R1. The final coding tree was checked by another member of our team to ensure trustworthiness.

2.8. Ethical Concerns and Data Management

The study participants were not at risk of any physical harm and did not directly benefit from the study. We conducted this study in compliance with the current version of the Declaration of Helsinki, the ICH-GCP, and ISO EN 14155 (as far as applicable), as well as all national legal and regulatory requirements. The study has been reviewed by the ethics review committee of the Canton of Zurich, which considered that it did not fall under the Swiss Law on Human Subjects Research. Therefore, after consultation with the national working group of Swiss ethics review committees, the committee issued a nation-wide waiver (BASEC-Nr. req-2018-00050).

We handled all data confidentially, and only persons who were directly involved in the data collection, transcription, or data analysis had access to them. The data were stored in a server provided by our institute, and we performed data anonymization, saving the data of each participant by giving them a code (e.g., P1, FC1...). We also deleted from the transcripts any information that could lead to the personal identification of participants [53]. Only R1 has access to the document with the identification of the participants, which is encrypted for added privacy protection. In order to present our results in this paper, we translated the selected quotations of the interviews that were not conducted in English using the DeepL Pro Translator. The translated data were not stored by DeepL, and all translations were compliant with our data protection regulations. The final translations were verified by a native speaker to ensure accurate translation of the original quotes.

3. Results

The study revealed seven overarching descriptive themes, which contain different subthemes. These themes can be found in Table 2.

3.1. Everyone's Parkinson's Is Different

PD was considered by virtually all the participants to be a disease that presents itself in a vastly different way to each person and to which everyone reacts differently.

3.1.1. Different Symptoms and Disease Progression

The symptoms experienced by the participants were very diverse and varied considerably from patient to patient. The most frequently mentioned symptoms were tremor, uncontrolled movements (dyskinesia), weight loss, fatigue, decreased facial expression, freezing of movement, sleeping disturbances, becoming slower, and having difficulties when walking (e.g., taking small steps) or talking (e.g., speaking too softly or not clearly). Many of the patients who experienced stiffness or walking difficulties did not experience tremors. Weight loss occurred more frequently in people who experienced dyskinesia. Other symptoms, reported by fewer people, were dizziness, shoulder pain, urinary incontinence, swallowing problems, and memory problems. Non-medication-related psychiatric symptoms and mood swings like touchiness, irritability, aggressivity, hallucinations, depressive episodes, and substance addiction were also reported.

> "I saw sand flowing from anywhere but in a closed circuit. It never stops (...) or I saw a black dog under the table at the hospital. There, I had a concentration of hallucinations from everyone. The doctors who came to see me at first that I was having these hallucinations, they had spaghetti hanging out". (P44)

Suffering from psychological or psychiatric manifestations of PD were pointed out as a concern that patients have:

> "Many people with Parkinson's disease say that if they have psychological problems from the disease, either from or with or because of the disease, it is much worse than if they tremble and cannot walk well. And I think that too". (P27)

One FC described how changes in mood can trigger PD motor symptoms:

> "About 15 years ago, she made a mistake with our boat and hit a buoy at high speed. Then the water police came (...) She was trembling all over her body and I have never seen her like this. That frightened me very much and since then, it happens whenever she gets upset (...) When she is tense, she has such uncontrolled movements. I first noticed in 2004 that when she is very excited or scared or something, she trembles". (FC13)

Not only do PD symptoms differ from patient to patient, but the disease progression also varies for each of them. Several participants explained that the progression of PD was very slow during the first decade. During this time, the disease was well controlled with low medication and, in one case, without taking any medication during the first ten years. All of them were grateful that they could continue doing things that were important to them (e.g., working or snowboarding) for a decade without experiencing many limitations. This period was referred to as "the honeymoon" by some participants. However, at a certain point, it came to an end, and the disease then progressed more rapidly, which required progressive increasing of medication over time. The worsening of the disease manifested in two different ways. Some patients experienced aggravation of symptoms that they already had (e.g., more fatigue or dyskinesias), while others noticed new symptoms (e.g., quieter voice, problems when walking). This progression brought new limitations on the patients that they did not have previously, such as being unable to continue working.

> "In the beginning, I experienced the honeymoon, it went great, and the more the disease progressed, the more the uncontrolled movement I had. (...) I lost 10 kilos in half a year because I couldn't sit quietly anymore". (P9)

Other patients experienced a much a faster PD progression from the beginning. The manifestation of new symptoms was very difficult for the FCs to cope with:

> "This has changed a lot, the disease. That is quite clear. Then, as you can see with the disease, where dyskinesia became more and more pronounced, comes the physiognomy change. I no longer knew my own wife by her face. It was so bad, the disfigurement that was caused by this illness that affects not only the movements but also the face". (FC22)

3.1.2. Different Perception of the Disease

Since every participant, both patients and FCs, was affected by PD in a different way, their perceptions of the disease varied greatly as well. Some participants have the impression that PD is not a fatal disease like cancer because it does not shorten life expectancy. PD was described by several participants as a disease for which physical activity was essential to relieve its symptoms. As sporting activity was one of the most important things in life for one of the patients, they explained that another disease would have been worse for them than PD. Other participants considered that many things are still unknown about PD. For many of the participants, PD marked a before and after point in their lives:

> "This is the life before and after the disease and then you learn to live with it. It is true that I have done a lot of research to find out where we were heading to (...) We were told that there are as many symptoms as there are sick people. And this is how it is". (P41)

In this sense, one of the participants defined PD as a family of diseases that affect every person differently rather than a just one disease:

> "I had the impression that Parkinson's itself does not exist and that it is a sum of factors that are individual. Therefore, they are really not understood, and they are mentioned below the name of Parkinson's (...) If there would be a better understanding of the whole mechanisms, one could finally say that there are many versions of Parkinson's, which are entirely related". (P1)

P1 also described PD as a disease that leads to the patient being automated and no longer in control of himself. Some patients depicted PD as a disease that evolves and worsens over time. Therefore, one needs to enjoy every day but also learn to cope with living with the disease every day.

> "I can just say that my attitude to life is like this, I fight as long as I can, but it's just getting harder and harder. It's really getting more and more difficult. (...) This disease is also very interesting in terms of what you forget when it changes again afterwards". (P12)

Some participants drawings reflected how it makes them feel to have PD or to have a loved one with PD. In Figure 1, we observe how P28 perceived PD as a succession of ups and downs that made him feel better or worse. To the patient the eye represents that both himself and the people around him can perceive the fluctuation of symptoms.

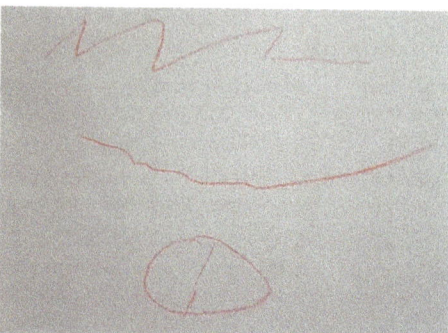

Figure 1. P28's perception of PD.

Figure 2 shows how the facial stiffness characteristic of PD makes relationships and communication difficult. The yellow waves symbolize the psychological, empathetic, and linguistic connection with her husband. The short vertical red lines reflect the loss of connection with her husband and the interruptions in their communication as a consequence of the disease. The blue wave represents her effort to maintain communication with her husband.

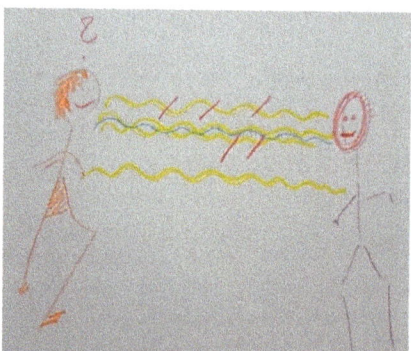

Figure 2. FC6's perception of PD.

"What I drew is what concerns me the most and touches me negatively, which is the effect as if he would have a mask on his face (...). I always have to think when I talk to him or when I get in touch with him whether there's something going on. He just looks glassy-eyed. It's not that there's something wrong or that something has happened (...) It is somehow difficult for him to express that he is there for the other person in an empathic way. And the connection is somehow interrupted. But maybe that has to do with me too. I react very personally". (FC6)

Several participants, both patients and FCs, represented PD in their drawings with different figures that show the impact of the disease on their lives. These figures are very varied and range from the representation of PD as a creature that is always there, like in Figures 3–5, to describing PD by analogy to the weather or the seasons of the year, like in Figures 6 and 7.

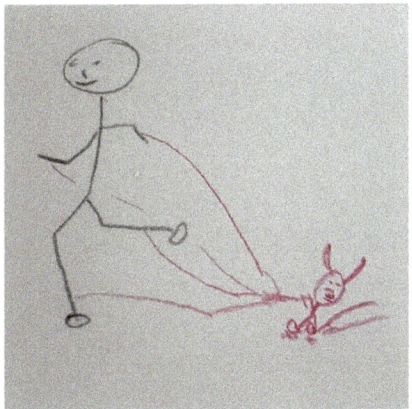

Figure 3. P5's perception of PD.

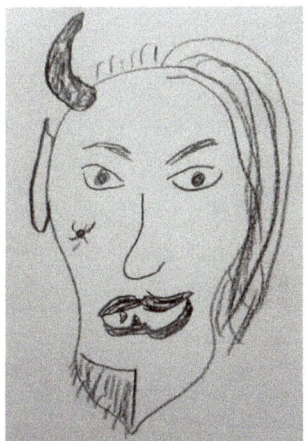

Figure 4. FC29's perception of PD.

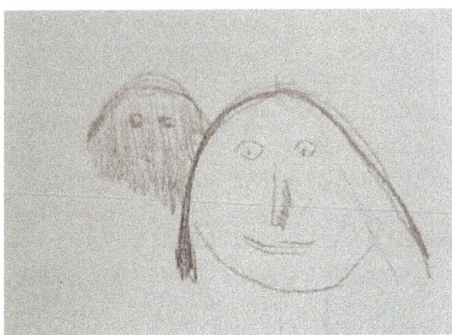

Figure 5. P35's perception of PD.

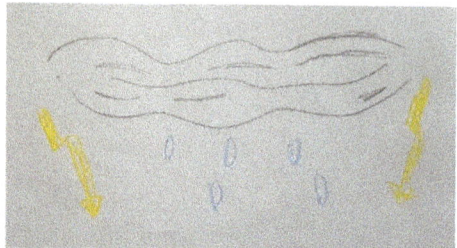

Figure 6. P40's perception of PD.

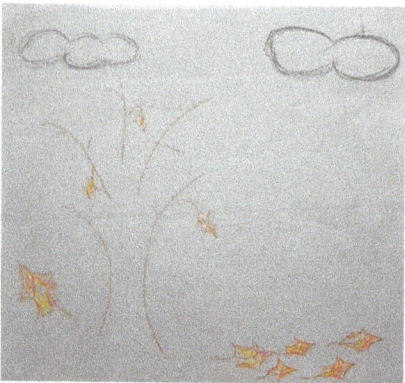

Figure 7. FC41's perception of PD.

"That's me. I have several ropes attached to my legs and arms and a little demon that holds me back. Then, my mobility is limited". (P5)

"I think the disease itself is the devil on one side and the beautiful fairy on the other side. It is entirely day-dependent, time-dependent. Sometimes you could almost despair about the disease and other times, everything it's quite normal and you can say to yourself that everyday life is actually quite normal. And then in the next half hour nothing works at all. What is also the problem is that we have to prepare every appointment very carefully". (FC29)

"This is me, actually a satisfied person. And he has a shadow. And he doesn't have an angry face, but he's looking to see how I am (...) I'm actually happy when he stays behind me, when he doesn't come in front of me (...) Whether I like it or not, he's always there. I can't turn him off". (P35)

"It's to explain the bad weather, the worst of the bad weather, for me. I was very active. I was really someone who was moving and all of sudden I had to stop because it was no longer possible, and my body wasn't following". (P40)

In Figure 7, we can observe how PD is perceived as a before and after in the lives of both patients and FCs.

"It [PD] is autumn. Autumn. The leaves falling is not the end of life, but it's the end of a life. It's the end of the life before illness. So, it's a time to mourn". (FC41)

Some patients visually perceive PD as the lack of movement or freedom (e.g., Figures 8 and 9), rather than as concrete and defined figures, whose symbolism explains the impact on their life (e.g., Figures 3–7).

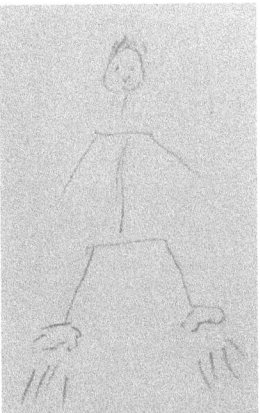

Figure 8. P21's perception of PD.

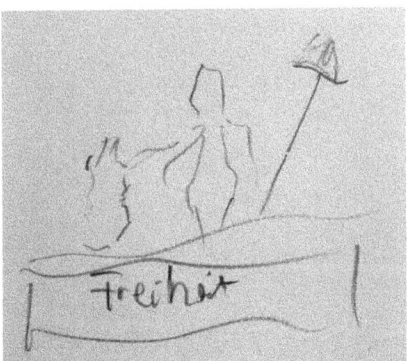

Figure 9. P8's perception of PD. The word "Freiheit" in German means freedom.

> "There's glue on your feet. You want to go somewhere, and you can't. In your head you are already there, but your body cannot go there because your feet are sticky. The dopamine is missing". (P21)

> "This freedom, I don't have it anymore, because I have Parkinson's disease and I've lost my freedom. I find that very bad. I find it so sad (...) Now I simply have a good life, a good care, but I do not have freedom anymore". (P8)

This feeling of loss of freedom has also been described by some FCs:

> "Parkinson's is like a cage for the person. The person is like in a cage for me and I can't get into this cage". (FC6)

3.1.3. Different Reaction to Drugs

Most participants had good experiences with the medication until it had to be increased. However, a few explained that the medication never helped to control the disease symptoms. While some participants found it difficult to distinguish between disease symptoms and side effects, others considered that certain effects were side effects of the medication and not PD symptoms. This impression is due to the disappearance of symptoms once the dosage of the medication was decreased at the start of treatment with DBS. A wide variety of side effects were reported, such as diarrhea, stomach pain, dry mouth, lost sense of taste, increased libido, various addictions (e.g., to sex or compulsive shopping), hyperactivity, aggressivity, and depression.

"Our friends also noticed that he was so uninhibited and always restless. He always had to be stimulated and always had to listen to music. He also bought a lot of things like cars. He had a different behavior". (FC2)

The experience of hallucinations was the most mentioned side effect. In some cases, hallucinations appeared to or became more frequent after increasing the medication. The side effects of medication also have a direct impact on the FCs:

"The increased libido is a problem after all. People don't talk about it so much, but it's a side effect of the medication and it's very demanding for the partner". (P1)

FC2 described her husband's difficulties in controlling his impulses due to the medication he received before starting DBS treatment. She explained that this side effect was very challenging for family life because they had very young children at that time:

"For example, when we were at the table with the children, he ate a lot and very quickly, and then stood up and went to his computer. And that's difficult with children, when you try to educate the children and say: wait until everyone has finished and then you can get up and leave the table. And he, he had no concept of parenting anymore". (FC2)

3.1.4. Different Difficulties and Changes That Led to Different Daily Routines

PD symptoms are limiting and lead to changes in life daily routine. For example, several of them had to change their routine and concentrate all their tasks and activities during the day because in the evening they had no energy. The pace of doing things and the perception of time also changes during the disease, which changes daily routines for patients and FCs:

"People with Parkinson's, they lose their sense of reality over time. For example, when she cooks something, it goes in slow motion. When I say: 'can't be done faster?'. She says: 'yes, I do work fast'. Or also with movements, when people with Parkinson's walk, it's centimeter by centimeter and when you ask them about it and say: 'why don't you take bigger steps? It's better', she says: 'yes, I do take big steps'. It's as if reality slowly disappears". (FC29)

Some patients also experienced difficulties such as being less productive than before, performing daily tasks much slower, being less flexible, or not being able to do certain activities such as traveling or driving. Most of the patients who were still working at the time of diagnosis reported some difficulties at work that caused them great stress (e.g., difficulties while typing on a computer, speaking in public, staying focused, or performing physically demanding work). Due to these difficulties, many of them reduced their working time, delegated some of their tasks to others, or stopped working.

Other difficulties in daily life expressed by some participants were the need to plan every little thing well in advance, the impossibility to stop thinking about the disease, or the loss of autonomy by needing the help of others in daily activities:

"I feel sometimes pressured because I make an appointment for her somewhere and calculate how long we need to get her ready and to be there. And then when we leave, it can happen that nothing works until we get to the station because it takes us a quarter of an hour to walk ten meters and then the train bye". (FC29)

"One loses independence and of course is somewhat limited. You're glad to have someone by your side to help you up, for example, on the edge of the bed to get up". (P9)

This dependence of some patients led to changes in the routine of FCs to be more available to their spouses. While some patients did not require much help from their spouses in daily life, in other cases, the FCs needed to take care of all the household chores or assist patients with personal hygiene. Both patients and FCs described feeling as if daily routine was marked by the disease. Another difficulty experienced by the participants was the necessity of preparing for the future changes and the uncertainty that PD entails, which is sometimes more difficult for FCs than for the patients themselves:

"What comes next? How much should I work? Should I take this job or better this one? (…) How will it go financially and how will it go later? How many years will it take before he needs care? What will I do then? Can I care for someone at all? I'm not the caring type of person. I noticed that a long time ago. Then I thought, oh my God, how do I do that then? It was always like a sword of Damocles hanging over you and you have to think, what's next?" (FC6)

3.1.5. Different Impact on Familial and Couple Relationships and on Social Life

While some participants did not observe changes in their lives as a couple, others reported large changes in their relationships:

"Something changed, I don't know (…) Over time he became more of a patient and I became more of a caregiver, but I wouldn't say from the beginning. It was over time, when more and more symptoms appeared (…) The illness has a strong influence on communication, because he often speaks very softly, because he speaks unclearly. Now, in the last few months, he is increasingly unable to express himself so well. The words don't come out or he no longer knows what he wants to say, and his range of interests is simply more limited". (FC17)

Many of our participants needed to adapt to great changes in their couple life including the impossibility of sharing their hobbies (e.g., travelling, skiing, taking long walks), having sex, or even sleeping together due to sleep disturbances caused by the patients' PD. A few participants described having gone through marital crises as the disease progressed. A couple of patients reported lack of support from their partners during the illness due to the burden it places on FCs:

"She does not want to talk about it [PD] (…) My wife is not understanding as others can be. It's always like that, an illness, it always affects both the relatives and the affected persons themselves (P7) (…) Would you say that your relationship with your wife changed after the diagnosis? (Researcher 1). "Yes, yes. I think it has. Yes, yes. She can't help like that either, can she? (…) There are some people who really still have complaints and I also have complaints, but those who can no longer walk or are really old people. And with such problems my wife simply has problems. She doesn't want to see them at all". (P7)

One of the patients explained that his second wife asked him for a divorce after finding out about the diagnosis.

"In our wedding day, she told me that you were limping (…) And then I went to the doctor, first to the general doctor and then to the neurologist. The second wife, she asked for divorce. I actually understood that, because she had already known my mother and seen how it is (…) And my second wife couldn't stand that". (P8)

One FC described the relationship between her son and daughter-in-law deteriorated because he lost patience.

"It's just that for many couples it's a big challenge. I see many who are trembling, and it's easy, it wouldn't work anymore if the partner didn't have more patience. It's tragic to see how that hurts you. There are so many different people. There are people who deal with it better and others who deal with it worse. You know, my son is washed up with it because he's always had Parkinson's around him. He experienced the grandfather yes. He came from school, he had to find the grandfather somewhere, he had to put him up again and bring him into the house. Then he experienced his father for 30 years. And now his partner and that is a lot for him at the moment and I think that often he just doesn't have the energy anymore (…) She was very unwell before the operation and I just felt she had a nervous breakdown (…) I just notice that when she gets stressed, it comes through, and she needs another day [to recover]. And my son is allergic to it. He just almost can't stand it. He didn't want to be there today" (FC24). "Can I ask why?" (R1). "Something

kind of broke" (FC24). "In the relationship you mean?" (R1). "Unfortunately. That hurts me a lot". (FC24)

PD also had an impact on the family life of several patients and their relationships with their children. In cases where children were very young, some patients tried to avoid mentioning the disease in front of them, but the children still sensed the disease and were affected by it.

"At one point he was quite affected, and I asked him the question. I said, but what's wrong? Then he looked to me in the eye and said: are you going to die daddy? I said no, but no, but no! It had nothing to do with it. In fact we hadn't explained it to him because we thought we were protecting him and then we realized that he was still worried about it". (P40)

In many cases, adult children were a support for their parents with the disease. However, in other cases, the illness was a rarely discussed topic between the patients with their adult children. One of the participants described the deterioration of the relationship with their children:

"It's quite difficult, it depends. My wife doesn't have a problem, but she understands everything. She has given herself body and soul for me. But the children are not the same at all. It has changed (...) let's just say that they don't understand so much that you're sick". (P44)

In relation to the impact of the disease on social life, some participants did not notice any changes in their friendships as a consequence of PD. While some of them consider that there were not changes because they did not talk about the disease with their friends, others thought that their friendships remained unchanged because they had talked openly about their illness from the very beginning. However, a few reported losing some friends due to the disease. Some also explained that due to the disease, they no longer felt comfortable organizing events, going out, or having too many people to visit, which greatly reduced their social life.

"I didn't want to show others this image of me, this image of the disease in fact" (P40). "So you didn't go out anymore?" (R2). "Very little (...) I have the impression that some people think that we are not the same because we are sick. I think there are many who think that because maybe I'm a little slower, I have more difficulty in talking, that inside we're not the same, whereas inside, when I think, I think very quickly". (P40)

3.1.6. Different Personal Coping Strategies

Most of our participants considered PD to be a disease that requires being addressed proactively, because they needed to do something to cope with it and make it more bearable. However, the same coping strategies did not work for all of them. For instance, while for some of them, looking for information about PD was a way of coping with the disease, others preferred not to know much about the illness to avoid feeling drowned by the situation:

"In fact, I preferred not to know anything (...) I told myself that if I didn't know anything, I wouldn't have symptoms that could happen later". (P40)

Coping strategies for PD described by the patients include practicing different sports or physical activities such as coordination training, walking, tai chi, snowboarding, dancing, or kickboxing; other activities such as starting a new hobby (e.g., doing a cooking course); or focusing on the family and specially playing with their grandchildren. Other helpful habits mentioned by the patients for coping mentally with PD were paying attention to diet or staying positive by valuing the small things of everyday life such as enjoying a sunny day or the forest colors. Other strategies to help patients cope with the physical symptoms of the disease were receiving daily leg massages in a massage chair, daily recording of the symptoms to keep track of them, reading aloud to train the voice, or resting the day before a social event to avoid being too tired. Strategies to help the patient walk included counting the steps or following someone while walking. The habits that help each patient with different aspects of the disease are very varied, but there is a consensus on the ideas that physical activity or being distracted contribute to the patient experiencing fewer symptoms while carrying out an activity. FCs also described several activities that helped them to cope better with their loved ones' illness such as praying, reading books with characters with whom they can identify, or doing things alone to clear their mind. Having time for themselves doing activities they enjoy such as sports or socializing was also seen as a way of coping with the illness of their loved ones.

The contact with other people who have PD or who have family members with PD was mentioned as a support in coping with the disease for both patients and FCs. Many of the participants attended self-help groups specifically for patients with PD treated with DBS or for their relatives:

> "That is also the purpose of this self-help group, because people meet there who know what it means to have experienced this operation, but also what it means to have survived it. And what it means when other people think you are healthy again". (P12)

Visiting a self-help group was an opportunity for the FCs to look after themselves by discussing their experiences and how they deal with the disease as FCs:

> "In my opinion, too much is said about the sick person in our self-help group and not about oneself in the relatives' group. So, I always bring that up there (...) I ask: 'how are you doing' and now they are starting to talk a bit more about themselves. (...) It helps to talk to people who have similar experiences. So, it's also like not being alone. Talking about it with other people is always a bit difficult if they judge how it should be (...) But with those who have the same experiences, you only say I do it this way or I do it differently. And, um, yes, you also have to look after yourself". (FC17)

However, some patients and FCs expressed that speaking about the disease or seeing people in the same situation as them would have not helped. Instead, some FCs, who did not want to join self-help groups, talked about the disease with relatives, friends, or acquaintances as a way of coping with their loved ones' disease. Sometimes, this was contrary to the individual patient's way of coping with PD:

> "He had the impression that we were seeing something [PD symptoms], when it wasn't at all (...) But he could see that, and he had the impression that everyone was paying attention to it. So, he didn't want to talk about it too much, and I was the opposite. For me, to talk about it was a way of trivializing this illness. It was like saying I have the flu, yes, he has Parkinson's, and then there you go. Then I talked a lot about it. It's true, I pushed him to do it because it's not keeping things inside that's going to help". (FC41)

3.2. Going through PD Together

As previously mentioned, FCs provide support in many aspects of daily life, such as help with getting out of bed, help with personal hygiene, accompanying patients to medical appointments, or doing activities with the PD patient to stimulate their memory or their motor skills:

> "I do everything for my partner. Doctor talks, everything, and I'm there and I want to know what's being done and yes. That's everything for me. And that's why, we manage, we do everything. It works". (FC14)

Although some patients were not supported by their spouses with the disease, most patients described the support and understanding provided by their spouses as invaluable for dealing with the disease:

> "I think I wouldn't have made it without her" (P44)

PD was a shared experience for several participants, as shown in Figure 10. This figure also portrays how some couples tried to enjoy as much as possible together despite one of them having PD.

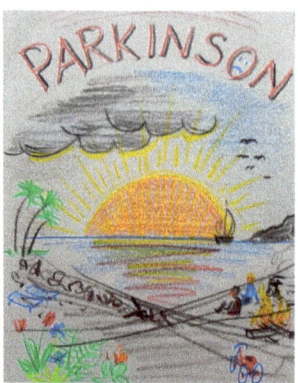

Figure 10. FC26's perception of PD as a joint journey for the couple.

> "It is a double-edged sword. Dark clouds and clear bright sky (...) I have painted a small campfire here, and my wife's tricycle, with the walker standing next to it. We live with these handicaps, with these difficulties, but we always enjoy the sea and the view. We see a horizon (...) The ship disappears in the horizon to unknown places. We don't see exactly where we are going but we are inside this ship and hope that it leads to a good destination towards the sun. The flowers at the beach indicate that we are also having a good time. We have experienced a lot of beautiful things, we were lying in the sun, here the chairs have become empty now, but we are still here (...). Seen from my point of view, it is a hopeful picture, which nevertheless has the shadows of everyday life, and it shows that there are also dark sides, stony paths, or you can be alone sometimes and still be together as a couple as long as it is possible. The fire is still burning, maybe a small one (...) Even our living together, our intimate life, that hasn't been extinguished". (FC26)

3.3. Changing as a Person during the Disease

A large number of participants explained that they perceived changing as a consequence of PD or noticing that their loved ones were no longer the same people they were before having PD. Some patients, despite noticing a change in their personality or character, were unable to put this change into words and considered their spouses better able to explain these changes. Some of the changes most frequently observed by patients or their FCs were the loss of a sense of reality and a decline in self-esteem, self-confidence, and initiative. Changes in personality including increased negativity, irritability, snappiness, selfishness, or impatience were reported by some participants:

> "I have the feeling that my personality has been turned around a bit. I am not the same person I was before. I was so friendly and nice before. And today I am almost toxic. Sometimes I also give poisonous answer to my husband. I feel like that's not very good. But I can't help it" (...) (P28). "And you think this change has to do with the disease?" (R1). "Sure, 100 per cent yes, because it has come more now" (P28). "Since when?" (R1). "Since I could no longer walk. That was the worst thing for me". (P28)

Both patients and FCs frequently mentioned increased introversion and decreased talkativeness. These kind of changes in behavior, character, or personality can be very challenging for FCs:

> "That's still a bit difficult for me now. Yes. In the past few years I had the feeling that he was somehow isolating himself and he is like in a cage with his illness. Somehow, I have the feeling that I can't get close to him anymore as if there would be like a Parkinson's wall between us". (FC6)

> "Before the illness, she was really energetic and always had to do something, and now with the illness, I almost have to force her to go somewhere, to the theatre or the cinema

or somewhere. She has all the excuses she needs not to be around many people. And yes, how should I put it, um, because of the illness she has also become more selfish. So, she comes first and then again and then maybe the others. Sometimes I've also said, I'm not a domiciliary care provider. You pay him and you can give him orders, but I don't get paid". (FC29)

One FC explained that her husband drastically changed during the illness due to the combination of the side effects of the oral medication and his way of coping with the disease:

"He was so hyperactive, and I didn't know if that was because he knew that he had a disease and he wanted to enjoy life (...) He was thinking more about himself, looking more for his own pleasure. He had no sense of time and he was looking for his pleasure. That was his first concern, to think of himself". (FC2)

Other changes observed were decreased spontaneity or concentration, becoming more forgetful or hesitant to do things, or developing risky behavior (e.g., riding a motorbike without a helmet). Some participants explained that aging plays a role in changing as a person during the illness. The above-mentioned changes were considered to be rather negative by both patients and FCs. Two of the participants described some positive changes in their way of being after the PD diagnosis. For instance, becoming more patient with others or being more able to enjoy the little things in life. A couple of participants identified changes in themselves but did not consider them to be either positive or negative. For example, one explained that since he had PD, he perceived emotions differently:

"On the one hand, you get emotional much more quickly. So, when there is an emotional situation, tears come immediately, even if I don't want them to come. Both positively and negatively. The emotionality is actually much greater. But conversely, in the perception of happiness and unhappiness, one becomes somehow like a little more indifferent. Everything is always a little more or less good. It's not extremely good and it's not extremely bad either". (P5)

3.4. DBS Improved My Life

Many participants reported that DBS greatly improved their motor skills. For instance, better body control and recovery of fine motor skills, experiencing fewer tremors, or decreased rigidity, dyskinesia, and freezing. The greater mobility from the decreased symptoms allows the patient to perform daily tasks (cooking, eating, going to bed, getting up, repairing things, walking without falling or working) more easily. This allowed them to enjoy greater autonomy and to be less afraid of doing things like going out or driving alone. Having more energy during the day, increased concentration, and being able to restart activities they were previously unable to do, such as doing sport or knitting, were also reported.

"Since then, she can use her hand completely again. She doesn't tremble. She can do different things by herself again. Before I had to cut the meat and everything for her, and today everything is back to normal". (FC29)

Due to this improvement in PD symptoms, many patients and FCs described DBS as the beginning of a new life, as shown in Figures 11 and 12:

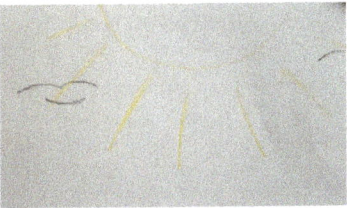

Figure 11. P40's perception of DBS's effect.

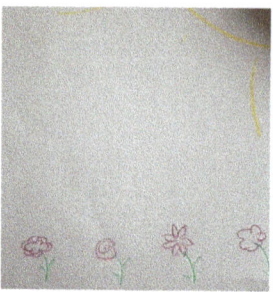

Figure 12. FC41's perception of DBS's effect.

"Well, there's a kind of rebirth, yes, with a few clouds, because it's not easy every day. But already much, much better than before". (P40)

"And then after I drew spring, because the stimulation (DBS) is hope, renewal, and then it's life that blooms again". (FC41)

Some participants believed that their physical condition would be much worse if they had not undergone DBS:

"If I hadn't had the operation, I might be in a nursing home or something (…) If I hadn't operated, I think it would probably be more difficult. Almost certainly. Anyway, my partner says that it has helped 100 per cent". (P9)

"I'm alive now and if I wouldn't have gone through it, I'd already be underground". (P21)

DBS also improved the FC's life quality as they felt relieved by the reduction in their loved ones symptoms and were able to have more time for themselves because they were not required to be as attentive to the patient. Likewise, the patients' motor improvement enabled them to resume hobbies with their FCs that they enjoyed doing together. The positive effects of DBS gave many participants hope and the possibility to plan for the future again:

"Do you now feel that deep stimulation has changed your life?" (Researcher 1). *"Yes, certainly, in the sense that I can do practically everything again. I have a perspective again, at least for the next ten years, a positive perspective. I can consciously plan things again that were previously written in the stars. I can now seriously plan them again. For example, going on a trip with my wife after retirement. We have so many plans that it makes a huge difference when you can plan again and assume that it will work out. We had all these uncertainties before. Before, I didn't even know if I would be able to work until retirement. That is no longer a question. I've already agreed with my colleague that I'll be available and able to work after retirement"*. (P5)

In addition to the improvements in the symptoms mentioned above, the ability to speak more clearly and loudly again improved both the patient's social life and their couple relationship.

"He is more at ease when speaking (…) He can stay standing or go with them [the neighbors] to see something. Whereas before he withdrew himself a little when he had so much dyskinesia. I do think that it's better now for the contact and the neighborhood network" (FC39)

"Now it's better after the deep brain stimulation. It is really better (…) The speaking part that is very important for me, that you can exchange and talk to each other. Of course, that became less. Parkinson's patients also speak less, of course. That was also a huge problem for me. I like to talk about everything. I want to exchange ideas. That was no longer possible. That is better now". (FC6)

Several FCs mentioned the recovery of facial expression as an important improvement seen with DBS. Figure 13 shows how facial expression of FC6's husband improved in comparison with Figure 2, which led to fewer interruptions in communication and improved their couple communication. Fewer short red lines are observed in Figure 13 than in Figure 2 because of this. The question mark in Figure 2 has disappeared because she no longer needs to try as hard to understand if something is happening to her husband. The speech of her husband improved, which allowed him to express himself better, showing more empathy when speaking and communicating more fluidly.

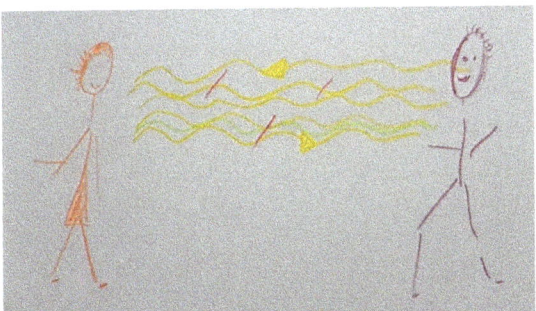

Figure 13. FC6's perception of DBS's effect.

The blue line symbolizing FC6's efforts to communicate properly with her husband from Figure 2 is substituted in Figure 13 by a green line, which represents the improved communication and connection between FC6 and her husband. The following reason was given:

"Now here I have the hope, partly after the deep brain stimulation, that even if it is a bit worse in between, it will get better again". (FC6)

The reduction of medication and its associated side effects (such as hyperactivity, stomach problems, or lack of taste), the possibility of controlling PD symptoms without having to increase medication, and no longer experiencing the on–off effect of the medication were considered positive aspects of DBS by several participants.

"One of my doctors described it [DBS effects], very well. He said that it's like sitting in a cold room and making a fire. The fire goes up, down up, down, and you are cold and then warm, and cold and warm. And the stimulator is like you install a central heating system. So, it's a continuous effect (...) Before [with oral treatment], it was high low high low, and the stimulation is straight. You have a constant effect with the stimulation". (P1)

"It doesn't always work out equally well, but as long as it is still possible to put the power up and then it works (...) Before, it was necessary to increase the meds, and now you can do the same much easier just using electricity". (P27)

A few patients mentioned the ability to modulate the amplitude of the stimulation with a remote control to better control certain symptoms as an advantage; however, most of the patients did not use it.

"Yes, I use it occasionally, so for control, but I don't change it every day or much. I think I'm actually not badly adjusted. What I'm going to do, maybe this week, is to lower it a bit on the other side because I'm having more and more cramps in this upper arm, which are very painful and that can help". (P12)

3.5. I Am Treated with DBS but I Still Have Parkinson's

Despite the improvements many patients noticed in their health, both patients and FCs highlighted that DBS is not a cure for PD. It is a therapy that can improve certain symptoms of PD but not all of them, and it does not halt the progression of the disease:

"The disease is progressing (...) It's going to get worse and worse" (P44)

"It's better, but you still live next to a sick person, and you sleep next to a sick person" (FC2)

"I have been given a new life. Another chance, so to speak. But this chance is now increasingly limited, of course, because I realize that I can't do many things any more (...) It's not a cure. That's precisely the problem (...) Other people think you are healthy again. That is a consequence of the operation, that many people in the circle of friends then thought, now you have had the operation, now you are as you were before, capable of performing, able to work under pressure. And that is simply not true (...) The effect [of DBS] was like getting a new life, but now the illness is coming back stronger". (P12)

Despite knowing that the disease is still present, Figure 14 shows how some patients have the impression that they can manage the disease better with DBS than with their previous treatment.

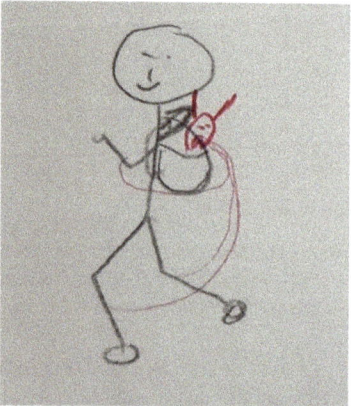

Figure 14. P5's perception of DBS's effect.

"I would say that the little devil is still there, but at the moment he is sitting in a backpack and is not hindering me (...) I know that [PD] is not gone. That must always be clear. Maybe it'll get out of the backpack again and lead back again. I don't know. The doctors think I could expect the effect of deep brain stimulation for about ten years". (P5)

Although some aspects have improved greatly with DBS, others may worsen as the disease progresses. As a result, some FCs ended up taking on more and more everyday tasks.

"It is noticeable today that everything has become a little slower (...) The asking back and forth, that has increased. In the past she cooked, I had no problem, I ate what she made. Today I have to ask her, what would you like for dinner today? That has become our daily routine, three times a day, or, in the morning, I say, what would you like, bread, everything, at noon and in the evening. Yes, that has become my task, to think a bit more for my wife as well" (FC26). "More after the intervention than before?" (Researcher 1). "Yes, before I didn't have to think for my wife anything. She organized everything herself and was independent in every way. She managed the household, but today we have to share everything". (FC26)

Figure 15 shows life of her husband since he is treated with DBS because the disease started to progress quickly:

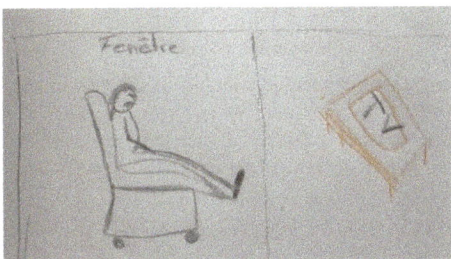

Figure 15. FC45's perception of DBS's effect.

"It simply means that life in society is different. It means that he is often in a chair at home, uh, because of fatigue. Fatigue and then walking, eh walking, it has decreased a lot too". (FC45)

Furthermore, being treated with DBS does not always mean the end of taking tablets; many of the participating patients had their medication dosage reduced but not stopped. Figure 16 shows how PD and the timing of medication still mark the daily routine for some patients and FCs.

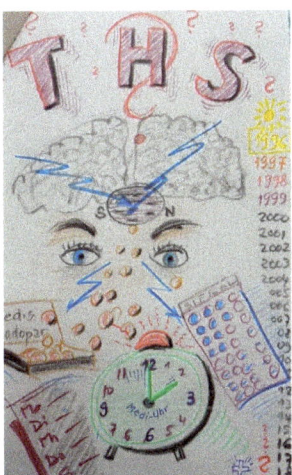

Figure 16. FC26's perception of DBS's effect.

"It is a picture full of confusion. You can see the brain and the lightning that works into the substantia nigra, those are the electronic currents. And that goes out again with these daily worries, with the medication, with the appointments you have, you always have to think about it, about all kinds of things. Time runs. It's ringing again, that's the alarm for the tablets intake that is at the center here. Today, it controls our everyday life quite strongly (...) The eyes are perhaps a little bit empty here (...). I would say they [the eyes] are hopeful for the future despite all the chaos, the lightning that comes at us every day, the question marks that surround everything here, DBS, the medications, yes, and so on". (FC26)

3.6. DBS Is Not Perfect

DBS did not work equally for all patients; many experienced great improvement from the start, while some only experienced good symptom control for a short period of time, and a minority observed little to no improvement with DBS.

"Does the medicine work right away? Doesn't it work yet? Uh, a lot of things are happening at the same time. It's very difficult and each person is very different". (FC45)

Although DBS contributed to improving the life quality of many of the patients, some mentioned that it is not a foolproof treatment because it can also worsen certain aspects. The worsened aspects included: their energy level, balance, speaking, coordination, or flexibility. This had an impact on the participants' social life and in some cases led to withdrawal from certain activities or hobbies.

"If he has to speak for a long time, usually his voice will diminish, he won't be able to (...) He enjoys going to restaurants, eating, something he didn't enjoy before. But on the other hand, he can't express himself when he is in society and has to speak when there are a lot of people (...) So that's one of the disadvantages". (FC41)

It was mentioned that some aspects cannot be controlled with DBS such as fatigue, freezing episodes, or experiencing difficulty in walking:

"Walking is going down, but the doctor surgeon, neurologist said that deep stimulation does nothing for walking or very little. We had the impression that it was very difficult to adjust it, to make a fine adjustment". (P39)

A few participants mentioned being somewhat disappointed with the treatment because they expected it to eliminate all symptoms permanently, and only partial improvement was achieved:

"I have to say, I expected more. I thought after the brain operation everything would be fine, yes, fine, the hope was there, now everything will be fine again. If I am stimulated every day afterwards it'll be like before. But that wasn't the case. That was only at the beginning. The shared joy (...) It's only possible to adjust it so that it is optimal (...) And that ideal point, was not always ideal. At the beginning, they had to change it a bit up, a bit down, and then it is found wasn't the best result. Ah, it's the best possible, but not what we had hoped for". (FC26)

One patient mentioned that her husband hoped to be able to travel more with her after the improvements achieved with DBS, whereas she did not feel able to:

"Yes, well my husband, he would rather go on holiday even more than I would. For me it's always in a new place is already a bit stressful. So I notice that. I told you, I'm not so resilient anymore. So packing, that's hard for me". (P35)

Figure 17 shows some of the negative experiences like the occurrence of infection due to the surgery or depression as a side effect of DBS, which some patients went through, even if they were satisfied with the treatment.

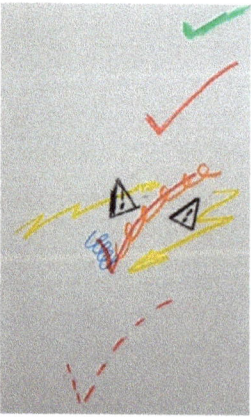

Figure 17. P1's perception of DBS effects.

"This is at the beginning, and there is no signal, or few signals before the DBS is implanted, and afterwards there is a positive V. It's a "big turn" but it is still fragile, and this is the infection [the triangles with the exclamation mark]. After the infection, it went well, but now, I have to say I always have the impression that in the depression, the stimulator is a very important element". (P1)

3.7. Being Different after DBS

A few participants described changes in their personality or their loved ones since the treatment with DBS started. The following changes were reported: impulsive behavior, irritability, excessive euphoria, or becoming more selfish, emotional, impatient, or withdrawn:

"He takes care of things he likes and doesn't need to have a lot of people around him" (FC45). "And that was also like that before the operation?" (Researcher 2). "There was already a little bit like that before the operation, but it was really minimal. It didn't happen daily or anything like that. (…) And then [after DBS intervention], he became much more sensitive. For example, if you watch a film and there are emotions involved in that film, he would cry straight away. You can see the tears. He was never like that". (FC45)

"I was irritable, belligerent, and freaked out. I drove everyone crazy in the hospital" (P23). "And this was immediately after the operation?" (Researcher 1). "Immediately? Yes. Maybe three weeks later as well" (P23). "And now do you still feel different?" (Researcher 1). "Yeah. Still not good". (P21)

Some of the described changes occurred in the first weeks or months after the surgery and disappeared after a few months, while in other cases, these changes in personality or behavior remained. In some cases, these changes were accentuations of personality traits that had developed during the course of disease. Sudden mood changes and manic or depressive episodes never experienced before DBS were also described by a few participants:

"He really had a personality change for a short period of time and also a manic phase. He was completely different for a while" (FC37). "What do you mean by manic phase?" (Researcher 1). "Yes, after the operation he was really changed in his manner, that he for example/that he complimented me or hugged me when greeting me, as he never did before (…) He bought an expensive watch and booked holidays, big holidays, without discussing it with my mother. And also wanted to write a book. Yes, things like that". (FC37)

Mood swings brought stress into the couple life of some participants:

"After DBS, she had a bit of trouble when I had so many ups and I made a lot of quick decisions. I invited people to our place and so on, and she didn't appreciate that so much. Just because she also didn't like it so much when it went down again after DBS. It wasn't depression, but depressive moods". (P27)

One of the FCs explained that they were not prepared for the occurrence of depressive episodes with DBS because they were not informed about it:

"And he had it again a fortnight ago. So, depression-like episodes (…) No one told me that could happen (…) He wasn't told either. We talked about it recently. I told him, why don't you ask that in the next consultation? I told him that when he has an examination in hospital, then he should ask whether this side effect is possible". (FC17)

One patient explained that being treated with DBS made her worry about things she didn't worry about before and that this led to arguments with her partner that she did not have before:

"My partner said, oh, you have to get an induction cooker. And then I immediately thought, magnetic fields. And then it was when I first googled that and it's a topic in the media and that's why I thought, I don't want it. I don't want that in ten years will be found out that it's harmful for the brain or the battery. And those are moments that are different with my partner". (P35)

Some perceived changes, such as finding themselves or their loved ones more relaxed, positive, disinhibited, or with a cheekier sense of humor were positively valued by a few participants. One patient explained that it was positive for him to be more open to talk to people he did not know, including strangers. A couple of patients explained that since they were treated with DBS, they felt like the person they were before the disease, while others described feeling like a new person because they have a new life. Some FCs also reported the impression that their loved ones resembled the people they were before the disease again or the feeling that both of them were given a new life after the improvement of PD symptoms due to DBS. One of the patients described not feeling like the same person as before DBS intervention differently to experiencing changes in personality or feeling like a new person:

> "I don't have the feeling that I've become a different person. I haven't but at the same time I'm not the same. I'm much more anxious. (...) It [DBS intervention] was certainly a borderline experience. It's a borderline experience like a birth. I also compare it to a new life that I got. Other people don't have this borderline experience, and that creates often a distance to others". (P12)

The presence of a device in the brain was not described as an element changing them as people, but as something that is now part of their lives. Although some of them could notice the device being inside their, or their partners, bodies, it was not a problem for them:

> "I don't have the feeling that there is something in there. I do notice it, of course it is a foreign body in my body, but I live with it now and not badly". (P7)

> "No, nothing bothers me about her, even that she has such a device above her chest that you can see and feel, that doesn't bother me. (...) That belongs to my wife. Exactly. It's not a foreign body from my point of view. I don't perceive her as my wife, who has electronics in her brain. I just don't think about it at all". (FC26)

One of the patients called himself a cyborg, explaining that this term did not have a negative connotation for him, although it did for other people:

> "I've always said I'm a so-called cyborg now. The funny thing was that I said this once to my neurologist that I would be a cyborg afterwards. Then he immediately objected and said, no, no, you are still a human being". (P5)

4. Discussion

Our study examines the perception of patients and FCs of PD and DBS and the changes in life that they face as a consequence. We observed great heterogeneity in PD symptoms, their progression, the effects of DBS, and the perception of patients and FCs of PD as a disease and DBS as a therapy. Therefore, "everyone's Parkinson is different" is the overarching theme. Each person has a different experience of the disease and reacts differently to it. This means that PD impacts their daily lives and relationships differently and that their experience with the treatment is different. Therefore, different coping strategies were described by patients and FCs. Our results show that what works for some does not work for others. However, there is one strategy that helps most patients cope with PD symptoms and that FCs recommend. This strategy involves patients doing physical activity or concentrating on something they enjoy, because they experience fewer symptoms while doing it. This information could be relevant for clinicians when they provide patients and FCs with strategies to cope with their symptoms in day-to-day life.

We decided to implement a multimodal approach with the aim of capturing a more detailed account of the participants' experiences [48]. Complementing the interviews with drawing gives participants the opportunity to convey their emotions through the use of color and shape, giving their words a new dimension. This provides the researcher with additional insights into their experiences [59,65,66]. The drawings allowed us to identify major difficulties and concerns that participants had in relation to PD, as well as the implications of DBS as a therapy on their lives. Drawing gives the participants in qualitative studies a tool to reveal feelings and aspects of their internal world that are not always visible [67]. For instance, in Figure 2, FC6 uses lines and curves of different colors and shapes to visually describe the impact of PD on her communication with her husband and the internal struggle she felt due the breaking of the emotional connection between her and her husband. The short lines in red that we saw earlier represented both the interruptions in communication and the emotional pain caused by this situation. This is similar to the representations of physical pain drawn by some participants in a study on the pictorial representation of chronic pain [66]. In this study, two participants represent the process of managing pain with blue as FC6 does when she draws a blue line to symbolize her efforts on maintaining the connection and communication with her husband.

Another study on chronic pain shows the how the participants associate pain with certain figures, in the same way that some of our participants did when they drew how they visually perceived PD [68]. For example, Figures 3 and 5 illustrate the feeling of PD being a constant presence in their lives either in the form of a shadow behind them or a devil pulling them along. Figure 4 represents the duality of PD as a demon and a fairy, showing the loss of control for both the patient and FC due to PD. In this drawing, normality is associated with the absence of symptoms, represented by the fairy, which allows the participants to carry out their daily routine without interruptions. However, this sense of normality disappears when the symptoms associated with the demon manifest themselves, which cannot always be foreseen or anticipated. Thus, Figure 4 shows us the unpredictability and uncertainty that characterize PD and how this is also a burden for the relatives.

In Figures 8 and 9, we see different symbolism for PD: the grim reaper who takes away the freedom of the person or the glue that does not allow the patient to lift their feet from the ground. They both represent the lack of freedom that PD enforces on the life of patients and FCs, which marks a turning point in the life of both patients and FCs. Therefore, DBS also marked a before and after point for those who had a good response to the treatment, which is represented through Figures 6, 7, 11 and 12. On the one hand, Figures 6 and 7 show the disease in the form of a storm and the autumn leaves denoting the end of summer. On the other hand, Figures 11 and 12 show the association between life with DBS and the resurgence of a sunny day or the blossoming of flowers in spring. Other studies also show how images of seasonal or weather change represent life transition for people with different health conditions [59]. In the case of our participants, the treatment with DBS implied a new period of life that brings better quality of life and a sense of greater control, as we can also see in Figure 14, where the devil is on the patient's back and no longer behind him pulling him back. However, this devil could get off and start holding the patient back again, which denotes the patients' concern about the evolution of PD and the awareness of PD not being a cure. Furthermore, not all participants benefited equally from the therapeutic effect of DBS. This is reflected in Figure 15, showing life with DBS when it does not have the expected effect or when the effect disappears due to the progression of the disease.

All these drawings, and the explanations that accompany them, show us the complexity of living with PD and receiving treatment with DBS. It is a shared experience between patients and their FCs, as Figures 10 and 16 show us. In these images, FC26 shows us how they go through PD and DBS together, which has been also described by other authors [69]. The FCs (especially in the case of spouses) are not only emotionally involved in the illness of their loved ones, but they also provide care at home. Not only do they need to learn to manage the internal impact on their lives that the fact that their spouses have a chronic illness has, in most cases, they also adapt their routines to assist their loved ones in different tasks, such as helping with personal care and hygiene, managing the patient's treatment, or organizing medical appointments [50,52,69]. In most cases, they are a great source of support and understanding for patients [49,70]. In addition, certain symptoms of PD disease (e.g., slowness of movement, fatigue, or psychiatric manifestations) or some side-effects of dopaminergic medication (e.g., hyperactivity or hypersexuality) or DBS (e.g., temporary mania or mood changes) add great pressure on the shoulders of FCs. Previous work highlights the need to consider the impact of PD on FCs' wellbeing and their need to receive support from health services to deal with the situation [70–72]. Self-help groups are an important source of support for some FCs because they allow them to find information about PD and DBS and emotional support by sharing experiences with other people in the same situation [73]. This is especially important because the burden of the disease on relatives does not disappear with DBS; nonetheless, it is mitigated for some time when DBS goes well [69,74]. Thus, it is important to help FCs, in addition to patients, to understand the implications and limitations of DBS in order to prevent unrealistic expectations (e.g., expecting life to be the same as before the disease) [75,76]. Both patients and FCs should also be prepared for the fact that DBS may not resolve certain PD symptoms or may cause side effects, affecting patients' personality or behavior [76].

We analyzed the patients' process of change during the disease and the treatment from their own perspective and that of their FCs. In order to assess the impact of both PD and DBS on patients' identity, personality, or behavior, we asked both patients and FCs whether they had the feeling that they or their loved ones had changed as people. This decision was made because the concepts of personality or identity do not have a universal meaning and depend on culture and individual evaluations [77]. We therefore consider that the idea of changing as a person could be understood in a more homogeneous way. While some participants did mention the concepts of personality or identity directly when answering this question, not all of them did. In the bioethics literature, it is common that the side effects of DBS are portrayed as a threat to patients' personality, identity, agency, and self-perception [32,78–80]. Although many of these articles are not based on firsthand studies, there are studies showing some post-operative changes that could negatively affect personality, behavior, or mood (e.g., impulsive behavior, depression, mania) [35,81–85]. While these may occur, it should not be forgotten that PD often presents with psychological and psychiatric manifestations (e.g., depression, anxiety, hallucination, apathy) [86] and dopaminergic medication like dopamine agonists can also lead to impulsive behavior such as compulsive buying, hyperactivity, or sexual behavior [87–90]. For instance, some of our participants described changes in their personality prior to undergoing the DBS intervention such as hypersexuality, compulsive shopping, or sudden changes in mood, which in the bioethics literature are normally associated with DBS. Given that many patients continue to require oral medication (at lower doses) and the disease keeps progressing, it is difficult for clinicians, researchers, and also patients to discriminate between PD symptoms and drug- or DBS-induced side effects. Examples of such difficulty may be the mention of anosmia as a side effect of the medication by the participants, although in fact it is an early symptom of PD, or the consideration of dyskinesia as a PD symptom, when it is a side effect of prolonged treatment with levodopa [91,92].

Furthermore, our study reveals that the patients' experiences with DBS are inherently entangled with their experience of suffering from PD, which is still present. Therefore, the whole experience of both suffering from a chronic disease and being treated for it has an impact on the patients' narrative and not just the fact of being treated with DBS, as is often portrayed in the literature on neuroethics [30,79,80,93]. Thus, patients and FCs have to integrate all these elements and changes, which requires a process of adaptation and adjustment that every person experiences in a different way. Whilst we did not identify severe problems with social adjustment as other authors did [31,46], we did observe that our participants went through a process of adaptation and adjustment that every person experienced in a different way. However, in general, patients with positive therapeutic results with DBS showed satisfaction with their life and the improvements in their symptoms.

Some authors address the issue of the burden of normality by describing it as the reconceptualization of the patient's identity from chronically ill to "cured" due to the disappearance or improvement of PD symptoms as a result of DBS [37,94–99]. According to our data, the patients who participated in our study did not consider themselves cured because they had fewer or no symptoms of the disease or as if they had lost the "disease label" [100]. All of them, including those with very positive experiences with the device, were aware that the disease was still there and could worsen again over time. This awareness of the presence of the disease is evident from Figure 15, in which the devil-shaped PD is under control in the backpack but has not disappeared and may come down to the ground again. Furthermore, some debilitating PD symptoms such as fatigue, freezing of gait, and balance impairment could not be targeted by DBS [76]. The closest experience we found to the burden of normality but without actually being so was the description of a patient of DBS as a "borderline experience" for two reasons: the experience of the surgery and the fact that she was given a new life that allowed her to do many things she could not do before. Although the reduction in symptoms was something she enjoyed, she reported feeling certain social distance from people who had not experienced undergoing DBS. Nevertheless, the improvement in PD symptoms did not led her to experience radical adjustment problems or behavioral changes negatively affecting her as shown in other studies [50,52,69].

In the bioethics literature, it has also been described how couples can find themselves under pressure following symptom improvement and relief from withdrawal or reduction of medication [32,97,100]. However, we have rather observed an improvement in spousal relationships as a result of motor improvement. What was a source of stress for a few couples were some of the side effects of DBS such as impulsivity or depressive episodes, which usually occur in the first few months with DBS and are often resolved by adjusting the stimulation parameters [46,100–102]. Nevertheless, PD symptoms, both motor and non-motor, as well as drug-induced side effects, pose important challenges for the couple's relationships. Nevertheless, PD symptoms, both motor and non-motor, as well as the side-effects of dopamine agonists, may be even more challenging for the couple's relationships [89,90,103]. In this regard, a number of participants reported a series of difficult situations they had experienced: the progressive change of the spouse's role from partner to caregiver, the lack of communication of some couples about the disease, the impossibility of sharing some hobbies or interests, the differences of opinion on whether or not to talk about the disease, the pressure on the partner dealing with episodes of addiction or hyperactivity caused by dopaminergic medication, and the marital crises, which in one case ended in divorce. Therefore, we consider that in the case of our participants, DBS improved their relationships due to the reduction of PD symptoms and lower medication, which decreased the side effects associated with it.

Based on our results, we do not share the idea defended by other authors that patients undergo DBS with the objective of changing or enhancing their personality or their way of being (at least not in the case of PD) [79,93,104,105]. Although some patients since being treated with DBS did experience some changes in their personality, behavior, or mood (e.g., being more positive, relaxed, or disinhibited) that were welcomed by them, this was not the aim of the therapy. It is also important to remark that different individuals may value the same side effect either as positive or negative depending on their character, life circumstances, or life narrative [39,106]. Our participants did not use the remote control with the aim of changing or stimulating their personality, as described in the literature in bioethics [104], but rather to better control or relieve certain motor symptoms.

Another aspect that has received much attention in the literature is the relationship between patients and the DBS device. As a device partially implanted in the brain and considering the close relationship between brain and mind, some authors have underlined the importance of carrying out an assessment of the psychosocial consequences of this treatment [107]. Other authors consider that DBS may induce self-estrangement as some patients struggle finding themselves after surgery [108]. It has been described that some patients had the feeling as if they had lost their true self or as if they would be a machine or a cyborg [31,32,46,95,109]. In contrast, our participants did not find it problematic having a device in their brain or their loved ones having it. Even one of our participants defined himself as a cyborg without feeling lost or alienated. He was therefore surprised by the reaction of his doctor, who emphasized that he was not a cyborg but a person. We believe that DBS (especially if it works well) may become a constitutive dimension of lived experience, which does not need to cause self-alienation in the person [109]. In fact, DBS can also have a restorative effect on the person [106]. Our participants had rather the feeling that they have become more themselves because they see themselves as more identified with the person they were before the disease. Others felt they had received a new life that could enjoy more than the one they had before the surgery, which is described in the medical literature as a "second honeymoon" [110]. The patient who described having undergone DBS as a "borderline experience" in her life described how she did not feel the same anymore after DBS without having become a different person. However, this feeling was not due to the fact that she had a device inside her brain but due to the experience of having undergone invasive surgery and having been given a new life. We believe that the embodiment of the device as a part of the patient's body may be the reason why our patients did not experience self-estrangement, even though they may have noticed changes in themselves during the time they have been treated with DBS.

In view of all the above, we did not observe a deteriorative post-DBS biographical disruption as other authors described [31,95]; nonetheless, we did observe a post-PD biographical disruption [111]. PD as chronic disease alters the structures of everyday life and affects self-perception, modifying patients' sense of self and agency [112,113]. It also challenges the interrelationship between mind and body because the body does not always act when and how the mind asks it to act [114,115]. Furthermore, the diagnosis of PD and its progression implies for both patients and FCs a continuous reinterpretation of the past, the present, and the future, and DBS is part of this reinterpretation but not the only cause [116].

Strengths, Limitations, and Future Directions

Our study applies the narrative DIPEx approach to explore how patients and FCs perceive and experience PD and DBS, which gives the participants a greater control over the structure, length, and content of the interview [57]. This facilitated long and in-depth discussions with the participants, which led to rich and credible results due to the strategies of prolonged engagement and persistent observation [117]. Furthermore, most participants, both patients and FCs, experienced a beneficial emotional effect from having been listened to and from their personal stories having been taken into account for research [52]. We consider that this feeling of being valued and trusted by us during the interview encouraged them to talk very freely about their emotions, fears, and needs. Another strength has been the inclusion of FCs in the study, which allowed us to examine their perception of PD and DBS and their role in supporting the management of the disease and the treatment at home. The account of FCs also served to complement the information given by the patients about their own experiences, especially in cases where the disease was more advanced, and hence, their inclusion provided us with valuable information that highly enriched our study. For data analysis, we have employed a hybrid process of inductive and deductive thematic analysis. This method has been adequate to categorize and analyze in depth a large number of experiences and to explore the differences between the patient's perspective and the concerns shown in the bioethics literature.

Furthermore, we consider our multimodal approach as a major strength of our study, which is the first one that has been conducted to explore the experiences of patients and FCs with both PD and DBS. Drawing has been explored as a possible tool for early diagnosis of PD but not as a qualitative method to analyze experiences with PD [118,119]. We believe that the collection of drawings as a complement to the interviews provided us with additional insights into the participants' internal world and their subjective experiences with PD and DBS. It offered us access to nonverbal meanings and to a qualitatively different aspect of the participants' experiences [53,120]. Furthermore, the action of drawing allowed our participants to reflect on their own narrative and visually show the impact of PD and DBS [121–123].

For all these reasons, we can argue that our study applied rigorous qualitative methodology in data collection and analysis that meet the criteria of credibility, transferability, dependability, confirmability, and reflexivity, ensuring the trustworthiness of our results [117].

We identified five possible limitations in our study due to its design and methodology:

- Firstly, our study was very comprehensive and did not focus specifically on one issue in relation to PD or DBS as other studies did. Therefore, some issues may have been missed during the interviews, such as the burden of normality, particularly in FCs. This particular topic should be investigated in more detail in the future as it is a very underrepresented topic in the medical literature.
- The participants were interviewed only after being treated with DBS and not before they started receiving this treatment. Although all participants were asked questions about their daily lives and how they were doing before treatment, those who have lived with PD and DBS for a longer period of time may have lost perspective on the before and after. This may have led to recall bias.
- Some patients who initially showed interest in the study finally decided not to participate because they were going through a difficult time with DBS side effects. Therefore, we missed some negative experiences with DBS due to the fact that people who have bad experiences are often more reluctant to share their experiences than those who have had positive experiences with the treatment.
- PD patients treated with DBS are a defined sub-cohort of PD and are not representative of the entire PD population. For example, patients within the first years after the first diagnosis (i.e., <5 years) are not represented, since DBS is usually not provided at this stage of the disease. Furthermore, patients experiencing moderate to severe dementia or with lack of physical or psychological resilience were excluded from the study. This means that the population of patients at a very advanced stage of the disease is not represented in our study either. We are aware that this exclusion may have led to inclusion bias. However, we could not include participants unable to hold a long conversation sharing stories over different time frames (e.g., before and after DBS), which is very difficult for patients with advanced PD. Therefore, we consider that despite the risk of inclusion bias, our study applied the best sampling strategy for the objectives of our study and its methodology.
- Only patients treated from 6 months to 10 years with DBS were included to have a broad spectrum of experiences with DBS at different stages. Further studies are needed to delve into the individual patients' difficulties and needs at each stage of the treatment. Other issues need further elucidation, such as patient and FC experiences with the side-effects resulting from dopaminergic treatment or the impact of memories of DBS surgery.

5. Conclusions

This study applied a multimodal approach through narrative semi-structured interviews and drawings to analyze the experiences of nineteen patients and seventeen FCs with PD and DBS. We explored the heterogeneity that defines PD, which is visible in both the manifestation of the disease and in the way of coping with it, as both aspects change from person to person. Although it does not affect everyone in the same way, our results show the great impact of PD on different aspects of daily life, including self-care, housework, hobbies, work, self-perception, plans for the future, and relationships with partners, family, and friends. Moreover, it does not only affect patients but also their FCs, who have to cope with a change in their role within the couple and/or the family and restructure their daily life to adapt to the patients' needs.

Our findings show how DBS, without being perceived as a cure for all PD symptoms or its progression, is a treatment that in many cases improves the motor skills of patients. This improvement translates into greater autonomy and a better quality of life for both patients and their families. However, in some cases, the desired therapeutic effect of DBS was not achieved or disappeared over time due to disease progression. Whilst possible DBS side effects may have an impact on the patients' personality and behavior, PD symptoms and dopaminergic medication side effects also have a great impact on personality and self-perception. Nevertheless, these aspects are less mentioned in the bioethics literature. Another aspect that deserves further investigation is the burden of normality not only in patients but also in FCs, as with regard to FCs, this topic is underrepresented in the literature. We suggest the use of multimodal research approaches to explore these aspects because it gives participants the opportunity both to convey emotions through the use of color and shape and to visually share their greatest struggles and concerns with the disease and the treatment. In this way, researchers will have access to valuable additional information on under-studied topics, which will allow healthcare professionals to better understand the specific concerns and needs of their patients with PD and their FCs. Our findings may moreover support clinicians in better informing patients and FCs about PD symptoms or DBS side effects in a way that is more focused on their needs, priorities, and fears. In addition, we believe that asking patients to draw can be a useful tool for clinicians when addressing sensitive topics during consultation to better understand the perspective of patients.

Author Contributions: Y.M.C.G.: set-up of the study, data collection and analysis, literature review, manuscript write-up, and manuscript editing; F.B.: research supervision, manuscript write-up, and manuscript editing; N.B.-A.: research supervision, manuscript write-up, and manuscript editing. All authors have read and agreed to the published version of the manuscript.

Funding: The Spanish foundation "La Caixa" has funded part of the study from which the data presented in this paper are drawn. The grant number is LCF/BQ/EU17/11590025.

Institutional Review Board Statement: The study was conducted according to the guidelines of the Declaration of Helsinki, ISO EN 14155 as well as all national legal and regulatory requirements. Ethical review and approval were waived (BASEC-Nr. req-2018-00050) for this study by the Ethics review Committee of the Canton of Zurich due to the study design does not fall under the Swiss Law on Human Subjects Research.

Informed Consent Statement: Informed consent was obtained from all subjects involved in the study to conduct the study and publish the results.

Data Availability Statement: Some of the data presented in this study will be made public in 2022 on the Website www.dipex.ch (accessed on 4 May 2021).

Acknowledgments: We would like to thank the Spanish foundation "La Caixa" for their economic contribution to our study; Stephan Bohlhalter, Stefan Hägele-Link, Benninger, and the self-help groups of the Association Parkinson Schweiz for their cooperation in our study and their help in the selection of participants; and Corine Mouton for her work in the collection and analysis of part of the data presented in this paper.

Conflicts of Interest: The funders had no role in the design of the study; in the collection, analyses, or interpretation of data; in the writing of the manuscript; or in the decision to publish the results.

Appendix A

- Do you notice any difference when you compare a day now with a day before DBS?
- Have you developed new interests after the operation?
- What support do you currently receive?
- Do you feel that DBS has improved your quality of life?
- Do you feel that DBS has changed you as a person in any way? Do you feel different?
- Have you experienced mood swings during treatment?
- Do you notice anything different in your body since you have been treated with DBS?
- Do you have the impression that you interact differently with other people since being treated with DBS?
- Do your relatives or friends think that DBS has changed you in some way?

Figure A1. Extract of the interview guide.

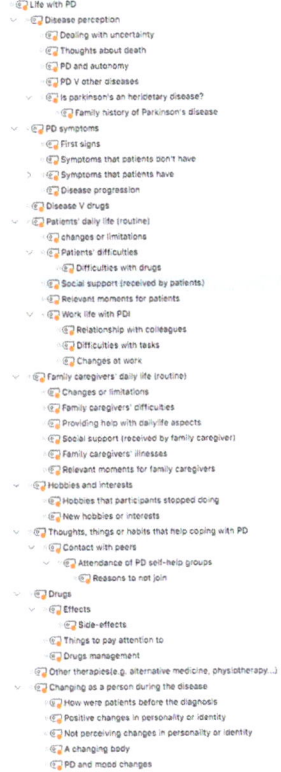

Figure A2. Extract of the coding three.

References

1. Rizek, P.; Kumar, N.; Jog, M.S. An update on the diagnosis and treatment of Parkinson disease. *Can. Med. Assoc. J.* **2016**, *188*, 1157–1165. [CrossRef] [PubMed]
2. Dorsey, E.R.; Sherer, T.; Okun, M.S.; Bloem, B.R. The Emerging Evidence of the Parkinson Pandemic. *J. Park. Dis.* **2018**, *8*, S3–S8. [CrossRef] [PubMed]
3. Casacanditella, L.; Cosoli, G.; Ceravolo, M.; Tomasini, E. Non-contact measurement of tremor for the characterisation of Parkinsonian individuals: Comparison between Kinect and Laser Doppler vibrometer. *J. Phys. Conf. Ser.* **2017**, *882*, 012002. [CrossRef]

4. Eeden, S.K.V.D.; Tanner, C.M.; Bernstein, A.L.; Fross, R.D.; Leimpeter, A.; Bloch, D.A.; Nelson, L.M. Incidence of Parkinson's Disease: Variation by Age, Gender, and Race/Ethnicity. *Am. J. Epidemiol.* **2003**, *157*, 1015–1022. [CrossRef]
5. Parkinson, J. An Essay on the Shaking Palsy. *J. Neuropsychiatry Clin. Neurosci.* **2002**, *14*, 223–236. [CrossRef]
6. Charcot, J.M. *Leçons du Mardi à la Salpêtrière: Policliniques 1887–1888*; Publications du Progrès Médical: Paris, France, 1887.
7. DeMaagd, G.; Philip, A. Parkinson's disease and its management: Part 1: Disease entity, risk factors, pathophysiology, clinical presentation, and diagnosis. *Pharm. Ther.* **2015**, *40*, 504.
8. Hawkes, C.H.; Del Tredici, K.; Braak, H. A timeline for Parkinson's disease. *Park. Relat. Disord.* **2010**, *16*, 79–84. [CrossRef] [PubMed]
9. Schrag, A.; Horsfall, L.; Walters, K.; Noyce, A.; Petersen, I. Prediagnostic presentations of Parkinson's disease in primary care: A case-control study. *Lancet Neurol.* **2015**, *14*, 57–64. [CrossRef]
10. Cronin-Golomb, A. Emergence of nonmotor symptoms as the focus of research and treatment of Parkinson's disease: Introduction to the special section on nonmotor dysfunctions in Parkinson's disease. *Behav. Neurosci.* **2013**, *127*, 135–138. [CrossRef]
11. Ortiz, K.Z.; Brabo, N.C.; Minett, T.S.C. Sensorimotor speech disorders in Parkinson's disease: Programming and execution deficits. *Dement. Neuropsychol.* **2016**, *10*, 210–216. [CrossRef]
12. Smith, K.M.; Caplan, D.N. Communication impairment in Parkinson's disease: Impact of motor and cognitive symptoms on speech and language. *Brain Lang.* **2018**, *185*, 38–46. [CrossRef]
13. Soundy, A.; Stubbs, B.; Roskell, C. The Experience of Parkinson's Disease: A Systematic Review and Meta-Ethnography. *Sci. World J.* **2014**, *2014*, 1–19. [CrossRef] [PubMed]
14. Yang, W.; Hamilton, J.L.; Kopil, C.; Beck, J.C.; Tanner, C.M.; Albin, R.L.; Dorsey, E.R.; Dahodwala, N.; Cintina, I.; Hogan, P.; et al. Current and projected future economic burden of Parkinson's disease in the U.S. *NPJ Park. Dis.* **2020**, *6*, 1–9. [CrossRef] [PubMed]
15. Noyes, K.; Liu, H.; Li, Y.; Holloway, R.; Dick, A.W. Economic burden associated with Parkinson's disease on elderly Medicare beneficiaries. *Mov. Disord.* **2005**, *21*, 362–372. [CrossRef]
16. Nutt, J.G.; Woodward, W.R.; Hammerstad, J.P.; Carter, J.H.; Anderson, J.L. The "On–Off" Phenomenon in Parkinson's Disease. *N. Engl. J. Med.* **1984**, *310*, 483–488. [CrossRef]
17. Wood, L.D. Clinical Review and Treatment of Select Adverse Effects of Dopamine Receptor Agonists in Parkinson's Disease. *Drugs Aging* **2010**, *27*, 295–310. [CrossRef] [PubMed]
18. Groiss, S.; Wojtecki, L.; Südmeyer, M.; Schnitzler, A. Review: Deep brain stimulation in Parkinson's disease. *Ther. Adv. Neurol. Disord.* **2009**, *2*, 379–391. [CrossRef]
19. Weaver, F.M.; Follett, K.A.; Stern, M.B.; Luo, P.; Harris, C.L.; Hur, K.; Marks, W.J.; Rothlind, J.C.; Sagher, O.; Moy, C.S.; et al. Randomized trial of deep brain stimulation for Parkinson disease: Thirty-six-month outcomes. *Neurology* **2012**, *79*, 55–65. [CrossRef]
20. Garcia-Ruiz, P.J. Impulse Control Disorders and Dopamine-Related Creativity: Pathogenesis and Mechanism, Short Review, and Hypothesis. *Front. Neurol.* **2018**, *9*, 1041. [CrossRef]
21. Martinez-Ramirez, D.; Hu, W.; Bona, A.R.; Okun, M.; Shukla, A.W. Update on deep brain stimulation in Parkinson's disease. *Transl. Neurodegener.* **2015**, *4*, 1–8. [CrossRef]
22. Tekriwal, A.; Baltuch, G. Deep Brain Stimulation: Expanding Applications. *Neurol. Med. Chir.* **2015**, *55*, 861–877. [CrossRef] [PubMed]
23. Sarem-Aslani, A.; Mullett, K. Industrial Perspective on Deep Brain Stimulation: History, Current State, and Future Developments. *Front. Integr. Neurosci.* **2011**, *5*, 46. [CrossRef] [PubMed]
24. Martinez-Ramirez, D.; Jimenez-Shahed, J.; Leckman, J.F.; Porta, M.; Servello, D.; Meng, F.-G.; Kuhn, J.; Huys, D.; Baldermann, J.C.; Foltynie, T.; et al. Efficacy and Safety of Deep Brain Stimulation in Tourette Syndrome. *JAMA Neurol.* **2018**, *75*, 353–359. [CrossRef]
25. Dandekar, M.P.; Fenoy, A.J.; Carvalho, A.F.; Soares, J.C.; Quevedo, J. Deep brain stimulation for treatment-resistant depression: An integrative review of preclinical and clinical findings and translational implications. *Mol. Psychiatry* **2018**, *23*, 1094–1112. [CrossRef]
26. Youngerman, B.; Chan, A.K.; Mikell, C.B.; McKhann, G.M.; Sheth, S.A. A decade of emerging indications: Deep brain stimulation in the United States. *J. Neurosurg.* **2016**, *125*, 461–471. [CrossRef] [PubMed]
27. Kahn, L.; Mathkour, M.; Lee, S.X.; Gouveia, E.E.; Hanna, J.A.; Garces, J.; Scullen, T.; McCormack, E.; Riffle, J.; Glynn, R.; et al. Long-term outcomes of deep brain stimulation in severe Parkinson's disease utilizing UPDRS III and modified Hoehn and Yahr as a severity scale. *Clin. Neurol. Neurosurg.* **2019**, *179*, 67–73. [CrossRef] [PubMed]
28. Lozano, A.M.; Lipsman, N.; Bergman, H.; Brown, P.; Chabardes, S.; Chang, J.W.; Matthews, K.; McIntyre, C.C.; Schlaepfer, T.E.; Schulder, M.; et al. Deep brain stimulation: Current challenges and future directions. *Nat. Rev. Neurol.* **2019**, *15*, 148–160. [CrossRef]
29. Elliott, M.; Momin, S.; Fiddes, B.; Farooqi, F.; Sohaib, S.A. Pacemaker and Defibrillator Implantation and Programming in Patients with Deep Brain Stimulation. *Arrhythmia Electrophysiol. Rev.* **2019**, *8*, 138–142. [CrossRef]
30. Baylis, F. "I Am Who I Am": On the Perceived Threats to Personal Identity from Deep Brain Stimulation. *Neuroethics* **2011**, *6*, 513–526. [CrossRef] [PubMed]
31. Gisquet, E. Cerebral implants and Parkinson's disease: A unique form of biographical disruption? *Soc. Sci. Med.* **2008**, *67*, 1847–1851. [CrossRef] [PubMed]

32. Kraemer, F. Me, Myself and My Brain Implant: Deep Brain Stimulation Raises Questions of Personal Authenticity and Alienation. *Neuroethics* 2011, *6*, 483–497. [CrossRef] [PubMed]
33. Gilbert, F.; Viaña, J.N.; Ineichen, C. Deflating the "DBS causes personality changes" bubble. *Neuroethics* 2018, 1–17. [CrossRef]
34. Lhommée, E.; Boyer, F.; Wack, M.; Pélissier, P.; Klinger, H.; Schmitt, E.; Bichon, A.; Fraix, V.; Chabardès, S.; Mertens, P.; et al. Personality, dopamine, and Parkinson's disease: Insights from subthalamic stimulation. *Mov. Disord.* 2017, *32*, 1191–1200. [CrossRef]
35. Pham, U.; Solbakk, A.-K.; Skogseid, I.-M.; Toft, M.; Pripp, A.H.; Konglund, A.E.; Andersson, S.; Haraldsen, I.R.; Aarsland, D.; Dietrichs, E.; et al. Personality Changes after Deep Brain Stimulation in Parkinson's Disease. *Park. Dis.* 2015, *2015*, 1–7. [CrossRef]
36. Kubu, C.S.; Ford, P.J.; Wilt, J.A.; Merner, A.R.; Montpetite, M.; Zeigler, J.; Racine, E. Pragmatism and the Importance of Interdisciplinary Teams in Investigating Personality Changes Following DBS. *Neuroethics* 2019, *2019*, 1–11. [CrossRef]
37. Thomson, C.J.; Segrave, R.A.; Racine, E.; Warren, N.; Thyagarajan, D.; Carter, A. "He's Back so I'm Not Alone": The Impact of Deep Brain Stimulation on Personality, Self, and Relationships in Parkinson's Disease. *Qual. Health Res.* 2020, *30*, 2217–2233. [CrossRef] [PubMed]
38. Haahr, A.; Kirkevold, M.; Hall, E.O.; Østergaard, K. From miracle to reconciliation: A hermeneutic phenomenological study exploring the experience of living with Parkinson's disease following Deep Brain Stimulation. *Int. J. Nurs. Stud.* 2010, *47*, 1228–1236. [CrossRef]
39. Chacón Gámez, Y.M. Deep brain stimulation and changes in personality and personal identity: The importance of qualitative studies. *Neuroethics* 2020, *6*, 486–492.
40. Armstrong, N.; Powell, J. Patient perspectives on health advice posted on Internet discussion boards: A qualitative study. *Health Expect.* 2009, *12*, 313–320. [CrossRef] [PubMed]
41. Jonasson, S.B.; Nilsson, M.H.; Lexell, J.; Carlsson, G. Experiences of fear of falling in persons with Parkinson's disease—A qualitative study. *BMC Geriatr.* 2018, *18*, 44. [CrossRef]
42. Renouf, S.; Ffytche, D.; Pinto, R.; Murray, J.; Lawrence, V. Visual hallucinations in dementia and Parkinson's disease: A qualitative exploration of patient and caregiver experiences. *Int. J. Geriatr. Psychiatry* 2018, *33*, 1327–1334. [CrossRef] [PubMed]
43. Cabrera, L.Y.; Kelly-Blake, K.; Sidiropoulos, C. Perspectives on Deep Brain Stimulation and Its Earlier Use for Parkinson's Disease: A Qualitative Study of US Patients. *Brain Sci.* 2020, *10*, 34. [CrossRef] [PubMed]
44. De Haan, S.; Rietveld, E.; Stokhof, M.; Denys, D. Effects of Deep Brain Stimulation on the Lived Experience of Obsessive-Compulsive Disorder Patients: In-Depth Interviews with 18 Patients. *PLoS ONE* 2015, *10*, e0135524. [CrossRef] [PubMed]
45. Lewis, C.J.; Maier, F.; Horstkötter, N.; Zywczok, A.; Witt, K.; Eggers, C.; Meyer, T.D.; Dembek, T.A.; Maarouf, M.; Moro, E.; et al. Subjectively perceived personality and mood changes associated with subthalamic stimulation in patients with Parkinson's disease. *Psychol. Med.* 2014, *45*, 73–85. [CrossRef] [PubMed]
46. Schupbach, M.; Gargiulo, M.; Welter, M.L.; Mallet, L.; Behar, C.; Houeto, J.L.; Maltete, D.; Mesnage, V.; Agid, Y. Neurosurgery in Parkinson disease: A distressed mind in a repaired body? *Neurology* 2006, *66*, 1811–1816. [CrossRef]
47. Liddle, J.; Phillips, J.; Gustafsson, L.; Silburn, P. Understanding the lived experiences of Parkinson's disease and deep brain stimulation (DBS) through occupational changes. *Aust. Occup. Ther. J.* 2017, *65*, 45–53. [CrossRef]
48. Jewitt, C. *The Routledge Handbook of Multimodal Analysis*, 2nd ed.; First Published in Paperback; Routledge: London, UK; Taylor & Francis Group: New York, NY, USA, 2017.
49. McLaughlin, D.; Hasson, F.; Kernohan, G.; Waldron, M.; McLaughlin, M.; Cochrane, B.; Chambers, H. Living and coping with Parkinson's disease: Perceptions of informal carers. *Palliat. Med.* 2010, *25*, 177–182. [CrossRef]
50. Rastgardani, T.; Armstrong, M.J.; Marras, C.; Gagliardi, A.R. Improving patient-centred care for persons with Parkinson's: Qualitative interviews with care partners about their engagement in discussions of "off" periods. *Health Expect.* 2019, *22*, 555–564. [CrossRef]
51. Hariz, G.-M.; Limousin, P.; Tisch, S.; Jahanshahi, M.; Fjellman-Wiklund, A. Patients' perceptions of life shift after deep brain stimulation for primary dystonia-A qualitative study. *Mov. Disord.* 2011, *26*, 2101–2106. [CrossRef]
52. Chacón Gámez, Y.M.; Mouton Dorey, C.; Biller-Andorno, N. Exploring the experiences of Parkinson's patients and their family caregivers with healthcare professionals: A qualitative assessment of unmet needs. *PLoS ONE* 2021, *14*, e0226916.
53. Gámez, Y.M.C.; Biller-Andorno, N. Living with Parkinson's disease and connected to the duodopa pump: A qualitative study. *Qual. Res. Med. Health* 2021, *4*. [CrossRef]
54. ERG. *Health Experiences Research Group, Researcher's Handbook Health Talk Online & Youth Health Talk Modules*; Department of Primary Health Care: Oxford, UK, 2018.
55. Creswell, W.J. *Qualitative Inquiry & Research Design. Choosing among Five Approaches*, 3rd ed.; SAGE: London, UK, 2013.
56. Ziebland, S.; McPherson, A. Making sense of qualitative data analysis: An introduction with illustrations from DIPEx (personal experiences of health and illness). *Med. Educ.* 2006, *40*, 405–414. [CrossRef]
57. Ziebland, S.; Herxheimer, A. How patients' experiences contribute to decision making: Illustrations from DIPEx (personal experiences of health and illness). *J. Nurs. Manag.* 2008, *16*, 433–439. [CrossRef]
58. Adami, E. *Multimodality*; Routledge: London, UK, 2015. [CrossRef]
59. Guillemin, M. Understanding Illness: Using Drawings as a Research Method. *Qual. Health Res.* 2004, *14*, 272–289. [CrossRef]
60. Eassey, D.; Reddel, H.K.; Ryan, K.; Smith, L. Living with severe asthma: The role of perceived competence and goal achievement. *Chronic Illn.* 2019. [CrossRef]

61. Fereday, J.; Muir-Cochrane, E. Demonstrating Rigor Using Thematic Analysis: A Hybrid Approach of Inductive and Deductive Coding and Theme Development. *Int. J. Qual. Methods* **2006**, *5*, 80–92. [CrossRef]
62. Costa, K. *Systematic Guide to Qualitative Data Analysis within the C.O.S.T.A Postgraduate Research Model*; OSF Preprints: Charlottesville, VA, USA, 2019. [CrossRef]
63. Roberts, K.; Dowell, A.; Nie, J.-B. Attempting rigour and replicability in thematic analysis of qualitative research data; a case study of codebook development. *BMC Med. Res. Methodol.* **2019**, *19*, 66. [CrossRef] [PubMed]
64. Nowell, L.S.; Norris, J.; White, D.E.; Moules, N.J. Thematic Analysis: Striving to meet the trustworthiness criteria. *Int. J. Qual. Methods* **2017**, *16*. [CrossRef]
65. Cheung, M.M.Y.; Saini, B.; Smith, L. Using drawings to explore patients' perceptions of their illness: A scoping review. *J. Multidiscip. Health* **2016**, *9*, 631–646. [CrossRef] [PubMed]
66. Kirkham, J.A.; Smith, J.A.; Havsteen-Franklin, D. Painting pain: An interpretative phenomenological analysis of representations of living with chronic pain. *Health Psychol.* **2015**, *34*, 398–406. [CrossRef] [PubMed]
67. McGowan, L.; Luker, K.; Creed, F.; Chew-Graham, C.A. 'How do you explain a pain that can't be seen?': The narratives of women with chronic pelvic pain and their disengagement with the diagnostic cycle. *Br. J. Health Psychol.* **2007**, *12*, 261–274. [CrossRef]
68. Phillips, J.; Ogden, J.; Copland, C. Using drawings of pain-related images to understand the experience of chronic pain: A qualitative study. *Br. J. Occup. Ther.* **2015**, *78*, 404–411. [CrossRef]
69. Haahr, A.; Kirkevold, M.; Hall, E.O.; Østergaard, K. 'Being in it together': Living with a partner receiving deep brain stimulation for advanced Parkinson's disease—A hermeneutic phenomenological study. *J. Adv. Nurs.* **2012**, *69*, 338–347. [CrossRef] [PubMed]
70. Theed, R.; Eccles, F.; Simpson, J. Experiences of caring for a family member with Parkinson's disease: A meta-synthesis. *Aging Ment. Health* **2016**, *21*, 1007–1016. [CrossRef]
71. Padovani, C.; Lopes, M.C.D.L.; Higahashi, I.H.; Pelloso, S.M.; Paiano, M.; Christophoro, R. Being caregiver of people with Parkinson's Disease: Experienced situations. *Rev. Bras. Enferm.* **2018**, *71*, 2628–2634. [CrossRef] [PubMed]
72. Martínez-Martín, P.; Forjaz, M.J.; Frades-Payo, B.; Rusiñol, A.B.; Fernández-García, J.M.; Benito-León, J.; Arillo, V.C.; Barberá, M.A.; Sordo, M.P.; Catalán, M.J. Caregiver burden in Parkinson's disease. *Mov. Disord.* **2007**, *22*, 924–931. [CrossRef] [PubMed]
73. Abendroth, M.; Greenblum, C.A.; Gray, J.A. The Value of Peer-Led Support Groups Among Caregivers of Persons With Parkinson's Disease. *Holist. Nurs. Pract.* **2014**, *28*, 48–54. [CrossRef]
74. Van Hienen, M.M.; Contarino, M.F.; Middelkoop, H.A.; Van Hilten, J.J.; Geraedts, V.J. Effect of deep brain stimulation on caregivers of patients with Parkinson's disease: A systematic review. *Park. Relat. Disord.* **2020**, *81*, 20–27. [CrossRef] [PubMed]
75. Joint, C.; Aziz, T.Z. Outcome After Deep Brain Stimulation Surgery of the Subthalamic Nucleus for Parkinson Disease: Do We Understand What Is Important to Our Patients? *World Neurosurg.* **2014**, *82*, 1035–1036. [CrossRef] [PubMed]
76. Rossi, M.; Bruno, V.; Arena, J.; Cammarota, Á.; Merello, M. Challenges in PD Patient Management After DBS: A Pragmatic Review. *Mov. Disord. Clin. Pract.* **2018**, *5*, 246–254. [CrossRef]
77. Müller, S.; Christen, M. Deep brain stimulation in parkinsonian patients—Ethical evaluation of cognitive, affective, and behavioral sequelae. *AJOB Neurosci.* **2011**, *2*, 3–13. [CrossRef]
78. Witt, K.; Kuhn, J.; Timmermann, L.; Zurowski, M.; Woopen, C. Deep Brain Stimulation and the Search for Identity. *Neuroethics* **2011**, *6*, 499–511. [CrossRef] [PubMed]
79. Hildt, E. Electrodes in the brain: Some anthropological and ethical aspects of deep brain stimulation. *Int. Rev. Inf. Ethics* **2006**, *5*, 33–38. [CrossRef]
80. Schechtman, M. Philosophical reflections on narrative and deep brain stimulation. *J. Clin. Ethics* **2010**, *21*, 133–139.
81. Voon, V.; Saint-Cyr, J.; Lozano, A.; Moro, E.; Poon, Y.Y.; Lang, A. Psychiatric symptoms in patients with Parkinson disease presenting for deep brain stimulation surgery. *J. Neurosurg.* **2005**, *103*, 246–251. [CrossRef] [PubMed]
82. Radziunas, A.; Deltuva, V.P.; Tamasauskas, A.; Gleizniene, R.; Pranckeviciene, A.; Surkiene, D.; Bunevicius, A. Neuropsychiatric complications and neuroimaging characteristics after deep brain stimulation surgery for Parkinson's disease. *Brain Imaging Behav.* **2018**, *14*, 62–71. [CrossRef]
83. Zarzycki, M.Z.; Domitrz, I. Stimulation-induced side effects after deep brain stimulation—A systematic review. *Acta Neuropsychiatr.* **2019**, *32*, 57–64. [CrossRef] [PubMed]
84. Christen, M.; Ineichen, C.; Bittlinger, M.; Bothe, H.-W.; Müller, S. Ethical Focal Points in the International Practice of Deep Brain Stimulation. *AJOB Neurosci.* **2014**, *5*, 65–80. [CrossRef]
85. Mosley, P.; Marsh, R. The Psychiatric and Neuropsychiatric Symptoms after Subthalamic Stimulation for Parkinson's Disease. *J. Neuropsychiatry Clin. Neurosci.* **2015**, *27*, 19–26. [CrossRef]
86. Han, J.W.; Ahn, Y.D.; Kim, W.-S.; Shin, C.M.; Jeong, S.J.; Song, Y.S.; Bae, Y.J.; Kim, J.-M. Psychiatric Manifestation in Patients with Parkinson's Disease. *J. Korean Med. Sci.* **2018**, *33*. [CrossRef]
87. Leeman, R.F.; E Billingsley, B.; Potenza, M.N. Impulse control disorders in Parkinson's disease: Background and update on prevention and management. *Neurodegener. Dis. Manag.* **2012**, *2*, 389–400. [CrossRef] [PubMed]
88. Corvol, J.-C.; Artaud, F.; Cormier-Dequaire, F.; Rascol, O.; Durif, F.; Derkinderen, P.; Marques, A.-R.; Bourdain, F.; Brandel, J.-P.; Pico, F.; et al. Longitudinal analysis of impulse control disorders in Parkinson disease. *Neurology* **2018**, *91*, e189–e201. [CrossRef] [PubMed]
89. Moore, T.J.; Glenmullen, J.; Mattison, D.R. Reports of Pathological Gambling, Hypersexuality, and Compulsive Shopping Associated With Dopamine Receptor Agonist Drugs. *JAMA Intern. Med.* **2014**, *174*, 1930–1933. [CrossRef] [PubMed]

90. Klos, K.J.; Bower, J.H.; Josephs, K.A.; Matsumoto, J.Y.; Ahlskog, J.E. Pathological hypersexuality predominantly linked to adjuvant dopamine agonist therapy in Parkinson's disease and multiple system atrophy. *Park. Relat. Disord.* **2005**, *11*, 381–386. [CrossRef] [PubMed]
91. Tarakad, A.; Jankovic, J. Anosmia and Ageusia in Parkinson's Disease. *Int. Rev. Neurobiol.* **2017**, *133*, 541–556. [CrossRef]
92. Pandey, S.; Srivanitchapoom, P. Levodopa-induced Dyskinesia: Clinical Features, Pathophysiology, and Medical Management. *Ann. Indian Acad. Neurol.* **2017**, *20*, 190–198. [CrossRef]
93. Glannon, W. Stimulating brains, altering minds. *J. Med. Ethics* **2009**, *35*, 289–292. [CrossRef]
94. Gilbert, F. The burden of normality: From 'chronically ill' to 'symptom free'. New ethical challenges for deep brain stimulation postoperative treatment. *J. Med. Ethics* **2012**, *38*, 408–412. [CrossRef]
95. Gilbert, F.; Goddard, E.; Viaña, J.N.M.; Carter, A.; Horne, M. I Miss Being Me: Phenomenological Effects of Deep Brain Stimulation. *AJOB Neurosci.* **2017**, *8*, 96–109. [CrossRef]
96. Costanza, A.; Radomska, M.; Bondolfi, G.; Zenga, F.; Amerio, A.; Aguglia, A.; Serafini, G.; Amore, M.; Berardelli, I.; Pompili, M.; et al. Suicidality Associated With Deep Brain Stimulation in Extrapyramidal Diseases: A Critical Review and Hypotheses on Neuroanatomical and Neuroimmune Mechanisms. *Front. Integr. Neurosci.* **2021**, *15*. [CrossRef]
97. Bell, E.; Maxwell, B.; McAndrews, M.P.; Sadikot, A.F.; Racine, E. A Review of Social and Relational Aspects of Deep Brain Stimulation in Parkinson's Disease Informed by Healthcare Provider Experiences. *Park. Dis.* **2011**, *2011*, 1–8. [CrossRef] [PubMed]
98. Baertschi, M.; Favez, N.; Radomska, M.; Herrmann, F.; Burkhard, P.R.; Weber, K.; Canuto, A.; Dos Santos, J.F.A. An Empirical Study on the Application of the Burden of Normality to Patients Undergoing Deep Brain Stimulation for Parkinson's Disease. *J. Psychosoc. Rehabil. Ment. Health* **2019**, *6*, 175–186. [CrossRef]
99. Baertschi, M.; Dos Santos, J.F.A.; Burkhard, P.; Weber, K.; Canuto, A.; Favez, N. The burden of normality as a model of psychosocial adjustment after deep brain stimulation for Parkinson's disease: A systematic investigation. *Neuropsychology* **2019**, *33*, 178–194. [CrossRef]
100. Accolla, E.A.; Pollo, C. Mood Effects after Deep Brain Stimulation for Parkinson's Disease: An Update. *Front. Neurol.* **2019**, *10*, 617. [CrossRef] [PubMed]
101. Mosley, P.E.; Robinson, K.; Coyne, T.; Silburn, P.; Breakspear, M.; Carter, A. 'Woe Betides Anybody Who Tries to Turn me Down.' A Qualitative Analysis of Neuropsychiatric Symptoms Following Subthalamic Deep Brain Stimulation for Parkinson's Disease. *Neuroethics* **2019**, 1–17. [CrossRef]
102. Bogdan, I.D.; Van Laar, T.; Oterdoom, D.M.; Drost, G.; Van Dijk, J.M.C.; Beudel, M. Optimal Parameters of Deep Brain Stimulation in Essential Tremor: A Meta-Analysis and Novel Programming Strategy. *J. Clin. Med.* **2020**, *9*, 1855. [CrossRef]
103. Brown, R.; Jahanshahi, M.; Quinn, N.; Marsden, C.D. Sexual function in patients with Parkinson's disease and their partners. *J. Neurol. Neurosurg. Psychiatry* **1990**, *53*, 480–486. [CrossRef] [PubMed]
104. MacKenzie, R. Who Should Hold the Remote for the New Me? Cognitive, Affective, and Behavioral Side Effects of DBS and Authentic Choices over Future Personalities. *AJOB Neurosci.* **2011**, *2*, 18–20. [CrossRef]
105. MacKenzie, R. Must Family/Carers Look after Strangers? Post-DBS Identity Changes and Related Conflicts Of Interest. *Front. Integr. Neurosci.* **2011**, *5*, 12. [CrossRef]
106. De Haan, S. Missing Oneself or Becoming Oneself? The Difficulty of What "Becoming a Different Person" Means. *AJOB Neurosci.* **2017**, *8*, 110–112. [CrossRef]
107. Mecacci, G.; Haselager, P. Stimulating the Self: The Influence of Conceptual Frameworks on Reactions to Deep Brain Stimulation. *AJOB Neurosci.* **2014**, *5*, 30–39. [CrossRef]
108. Gilbert, F. Deep Brain Stimulation: Inducing Self-Estrangement. *Neuroethics* **2017**, *11*, 157–165. [CrossRef]
109. Pateraki, M. The multiple temporalities of deep brain stimulation (DBS) in Greece. *Med. Health Care Philos.* **2018**, *22*, 353–362. [CrossRef]
110. Tanner, C.M. A second honeymoon for Parkinson's disease? *N. Engl. J. Med.* **2013**, *368*, 675–676. [CrossRef]
111. Charmaz, K. *Good Days, Bad Days: The Self in Chronic Illness and Time*; Rutgers University Press: New Brunswick, NJ, USA, 1991.
112. Vann-Ward, T.; Morse, J.M.; Charmaz, K. Preserving Self: Theorizing the Social and Psychological Processes of Living with Parkinson Disease. *Qual. Health Res.* **2017**, *27*, 964–982. [CrossRef]
113. Pesantes, M.A.; Somerville, C.; Singh, S.B.; Perez-Leon, S.; Madede, T.; Suggs, S.; Beran, D. Disruption, changes, and adaptation: Experiences with chronic conditions in Mozambique, Nepal and Peru. *Glob. Public Health* **2019**, *15*, 372–383. [CrossRef]
114. Bramley, N.; Eatough, V. The experience of living with Parkinson's disease: An interpretative phenomenological analysis case study. *Psychol. Health* **2005**, *20*, 223–235. [CrossRef]
115. Williams, S. Chronic illness as biographical disruption or biographical disruption as chronic illness? Reflections on a core concept. *Sociol. Health Illn.* **2000**, *22*, 40–67. [CrossRef]
116. Barken, R. Caregivers' Interpretations of Time and Biography. *J. Contemp. Ethnogr.* **2014**, *43*, 695–719. [CrossRef]
117. Korstjens, I.; Moser, A. Series: Practical guidance to qualitative research. Part 4: Trustworthiness and publishing. *Eur. J. Gen. Pract.* **2017**, *24*, 120–124. [CrossRef]
118. Danna, J.; Velay, J.-L.; Eusebio, A.; Véron-Delor, L.; Witjas, T.; Azulay, J.-P.; Pinto, S. Digitalized spiral drawing in Parkinson's disease: A tool for evaluating beyond the written trace. *Hum. Mov. Sci.* **2019**, *65*, 80–88. [CrossRef] [PubMed]
119. Shimura, H.; Tanaka, R.; Urabe, T.; Tanaka, S.; Hattori, N. Art and Parkinson's disease: A dramatic change in an artist's style as an initial symptom. *J. Neurol.* **2011**, *259*, 879–881. [CrossRef] [PubMed]

120. Brailas, A. Using Drawings in Qualitative Interviews: An Introduction to the Practice. *Qual. Rep.* **2020**, *25*, 4447–4460. [CrossRef]
121. Broadbent, E.; Petrie, K.J.; Ellis, C.J.; Ying, J.; Gamble, G. A picture of health—Myocardial infarction patients' drawings of their hearts and subsequent disability. *J. Psychosom. Res.* **2004**, *57*, 583–587. [CrossRef]
122. Thorpe, C.; Arbeau, K.J.; Budlong, B. 'I drew the parts of my body in proportion to how much PCOS ruined them': Experiences of polycystic ovary syndrome through drawings. *Health Psychol. Open* **2019**, *6*. [CrossRef]
123. Broadbent, E.; Niederhoffer, K.; Hague, T.; Corter, A.; Reynolds, L. Headache sufferers' drawings reflect distress, disability and illness perceptions. *J. Psychosom. Res.* **2009**, *66*, 465–470. [CrossRef] [PubMed]

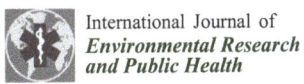

Article

First Insights into Barriers and Facilitators from the Perspective of Persons with Multiple Sclerosis: A Multiple Case Study

Joelle Ott [1], Nikola Biller-Andorno [1] and Andrea Glässel [1,2,*]

[1] Institute of Biomedical Ethics and Medical History, University Zurich, Winterthurerstrasse 30, CH-8006 Zurich, Switzerland
[2] Institute of Public Health (IPH), Department of Health Sciences Katharina-Sulzer-Platz 9, Zurich University of Applied Studies (ZHAW), CH-8401 Winterthur, Switzerland
* Correspondence: andrea.glaessel@ibme.uzh.ch; Tel.: +41-58-934-4397

Abstract: Multiple Sclerosis (MS) is a complex, lifelong disease. Its effects span across different areas of life and vary strongly. In Switzerland, there is an intense discussion on how to optimize quality of care and patient safety. Patients should be more involved in the management of health care to improve the quality of care from the patient's perspective and form a more comprehensive perspective. This multiple-case study explores the question of how persons with MS experience and describe functioning related barriers, facilitating factors, and ethically relevant conflicts. To address this from a comprehensive perspective, the MS core set of the International Classification for Functioning, Disability, and Health (ICF) is used as theoretical framework. To explore barriers, facilitators, and relevant ethical issues, different narrative sources were used for thematic analysis and ICF coding: (a) MS transcripts from DIPEx interviews and (b) an autobiographical book of persons living with MS. Insights that were meaningful for daily practice and education were identified: (a) understanding the importance of environmental circumstances based on narrative sources; (b) understanding the importance of a person's individual life situation, and the ability to switch perspectives in the medical field; (c) respect for PwMS' individuality in health care settings; (d) creating meaningful relationships for disease management and treatment, as well as building trust.

Keywords: multiple sclerosis; patient perspective; qualitative research methods; thematic analysis; ICF; DIPEx; patient experience; ethics; narration; multiple case study; source analysis

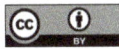

1. Introduction

1.1. Multiple Sclerosis

Multiple Sclerosis (MS) is one of the most common organic diseases of the central nervous system. Worldwide, 2.5 million people have been diagnosed with MS. Almost 70% of persons with MS are women [1]. In 2020, nearly 15,000 persons with MS (PwMS) lived in Switzerland [2]. This amounts to 180 affected people per 100.000 of the population. The disease burden of MS was previously estimated for Switzerland in the context of a larger, international consortia. More detailed, subgroup-specific burden estimates are lacking. This knowledge gap is regrettable from a public health perspective. More detailed findings reflecting the disease–severity distribution and age structure of the population of persons with MS (PwMS) are of high relevance for health policy and care providers [3].

The first symptoms develop between the ages of 20 and 40, but MS can also develop in children and people over 40, although this is less common [4]. Depending on the form, women can be up to three times as likely to be affected as men. Prevalence rises as one goes north from the equator.

MS is characterized by demyelination caused by local inflammation. This leads to a decrease in or loss of function of the affected nerve cells. MS is a chronic disease that represents an irreversible presence of disease conditions or damage to the nervous system.

The location of these lesions influences the symptoms. The symptoms can be motor, visual, psychological, cognitive, sensibility disorders or many other neurological symptoms. There is a large variation between patients and disease course [4]. Since the progression of the disease, as well as the presentation of symptoms, is very case-specific, the impact of the disease on daily life varies from person to person [5]. One important aspect of how strongly people are affected is how much their mobility is limited and their autonomy is restricted. Ambulation has been self-declared to be the most important body function that is impacted by PwMS. An estimated 75% of PwMS have walking disturbances. This can limit their participation in activities. Environmental factors and personal factors can lighten or exacerbate the impact of these limitations. Numerous devices can aid impaired mobility. These range from canes to motorized scooters to braces that assist ambulation. There are also numerous devices to assist in activities of daily living. These can make it possible for PwMS to retain their independence [5].

A diagnosis of MS fundamentally changes one's life and often requires a reorganization of many aspects of life [6]. Topics range from rethinking mobility to dealing with personal anxiety as to what the future might hold and do not leave much out in between. To ensure that those affected can gain or retain the best possible quality of life and patient security, a person-centered point of view, a comprehensive bio-psycho-social perspective on health and health care, is needed [7]. In Switzerland, there is an intense ongoing discussion regarding how quality of care and patient safety can be optimized and guaranteed in the future. A "National Report on Quality and Patient Safety in the Swiss Health care System", commissioned by the Federal Office of Public Health concludes, among other things, that patients should be more involved in their health care management and that the quality of treatment and care should be assessed and improved from the patient's perspective and from a more comprehensive perspective of health care [8].

1.2. International Classification of Functioning, Disability and Health (ICF)

Based on the bio-psycho-social model of health, which stipulates that a health condition is not an isolated entity but needs to be seen in its psycho-social context, the World Health Organization (WHO) developed the International Classification of Functioning, Disability and Health (ICF) (see Figure 1) [7]. This framework and its predecessor focus on functional management and individual chronic disease experiences by considering the whole life situation of a person and aims to provide a standardized language for this purpose. The ICF is based on a model of interaction that provides a system of classification for long-term, non-fatal effects of diseases. Human functioning, or a decrease in human functioning, is portrayed as an interaction between health conditions and contextual factors, which include environmental and personal factors. The different categories of the ICF are related and influence each other in different ways. They can even influence health conditions.

The ICF is organized into two parts: (a) functioning and disability and (b) contextual factors. Contextual factors are divided into environmental factors and personal factors. These components are divided into domains. These domains are further subdivided. Each term is defined starting at the level of the domain and has an alphanumerical code. The environmental factors, which are the focus of this paper, have five domains:

- e1 Products and Technology;
- e2 Natural Environment and Human-Made Changes to Environment;
- e3 Support and Relationships;
- e4 Attitudes;
- e5 Services, Systems and Policies.

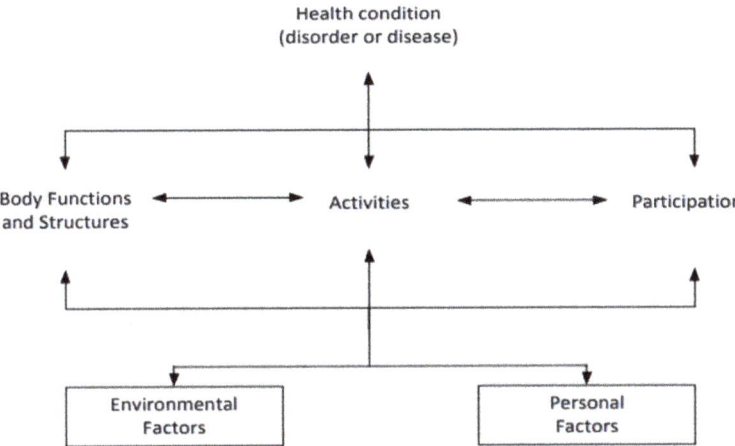

Figure 1. Bio-psycho-social model: This is an open access article distributed under the Creative Commons Attribution License, which permits unrestricted use, distribution, and reproduction in any medium, provided the original work is properly cited [7].

These can be qualified as facilitators or barriers depending on whether they support or hinder the person. The same domain or code occurring further down the tree can be a facilitator to one person and a barrier to another, depending on the person's needs and availability. In this study, the qualification of barrier or facilitator is made based on the PwMS's description.

This means an environmental factor such as medication (e1101 Drugs) can either be a barrier or facilitator, depending on the availability, impact, and its side-effects. Barriers are defined by the ICF as: "factors in a person's environment that, through their absence or presence, limit function or create disability. These include aspects such as a physical environment that is inaccessible, lack of relevant assistive technology, and negative attitudes of people towards disability, as well as services, systems and policies that are either nonexistent or that hinder the involvement of all people with a health condition in all areas of life" [7] (p. 222).

Facilitators are described as: "factors in a person's environment that, through their absence or presence, improve functioning and reduce disability. These include aspects such as a physical environment that is accessible, the availability of relevant assistive technology, and positive attitudes of people towards disability, as well as services, systems and policies that aim to increase the involvement of all people with a health condition in all areas of life. Absence of a factor can also be facilitating, for example the absence of stigma or negative attitudes. Facilitators can prevent an impairment or activity limitation from becoming a participation restriction, since the actual performance of an action is enhanced, despite the person's problem with capacity" [7] (p. 222).

Personal factors are defined as: "the particular background of an individual's life and living, and compromise features of the individual that are not part of a health condition or health states" [7] (p. 17), which are so far not classified.

Since the ICF is very extensive, so-called core sets have been developed for different health conditions and health-related situations [7,9–12]. Condition-specific ICF Core sets for MS were developed by Coenen et al. 2011 [11]. This standard allows for a structured description of persons with specific health conditions, using widely accepted terminology, without the need to navigate the whole ICF [11]. For clinical practice, a case example for PwMS on how to apply the ICF core sets for MS in long-term care, including the context-related factors and the interprofessional treatment team involved, is already available in Switzerland [12]. This paper uses the environmental factors of the comprehensive core set for MS as basis to evaluate barriers and facilitators from two different narrative sources of data: source (1) transcripts of two semi-structured Database of Individual Patients' Experiences (DIPEx) interviews, and source (2) a literary autobiographical representation of a person's life with MS.

1.3. Ethical Considerations and Aims of This Case Study

The ICF is a comprehensive theoretical framework for describing and categorizing function, disability, and health, but does not provide a detailed structure for ethical considerations. To strengthen these considerations, this paper uses the four ethical principles of Beauchamp and Childress's [13], which are widely established and applied in the medical field and health care sector: (a) respect for autonomy, (b) nonmaleficence, (c) beneficence and (d) justice. These principals are not a manual on how to solve a medical ethical dilemma, but a framework that can help to structure a decision-making process. When grappling with an ethical dilemma, it can help to determine which underlying principles are conflicting [14].

The aim of this multiple-case study, designed as a qualitative analysis of narrative sources, is to assess barriers, facilitators, and ethically relevant aspects from the perspective of PwMS, using the common language of the ICF and the MS-specific core set to derive important aspects in PwMS health care. The general research question of this paper is:

"How do PwMS experience and describe barriers, facilitators and ethically relevant conflicts?"

Our research question will be specified as follows:

(a) Which causes are identified, what could possible solutions to functioning-related barriers look like, and which ethical aspects become recognizable?
(b) What consequences and benefits can be found for the collaborative practice in the care of PwMS?

2. Materials and Methods

2.1. Study Design and Methodology

Our research question is based on a multiple-case study design, as described by Yin 2003 [15], to explore differences within and between cases and enhance data credibility. To make comparisons, the cases were carefully selected so that similar outcomes or contrasting outcomes could be predicted based on theory. In our study, the biopsychosocial model of the ICF was used. We examined three different cases to understand the similarities and differences between the cases. Yin (2003) describes how using multiple case studies either, "(a) predicts similar results (a literal replication) or (b) predicts contrasting results but for predictable reasons (a theoretical replication)" [15] (p. 47).

This work is based on the approach to meanings and understanding focusing on the lived experiences of individuals within a social and personal world. Thus, we follow the interpretive phenomenological analysis (IPA) approach of Smith and Osborn, 2003 [16,17]. IPA is appropriate for discovering how individuals "perceive certain situations they face as they perceive them" [18] (p.429). IPA goes back to Husserl (1913/1983) and his phenomenological position [19].

Therefore, in this multiple-case study, we focused on mixed methods to analyze contextual factors of the ICF. This analysis does not include the whole spectrum of functioning and disability. Additionally, our research questions will be answered using qualitative research methods based on a thematic analysis by Braun and Clarke [20,21] of two different narrative sources:

(1) Two narrative interviews: *Interview A* and *Interview B*.
(2) A literary autobiographical representation: *Book C*.

Interviews A and B are semi-structured narrative interviews, conducted for the MS module of the Swiss DIPEx project (www.DIPEx.ch (accessed on 21 August 2022)). The persons being interviewed were informed that the primary use of the interviews was for a website portraying MS, but that they might also be used anonymously for research.

DIPEx is an association of researchers conducting qualitative research into people's personal experiences of health and illness with a common methodology for conducting semi-structured interviews [22,23]. This narrative method was developed by the Health Experiences Research Group at the Nuffield Department of Primary Care at the University of Oxford. The international DIPEx network comprised thirteen countries implementing their own national DIPEx platforms, based on qualitative studies. The aim of DIPEx is to present a wide spectrum of diverse perspectives on different diseases and health conditions to the public (patients, family caregivers, health professionals, and students) [22,23]. To explain how we use the terms health, disease and illness in this study, we follow the definition of Rovesti et al.: "in the English language, there are three terms to indicate a pathological state: illness, which identifies the personal emotional state connected to the loss of health; disease, which refers to the objective, biological and measurable di-mension of it-strictly linked to the physician's activity-and sickness, which refers in-stead to the public dimension of the disease and highlights the link between illness and society" [24] (p. 163).

Book C is an autobiographical text published in 2019, which describes the author's journey from Switzerland to Venice in a wheelchair and his inner journey of learning to accept his need for a wheelchair. He writes about his individual experiences living with MS and tells stories about how his wheelchair makes his life easier and more complicated at the same time [25] (see Figure 2).

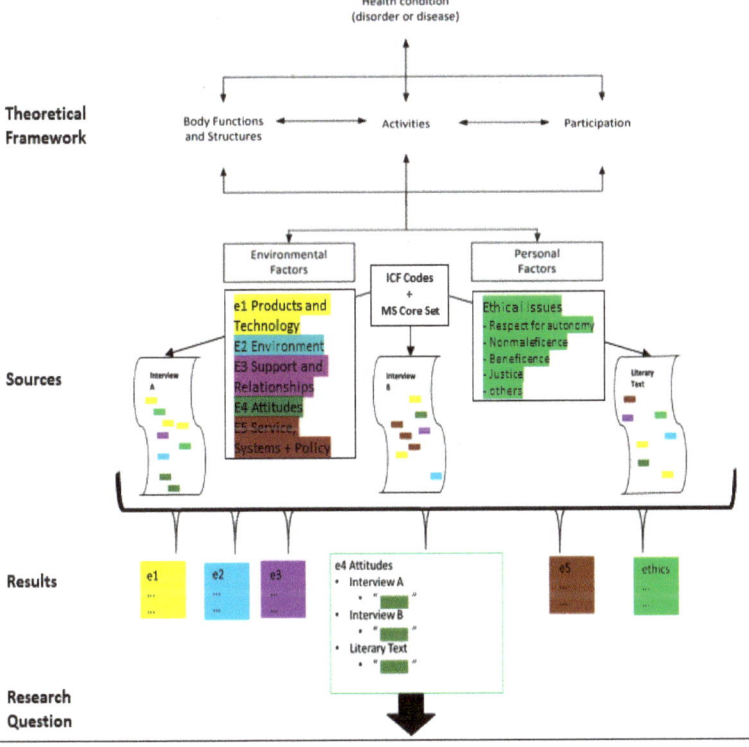

Figure 2. Flowchart and overview of paper's methods and their integration into the theoretical framework of the bio-psycho-social model of disease and the ICF.

This multiple-case study was conducted at the University of Zurich in Switzerland from September 2019 to July 2021, and structured in the following steps: selection of cases from the 30 interviews conducted by this point; reading of the book; introduction to the theoretical framework of the ICF and the ICF core sets for MS; training in ICF coding, especially focusing on contextual factors; introduction to the biomedical principles according to Beauchamp and Childress; qualitative research based on thematic analysis according to Braun and Clarke [20,21] to explore the narrative content; structuring and writing the manuscript.

Using a combination of inductive and deductive coding, the barriers, facilitators and ethical aspects mentioned were extracted. The deductive coding derived codes from the comprehensive MS core set developed by Coenen, et al. [11]. As inductive coding, non-core set codes were added where needed.

The ICF is anchored in the bio-psycho-social model for understanding diseases and their effects in daily life situations and their interactions. Additionally, ethical issues, which are part of the personal factors in the ICF, were coded using Beauchamp and Childress's [13] principles. The results were sorted by ICF domain and used to answer the research question (see Supplementary Materials—as a video presentation).

2.2. Role of Researchers

The first author (JO) is a medical student. Her background is focused on more the biological aspect of a disease and less on experiences of illness and the psychosocial evaluation thereof. Her learning has mainly concentrated on objective data and facts. These are an important basis for medical decision-making, and are what medical students are tested on throughout their studies. However, the doctor–patient relationship is also thought to have a significant influence on the treatment outcome. She (JO) is convinced that the doctor's understanding of a patient's situation will improve the relationship. This is her motivation for this project. She has never met any of the participants in the DIPEx study, she has never been involved in the treatment of a patient with MS, nor does she have any personal experience with the disease: not as a patient herself, not as friend, and not as a family member of a person diagnosed with MS. The interviewer of these DIPEx interviews is the last author (AG). She is leading the MS DIPEx module with a research background in public health, rehabilitation sciences, and applied ethics. In addition, she has years of experience in a neurorehabilitation setting as a physiotherapist. She is co-supervising this master project. She was not involved in the treatment of the individuals. NBA co-designed the larger study (the DIPEx Module) of which the presented sample is a subset.

2.3. Ethics

In response to ethics applications with BASEC-Nr. Req-2018-00050, the Ethics Commissions in Switzerland issued a declaration of non-jurisdiction. This paper is part of the project, that, in accordance with this decision, does not need sanctioning by an ethics commission. The persons interviewed agreed to have their testimonials used for research purposes.

2.4. Source Criticism

The narrative sources are first-person accounts, which gives us unfiltered access to the PwMS's accounts. The semi-structured form of the interviews enhances the comparability, while still leaving room for individual accounts. The literary text does not have predetermined topics, and thus leaves more room for the author to set priorities. All narrative sources are written in German and strongly colored by the narrators and their motivations for creating these sources. The interviews each lasted for about 2 h. The literary text covers 123 pages.

Source 1: Transcripts of two narrative semi-structured DIPEx interviews. The person in *Interview A* is asked how MS has influenced her and her personality; she answers: "completely" and that this is difficult for her. She references barriers more often than facilitators. Her motivation for participation seems to be to show the barriers and to give

MS a face, so that one does not only think of a disease, but of the persons affected by the disease.

The person in *Interview B* is more focused on the positive. She gives examples of ignoring inconveniences. This gives the impression that, while she might not leave out the hardships, she might underrepresent their influence. I think that her motivation for participating in this interview was to show that life with MS is still worth living. She says she has good quality of life.

Source 2: A literary autobiographical representation of a person's life with MS (Book). The author of *Book C* wrote this text to help himself reflect on his experiences with starting to need a wheelchair. While he focuses on tangible barriers and facilitators, he also writes about joy and hardships. This is presented in a rather matter-of-fact manner of writing, which still manages to convey emotions. His main motivation seems to be to foster understanding. Unlike interviews, all his words are deliberately chosen, reread, and then decided upon. This makes for easier reading and clearer lines of thought than an interview.

2.5. Data Analysis

The secondary analysis of both narrative sources (DIPEx interviews and book) is based on the thematic analysis by Braun and Clarke [20,21], which is conducted in six phases. The basic idea of the inductive coding is that the procedures of summarizing content analysis are used to develop categories from the material in a step-by-step process. With the inductive approach, the categories are not created before the material is inspected but are derived directly from the material without referring to the theoretical concepts used beforehand. The content analysis in this work aims to explore the barriers, facilitators and ethical aspects that are mentioned. A combination of inductive and deductive approach was chosen to anchor the findings in previous research and to obtain a framework for comparison.

For the deductive part of the coding, the codes were derived from the comprehensive MS core set developed by Coenen, et al. [11] (hereafter referred to as the MS core set). Since the subject was barriers and facilitators, only the ICF codes for environmental factors were used, because the other domains cannot be qualified as facilitators or barriers. Ethically relevant situations were also coded. These MS core-set-derived codes were created as the subject was referenced, as were ICF codes not from the core set when subjects of discussion fell into these categories. All the coding was carried out using the MAXQDA software [26].

2.6. Quality Assurance Methods

For quality assurance purposes, communicative validation was used for each step of the process, from developing the research question to the interpretation of the results. The first steps in coding were completed after a training (JO&AG) and peer-reviewing process, coding the content and processing it to ICF categories. The interviews were conducted according to the validated DIPEx methodology [23]. All statements made regarding the content of the narrative sources are directly tied to excerpts from the sources.

3. Results

Both narrative sources (*Interview A and B and Book C*) were coded with all five ICF domains of environmental factors and the environmental categories included from the ICF core set. Additional ICF categories from the environmental factors of the whole ICF were added when necessary. The ICF was anchored in the bio-psycho-social model for understanding diseases and their effects in daily life situations and their interactions. Additionally, ethical issues, which are part of the personal factors included in the ICF, were coded using Beauchamp and Childress's principles [13]. The results were ordered by ICF domain and used to answer the research question. There are a total 314 references throughout the narrative sources, which were translated into ICF language to provide a common basis for comparison.

3.1. Overview of Identified Barriers and Facilitators of Environmental Factors

Overall, more facilitators (184) were referenced than barriers (129). The ICF categories e1 Products and Technology (115) and e120 Support and Relationships (120) each received quite a few more references than the e2 Natural Environment and Human-Made Changes to Environment (12) or e4 Attitudes (9), the ICF domains with the fewest references. *Interview A* was the only source which referenced more barriers than facilitators, with almost 60% barriers. Only 17% of *Interview B*'s codes were barriers. In *Book C*, just over a third of all references were barriers.

The distribution of code by narrative sources and between barriers and facilitators is shown in Figure 3.

Nr	Domain	Facilitators				Barriers				Total Mentions
		Interview A	Interview B	Book C	Total Facilitators	Interview A	Interview B	Book C	Total Barriers	
e1	Products and Technology	11	16	36	63	19	4	29	52	115
e2	Natural Environment and Human-Made Changes to Environment	2	4	0	6	4	2	0	6	12
e3	Support and Relationships	16	26	44	86	20	1	13	34	120
e4	Attitudes	0	0	1	1	4	3	1	8	9
e5	Services, Systems and Policies	12	7	17	36	7	1	14	22	58
	Sum	41	53	98	192	54	11	57	122	314

Figure 3. Distribution of codes by ICF domains: This figure shows the frequency of references by domains as facilitators and as barriers. Additionally, it tallies all references as facilitators or as barriers by source, as well as facilitators and barriers both separately and together by domain.

3.2. Barriers and Facilitators Identified in ICF Domain e1: Products and Technology

Domain *e1: Products and Technology* has a significant impact on the quality of life of PwMS. This domain is defined by the ICF and includes: "natural or human-made products or systems of products, equipment and technology in an individual's immediate environment that are gathered, created, produced or manufactured." The ISO 9999 classification of technical aids defines these as "any product, instrument, equipment or technical system used by a disabled person, especially produced or generally available, preventing, compensating, monitoring, relieving or neutralizing" disability. Any product or technology can be assistive. (See ISO 9999: Technical aids for disabled persons-Classification (second version); ISO/TC 173/SC 2; ISO/DIS 9999 (rev.).) For the purposes of this classification of environmental factors, however, assistive products and technology are defined more narrowly as "any product, instrument, equipment, or technology adapted or specially designed for improving the functioning of a disabled person" [7] (p. 173).

This ICF domain *e1: Products and Technology* indicates, as shown in Figure 4, that the same environmental factor, such as the wheelchair, can be both a barrier and a facilitator depending on the perspective and time-related context. An important facilitator that both *Interview B* and *Book C* mention is the wheelchair. They both struggled to accept that they needed one. *Interview B* does not go into detail as to why that was the case for her, but she refused to use one for long after it would have been helpful. When she did start to use it, she saw the difference it made to her quality of life. *Book C* and his daughter saw the wheelchair as a symbol of sickness and dependence. When trying one out for the first time, though, he describes as a sense of freedom. He writes:

"A feeling of freedom overcame me. I moved effortlessly. I had completely forgotten what freedom of movement felt like. So far, I had only been able to move forward extremely slowly and clumsily. But now? In comparison to before it was like flying." (Book C)

Nr	Code	MS Core Set	ICF	Facilitators Interview A	Facilitators Interview B	Facilitators Book C	Total Facilitators	Barriers Interview A	Barriers Interview B	Barriers Book C	Total Barriers	Total Mentions
e120	Products and Technology for Personal Indoor and Outdoor Mobility and Transportation	x	x	0	10	21	31	0	2	11	13	44
e150	Design, Construction und Building Products and Technology of Buildings for Public Use	x	x	0	0	11	11	1	0	16	17	28
e1101	Drugs	x	x	6	2	0	8	7	1	0	8	16
e115	Products and Technology for Personal Use in Daily Living	x	x	3	1	0	4	5	0	1	6	10
e165	Assets	x	x	0	0	4	4	4	0	0	4	8
e155	Design, Construction und Building Products and Technology of Buildings for Private Use	x	x	0	2	0	2	1	1	0	2	4
e125	Products and Technology for Communication	x	x	0	1	0	1	1	0	0	1	2
e199	Products and Technology Unspecified		x	1	0	0	1	0	0	1	1	2
e1100	Food		x	1	0	0	1	0	0	0	0	1
e135	Products and Technology for Employment	x	x	0	0	0	0	0	0	0	0	0
			Sum	11	16	36	63	19	4	29	52	115

Figure 4. Distribution of codes in the domain *e1 Products and Technology*: This figure shows the frequency of MS core set codes and non-core set codes of this domain, referenced in each source as a facilitator and as a barrier. Additionally, it tallies all references throughout the domain as facilitators or as barriers by source, as well as tallying facilitators and barriers separately and together by code.

Interview B attributes some of her quality of life to the wheelchair. Many other large and small tools, such as maps of Venice that showed wheelchair accessibility, a comic that explains MS to children and many more, made the lives of all three persons easier. While the wheelchair is a facilitator for the participants from *Interview B* and *Book C*, *Interview A* does not need one. Most of the tools are only mentioned in one of the sources. Not all tools that are meant to help are helpful, such as the shopping cart for persons in a wheelchair mentioned by *Book C*. This shopping cart did not work for the person in *Book C's* circumstances. He was shopping with his daughter, for whom the shopping cart was very heavy, especially in addition to him, in his wheelchair, who she also had to push. Additionally, the shopping kept pulling to the side.

The design of rooms in the rehabilitation center that the person in *Interview A* attended had a considerable influence on her. Having her own room was very facilitating for her.

Having to share her room on later visits was not ideal for her. As with the barriers the person in *Book C* describes, this barrier is not insurmountable but makes life harder for persons who are not the standard user. There are many ways for persons not to be the standard user. The person in *Interview A* most likely had a stronger desire for privacy and profited less from being around other persons than the standard user that the architects had in mind. Person *Book C* was often not the standard user, because of his wheelchair.

They benefited from or were hampered by things that are inconsequential to other people, such as having a private room in a rehabilitation facility or the slope of a ramp to the train tracks being slightly too steep to push oneself up.

The person in *Interview A* laments not having adequate vocabulary to describe her fatigue. In German, she feels that there is only one word for tired, while she feels several types of tiredness. What she experiences with her fatigue is different from when other people have a strenuous day and is not always the same for her either. Not having different words for these different experiences is a barrier. It makes it harder for her to communicate what is going on to other people. This makes it harder for these people to understand her situation. She says:

"Sometimes I sleep and am just as tired when I wake up. Fatigue is like that. It is a malfunction and not a usual tiredness. There are different types of tiredness, totally paralyzing, heavy weighing, every movement is hard work, you know? As if you had hung weights, so ehm, against resistance. Or tiredness that is maybe more in your head, kind of a "prrr fog", but otherwise one is actually, physically not as much, but up here (the head) is just not useable. Ehm, there are such big differences, are there not?" (Interview A)

Facilitators do not need to be related a diagnosis or consequences of a disease, such as when *Interview A* talks about food being a thing that brings her happiness and moments of joy. Additionally, sometimes, tools can have unwelcome effects, such as the sanitary napkins that the person in *Interview A* uses for her urinary incontinence. She says that these products influence her vanity and her femininity.

3.3. Barriers and Facilitators Identified in ICF Domain e2: Natural Environment and Human-Made Changes to Environment

The domain *e2: Natural Environment and Human-Made Changes to Environment* discusses "animate and inanimate elements of the natural or physical environment, and components of that environment that have been modified by people, as well as characteristics of human populations within that environment" [7] (p. 182).

Temperature was shown to be an influence in both *Interview A* and *Interview B* (please see Figure 5) For *Interview A* it is mainly heat that she has trouble with. She describes it as feeling *like having hot water pored over oneself*.

				Facilitators				Barriers				
Nr	Code	MS Core Set	ICF	Interview A	Interview B	Book C	Total Facilitators	Interview A	Interview B	Book C	Total Barriers	Total Mentions
e2	Natural Environment and Human-Made Changes to Environment Unspezified		x	1	4	0	5	2	1	0	3	8
e2250	Temperature	x	x	1	0	0	1	1	1	0	2	3
e2251	Humidity	x	x	0	0	0	0	1	0	0	1	1
e2253	Precipitation		x	x	0	0	0	0	0	0	0	0	0
			Sum	2	4	0	6	4	2	0	6	12

Figure 5. Distribution of codes in the domain *e2 Natural Environment and Human-Made Changes to Environment*: This figure shows the frequency of MS core set codes and non-core set codes of this domain referenced in each source as a facilitator and as a barrier. Additionally, it tallies all references throughout the domain as facilitators or as barriers by source, as well as tallying facilitators and barriers separately and together by code.

Interview A's intolerance for heat and humidity make summers hard, especially because others like to spend time outside during this time of year. Being out of sync this way is a barrier to nurturing friendships. For Interview B the cold is the bigger issue.

Both women find being in nature helpful. Interview B finds it reenergizing, saying:

"Then I go to a pond, sit down, stay for a quarter of an hour and there I notice, when I've been out in the fresh air. It isn't like that inside, but water has a calming effect. I recuperate quickly by the ponds." (Interview B)

Interview A associates it with happiness. The same facilitator brings different benefits to different persons, and this facilitator does not seem to have a direct connection to the disease that these women both have.

3.4. Barriers and Facilitators Identified in ICF Domain e3: Support and Relationships

The stories portray *e3: Support and Relationships* as facilitators almost twice as often as barriers (78:42). Per definition this domain is "about people or animals that provide practical physical or emotional support, nurturing, protection, assistance, and relationships to other persons, in their home, place of work, school or at play or in other aspects of their daily activities. The chapter does not encompass the attitudes of the person or people that are providing the support. The environmental factor being described is not the person or animal, but the amount of physical and emotional support the person or animal provides" [7] (p. 187).

The domain *e3 Support and Relationships* is referenced the most as a facilitator (please see Figure 6). In *Interview A*, it is also the domain that is mentioned the most as a barrier. The example of *Interview A's* relationship shows that a diagnosis such as MS, with the changes it brings, can strain a relationship. In this example the relationship possibly became a barrier, because it did not survive the changes.

Nr	Code	MS Core Set	ICF	Interview A (F)	Interview B (F)	Book C (F)	Total Facilitators	Interview A (B)	Interview B (B)	Book C (B)	Total Barriers	Total Mentions
e310	Immediate Family	x	x	2	10	14	26	5	0	5	10	36
e355	Health Professionals	x	x	5	9	0	14	7	0	0	7	21
e330	Acquaintances, Peers, Colleagues, Neighbours and Community Members	x	x	1	0	11	12	5	0	3	8	20
e345	Strangers		x	0	0	14	14	0	0	1	1	15
e320	Friends	x	x	6	3	1	10	3	1	0	4	14
e360	Other Professionals	x	x	0	1	4	5	0	0	4	4	9
e350	Domesticated Animals		x	2	3	0	5	0	0	0	0	5
e315	Extended Family	x	x	0	0	0	0	0	0	0	0	0
e340	People in Positions of Authority	x	x	0	0	0	0	0	0	0	0	0
e355	Personal Care Providers and Personal Assistants	x	x	0	0	0	0	0	0	0	0	0
	Sum			16	26	44	86	20	1	13	34	120

Figure 6. Distribution of codes in the domain *e3 Support and Relationships*: This figure shows the frequency of MS core set codes and non-core set codes of this domain referenced in each source as a facilitator and as a barrier. Additionally, it tallies all references throughout the domain as facilitators or as barriers by source, as well as tallying facilitators and barriers separately and together by code.

Interview A's conversation about husbands leaving wives after such a diagnosis goes to show that she was aware that the continuation of her marriage was not guaranteed.

Book C's relationship with his children plays a central role in his book. He writes about two of his children:

> "Joy and Charley < ... > helped significantly, that I do not see the wheelchair as a dis-aster anymore, but as a tool, that is sometimes needed." (Book C)

All also mentioned persons outside of their family. For *Interview A*, these are mainly friends. These are facilitators in 6 out of 9 references. For *Interview B*, her neurologist played an important facilitating role in her journey with MS. All references to him are as a facilitator. *Book C* talks about strangers and work colleagues. The strangers were facilitators 14 out of 15 times. These strangers told him about routes that were more wheelchair accessible, and strangers helped him get up after he fell. Colleagues were facilitators in 11 out of 14 references. He writes about them jumping up to offer him help and making sure he is seen when moving through a crowd.

For *Interview A*, many relationships with doctors were barriers because they did not take her needs into account, apart from her direct medical needs. These stories give the impression of her being reduced to her diagnosis. This is in stark contrast to the person in *Interview B's* relationship with her neurologist, where she feels that he knows what she wants and what she needs. She describes them deciding whether she needs to take cortisone as follows:

> "Sometimes he looks at me and he knows that I don't really like cortisone. But when he says there is nothing else, we need to do it, then I know, he isn't just doing this, he's prescribing it for a certain reason. < ... > he says: "I know you don't like it, but ..." Then I say, well, then we're doing it." (Interview B)

Book C presented two quite different experiences in two different stores that sold wheelchairs. The main differences seemed to be customer friendliness and competence. Additionally one of the salespeople talked about AHV (old age and survivors' insurance) wheelchairs. The person in *Book C* really did not like this. How things are named has an impact on people. The person in *Book C* is not old enough to receive AHV, but needs a wheelchair. The salesperson in the store where the author of *Book C* had the unpleasant experience seemed to have a standard user in mind, who was different from the one standing in front of him. Still he did not change his approach. He also did not seem to consider or ask about the needs of this customer.

Being reduced to someone who needs a wheelchair is shown as a barrier more than once in *Book C*. On the other hand, people being considerate that he is in a wheelchair, for example sitting down to be on eye level, was described as a facilitator. The statement, shows that people take his wheelchair into account:

> "Surprisingly there was always someone there, that helped me with my wheelchair. Usually people offered help, without me asking." (Book C)

Both *Interview A and B* described pets that are facilitators. Their being facilitators does not directly have anything to do with their MS. They enjoy the animals' company, like many people without MS.

Interview A, Interview B and *Book C* all put great emphasis on the people around them. The 120 references to this domain show this. People can be great facilitators, but unfortunately also barriers.

3.5. Barrieres and Facilitators Identified in ICF Domain e4: Attitudes

The domain *e4: Attitudes* includes the following aspects and is defined by the ICF as follows: "attitudes that are the observable consequences of customs, practices, ideologies, values, norms, factual beliefs and religious beliefs. These attitudes influence individual behavior and social life at all levels, from interpersonal relationships and community associations to political, economic, and legal structures; for example, individual or societal attitudes about a person's trustworthiness and value as a human being that may motivate positive, honorific practices or negative and discriminatory practices (e.g., stigmatizing, stereotyping, and marginalizing or neglect of the person). The attitudes classified are those of people external to the person whose situation is being described. They are not those of the person themselves. The individual attitudes are categorized according to the kinds of relationships listed in Environmental Factors Chapter 3. Values and beliefs are not coded separately from the attitudes as they are assumed to be the driving forces behind the attitudes" [7] (p. 190).

The woman in *Interview A* describes one specific attitude that has been a large barrier for her: society's focus on work as a central element of who we are. This leads people to ask strangers what they do for a living to get to know them. This can quickly lead to persons who do not work feeling othered, which, in person *Interview A's* example, led to her isolating herself from strangers, so she did not have to explain why she does not work to strangers during small talk. She says:

> "Yes, after years of avoiding new contacts, among other things simply because I. Yes, just like that, always MS, everywhere MS. Somehow the first question when you get to know someone new is always, what do (you) do in our culture. And then you are always there very quickly, you don't work, and you don't see my MS anymore when you look at me, so what is the problem? Well, then I am already explaining again." (Interview A)

Person *Book C* gives numerous examples of people seeing him in his wheelchair and offering help, from clearing a path for him in a crowd to bringing him food from a buffet. While this description of society's attitude towards persons who visibly have special needs is a facilitator for him, it could also become a barrier for persons whose needs are not as obviously visible.

The distribution of codes quite clearly shows that attitudes were referenced as barriers a lot more than as facilitators (8/9). This could be interpreted as attitudes tending to be barriers more often than facilitators. It is also possible, and maybe even more likely, that attitudes that hinder are easier to name than those that help.

No codes outside of the MS core set were used. A total of 4/7 of the MS core set codes were referenced; please see Figure 7.

Nr	Code	MS Core Set	ICF	Facilitators Interview A	Interview B	Book C	Total Facilitators	Barriers Interview A	Interview B	Book C	Total Barriers	Total Mentions
e450	Individual Attitudes of Health Professionals	x	x	0	0	0	0	3	0	1	4	4
e460	Societal Attitudes	x	x	0	0	1	1	1	1	0	2	3
e415	Individual Attitudes of Immediate Family Members	x	x	0	0	0	0	0	1	0	1	1
e425	Individual Attitudes of Acquaintances, Peers, Colleagues, Neighbors and Community Members	x	x	0	0	0	0	0	1	0	1	1
e420	Individual Attitudes of Friends	x	x	0	0	0	0	0	0	0	0	0
e430	Individual Attitudes of People in Positions of Authority	x	x	0	0	0	0	0	0	0	0	0
e440	Individual Attitudes of Personal Care Providers and Personal Assistants	x	x	0	0	0	0	0	0	0	0	0
			Sum	11	16	36	63	19	4	29	52	115

Figure 7. Distribution of codes in the domain *e4 Attitudes*: This figure shows the frequency of MS core set codes and non-core set codes of this domain referenced in each source as a facilitator and as a barrier. Additionally, it tallies all references throughout the domain as facilitators or as barriers by source, as well as tallying facilitators and barriers separately and together by code.

3.6. Barrieres and Facilitators Identified in ICF Domain e5: Services, Systems and Policies

This section leads into domain *e5: Services, Systems and Policies*, the contents of which are described as follows: "1. Services that provide benefits, structured programs and operations, in various sectors of society, designed to meet the needs of individuals. (Included in services are the people who provide them). Services may be public, private, or voluntary, and may be established at a local, community, regional, state, provincial, national, or international level by individuals, associations, organizations, agencies, or governments. The goods provided by these services may be general or adapted and especially designed. 2. Systems that are administrative control and organizational mechanisms, and are established by governments at the local, regional, national, and international levels, or by other recognized authorities. These systems are designed to organize, control, and monitor services that provide benefits, structured programs, and operations in various sectors of society. 3. Policies constituted by rules, regulations, conventions, and standards established by governments at the local, regional, national, and international levels, or by other recognized authorities. Policies govern and regulate the systems that organize, control, and monitor services, structured programs, and operations in various sectors of society [7] (p.192)".

Book C shows many examples of public transportation being adapted to his needs sitting in a wheelchair. Having a hotline to organize assistance for getting into specific trains is one of the many cases where these adaptions were facilitators. When it was unclear where his reserved seat was, because of a not-documented seat change due to his wheelchair and other such examples, imperfections in the adaptations to his needs were barriers. In this example he switched train cars twice with children, luggage, and a wheelchair. For the person in *Interview B*, public transportation where she lives is not good enough for her to solely rely on it.

Nobody described *e580 Health Services, Systems and Policies* as not being functional. *Interview A* and *Interview B* have different experiences with the degree of personalization. *Interview B* discusses the rehabilitation center she attended at the time of the interview:

> "Here it's good in any case. If something were not to work, or is too strenuous, then I can say so. I think, up here everyone can say so, and then you do something else." (Interview B)

All three narrative sources (A, B, C) report receiving financial support from different forms of insurance, without claiming it to beinsufficient.

Most codes of the MS core set in this domain were not referenced (*e550 Legal Services, Systems and Policies e515, e525 Housing Services, Systems and Policies, e575 General Social Support Services and Policies, e585 Education and Training Services, Systems and Policies*); please see Figure 8.

3.7. Identified Ethical Issues

Unlike the other topics, this chapter does not follow the ICF, since the ICF does not explicitly take ethical issues into account. Instead this chapter discusses ethical issues as conflicts between Beauchamp and Childress's four ethical principles, [13] which are widely established and applied in the bio-medical field and health care sector:

1. Respect for autonomy.
2. Nonmaleficence.
3. Beneficence.
4. Justice.

This chapter indicates the situations described in the interviews and the literary text, where not all of Beauchamp and Childress's ethical principles were acted upon.

Only *Interview A* describes a lack of beneficence. In two examples, situations made her uncomfortable and kept her from obtaining the optimum amount out of either setting, even though both were meant to be for her benefit. In the third example, the neurologist did not make a diagnosis, because he did not find it medically relevant. He did not see the benefits that it could have had for her psychologically.

In both *Interviews A* and *B*, situations are described where *e355 Health Professionals* do not fulfill the principle of autonomy. In one example, they do not allow the PwMS to set her own goals. In another, they override the PwMS's preferences. In *Book C*, the *e540 Transportations Services, Systems and Policies* tried to take away the author's autonomy by telling him where to spend his layover.

Both instances mentioned persons not adhering to the principle of nonmaleficence: e355 Health Professionals said inopportune things. When the person in *Interview B* asked whether she had MS, she was told it could also be a brain tumor. The person in *Interview A* was told:

"Ach, if you did not always cry, you would be a pretty woman ..." (Interview A)

Nr	Code	MS Core Set	ICF	Facilitators				Barriers				Total Mentions
				Interview A	Interview B	Book C	Total Facilitators	Interview A	Interview B	Book C	Total Barriers	
e540	Transportation Services, Systems and Policies	x	x	0	0	16	16	0	1	14	15	31
e580	Health Services, Systems and Policies	x	x	10	3	0	13	7	0	0	7	20
e570	Social Security Services, Systems and Policies	x	x	2	2	1	5	0	0	0	0	5
e590	Labour and Employment Services, Systems and Policies	x	x	0	2	0	2	0	0	0	0	2
e515	Architecture and Constrction Services, Systems and Policies	x	x	0	0	0	0	0	0	0	0	0
e525	Housing Services, Systems and Policies	x	x	0	0	0	0	0	0	0	0	0
e550	Legal Services, Systems and Policies	x	x	0	0	0	0	0	0	0	0	0
e555	Associations and Organizational Services, Systems and Policies	x	x	0	0	0	0	0	0	0	0	0
e575	General Social Support Services, Systems and Policies	x	x	0	0	0	0	0	0	0	0	0
e585	Education and Training Services, Systems and Policies	x	x	0	0	0	0	0	0	0	0	0
			Sum	12	7	17	36	7	1	14	22	58

Figure 8. Distribution of codes in the *domain e5 Services, Systems and Policies*: This figure shows the frequency of MS core set codes and non-core set codes of this domain referenced in each source as a facilitator and as a barrier. Additionally, it tallies all references throughout the domain as facilitators or as barriers by source, as well as tallying facilitators and barriers separately and together by code.

4. Discussion

With this multiple-case study, we explored the following question: "How do persons with MS experience and describe barriers, facilitators and ethically relevant conflicts?" We looked at the backgrounds that are discernible in this by means of narrative source analysis of experiences of PwMS, and the consequences for health care management for persons with MS. Based on the translation of these narrative sources into the common language of the systematic bio-psycho-social structure of the ICF, it was possible to identify patient-health-care-relevant context factors as barriers and facilitating factors and to compare them to the MS ICF core sets as a practical tool for a comprehensive health care management. There are several aspects that we would like to discuss here.

4.1. Quantitative Distribution

For most comparisons between the number of barriers and facilitators referenced per code, there were more facilitators (13:9). The categories where barriers outweighed facilitators tended to have fewer references than those where facilitators outweighed barriers. There was an average of almost 18 references per code where facilitators outweighed barriers and an average of almost 8 where barriers outweighed facilitators.

4.2. Ethical Issues

Based on the systematic coding of the narrative sources with the ICF, ethically relevant aspects of the PwMS became clear, which can generally be assigned to the contextual factors. A detailed description of this is not found in the ICF. Based on the four biomedical principles, a classification became possible.

The focus of the ethical issues was *e355 Health Professionals* not respecting autonomy or not fulfilling the potential for beneficence. The principle of justice was not touched upon, perhaps because the focus in all three accounts was very much on the individual. The portrayed circumstances were varied and the underlying causes were not always entirely clear. Chu's research also emphasizes that ethical thinking and acting are important components of narrative subjectivity, including the ability to understand others and overcome differences, understand and reflect on values, to compromise, to reach a trade-off between different values, and, finally, to undergo an interdisciplinary collaboration with different professions [27].

Still some inferences and suggestions to circumvent such incidents can be made and similar ideas are portrayed in the following chapters.

4.3. Lessons Learned Based on an Analysis of Narrative Sources of PwMS

Based on the results of this multiple-case study, the first insights of lessons learned from the Swiss experiences of PwMS regarding barriers and facilitators are postulated in the following sub-chapters. To indicate the Swiss perspective, we connect our results to the findings of Bechtold's et al., as shown in their study "Quality through patients' eyes" [28].

One of our goals is to describe the factors we explored, and whether they had a positive influence as a facilitator or a negative influence as a barrier, in collaboration with the interdisciplinary treatment of PwMS, which is addressed where suitable in the following sub-chapters. For this the descriptions in these narrative sources were used to make inferences as to why some aspects were barriers and others were facilitators, and why the same aspects could be a barrier for one person and a facilitator for another person, or in a different circumstance.

4.3.1. Understanding the Importance of Environmental Circumstances Based on Narrative Sources

As shown in the study of Chu et al., narrative thinking is not meant to arrange events in chronological order, but to place the disease/hospitalization in the context of life to construct the temporality of the disease [27]. In Chu's words: traditional "biomedicine orientation (is) seeking the truth and facts, narrative thinking focuses on the authenticity of patients and diseases, which refers to touching stories and revelations in medical care, including the value of life, the beauty of human nature, selfless dedication, resistance to disease, family emotions, loss, rebirth, etc." [27]. This aspect is also presented by Chiu et al. They identified barriers to health care, which they divided into three phases of utilization: (a) in the pre-visit phase, the most frequently cited barrier was transportation; (b) in the phase during the visit, the quality of communication was the biggest problem; (c) in the phase after the visit, the failure to refer for follow-up treatment was what the biggest barrier [29].

The importance of understanding individual circumstantial experiences of illness became especially clear when the PwMS telling their stories in these sources spoke of the tools they used and their strategies for managing life with a chronic disease. The better adapted the strategies were to the individual's circumstances, the more beneficial they were. This ranged from a comic book that was ideal to explain MS to children to wheelchair shopping carts that were too heavy to push in addition to a wheelchair. They also included sanitary napkins designed for menstruation that also work for incontinence, but leave much to be desired.

Understanding circumstances is not only important for providing tangible aid, but also when lending a helping hand. When it is overdone, it can diminish a person's autonomy and the necessary degree of care turns into over-care or even paternalism. It is always important to consider the individual and his or her subjective experiences and needs, and not to reduce persons with MS to their diagnosis.

Facilitators do not have to be connected to the person's MS. The person in *Interview A* finds that food brings her joy. *Interview A* and *B* both describe pets as facilitators. Research has shown that pets can have positive effects on psychological as well as physical wellbeing [30]. There is no impression that either of these facilitators have anything to with them having MS or any disabilities resulting from this. This does not make their effect less valuable. Broadening our view of what can help somebody to include things that are not disease- or disability-specific could allow us to think of such things. It could also help the affected people look for facilitators further away from their ailment or find tools that are especially helpful to them even if they are not specifically designed for PwMS, such as the easy-to-clean kitchen mentioned in *Interview B*.

Both *Interview A* and *Book C* describe finding it uncomfortable when they get the impression of being reduced to a PwMS or a person in a wheelchair.

Researchers have investigated different circumstances to try and find solutions. This includes researchers who explored the circumstances of falls in wheelchair users [31], but also topics that are far from from this paper's topic and focus on very different circumstances, such as a paper that investigated the circumstances around women's entry into sex work to find ways to help targeted HIV prevention [32,33]. Sometimes it is small things that can have a large impact. Hammel et al. gives examples of simple devices, such as remote controls or pagers, which have a large benefit, because they meet a person's needs [34].

4.3.2. Understanding the Importance of Person's Individual Life Situation–Ability to Switch Perspectives in the Medical Field

The sources show multiple examples of persons seeking to understand. This ranges from criticism of medical jargon that is difficult to understand to grandchildren informing themselves about what is going on with their grandmother using comic books, as well as to the person in *Interview A* wanting a diagnosis whether it was relevant to the treatment or not. The sources also show the importance of being understood. The person in *Interview B* feels judged for her unsteady gait. She also feels her doctor knows that she does not like taking cortisone. She describes him prefacing his recommendation that she take cortisone with: "I know you don't like it, but ..." This makes her more receptive when he does suggest she take it. This reciprocal understanding makes for a good working relationship between patient and doctor.

While a PwMS will undoubtedly play a large role in their treatment, one needs to make sure not to reduce the person or the treatment to the diagnosis. As much as a there is a person sitting in the wheelchair in person *Book C's* story, not just a purse, there is more to each PwMS than their diagnosis. This line of thinking can lead to other ways to help and increase understanding for the person. In the Swiss context Berchtold et al. were able to show, in their study on health care quality in Switzerland, that "professionally perceived quality on the one hand and patient experience in spoken and written narratives on the other hand represent two fundamentally different perspectives: It is precisely this difference in perspective that patients address in the narrative interviews" [28] (p. 13). As Berchtold et al. show that no one doubts the basic competence of the physicians. Not even the young woman who had to wait seven years for her diagnosis. However, all of them react with unease when they do not find their questions and concerns taken up, when they feel pressed into medical categories and when they do not feel perceived as individuals [ibid].

Furthermore, as explored by Schmid et al., the patient's perspective plays a critical role in health care and quality assurance. During an episode of a disease, patients come into contact with many therapists involved in inpatient and/or outpatient care. They can review the entire chain of care. As a therapist one must learn to understand the patient's point of view and put oneself in his or her shoes. PwMS often try to do their best or to improve or maintain their quality of life by themselves. Patients develop coping skills; therefore, healthcare professionals mentioned coping strategies for everyday actions [35].

4.3.3. Respect for PwMS' Individuality in Health Care Settings

Not everyone is alike. Just because someone fits into a category, this does not stop them from being individual. For example people presumed that the person in *Interview A* needed company, because others had. Wheelchair accessibility did not mean the same thing for the author *Book C* as it did for the people declaring whether trains were wheelchair accessible or not. While 75% of PwMS have impaired mobility, this also means that 25% do not. As with this symptom, the whole clinical presentation differs from patient to patient [32]. In Fakolade et al.'s research over 70% of participants with MS cited lack of choice and control of physical activity and level of engagement as a barrier to participation in physical activity programs [36]. This is just one example for a possibility to increase the impact and accessibility of valuable programs by increasing their adaptability to individual needs. For example, Kayes et al. [37] looked at what helped or hindered physical activity in PwMS. While they also found disease-related variables that had an influence, they found barriers that had no direct link to the disease. They propose that health professionals gaining an understanding of these individual barriers could improve the PwMS' physical activity and barriers to accessibility. The literature review of Chiu et al. recommend that clinicians find individualized solutions with PwMS who face transportation barriers to care, including reimbursements for travel and home medication delivery [29]. In other words seeing the PwMS as a person with attributes not related to the disease allows for health professionals to be more effective, since their patient might have barriers that are not related to the disease.

From a more general and Swiss health care perspective, the findings of Berchtold et al. show that one important, issue when building trust and increasing the understanding of good health care, is offering sufficient space, attention, and appreciation to the individual patient's situation [28]. They show that patients find it very unpleasant to be perceived only as an object instead of as a "whole person" and to be pressed into medical categories as quickly as possible. This is important in the acute setting, but especially in the aftercare setting, where the patient's needs are manifold. In principle Berchtold et al. recommend that medical and nursing professionals are more systematically trained to deal with differences in perspective than is currently the case in Switzerland [ibid]. Specifically in relation to MS, Mayo et al. (2021) substantiate Bechtold's claims and emphasize that PwMS and their health care professionals can benefit from a structured and comprehensive MS-specific education. Education can address the process of addressing unmet health care needs in health care settings and ultimately lead to a higher quality of life for people with MS [38].

4.3.4. Relationships Are Meaningful for the Disease Management and Treatment to Build Trust

All three narrative sources of PwMS, that were studied in this paper, provide multiple examples of facilitating relationships and indicate the meaning and relevance of these relationships for PwMS. These range from *Interview B's* neurologist to *Book C's* children. e3 *Support and Relationships* is the domain with the most references and the domain that most strongly favors facilitators. The hardships that arise in a relationship when one partner is diagnosed with MS and how these relationships can be helpful has been researched previously [39–41]. As shown by Fakolade et al., when PwMS and their caregivers ranked what they most needed to participate in physical activities, programs that included the family caregivers ranked first for family caregivers and second for PwMS, showing the central role that relationships play [36]. Kassie et al. found that social support or lack thereof was mentioned in almost all the interviews, demonstrating the importance given to this topic. Those who had support viewed it as indispensable to the management of their disease [42]. For PwMS, relationships are an important factor in managing their disease.

The importance of relationships has also been pointed out by Haubrick et al., who explored the lived experience of adults with MS. It became clear that while medical professionals and family members do not always offer support, respondents indicated that, in contrast, they find help and friendship in MS support groups. One woman stated, "I've become an outcast to most of the people I knew before." Participants unanimously valued social engagement when coping with illness [43].

Obtaining insight into significant factors of PwMS also requires good medical relations, according to Chu. This includes communication between doctors and patients, as well as across medical professions. The exchange of life experiences and dialogue between doctors and patients is one of the steps in the promotion of good medical care [27].

4.4. Potential Benefits from a Methodological Point of View

What do the insights based on this multiple-case study from a methodological and learning theory perspective indicate for medical students? They offer various benefits due to their systematic, structured approach using different narrative sources: (1) *interview (A and B)* and (2) a literary autobiographical representation by a *book (C)*. These insights can sharpen reflections regarding:

(a) The contextual reference, starting from a diagnosis-related focus and demonstrated by the real-life situations of the personal accounts of PwMS in the DIPEx interviews.
(b) The intensity of the in-depth content analysis of ICF's (interaction model and classification for functioning and disability) real-life descriptions on a bio-psycho-social basis.
(c) The systematic consideration of different factors favoring or aggravating the life situation from the perspective of persons affected by MS and its influence on health care.
(d) A potential comparability of statements based on a common language, known for the clinical picture (ICF) in rehabilitation and standards developed for this purpose to describe functioning and disability (ICF core set for MS) as a reference.
(e) The inclusion of biomedical principles as an analysis, aiding in the recognition of ethically relevant aspects, that are woven into real-life situations.

4.5. Limitations

This multiple case-study offers some initial insights into the barriers and facilitators for PwMS and does not allow us to generalize, but can be assumed to provide a basis for initial hypotheses. The methodology aims to show areas of interest without claiming to assess their transferability to other situations. This includes this paper's focus on PwMS. This qualitative approach, based on a case study design and without saturation of data, does not allow for generalization, but it provides a basis for developing initial hypotheses.

Our three narrative sources focusing on barriers and facilitators do not reference all the topics of functioning and disability in the MS core set. This does not provide a complete view of the PwMS's situations. The payoff is that this methodology is more open to topics that would not have come up if the MS ICF core set had been used as a questionnaire. Another limitation for the scope of the statements for Switzerland, with its three national languages, German, French and Italian, is that the three sources (A–C) were German-speaking and do not allow for transference to the other two language regions.

All three narrative sources are from a PwMS's perspective. To obtain an objective picture of a situation, one needs multiple points of view. Obtaining such an objective picture was never the objective of this paper. MS is also called the disease with a thousand faces for a reason. The goal was to explore the PwMS's perspectives based on their subjective experiences regarding barriers and facilitators, which are ethical issues for those living with MS, to receive an initial overview.

5. Conclusions

Barriers and facilitators impact the success of health care and are, therefore, significant in medicine. This paper, whose method is strongly influenced by the humanities, while still being a medical master's thesis, should be seen as a supplement to the more deficit-oriented way that medicine is often practiced. It is not a criticism of this way of looking at disease, but an additional perspective. In addition to the more standard interventions, such as medication, it is important to be aware of environmental factors and their impact on a PwMS's life. Putting all this together is a challenge that medical professionals face every day. This paper lists four lessons that are meaningful for the daily practice and education of medical and health professional students:

- Understanding and importance of environmental circumstances based on narrative sources.
- Understanding and importance of a person's individual life situation and ability to switch perspectives in the medical field.
- Respect for PwMS' individuality in a health care setting and not reducing persons to their diagnosis.
- Constructing meaningful relationships and building trust for the disease management and treatment.

These are not entirely novel, but are important to reiterate and could use additional research, especially to reconsider these aspects' inclusion in medical and health care education programs and learning plans, as suggested by Chu [27]. With our insights, we join Berchtold [28] and invite medical professionals to switch their perspective of the medical field to that of a person being treated instead of the person providing the treatment. The factors explored here can be supported by tools such as DIPEx, which share a wide variety of patients' perspectives. Important questions include their transferability to other PwMS and possibly to persons with other chronic diseases, as well as the possibility of deepening medical students' reflections, looking beyond diagnosis towards a bio-psycho-social perspective. Even if many of these obstacles ultimately require the implementation of lasting policy changes, others can be more easily removed by increasing awareness among health care professionals and responding to patients' needs.

Supplementary Materials: The following supporting information can be downloaded at: https://www.mdpi.com/article/10.3390/ijerph191710733/s1, Video S1: English presentation of study: "Barriers and facilitators from person's perspective with multiple sclerosis—A case-based source analysis" at European Congress of NeuroRehabilitation (ECNR) 2021 jointly with 27. Jahrestagung der Deutschen Gesellschaft für Neurorehabilitation (DGNR) 08–11 December 2021.

Author Contributions: J.O.: reviewed the literature; study administration; data collection and analysis; wrote manuscript; edited manuscript; A.G.: conceptualization, study design and methodology; partly involved in data collection and analysis for training and validation; partly involved in visualization; research co-supervision, manuscript write-up, manuscript editing. N.B.-A.: research supervision; manuscript write-up. All authors have read and agreed to the published version of the manuscript.

Funding: This research for this Master Thesis received no external funding. Data collection of Interview A and B was financially supported by the Swiss Multiple Sclerosis Foundation—Grant Quality of Life (10 July 2017).

Institutional Review Board Statement: The DIPEx Switzerland project was conducted in accordance with the Declaration of Helsinki and received Swiss-wide approval from the cantonal ethics committee (University of Zurich) with the number BASEC Req-Nr. 2018-00050.

Informed Consent Statement: In the DIPEx project, informed consent was obtained from all subjects involved in the study.

Data Availability Statement: Not applicable.

Acknowledgments: The authors would like to thank all participants for their support and contribution to this study. Without their voluntary participation and openness to discuss personal experiences and opinions, it would not have been possible to achieve these results.

Conflicts of Interest: The authors declare no conflict of interest.

References

1. Kaufmann, M.; Puhan, M.A.; Kuhle, J.; Yaldizli, O.; Magnusson, T. A framework for estimating the burden of chronic diseases: Design and application in the context of multiple sclerosis. *Front. Neurol.* **2019**, *10*, 953. [CrossRef] [PubMed]
2. Kaufmann, M.; Puhan, M.A.; Salmen, A.; Kamm, C.P.; Manjaly, Z.-M.; Calabrese, P.; Schippling, S.; Müller, S.; Kuhle, J.; Pot, C.; et al. 60/30: 60% of the Morbidity-Associated Multiple Sclerosis Disease Burden Comes From the 30% of Persons With Higher Impairments. *Front. Neurol.* **2020**, *11*, 156. [CrossRef] [PubMed]
3. Recommendations on Rehabilitation Services for Persons with Multiple Sclerosis in Europe Endorsed by RIMS, Rehabilitation in Multiple Sclerosis European Multiple Sclerosis Platform (EMSP). 2012. Available online: https://www.google.com.hk/url?sa=t&rct=j&q=&esrc=s&source=web&cd=&cad=rja&uact=8&ved=2ahUKEwiK06zsrN75AhUKEYgKHWrLAkcQFnoECAMQAQ&url=https%3A%2F%2Fwww.emsp.org%2Fwp-content%2Fuploads%2F2015%2F11%2F12-0431_Henze-30-04-12.pdf&usg=AOvVaw3ZptZc45KRCoVPhZE4i67A (accessed on 21 August 2022).
4. Bennet, S.E.; Bednarik, P.; Bobryk, P.; Smith, C. *A Practical Guide to Rehabilitation in Multiple Sclerosis*; AIMS: Townsville Queensland, Australia, 2015.
5. Delle Fave, A.; Bassi, M.; Allegri, B.; Cilia, S.; Falautano, M.; Goretti, B.; Grobberio, M.; Minacapelli, E.; Pattini, M.; Pietrolongo, E.; et al. Beyond Disease: Happiness, Goals, and Meanings among Persons with Multiple Sclerosis and Their Caregivers. *Front. Psychol.* **2017**, *8*, 2216. [CrossRef] [PubMed]
6. Donisi, V.; Gajofatto, A.; Mazzi, M.A.; Gobbin, F.; Busch, I.M.; Ghellere, A.; Klonova, A.; Rudi, D.; Vitali, F.; Schena, F.; et al. A Bio-Psycho-Social Co-created Intervention for Young Adults with Multiple Sclerosis (ESPRIMO): Rationale and Study Protocol for a Feasibility Study. *Front. Psychol.* **2021**, *12*, 598726. [CrossRef]
7. WHO. *International Classification of Functioning, Disability and Health: ICF*; World Health Organization: Geneva, Switzerland, 2001.
8. Vincent, C.; Staines, A. *Verbesserung der Qualität und Patientensicherheit im Schweizer Gesundheitswesen*; Bundesamt für Gesundheit: Bern, Switzerland, 2019.
9. Bickenbach, J.; Cieza, A.; Rauch, A.; Stucki, G. *ICF Core Sets: Manual for Clinical Research*; Hogrefe Publishing: Göttingen, Germany, 2012.
10. Selb, M.; Escorpizo, R.; Kostanjsek, N.; Stucki, G.; Üstün, B.; Cieza, A. A guide on how to develop an International Classification of Functioning, Disability and Health Core Set. *Eur. J. Phys. Rehabil. Med.* **2015**, *51*, 105–117.
11. Coenen, M.; Cieza, A.; Freeman, J.; Kahn, F.; Miller, D.; Weise, A.; Kesselring, J. The development of ICF Core Sets for multiple sclerosis: Results of the International Consensus Conference. *J. Neurol.* **2011**, *259*, 1477–1488. [CrossRef]
12. Glässel, A.; Lückenkemper, M. Case Example 3: Applying the ICF Core Set for Multiple Sclerosis in Long-Term Care. In *ICF Core Sets: Manual for Clinical Practice*; Bickenbach, J., Cieza, A., Rauch, A., Stucki, G., Eds.; ICF Research Branch, in Cooperation with the WHO Collaborating Centre for the Family of International Classifications in Germany (DIMDI); Hogrefe Publishing: Göttingen, Germany, 2012.
13. Beauchamp, T.L.; Childress, J.F. *Principles of Biomedical Ethics*; Oxford University Press: New York, NY, USA, 2001.
14. Marckmann, G. *Was Ist Eigentlich Prinzipienorientierte Medizinethik*; Ethik in der Medizin: Stuttgart, Germany, 2000.
15. Yin, R.K. *Case study Research: Design and Methods*, 3rd ed.; Sage: Thousand Oaks, CA, USA, 2003.
16. Baxter, P.; Jack, S. Qualitative Case Study Methodology: Study Design and Implementation for Novice Researchers. *Qual. Rep.* **2008**, *13*, 544–559. [CrossRef]
17. Smith, J.A.; Osborn, M. Interpretive phenomenological analysis. In *Qualitative Psychology: A Practical Guide to Research Methods*; Smith, J.A., Ed.; Sage: London, UK, 2003; pp. 51–80.
18. Borkoles, E.; Nicholls, A.R.; Bell, K.; Butterly, R.; Polman, R.C.J. The lived experiences of people diagnosed with multiple sclerosis in relation to exercise. *Psychol. Health* **2008**, *23*, 427–441. [CrossRef]
19. Husserl, E. *Ideas Pertaining to Pure Phenomenology and to a Phenomenological Philosophy*; Original Work Published 1913; Martinus Nijhoff: The Hague, The Netherlands, 1983.
20. Braun, V.; Clarke, V. Using thematic analysis in psychology. *Qual. Res. Psychol.* **2006**, *3*, 77–101. [CrossRef]
21. Braun, V.; Clarke, V. *Successful Qualitative Research: A Practical Guide for Beginners*; Sage: London, UK, 2013; ISBN 1446289516.
22. DIPEx Switzerland. Available online: http://dipex.ch (accessed on 29 July 2022).
23. DIPEx International. Available online: https://dipexinternational.org/ (accessed on 29 July 2022).
24. Rovesti, M.; Fioranelli, M.; Petrelli, P.; Satolli, F.; Roccia, M.G.; Gianfaldoni, S.; Tchernev, G.; Wollina, U.; Lotti, J.; Feliciani, C.; et al. Health and Illness in History, Science and Society. *Open Access Maced. J. Med. Sci.* **2018**, *6*, 163–165. [CrossRef]
25. Oppliger, M. *Mit Dem Rollstuhl Nach Venedig Oder Wie Eine Reise Zum Mond*; Markus Oppliger: Burgdorf, Switzerland, 2019.
26. Software Version. *MAXQDA*, 18.2.5; The Software for Qualitative and Mixed Methods Research: Berlin, Germany, 2018.
27. Chu, S.Y.; Wen, C.C.; Lin, C.W. A qualitative study of clinical narrative competence of medical personnel. *BMC Med. Educ.* **2020**, *20*, 415. [CrossRef]

28. Berchtold, P.; Gedamke, S.; Schmitz, C.H. Quality Through Patients' Eyes. 2020. Available online: https://www.bag.admin.ch/dam/bag/de/dokumente/kuv-leistungen/qualitaetssicherung/quality-through-patients-eyes.pdf.download.pdf/Bericht%20Quality%20through%20patients\T1\textquoteright%20eyes.pdf (accessed on 29 July 2022).
29. Chiu, C.; Bishop, M.; Pionke, J.J.; Strauser, D.; Santens, R.L. Barriers to the Accessibility and Continuity of Health-Care Services in People with Multiple Sclerosis: A Literature Review. *Int. J. MS Care* **2017**, *19*, 313–321. [CrossRef]
30. Sable, P. The Pet Connection: An Attachment Perspective. *Clin. Soc. Work J.* **2013**, *41*, 93–99. [CrossRef]
31. Sung, J.; Trace, C.; Peterson, E.W.; Sosnoff, J.J.; Rice, L.A. Falls among full-time wheelchair users with spinal cord injury and multiple sclerosis: A comparison of characteristics of fallers and circumstances of falls. *Disabil. Rehabil.* **2019**, *41*, 389–395. [CrossRef]
32. Zhai, Y.; Nasseri, N.; Pöttgen, J.; Gezhelbash, E.; Heesen, C.; Stellmann, J.P. Smartphone Accelerometry: A Smart and Reliable Measurement of Real-Life Physical Activity in Multiple Sclerosis and Healthy Individuals. *Front. Neurol.* **2020**, *11*, 688. [CrossRef]
33. McClarty, L.M.; Bhattacharjee, P.; Blanchard, J.F.; Lorway, R.R.; Ramanaik, S.; Mishra, S.; Isac, S.; Ramesh, B.M.; Washington, R.; Moses, S.; et al. Circumstances, experiences and processes surrounding women's entry into sex work in India. *Cult. Health Sex.* **2014**, *16*, 149–163. [CrossRef]
34. Hammel, J. Technology and the environment: Supportive resource or barrier for people with developmental disabilities? *Nurs. Clin. N. Am.* **2003**, *38*, 331–349. [CrossRef]
35. Schmid, F.; Rogan, S.; Glässel, A. A Swiss Health Care Professionals' Perspective on the Meaning of Interprofessional Collaboration in Health Care of People with MS-A Focus Group Study. *Int. J. Environ. Res. Public Health* **2021**, *18*, 6537. [CrossRef]
36. Fakolade, A.; Latimer-Cheung, A.; Parsons, T.; Finlayson, M. A concerns report survey of physical activity support needs of people with moderate-to-severe MS disability and family caregivers. *Disabil. Rehabil.* **2019**, *41*, 2888–2899. [CrossRef]
37. Kayes, M.N.; McPherson, K.M.; Taylor, D.; Schlüter, P.J.; Kolt, G.S. Facilitators and barriers to engagement in physical activitiy for people with multiple sclerosis: A qualitative investigation. *Disabil. Rehabil.* **2011**, *33*, 625–642. [CrossRef]
38. Mayo, C.D.; Farzam-Kia, N.; Ghahari, S. Identifying Barriers to and Facilitators of Health Service Access Encountered by Individuals with Multiple Sclerosis. *Int. J. MS Care* **2021**, *23*, 37–44. [CrossRef] [PubMed]
39. Neate, S.L.; Taylor, K.L.; Jelinek, G.A.; De Livera, A.M.; Simpson, S.; Bevens, W.; Weiland, T.J. On the path together: Experinces of partners of people with multiple sclerosis of the impact of life-style modification on their relationship. *Health Soc. Care Community* **2019**, *27*, 1515–1524. [CrossRef] [PubMed]
40. Killner, L.; Soundy, A. Motivation and experiences of role transition in spousal caregivers of people with multiple sclerosis. *Int. J. Ther. Rehabil.* **2018**, *25*, 405–413. [CrossRef]
41. Bogosian, A.; Ross-Morris, R.; Yardley, L.; Dennsion, L. Experiences of partners of people in the early stages of multiple sclerosis. *Mult. Scler. J.* **2009**, *15*, 876–884. [CrossRef]
42. Kassie, S.A.; Alia, J.; Hyland, L. Biopsychosocial implications of living with multiple sclerosis: A qualitative study using interpretative phenomenological analysis. *BMJ Open* **2021**, *11*, e049041. [CrossRef]
43. Haubrick, K.K.; Gadbois, E.A.; Campbell, S.E.; Young, J.; Zhang, T.; Rizvi, S.; Shireman, T.I.; Shield, R.R. The Lived Experiences of Adults with Multiple Sclerosis. *Rhode Isl. Med. J.* **2021**, *104*, 38–42.

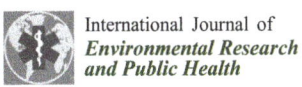

Article

A Swiss Health Care Professionals' Perspective on the Meaning of Interprofessional Collaboration in Health Care of People with MS—A Focus Group Study

Fabienne Schmid [1], Slavko Rogan [1,2] and Andrea Glässel [3,4,*]

1. Department of Health Professions, Division of Physiotherapy Bern, Bern University of Applied Sciences, 3008 Bern, Switzerland; avril_schmid@hotmail.com (F.S.); slavko.rogan@bfh.ch (S.R.)
2. Faculty of Physical Education and Physiotherapy, Vrije Universiteit Brussel, 1050 Brussel, Belgium
3. Institute of Biomedical Ethics and Medical History, University Zurich, Winterthurer Strasse 30, 8006 Zurich, Switzerland
4. Institute of Health Sciences, Zurich University of Applied Sciences, Katharina-Sulzer-Platz 9, 8401 Winterthur, Switzerland
* Correspondence: andrea.glaessel@ibme.uzh.ch; Tel.: +41-58-934-4397

Abstract: Multiple sclerosis (MS) is a chronic, inflammatory autoimmune disease of the central nervous system mainly of adults ranging from 20 to 45 years of age. The risk of developing MS is 50% higher in women than in men. Most people with MS (PwMS) experience a spectrum of symptoms such as spasticity, continence dysfunctions, fatigue, or neurobehavioral manifestations. Due to the complexity of MS and the variety of patient-centered needs, a comprehensive approach of interprofessional collaboration (IPC) of multiple health care professionals (HCP) is necessary. The aim of this qualitative study was to explore the meaning of IPC in the comprehensive care of PwMS from a HCP perspective. Focus groups (FG) with HCP were conducted, recorded, and transcribed verbatim. The sample contained HCP from three MS clinics in different phases of care and rehabilitation. Four main categories emerged: (a) experience with IPC, (b) relevant aspects for IPC in patients' treatment, (c) differences in in- and outpatient settings, and (d) influence of patient perspective. IPC plays a crucial role in HCP perspective when treating PwMS, which can benefit from an IPC therapeutic approach because HCP work together in a patient-centered way. The inpatient setting of HCP strongly supports the implementation of IPC. This prerequisite does not exist in outpatient settings.

Keywords: multiple sclerosis; health care professionals; qualitative research; focus groups; narration; interprofessional collaboration

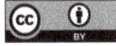

1. Introduction

Worldwide, 2.5 million people have been diagnosed with MS [1]. In Switzerland around 15,000 people are affected, mainly adults between 20 and 45 years. The risk of developing MS is 50% higher in women than in men [2]. The diagnosis of MS changes a life fundamentally and often requires a restructuring of life. MS is a chronic disease that represents an irreversible presence of disease conditions or damage of the nervous system. In order to promote self-sufficiency, maintain functional ability and prevent further disabilities, the entire environment of the person is rearranged [3] and people-centered care is needed. Rehabilitation is a people-centered health strategy with a set of interventions designed to optimize functioning and reduce disability of patients. The World Health Organization (WHO) integrated people-centered care concept places humans rather than their disabilities and diseases at the center of health care delivery [4]. To better explain the spectrum of limited disability and functioning of people with MS (PwMS), the help of the biopsychosocial model is used. The biopsychosocial model (Figure 1) forms the basis for International Classification of Functioning, Disability, and Health (ICF) [5]. ICF was designed as a common language and data standard that can be used for multiple purposes and in different environments [6].

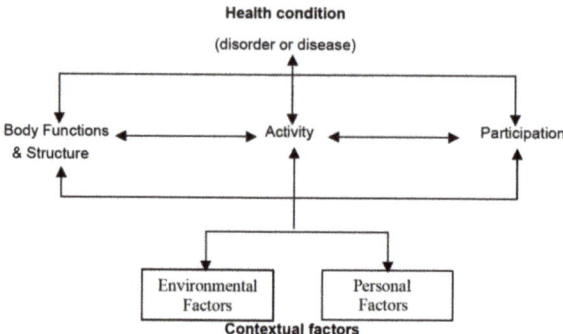

Figure 1. International Classification of Functioning, Disability, and Health (ICF) model of the World Health Organization [5].

MS, a chronic disease, is often called "the disease of a thousand faces" [7], which underlines the complexity of MS and the broad variety of patient-centered needs which addresses all dimensions of the ICF model. To achieve comprehensive health care management of PwMS, an approach of interprofessional collaboration (IPC) and comprehensive health care management is necessary. To provide comprehensive health care management from the patient perspective, individual preferences, requirements, and moral concepts which ensure that the patient guides all health decisions should be included. The patient's perspective and associated quality of life serves as a guide for designing further procedures and MS treatment strategies.

Successful patient-centered management of a complex neurological disease such as MS requires ongoing interactive relationships between the patient and multiple health professionals to take care of different needs. As it is unusual for one profession to deliver a complete program of care in isolation, high-quality care depends upon professions working together in interprofessional teams [8] (p. 1). There is an increasing interest in the ability of health care professionals (HCP) to work together, and in understanding how such collaborative practice contributes to primary health care. The WHO [9] (p. 4) defines IPC practice as "multiple health workers from different professional backgrounds working together with patients, families, caregivers, and communities to deliver the highest quality of care". Due to the multifaceted and complex nature of MS, an IPC approach is necessary to offer high-quality patient-centered care. Physiotherapists (PT), speech and language therapists (SLT), and occupational therapists (OT) play a key role in the comprehensive MS therapy team. Qualitative studies have explored the perspective of PwMS and their views on IPC access and, in general, their view on MS [10–14]. In general, studies which discuss health care in its pure form focus on competencies, implications, roles, education, and costs but do not specifically address different diagnoses such as of MS [15,16]. The few studies concentrating on the health care professionals working with PwMS address the following topics: needs of patients, and health care professionals' beliefs, treatments, and education [17–20]. These studies investigate the views and experiences of different health care professionals who work with modified treatments or exercise interventions for PwMS.

The aim of this study was to explore the perspective of specific health care professionals and their perception of IPC in comprehensive health care of PwMS. It will be specified by the following research questions:

(a) What is the perspective of health care professionals regarding the meaning of IPC in comprehensive health care of PwMS?
(b) How does experience with PwMS affect the health care professional's IPC?

2. Materials and Methods

To answer the research questions from the perspective of specific health care professionals and their perception of IPC in comprehensive health care of PwMS, we decided on a qualitative methodology by using focus groups in an outpatient setting.

2.1. Study Design

The reporting of this study was in accordance with consolidated criteria for reporting qualitative research (COREQ) [21]. To answer the research questions, a qualitative study based on a phenomenological approach and including focus groups was conducted between August and September 2018 with health care professional staff from three MS clinics specializing in different phases of care and rehabilitation, in three cantons, in the German speaking part of Switzerland. The methodology explored experiences and attitudes of research participants and depicted objects from the perspective of how they are experienced, thus allowing a search for the essence of the phenomenon [22]. Life conditions become relevant for the world when described by subjective meanings, which can be recorded in qualitative studies [23]. Qualitative research has an openness to the field of research, which enables knowledge gaps to be closed and new fields to be opened.

A characteristic of qualitative research is the studied reflexivity of the researcher's actions and perceptions in the field, understood as an essential part of the knowledge and not as a source of disturbance to be controlled. As physiotherapists, the authors of this study have a knowledge background as health care professionals but not as physiotherapy specialists in the treatment of PwMS, in contrast to the interviewed health care professionals. Nevertheless, the authors' own experience in relation to IPC in the inpatient as well as in the outpatient setting naturally brings with it a prior understanding on the part of the researchers. In qualitative research, the subjective perception of the researcher as a component of knowledge is used. The cognitive principle of qualitative research is the understanding of complex contexts rather than explanation by isolating an individual relationship [23].

In order to obtain some broader insights into the perspective of health care professionals' experiences, focus groups were conducted. This approach encouraged participants to consider the views and opinions of other participants because it was presented in a more natural environment than that of an individual interview, because participants influenced each other just as they do in their daily life [24] (p. 7).

The current study was approved by the cantonal Ethics Committee of Zurich, Switzerland (BASEC Nr.: Req-2018-00440, 14 June 2018). An approval by the ethics committee was not required because the project does not fall within the scope of the Human Research Act (HRA). A declaration of non-responsibility for this study was obtained. The study was performed in accordance with the Declaration of Helsinki [25]. All participants signed written informed consent. Personal data of participants were anonymized in all transcripts.

2.2. Sampling and Participants

To recruit health care professionals from in- and outpatient settings in the German-speaking part of Switzerland, different strategies to contact potential participants were applied: we acquired an open-access contact list of MS associations Switzerland, and contacted health care professional associations specializing in MS, specialized clinics for PwMS, and looked at specific outpatient settings for PwMS. Krueger [26] (p. 83) states that the best strategies for finding participants are existing lists of people fitting at least some of the predefined criteria. The goal was to have at least one person per focus group from each profession (PT, SLT, OT). Potential participants were contacted by mail or phone. A purposive sampling selection of the most productive sample was used to answer the research questions. Physiotherapists, speech and language therapists, and occupational therapists aim to enhance the daily living for persons with and without health restrictions through specific interventions which have an impact on a biological, psychosocial, and social levels. All three professions integrate both the material and the social environments of their clients in this transformation process [27] by supporting cognitive, sensory, and motor development. While other health care professionals, such as doctors, neuropsychologists and nurses, play an important role for PwMS, these professions are entrusted with other tasks.

2.3. Data Collection

To capture health care professionals' experiences, a semi-structured interview guide with open questions was developed to give participants the opportunity to describe and deepen their opinions more flexibly, led by topics. In contrast to standardized questionnaires and interviews, with this approach the moderator has the option to inquire about and clarify unclear statements [28] and a specific dynamic group interaction is created [26]. The semi-structured interview guide for focus groups was pre-tested and was based on a literature search to contextualize the theme of IPC with PwMS and contained the lead questions listed in Table 1. Questions were asked in positive and negative ways, e.g., supportive factors, chances and barriers, directions. Each focus group was led by two researchers and a moderator (AG/FS); furthermore, one researcher (FS/AG) took notes. For sociodemographic data, participants filled in a questionnaire.

Table 1. Questions of focus group interview guide.

Question Order	Questions of Focus Groups Interview Guide
A	**What experiences have you had with interprofessional cooperation (IPC) in the treatment of patients (positive and negative)?** Possible stimulus question: - What do you understand by interprofessional cooperation?
B	**What positive and/or negative aspects do you consider relevant from your perspective as a therapist for interprofessional treatment of PwMS?** Possible stimulus questions: - What is your experience with patients with MS compared to other patients? - What obstacles/challenges can you describe in terms of comprehensive treatment as a therapist in treating patients with MS? - What aspects do you think facilitate/hinder IPC in your work with patients with MS? - What role do you think the patient perspective plays for IPC? - What are the advantages/disadvantages of IPC in your opinion? - What experience do you have with regard to training in IPC?
C	**Do you think there are differences in IPC (knowledge and application) in inpatient and outpatient care?** Possible stimulus questions: - Are there any professional groups with whom more IPC takes place? - What opportunities and challenges can you see for IPC in the provision of health care for people with MS? - What are you personally doing to achieve better IPC? - In your opinion, is IPC demanded and necessary, or superfluous for MS patients?
D	**How do your experiences with PwMS influence the IPC of different health professionals?**
E	**Do you have additional aspects which are relevant from your perspective to add to IPC?**

2.4. Data Analysis

Focus groups discussions were in Swiss German (Swiss dialect), audio-recorded and transcribed verbatim into High German based on rules by Dresing and Pehl [29] by using the software program F5 (2004–2007—version 2.0.2). All focus groups transcripts were coded by using the software MAXQDA program (10.0 Standard 2018/04) based on the six phases of Braun and Clarke's thematic analysis [30,31]. The aim of qualitative thematic analysis is to process communication material, which was performed by an inductive and deductive categorization (Table 2).

2.5. Quality Assurance

For data quality assurance, the COREQ checklist was applied [21] and criteria of Flick, Kardorff, and Steinke [23] were considered: data security regulations regarding data storage were observed throughout the study. For peer-review, a pre-test for obtaining feedback on the focus group questions in the topic guide was conducted twice. Multiple strategies to capture the data were applied [26] (p. 145). Beside audio-recording and the minutes during all focus groups, field notes were collected by a second researcher. After each focus group, both researchers reflected on the process for potential improvements by written debriefing. Before starting data analysis, both researchers conducted training and drafted a coding scheme based on the questions. To ensure trustworthiness of data, the accuracy of the transcriptions was reviewed including application of rules and writing memos. For peer review, a second researcher coded 25% of data of the transcripts. Both researchers discussed the coding results for common agreement on each concept. For member checking, all participants were offered the transcripts. A plain language summery of the results was sent via email.

Table 2. Six phases of a thematic analysis of focus groups with health care professionals based on Braun and Clarke (own presentation) [30].

Phases 1–6:	Tasks of Thematic Analysis of Focus Groups
Phase 1: Familiarsing yourself with your data:	At the beginning, all transcripts were read and initial ideas were written down.
Phase 2: Generating initial codes:	Text passages were extracted from all three focus groups and provided with codes that were relevant for the research questions. This coding was inductive, and data controlled. Transcripts of all three groups were independently coded by a second researcher (AG) to improve research rigor. Created codes were compared and discussed by the research team (FS and AG). After coding all three focus groups, one researcher (FS) went through all coded transcripts again for reviewing and competition. Ideas and thoughts relating to every code were written down in memos. After a reviewing evaluation all statements were condensed to one code.
Phase 3: Searching themes:	Codes were collected to identify potential themes. For this, the written memos were used.
Phase 4: Reviewing themes:	The created themes and the associated codes were checked. Memo function was again used to refine definitions of the themes.
Phase 5: Defining and naming themes:	Themes were checked again and then divided into sets based on the questions.
Phase 6: Producing the report:	The individual sets were assigned to categories. A visual representation was carried out of code, topic, and sets.

3. Results

3.1. Sampling and Participants

Three focus groups were conducted with 13 health care professionals represented by six PTs, four OTs, and three SLTs in three German-speaking neuro-rehabilitation centers from July 2018 to April 2019. None of the participants dropped out. The average duration of the focus groups was 53 min, with a range from 33 to 77. Contacts to clinics resulted from a therapist list of the Swiss MS Society and from directly writing to leading clinic specialists. Answers were obtained from inpatient and semi-inpatient institutions. With a total of three persons, i.e., one person per focus group, SLTs were slightly underrepresented. Sociodemographic data of focus group participants are presented in Table 3.

All participating health care professionals had MS specific training; most frequently mentioned (7/13) were being trained in the Bobath concept or having obtained a Swiss Certificate of Advanced Studies (CAS) in MS (3/13). Regarding specific training in IPC, only three out of 13 participants had undergone external training. Internal training on IPC takes place in all visited clinics. The health care professionals were not evaluated individually according to their profession. As [26] states, caution must be exercised when focus group participants represent different categories of people as is the case in this study. If opinions of a single category of people are to be determined, a focus group with that specific category of people is needed. Krueger further testifies that a focus group of diverse people is not sensitive enough to discover trends of subcategories of people.

Table 3. Sociodemographic data of participants from the focus groups.

Demographics		Number of Participants
Age	20–30 years	2
	31–40 years	5
	41–50 years	4
	51–60 years	1
	No details	1
Gender	Male	1
	Female	12
Profession	Physiotherapy	6
	Occupational Therapy	4
	Speech and Language Therapy	3
Work field	Outpatient setting	1
	Inpatient setting	5
	both	7
Work experience with PwMS	<1 year	0
	1–2 years	1
	5–10 years	7
	10–20 years	4
	>20 years	1

3.2. Data Analysis

The codes that were generated were grouped into themes and categories. The following four main categories emerged from the data out of three focus groups: (a) experience with IPC, (b) relevant aspects for IPC on patients' treatment, (c) differences in in- and outpatient settings and (d) influence of the patient perspective (Figure 2). Sub-categories are described as follows, including sections and examples of health care professionals' quotations (see also Supplementary Figures S1 and S2).

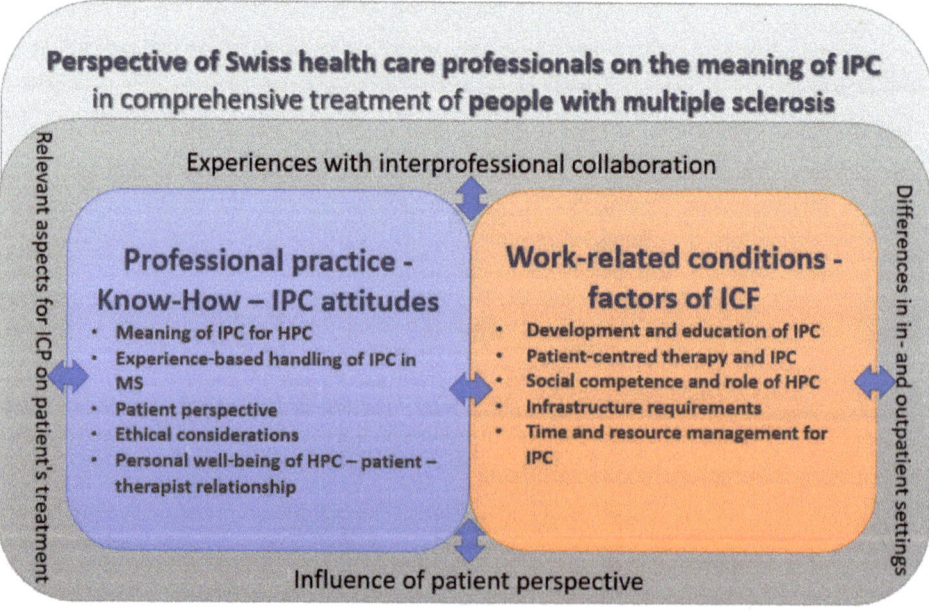

Figure 2. Overview of results from a health professional perspective (health care professionals = HCP).

3.2.1. Professional Practice—Know-How—IPC Attitudes

Meaning of IPC for Health Care Professionals

This section describes health care professionals' statements about their individual definitions, understanding, and relevance of IPC in managing a comprehensive health care situation of PwMS. Collaborative agreements between individual professions facilitate the achievement of goals.

«For me, interprofessional means pulling together on the same rope and if possible, being able to do inpatient work on the same goals in a discipline-specific way (–) and not sinking into parallel worlds where everyone works in a different direction». (FG03; 118)

«But the goal or the patient should actually be in the center. And the goal should be defined as realistically as possible. And, of course, we also need to talk to each other. But that's what I understand by the definition of interprofessional cooperation». (FG01; 114)

Participants discussed IPC as a huge benefit both for the patient and for the health care professionals themselves to work together for and follow the same goals. IPC gives the health care professionals a holistic picture of the patient based on ICF. By bringing together a large number of health care professionals with a highly specific training in MS, not only can the patient benefit but also the therapist. IPC also means an accumulation of knowledge and experience in one place.

«You also know who works a lot with PwMS, who can I ask, if this is not my subject. For example, if someone has breathing problems, I can ask this therapist». (FG01; 94)

«But we also have a holistic picture of our patients, it is not simply enough just to check out our own professional area. We are also always in contact with the physiotherapy, how far they can go. Because this also has a direct impact on patients' leisure time and independence and daily routine». (FG02; 21)

Experience and Handling of IPC in MS

Over the years in specific health care of PwMS, the participants were able to experience and learn a great deal about IPC. The exchange among the health care professionals gives them insights not only into their own specialist area but also into that of the other professionals involved. By forming mixed discussion groups, the risk of focusing too much on one's own profession-specific goal and thus possibly losing the overarching goal can be reduced.

«I think it makes it a lot easier. IPC is important to look and see, maybe I have forgotten something. There are cognitive problems for example, and there are also other problems. And that's where I see the importance of working together in addition to my own work». (FG03; 120)

Participants learn to see the treatment of PwMS in a broader and more comprehensive context as many people are involved. IPC is described by the health care professionals as a process to be learnt which one needs to grow into. As an employee, people will also learn the employer's philosophy regarding IPC and the corresponding approach to IPC. At best, you will learn to identify yourself with this approach of the house. The health care professionals experience how all the other professions contribute towards reaching the patient's goal.

«That you can only really work at its optimum if you work interprofessionally. And this fundamental attitude that I believe you have to learn to live». (FG01; 47).

Conducting a conversation with a person who has a chronic disease is complex. Participants said that experience with PwMS has shown that especially if you have got to know each other so well over the years due to this chronic illness, it is essential to take a clear stand and to be honest with patients. It is considered important to apply a common communication as an interprofessional team.

«You have to be clear about what you say, so that the patients understand. That they can understand when you do a lot of therapy for three weeks, but no progress shows up». (FG02; 54)

«Then you quickly reach limits of what you can do in the conversation with the patient, for example, how can I tell him that now? These are special challenges. So, the topic of conversation somehow, how can I justify myself? ». (FG01; 74)

Patient Perspective

The patient perspective plays a crucial role in health care and quality assurance. During a disease episode, patients get in contact with all therapists involved in care on an in- and/or outpatient basis. They can review the entire care chain. During their therapies, health care professionals perceive or provoke emotions from patients. They get insights into the patients' personal views, experiences, and life stories. The patient also enters the therapy with a form of expectation regarding, for example, the quality or type of therapy (treatment approach). The PwMS experience contact with other patients in the specialized clinics who are diagnosed with the same illness but possibly being at a different stage. This is perceived by therapists as both an advantage and a disadvantage.

«Yes, patients see their own future». (FG02; 94) «That is another condition to live clearly in the context I am getting worse and worse, I have a chronic illness, what awaits me, even young people with family». (FG01;67)

«For example, during the first stay, if the therapist recommends a foot lifter splint, they say no and generally reject everything. And over time, during the second or third stay, they see that other PwMS are better off with the same aids and then they accept it. They profit very much from each other». (FG02;71)

As a therapist, one must learn to understand the patient's point of view and to be able to take their position. On their own initiative, PwMS often try to get the best out of themselves or to improve or maintain their quality of life as well as possible. Patients develop coping skills; thus, the health care professionals mentioned coping strategies for everyday actions.

«For example, we have a patient who drives her wheelchair with a self-made mouth stick when her hand gets tired». (FG02; 66)

«Yes, they have surprising coping skills, also to some extent self-destructive. How they deal with their problems». (FG02; 62)

«And there they come up with their own ideas and you reflect and think together. You can't get such knowledge out of textbooks and reference books. For me, that has actually a lot of value as a therapist». (FG02; 66)

Ethical Considerations

The four biomedical principles of Beauchamp and Childress (2001) [32], which are (a) respect of autonomy, (b) justice, (c) beneficence, and (d) non-maleficence, are an established, widespread framework applied in challenging ethical questions of health care. When working with PwMS, health care professionals can sometimes find themselves in difficult ethical situations and are required to make adequate decisions, especially in difficult cases when two principles seem to be conflicting or even exclude each other. In MS changes in cognitive abilities are not infrequent, limiting patients in making autonomous and self-determined decisions. Therapists are faced with ethical challenges because the questioning of important topics can often not be made by explicitly asking the patient. When does it make sense to decide something for the patient that takes away a part of his or her quality of life, but is no longer acceptable for safety reasons? Balancing damage and benefit put health care professionals and PwMS in a conflict situation.

«And with PwMS, it's often the case that you don't want to take anything away from them. So, you know, it's probably already dangerous if he eats the peanuts now. But he loves them more than anything else and that would be a big incision for him now, if I said that he shouldn't eat them anymore. And then what does this neuropsychological clarification mean? That would mean in three quarters of the cases that they can no longer drive». (FG01; 71-83)

From the therapist's point of view, there is a need to be able to assess the change in individuals due to MS because there is a risk that cognitive limitations of PwMS can also be misinterpreted as patient reluctance or lack of motivation. The principle of autonomy often conflicts with beneficence. Health care professionals do not want to take anything from the patient that limits his or her autonomy but at the same time they want the best for him or her.

«...but if you are not that aware of the cognitive limitations, you often ask the patient and think the patient does not want that. But often the patient can't really estimate». (FG01; 79)

Personal Well-Being of Health Care Professionals/Patient–Therapist Relationship

Health care professionals reported that at some points they reached their personal limits in dealing with PwMS. What makes the therapeutic work successful? It is not only about well-founded training and the professional approach. Personal commitment and engagement are key requirements for working in an IPC environment. For successful treatment, the health care professionals have to take an individual approach tailored to the personality and peculiarities of this specific PwMS. This means being touched by the fate of this person, adding ideas, developing an image of this person and getting emotionally involved. It is an intense and close relationship. This patient–therapist relationship offers possibilities for disagreement and points of conflict.

«And then you feel very stupid. And I like to think I'm over 30 years old and he insults me like a little girl. I know how to react to it. I also see him as a patient who has a terrible illness, who can't deal with it. His illness changes him, we just treat him, but yes. Maybe he will be nice someday». (FG02; 80)

«I am overwhelmed when a patient approaches me very negatively or very impudently. That is difficult for me. There I am.... I already have a few strategies, but if all this is useless to me, if I am only loaded, then I know that my therapy has absolutely no effect at that moment. And then I also take the liberty to stop it. Yes, I have to explain that to my colleagues afterwards». (FG02; 77)

3.2.2. Work-Related Conditions—Factors of IPC

Development and Education of IPC

IPC has undergone a big change in recent years. Most rehabilitation clinics work interprofessionally and have developed and implemented organizational structures to offer IPC educational concepts. All participants explained they have gained more and more insight into the other professions, demonstrated by the fact that one professional group knows MS-specific instruments from another group of health care professionals.

«I can really see that in MS these are the pioneers of interprofessional cooperation». (FG01; 25)

«It has improved more and more over the last 10 to 15 years. It already starts with recording reports. All professions are present together and they are checking among each other what is the focus of this clinic stay. The therapy package will be put together accordingly. In the last two, three years, collaborations have become better, since we have a common team room.... On the other hand, when aids are needed or when positioning is required for the more severely affected patients, intensive collaboration is required. Or you make splints and we do the positioning together». (FG02; 18)

«For me, insights into job descriptions of the individual professionals are important. Because in recent years we have been able to gain insights from time to time. For example, we had a detailed explanation of how to swallow and how important that is. And if I have a good insight, I can put myself better into it. We had gotten further training; and mutually I know more about occupational therapy and speech therapy than if I didn't work here. (FG02; 38)

Patient-Centered Therapy in IPC

This section presents statements about the patient being the center of therapy and decision-making. IPC is a collaborative exchange that is carried out for the patients' benefit. A key statement of the health care professionals was to focus on the patient's view or him- or herself as a human being.

«But I think the goal should be that the patient's view of what he wants always comes first». That's how you should put it. And then perhaps a therapeutic goal can result from it». (FG01; 123) (FG01; 123)

«The fact that the patient is also a component of this interprofessional team includes him as a partner». (FG01; 106)

Additionally, challenges were mentioned. Health care professionals try to respond to wishes and specific needs of individual patients as far as possible.

«But it's just like doing a balancing act to say that is what the patient wants to do, but that is what I want to work towards now, something different». (FG01; 128)

«These people also usually come into therapy with a very precise idea of what to do now, what the next step could be and what they need. And picking them up, what they imagine and at the same time being able to bring in the therapeutic expertise is a bit of a balancing act». (FG01;64)

Social Competence and the Role of the Health Care Professionals

In the focus groups, participants discussed in depth the influence of the health care professional's own personality and social competences. The personal background (beliefs, education), motivation, mood, empathy, and perception of situations were all mentioned as factors that can have a positive and negative impact on IPC. IPC also means a division of labor, making joint cross-disciplinary agreements, having good communication between each other and knowing one's own role and importance in this interprofessional health care team.

«The one who sees a need addresses it». (FG03; 41) and «Communication is everything». (FG02; 107)

«...Should I do it now or will the SLTs do it? Regarding aids with communication devices, who does what? So simply that it does not run twice or that it will not get forgotten. There are both possibilities here». (FG01; 49).

Health care professionals stated that they have to be able to step back within the team and also to possess the ability to perceive when their role is needed and when not. It takes a high degree of reflexivity to work in this environment in order to be, and continue to be, able to cooperate. At the same time, a certain instinct is required to know when to resign and to commit oneself to represent the patient's goals in one's own therapy.

«To make arrangements and to be able to withdraw. If necessary, to be able to withdraw and remember that I may not be the main person (therapeutic discipline) who has to contribute something». (FG01; 155)

« I also think that one can ask easily and admit oneself, when I need help». (FG01; 94)

Connected to social competence, expressions such as emancipation, hierarchical structures, communication at head level, and rivalry were mentioned. IPC means to see the holistic picture of the patient and to look beyond one's own professional area.

«That you can also say, yes I step back now because the patient does not want my therapy. That you are also flexible with structures and hierarchies. That you have a level where you can really communicate with your team». (FG01; 118)

«I think this is very important, the emancipation from these old structures where the doctor was the leader who always knew everything. Which may be partly true, but often not, because it's actually not possible to know everything in such complex settings». (FG01; 119)

The personality of the therapist regarding the interest in implementing IPC is a basic condition. IPC means being able to work in a team and being interested in areas other than one's own. The fact that someone who works in the health care sector already has a high degree of social competence is a good prerequisite. Identification with IPC is an important factor for working successfully and for long-term satisfaction.

«I think similarly, one must have an interest. I wonder what patients do in speech therapy, what their cognitive abilities are and what they do in physiotherapy. I need to have an interest. It always takes self-initiative» (FG02; 42)

«...and we read each other's reports or then just go and ask or discuss when we have a concern». (FG03; 30)

Infrastructure Requirements

An often-cited topic was conditions or infrastructure of the employer. Clinic internal online networks provide health care professionals with information concerning treatments of all professions working around with a patient. Additionally, sharing treatment or break rooms among different health care professionals can stimulate IPC.

«What makes it easier is our process in the "Phoenix" system. We have made it very professional and now we have a sheet where all disciplines note their current state of therapy». (FG02; 92)

«Our infrastructure makes it easier to reach our destinations. Plus, that new ideas are implemented relatively quickly here. We therapists work door-to-door with each other, there is a lot of exchange». (FG02; 94)

Larger centers have a local advantage; all disciplines are combined in one place. This makes it more efficient for having conversations in specific time slots for meetings or in the corridor. Spontaneous meetings of two disciplines were especially mentioned as supportive and productive in relation to keeping on track to reach patient-oriented treatment goals.

«Or when we walk through a therapy room and see the colleagues from the physiotherapy treating the patient right now and we have a few minutes, then we observe briefly or can then use time for a brief exchange». (FG02; 22)

Health care professionals also mentioned that in controlled settings, as is the case in inpatient care, IPC is clearly easier to access compared to outpatient settings. Costs (time is money) for exchange, conversations, and documentation with other health care professionals regarding patient-specific needs for therapists who are working in strictly outpatient centers are higher and financially more difficult to bear. In the outpatient area, for example, only reports for accident insurance, disability insurance, and military insurance can be billed, and this only if the insurance company explicitly requested a report.

«Because the case with us in the outpatient clinic is that I have to consider whether I can find time for a phone call. I cannot charge this time as physiotherapy. And a lot of things that you normally wanted to contribute to quality just will be dropped and left away». (FG01; 110)

«You might be a bit more in your chamber and working on your own thing if you do it on external outpatient care. It rarely happens that I consult the responsible doctor for an outpatient patient». (FG03; 137; FG03; 158)

Time and Resource Management for IPC

Structured time frames for interprofessional patient meetings were emphasized to be important. Meetings are held at regular intervals and are a great facilitation to maintain IPC. Through shared discussion time, individual perspectives of disciplines on problems and goals can be reflected. This applies primarily to inpatient and semi-inpatient facilities but not to strictly outpatient settings. IPC needs a lot of time, thus also causing costs, which is seen as a risk for developing IPC.

«Yes, and I think the big difference for me is that there are also structures provided for this exchange in the inpatient sector». (FG03; 139)

«In the day clinic they take place every week, but each time different patients are discussed. Then one has 10 to 20 min time, where one discusses the patient with the interprofessional goals, agrees on these and names the main problems». (FG01; 45)

4. Discussion

This current study focused on exploration of the Swiss health care professionals' perspectives regarding the meaning of IPC in comprehensive health care of PwMS and what influence the experience with PwMS has on IPC of the health care professionals. This study highlighted that a patient-centered therapy in IPC means that PwMS are placed in the middle and their needs and demands are incorporated into the therapy and structure it. The importance of the patient perspective in the rehabilitation process manifests itself and corroborates the findings of other studies. Heesen et al. [33] concluded that 80% of PwMS require an autonomous role in treatment decisions. Moreover, Tractenberg et al. [34] concluded that there are qualitative differences in therapy outcomes that are using a patient-centered approach. Cutler et al. [35] summed up that including the patient in the health care professionals team makes sense for long-lasting treatments such as physiotherapy or mental health services but less for acute treatment like emergency care.

However, the ideas of PwMS and health care professionals can also diverge. The study of Rothwell et al. [36] could already show that the understanding of disability in MS differs between doctors and PwMS. So identifying needs and demands of PwMS is crucial for a comprehensive IPC. This highlights the aspect that the meaning of IPC for a health care professional can also be understood in different ways. As demonstrated in patient perspectives in this study, patients are increasingly searching the internet for information. With a diagnosis of a lifelong disease, PwMS inform themselves in depth about their symptoms and disease progression.

The findings in the section on personal well-being of health care professionals and the patient–therapist relationship in this study demonstrated that personal commitment and engagement are always required. However, there are situations as a health care professional treating a patient with MS in which one reaches personal limits and even has to stop his or her therapy. In such cases it is important for therapists to distance themselves from these high and difficult-to-reach expectations and hopes of PwMS. It challenges therapeutic success when people are denied reaching common defined treatment goals.

For the successful implementation of IPC, certain conditions are needed. Study results about infrastructure, time and resource management requirements are consistent with those in the literature, which states that the use of technology for the implementation of effectual IPC is traced as a core element [37,38]. A lack of compensation for interprofessional collaboration services is considered an influential hindering factor. Interprofessional collaboration among stakeholders has so far been based on the commitment of individuals. Remuneration is provided in the outpatient setting for physicians, but not for health care professionals [39]. Further elements, such as the geography of workplace and schedule, can have an influence on IPC. There is a need for tools to share and support face-to-face communication with institutions or teams [8]. The literature states that hierarchies can suppress IPC [40]. This can also be found in the results concerning the social competence and role of health care professionals. Important key factors are to ensure that every team member understands his or her own role, his or her field of work and to enhance respect for each other within the IPC team [15]. Therefore, it is crucial that members of the IPC team show respect for the competences of other health care professionals within the team and work together to achieve common patient goals. Health care professionals must also be able to admit a lack of knowledge without losing trust of PwMS. In the literature, skills and competences within teams are defined as key requirements for an effective work performance [15].

However, not only do health care professionals have roles, but patients and their engagement are also important within IPC, which is indicated in the category ethical considerations. Engagement of a patient has the potential to increase a health care professional's awareness that their actions can have real consequences for individuals, which in turn leads to moderate risk-taking behavior [41]. Still, as can be seen in the example of PwMS, effects of a disease can have an impact on patient engagement with health care professionals. Their illness, mental state, ethnicity, language spoken, and mental capacity can significantly affect their ability to engage themselves with the health care professional.

The experience and handling of IPC in the MS work field shows that the neurological disease provokes coping skills from a patient perspective but also in health care professionals dealing with PwMS. Coping was first specified in the 1960s as the effort of cognition and behavior to handle, reduce, or tolerate inside and outside demands which cannot be handled with one's own available resources [42]. In the literature the term is not only used in connection with positive results. This was also the case with the participants in this study. The health care professionals stated that PwMS partly react with the suppression of the problem. This suppression coping reaction stays in line with typical psychological adjustments among PwMS [43].

The Swiss Federal Office of Public Health (FOPH) also recognized the need for IPC. By means of a support program called "Interprofessionality in Healthcare 2017–2020" they try to improve IPC in the Swiss health care system and increase its efficiency [44]. Based on the program outcomes of interprofessional collaboration in health care, four policy briefs—findings and recommendations for target group-specific implementation (a) interprofessional education, (b) inpatient setting, (c) outpatient setting and (d) psychosomatic setting and interfaces—were published in May 2021 [45]. The findings are intended to be used by persons responsible at a local, cantonal, and national level, by communities, as well as private and public organizations, to promote interprofessional education and practice in the health care system in Switzerland.

Limitations

For a comprehensive in- and outpatient health care setting for PwMS, different health professions are relevant for IPC based on the need of care and depending on the phase of this life-long disease as physicians, neurologists, psychologists, nurses, pharmacists, podiatrists, and others including therapists. Our study was focusing on IPC in health care professionals; as therapists this means physiotherapists, occupations therapists and speech therapists. By reflection on the results, this will limit this study related to the comprehensive outpatient health care setting for PwMS. The findings of this study cannot answer the question of what the IPC experience in a strictly outpatient setting is, and how its implementation takes place. Although attempts were made to obtain outpatient results, outpatient health care professionals were not willing to make themselves available for focus groups or even individual interviews. The reason consistently given was a lack of time. To minimize the risk of losing the voice of outpatient health care professionals, one strategy was to conduct individual interviews with health care professionals in the outpatient setting before losing this information completely. However, the outpatient health care professionals were not supported to participate in a focus group during their working hours and outside their working hours they were not willing. Furthermore, the creation of outpatient focus groups was made more difficult by the different local workplaces. For future project methods, an online focus group approach could be a useful tool to include hard-to-reach health care professionals to facilitate their participation. All health care professionals who were included worked in inpatient rehabilitative settings and were thus locally limited. The most noticeable aspect when writing to outpatient health care professionals was that it was extremely rare that PT, SLT, and OT worked all together in a strictly outpatient practice. This may indicate further organizational problems for PwMS who depend on all three forms of therapy.

By reflecting the results, we would like to acknowledge that only some of the health care professionals approached for the study agreed to participate. This means we do not know the opinion and attitudes toward IPC of those who declined.

A critical look at this work reveals that the interviews were conducted by a professional colleague and master student. This position is, in fact, an insider position, which can be advantageous, for instance, because both sides share a common language and nomenclature. In a focus group setting, the researcher has several functions such as moderator, listener, observer, and eventually analyst [26]. A disadvantage is that the interviewer's own experiences, norms, and values regarding the phenomenon to be investigated are involved. In this study, health care professionals working in inpatient, semi-inpatient and rehabilitative settings were interviewed. In contrast the personal perceptions of the author herself, working in a strictly outpatient setting, is that IPC does not exist in the outpatient care of PwMS in Switzerland. However, this observation could only be compared to a limited extent with results from this study.

5. Conclusions

The study wanted to examine two research questions. On the one hand, 'What is the health care professionals' perspective regarding the meaning of IPC in a comprehensive health care of PwMS'? The findings suggest that IPC plays a crucial role in specific inpatient MS clinics in Switzerland. Moreover, it was revealed that overall PwMS can only benefit from an IPC therapeutic approach because health care professionals work together in a goal-oriented and patient centered way. It could be shown that close location (inpatient setting) of health care professionals strongly supports the implementation of IPC.

On the other hand, the second research question, 'How does the experience with PwMS affect the health care professional's IPC?' could be answered as follows: This is a disadvantage for PwMS in outpatient settings because this possibility does not exist in Switzerland so far. In settings where individual professions work at larger distances, less or no IPC seems to take place. Further research in outpatient settings about the implementation prerequisites of IPC for PwMS and health care professionals' views is needed. The outpatient sector shows a strong dispersion of the professions, which may also make it difficult for the PwMS if an interprofessional approach should be desired. Incentives for cooperation in the outpatient sector should be created from the field of politics in order to be able to connect health care professionals caring for PwMS in Switzerland.

Health care professionals themselves and health institutions can benefit from these findings to gain an overview of their processes and possible missing contacts for outpatient IPC.

Supplementary Materials: The following are available online at https://www.mdpi.com/1660-4601/18/12/6537/s1, Figure S1: Extract from MAXQDA Coding, Figure S2: MAXQDA Main Sets.

Author Contributions: F.S.: reviewed the literature; study administration; data collection and analysis; wrote manuscript; edited manuscript; S.R.: research supervision; manuscript write-up; A.G.: conceptualization; methodology; partly involved in data collection and analysis for training and validation; visualization; research supervision, manuscript write-up, manuscript editing. All authors have read and agreed to the published version of the manuscript.

Funding: This research received no external funding.

Institutional Review Board Statement: The study was conducted according to the guidelines of the Declaration of Helsinki and approved by the Institutional Review Board of the cantonal Ethics Committee of Zurich, Switzerland, University of Zurich (BASEC Nr.: Req-2018-00440, 14th of June 2018).

Informed Consent Statement: Written informed consent has been obtained from the participants for the interviews and to publish the study.

Data Availability Statement: Data are stored at the Institute of Biomedical Ethics and medical History, University of Zurich.

Acknowledgments: The authors would like to thank all participants for their support and contribution to this study. Without their voluntary participation and openness to discuss personal experiences and opinions it would not have been possible to achieve these results. We also thank our colleague David Stamm for proofreading the manuscript.

Conflicts of Interest: The authors declare no conflict of interest.

References

1. Multiple Sclerosis. Who Gets MS? Multiple Sclerosis (MS) Better Questions Lead to Better Answers. 2021. Available online: https://www.multiplesclerosis.com/global/about_ms.php (accessed on 24 May 2021).
2. Multiple Sklerose. Vorkommen. Schweizerische Multiple Sklerose Gesellschaft. 2021. Available online: https://www.multiplesklerose.ch/de/ueber-ms/multiple-sklerose/vorkommen/ (accessed on 24 May 2021).
3. Calabresi, P.A. Diagnosis and management of multiple sclerosis. *Am. Fam. Phys.* **2004**, *70*, 1935–1944.
4. Gimigliano, F.; Negrini, S. The World Health Organization "Rehabilitation 2030—A call for action". *Eur. J. Phys. Rehabil. Med.* **2017**, *53*, 155–168. [CrossRef]
5. World Health Towards a Common Language for Functioning, Disability, and Health: ICF. The Organization. International Classification of Functioning, Disability and Health. 2021. Available online: https://www.who.int/classifications/icf/en/ (accessed on 24 May 2021).
6. Kostanjsek, N. Use of The International Classification of Functioning, Disability and Health (ICF) as a conceptual framework and common language for disability statistics and health information systems. *BMC Public Health* **2011**, *11* (Suppl. 4), S3. [CrossRef] [PubMed]
7. Van Bochove, B. Multiple Sclerosis—The Disease with a Thousand Faces. *Commer. Ger.* **2015**, *13*, 9. Available online: https://www.amcham.de/publications/commerce-germany/ (accessed on 24 May 2021).
8. Reeves, S.; Lewin, S.; Espin, S.; Zwarenstein, M. *Interprofessional Teamwork for Health and Social Care*; Blackwell-Wiley: London, UK, 2010.
9. World Health Organization. Interprofessional Collaboration Practice in Primary Health Care: Nursing and Mid-wifery Perspectives. Human Resources for health Observer (13). 2013. Available online: https://www.who.int/hrh/resources/observer13/en/ (accessed on 24 May 2021).
10. Galushko, M.; Golla, H.; Strupp, J.; Karbach, U.; Kaiser, C.; Ernstmann, N.; Pfaff, H.; Ostgathe, C.; Voltz, R. Unmet Needs of Patients Feeling Severely Affected by Multiple Sclerosis in Germany: A Qualitative Study. *J. Palliat. Med.* **2014**, *17*, 274–281. [CrossRef] [PubMed]
11. Hepworth, M.; Harrison, J.; James, N. Information needs of people with multiple sclerosis and the implications for information provision based on a national UK survey. *Aslib Proc.* **2003**, *55*, 290–303. [CrossRef]
12. Kantor, D.; Bright, J.R.; Burtchell, J. Perspectives from the Patient and the Healthcare Professional in Multiple Sclerosis: Social Media and Participatory Medicine. *Neurol. Ther.* **2018**, *7*, 37–49. [CrossRef]
13. Kirk, S.; Hinton, D. "I'm not what I used to be": A qualitative study exploring how young people experience being diagnosed with a chronic illness. *Child Care Health Dev.* **2019**, *45*, 216–226. [CrossRef]
14. Somerset, M.; Campbell, R.; Sharp, D.J.; Peters, T. What do people with MS want and expect from health-care services? *Health Expect.* **2001**, *4*, 29–37. [CrossRef]
15. Bainbridge, L.; Nasmith, L.; Orchard, C.; Wood, V. Competencies for Interprofessional Collaboration. *J. Phys. Ther. Educ.* **2010**, *24*, 6–11. [CrossRef]
16. Delva, D.; Jamieson, M.; Lemieux, M. Team effectiveness in academic primary health care teams. *J. Interprof. Care* **2008**, *22*, 598–611. [CrossRef]
17. Cameron, E.; Rog, D.; McDonnell, G.; Overell, J.; Pearson, O.; French, D.P. Factors influencing multiple sclerosis disease-modifying treatment prescribing decisions in the United Kingdom: A qualitative interview study. *Mult. Scler. Relat. Disord.* **2019**, *27*, 378–382. [CrossRef]
18. Smith, C.M.; Hale, L.A.; Olson, K.; Baxter, G.D.; Schneiders, A.G. Healthcare provider beliefs about exercise and fatigue in people with multiple sclerosis. *J. Rehabil. Res. Dev.* **2013**, *50*, 733. [CrossRef]
19. Turner, A.P.; Martin, C.; Williams, R.M.; Goudreau, K.; Bowen, J.D.; Hatzakis, M., Jr.; Whitham, R.H.; Bourdette, D.N.; Walker, L.; Haselkorn, J.K. Exploring educational needs of multiple sclerosis care providers: Results of a care-provider sur-vey. *J. Rehabil. Res. Dev.* **2006**, *43*, 25–34. [CrossRef]
20. Upton, D.; Taylor, C. What Are the Support Needs of Men with Multiple Sclerosis, and Are They Being Met? *Int. J. MS Care* **2015**, *17*, 9–12. [CrossRef]

21. Tong, A.; Sainsbury, P.; Craig, J. Consolidated criteria for reporting qualitative research (COREQ): A 32-item checklist for interviews and focus groups. *Int. J. Qual. Health Care* **2007**, *19*, 349–357. [CrossRef]
22. Malterud, K. Systematic text condensation: A strategy for qualitative analysis. *Scand. J. Public Health* **2012**, *40*, 795–805. [CrossRef]
23. Flick, U.; Kardorff, E.V.; Steinke, I. *Qualitative Forschung*, 12th ed.; Rowohlt: Reinbek, Germany, 2017.
24. Robson, C. *Real World Research: A Resource for Social Scientists and Practitioner—Researchers*, 2nd ed.; Blackwell Publishing: Oxford, UK, 2002.
25. World Medical Association. World Medical Association Declaration of Helsinki. Ethical principles for medical research involving human subjects. *Bull. World Health Organ.* **2001**, *79*, 373–374.
26. McQuarrie, E.F.; Krueger, R.A. Focus Groups: A Practical Guide for Applied Research. *J. Mark. Res.* **1989**, *26*, 371. [CrossRef]
27. Wechselwirkung auf die Versorgung von Berufszufriedenheit—Akademischer Erstqualifizierung und der Bedarfsentwicklung in der Ergotherapie. Available online: http://bdsl-ev.de/wp-content/uploads/2019/11/probst_bmg_14.11.2018.pdf (accessed on 16 June 2021).
28. Merriam, S.B. *Qualitative Research and Case Study Applications in Education. Revised and Expanded from "Case Study Research in Education"*; Jossey-Bass: San Francisco, CA, USA, 1998.
29. Dresing, T.; Pehl, T. *Praxisbuch Interview, Transkription & Analyse. Anleitungen und Regelsysteme für Qualitativ For-Schende*, 8th ed.; Eigenverlag: Marburg, Germany, 2018; Available online: https://www.audiotranskription.de/downloads#praxisbuch (accessed on 24 May 2021).
30. Braun, V.; Clarke, V. Using thematic analysis in psychology. *Qual. Res. Psychol.* **2006**, *3*, 77–101. [CrossRef]
31. Clarke, V.; Braun, V. *Successful Qualitative Research: A Practical Guide for Beginners*; Sage: London, UK, 2013.
32. Beauchamp, T.; Childress, J. *Principles of Biomedical Ethics*, 7th ed.; University Press: Oxford, MO, USA, 2001. [CrossRef]
33. Heesen, C.; Köpke, S.; Richter, T.; Kasper, J. Shared decision making and selfmanagement in multiple sclerosis—A consequence of evidence. *J. Neurol.* **2007**, *254*, II116–II121. [CrossRef] [PubMed]
34. Tractenberg, R.E.; Garver, A.; Ljungberg, I.H.; Schladen, M.M.; Groah, S.L. Maintaining primacy of the patient perspective in the development of patient-centered patient reported outcomes. *PLoS ONE* **2017**, *12*, e0171114. [CrossRef] [PubMed]
35. Cutler, S.; Morecroft, C.; Carey, P.; Kennedy, T. Are interprofessional healthcare teams meeting patient expectations? An exploration of the perceptions of patients and informal caregivers. *J. Interprof. Care* **2018**, *33*, 66–75. [CrossRef] [PubMed]
36. Rothwell, P.M.; McDowell, Z.; Wong, C.K.; Dorman, P.J. Doctors and patients don't agree: Cross sectional study of patients' and doctors' perceptions and assessments of disability in multiple sclerosis. *BMJ* **1997**, *314*, 1580. [CrossRef]
37. James, T.A.; Page, J.S.; Sprague, J. Promoting interprofessional collaboration in oncology through a teamwork skills simulation programme. *J. Interprof. Care* **2016**, *30*, 1–3. [CrossRef]
38. McLoughlin, C.; Patel, K.D.; O'Callaghan, T.; Reeves, S. The use of virtual communities of practice to improve interprofessional collaboration and education: Findings from an integrated review. *J. Interprof. Care* **2017**, *32*, 136–142. [CrossRef]
39. Stakeholders' Perspectives on Innovative Models of Interprofessional Collaboration in Community-Based Care. Available online: https://www.cnhw.ch/fileadmin/user_upload/Abstract_ID_2.pdf (accessed on 16 June 2021).
40. Soklaridis, S.; Romano, N.; Fung, W.L.A.; Martimianakis, M.A.; Sargeant, J.; Chambers, J.; Wiljer, D.; Silver, I.; Fung, A.W.L. Where is the client/patient voice in interprofessional healthcare team assessments? Findings from a one-day forum. *J. Interprof. Care* **2016**, *31*, 1–3. [CrossRef]
41. Howe, A. Can the patient be on our team? An operational approach to patient involvement in interprofessional approaches to safe care. *J. Interprof. Care* **2006**, *20*, 527–534. [CrossRef]
42. Goretti, B.; Portaccio, E.; Zipoli, V.; Hakiki, B.; Siracusa, G.; Sorbi, S.; Amato, M.P. Coping strategies, psychological variables and their relationship with quality of life in multiple sclerosis. *Neurol. Sci.* **2009**, *30*, 15–20. [CrossRef]
43. McCabe, M.P.; McKern, S.; McDonald, E. Coping and psychological adjustment among people with multiple sclerosis. *J. Psychosom. Res.* **2004**, *56*, 355–361. [CrossRef]
44. FOPH. Förderprogramm Interprofessionalität im Gesundheitswesen 2017–2020. 2018. Available online: https://www.bag.admin.ch/bag/de/home/strategie-und-politik/nationale-gesundheitspolitik/foerderprogramme-der-fachkraefteinitiative-plus/foerderprogramme-interprofessionalitaet.html (accessed on 24 May 2021).
45. FOPH. Policy Briefs—Findings and Recommendations for Target Group-Specific Implementation. 2021. Available online: https://www.bag.admin.ch/bag/de/home/strategie-und-politik/nationale-gesundheitspolitik/foerderprogramme-der-fachkraefteinitiative-plus/foerderprogramme-interprofessionalitaet/policy-briefs-interprof.html#704340575 (accessed on 24 May 2021).

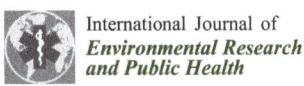

Article

Preventive Counseling in Routine Prenatal Care—A Qualitative Study of Pregnant Women's Perspectives on a Lifestyle Intervention, Contrasted with the Experiences of Healthcare Providers

Laura Lorenz *, Franziska Krebs, Farah Nawabi, Adrienne Alayli and Stephanie Stock

Institute of Health Economics and Clinical Epidemiology (IGKE), Faculty of Medicine and University Hospital Cologne, University of Cologne, 50935 Cologne, Germany; franziska.krebs@uk-koeln.de (F.K.); farah.nawabi@uk-koeln.de (F.N.); adrienne.alayli@uk-koeln.de (A.A.); stephanie.stock@uk-koeln.de (S.S.)
* Correspondence: laura.lorenz@uk-koeln.de

Abstract: Maternal lifestyle during pregnancy and excessive gestational weight gain can influence maternal and infant short and long-term health. As part of the GeMuKi intervention, gynecologists and midwives provide lifestyle counseling to pregnant women during routine check-up visits. This study aims to understand the needs and experiences of participating pregnant women and to what extent their perspectives correspond to the experiences of healthcare providers. Semi-structured interviews were conducted with 12 pregnant women and 13 multi-professional healthcare providers, and were analyzed using qualitative content analysis. All interviewees rated routine check-up visits as a good setting in which to focus on lifestyle topics. Women in their first pregnancies had a great need to talk about lifestyle topics. None of the participants were aware of the link between gestational weight gain and maternal and infant health. The healthcare providers interviewed attributed varying relevance regarding the issue of weight gain and, accordingly, provided inconsistent counseling. The pregnant women expressed dissatisfaction regarding the multi-professional collaboration. The results demonstrate a need for strategies to improve multi-professional collaboration. In addition, health care providers should be trained to use sensitive techniques to inform pregnant women about the link between gestational weight gain and maternal and infant health.

Keywords: patient experience; prevention; qualitative research; pregnancy; gestational weight gain; maternal health; lifestyle intervention

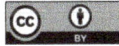

1. Introduction

Overweight and obesity are major public health challenges and risk factors for subsequent diseases in both children and adults [1,2]. The foundations for overweight and obesity are established early in life. There is growing evidence that excessive gestational weight gain and the maternal lifestyle during pregnancy can influence the child's risk of obesity and chronic disease in the long term [3–5]. Furthermore, excessive gestational weight gain is a risk factor for pregnancy and birth complications, such as preeclampsia, macrosomia, cesarean section, gestational diabetes mellitus (GDM), and Large for Gestational Age (LGA) [3,4,6–12].

Due to this, pregnancy is described as a unique "window of opportunity" for preventive interventions aimed at improving maternal and child health [13]. Modifiable behavioral risk factors for adverse pregnancy outcomes and lifelong non-communicable diseases include a lack of physical activity, unhealthy diet, alcohol consumption, and smoking during pregnancy [14]. Even though adopting a healthy lifestyle before pregnancy is beneficial for the health of the mother and child [15,16], the period of pregnancy is discussed as a "teachable moment" and may, therefore, be a favorable time for interventions. This is because pregnant women may be particularly motivated toward ensuring that they are in good health, and the importance of risk factor modification and healthy lifestyles can be reinforced effectively [17,18]. There is evidence that lifestyle interventions can be effective in improving maternal lifestyle and limiting excessive gestational weight gain [14,19–23].

The percentage of women experiencing excessive weight gain during pregnancy based on National Academy of Medicine (NAM; formerly known as the Institute of Medicine, IOM) guidelines [24] ranges from 47 to 68.5% across various studies and countries [3,7,10,25–28]. These figures highlight the urgent need for preventive intervention. The International Weight Management in Pregnancy (i–WIP) Collaborative Network published a "statement on tackling obesity in pregnancy", in which it called for the incorporation of lifestyle counseling into routine prenatal care [29].

In Germany, lifestyle topics are not discussed consistently in the context of prenatal care [30,31]. Prenatal care in Germany is provided by office-based gynecologists and midwives, and focuses mainly on the early identification of diseases and developmental problems in the fetus [30,31]. While prenatal care can, in principle, be provided by midwives and gynecologists individually, it should preferably be administered in a complementary manner [31]. Almost all pregnant women in Germany utilize prenatal screening appointments, which are paid for by the Statutory Health Insurance. As a result, they are monitored closely throughout the entire course of their pregnancies [31]. In addition to this, gynecologists are often the main healthcare providers (HCPs) for women of childbearing age and accompany these women for many years during regular preventive check-ups [32]. As such, routine prenatal care provides an ideal setting for lifestyle intervention. The GeMuKi intervention (acronym for "Gemeinsam gesund: Vorsorge plus für Mutter und Kind"—Strengthening health promotion: enhanced check-up visits for mother and child), carried out in Germany, uses this setting to address lifestyle topics and to involve multiple HCPs who consistently complement each other [33,34].

In order for lifestyle interventions to be effective and sustainable, they must be adapted to the needs of pregnant women. At the same time, HCPs who implement these in routine care need to find the interventions acceptable and feasible [35]. A qualitative study conducted in the U.S. showed that most women had a positive attitude toward counseling during pregnancy, while HCPs discussed barriers to counseling, including, among others, a lack of time, lack of patient interest, or inadequate training [36]. A German study revealed information gaps among pregnant women in the fields of healthy eating and weight gain, as well as the need for information and motivation regarding suitable forms of exercise during pregnancy [37]. As demonstrated by an integrative review, evidence regarding women's overall experience with regard to prenatal care is currently limited and further research is needed to enable HCPs to modify their care to more adequately fit women's needs [38].

In light of this, this study aims to answer the following research questions: What needs, demands, and experiences do women have with regard to the preventive lifestyle counseling provided in the GeMuKi intervention? How do their perspectives correspond to the experiences of HCPs? The results can be used to develop strategies for adapting and improving prenatal care service structures.

2. Materials and Methods

2.1. Backrgound of This Study: The GeMuKi Intervention

This qualitative study was conducted as part of the process evaluation of the GeMuKi trial. The GeMuKi trial implemented a computer-assisted multi-professional intervention in order to address the lifestyle-related risk factors for overweight and obesity in expecting mothers and their infants. The intervention was carried out in five intervention regions of the southern German state of Baden-Wuerttemberg between January 2019 and January 2022 [33,34].

Embedded into regular check-up visits during pregnancy, six additional preventive counseling sessions were provided: four by trained gynecologists and two by trained midwives. All HCPs who delivered the intervention received eight hours of training in advance on lifestyle topics and on motivational interviewing (MI) techniques. MI is a client-centered approach designed to evoke intrinsic motivation for behavioral change [39,40]. The counseling topics were based on the national recommendations for a healthy lifestyle during pregnancy issued by the 'Healthy Start—Young Family Network' ("Netzwerk Gesund ins Leben") [41]. During each counseling session, the women were asked to choose from the following topics: nutrition, water intake, physical activity, breastfeeding, alcohol, nicotine, and drug use. At the end of each session, the women and HCPs agreed on jointly set SMART (Specific, Measurable, Achievable, Reasonable, Time-Bound) goals for lifestyle changes. The achievement of these goals was then discussed in the next counseling session. The GeMuKi intervention included a novel shared telehealth platform that aids multi-professional HCPs during the counseling process (the GeMuKi-Assist counseling tool) and a corresponding app (the GeMuKi-Assist app) for the women participating in the intervention. One of the features used allowed HCPs to enter each women's jointly agreed SMART goals into the GeMuKi-Assist counseling tool. After each counseling session, the participants received a reminder (push notification) of their lifestyle goals in their GeMuKi-Assist app. Further details on the GeMuKi trial and the GeMuKi intervention can be found elsewhere [33,34,42]. The GeMuKi trial was designed as a hybrid effectiveness–implementation trial, meaning that data on effectiveness and implementation were collected simultaneously [43]. The results on the effectiveness of the intervention, which was evaluated using a cluster randomized controlled design, are yet to be published.

2.2. Study Design

The report and conduct of this study are based on the 'COnsolidated criteria for REporting Qualitative research' (COREQ) (Figure S1) [44].

Qualitative interviews were conducted alongside the GeMuKi trial as part of the process evaluation during the first year of implementation. In order to answer the research question, an in-depth perspective from both the participating pregnant women and the HCPs was required. The use of qualitative methods appeared to be most appropriate, since this allowed an intensive description of the needs and perceptions of the interviewees.

Ethical approval was obtained from the University Hospital of Cologne Research Ethics committee on 22 June 2018 (ID: 18-163) and from the State Chamber of Physicians in Baden-Wuerttemberg on 28 November 2018 (ID: B-F-2018-100).

The interviews were conducted using semi-structured interview guides, which can be found in the Supplementary Materials (Table S1). To systematize the research interest, the development of the interview guides was informed by theoretical frameworks for the factors that influence implementation. The frameworks included were the 'Implementation outcomes' developed by Proctor et al. 2011 [45] and the 'Tailored Implementation for Chronic Diseases (TICD) checklist' [46], which is based on a synthesis of frameworks and taxonomies for determinants of professional practice. The interview guides contain open-ended questions regarding the procedure and the topics of the counseling sessions, as well as the participants' satisfaction with the intervention and the needs of the pregnant women and HCPs. Depending on the flow of the conversation, the open-ended questions allowed individuals to bring up topics not covered by the interview guides.

At the end of the interviews, once the closing question had been answered, the pregnant women were asked to answer some questions related to sociodemographic factors and their pregnancy, while HCPs were asked about their professional experience and working environments. The interview guides were tested and discussed with women of childbearing age, experts from professional associations of gynecologists and midwives, and the project's scientific advisory board.

2.3. Recruitment and Sample

The sample for this study was drawn from women and HCPs who were enrolled in the GeMuKi-trial. HCPs and pregnant women were invited to participate if they had undergone at least two counseling sessions. This applied to 23 gynecologists and their medical assistants from 17 gynecologic practices, 7 midwives, and 59 pregnant women. Pregnant women, gynecologists, and medical assistants were invited by postal mail to participate in the interviews. Letters of invitation were sent out to the women in June 2019, while invitations to the gynecological practices were sent out in October 2019 (in one of the five regions, the recruitment of interviewees was carried out one year later, as the implementation of the intervention in this region started one year later. This involved only one pregnant woman and two medical assistants). Midwives were recruited exclusively via telephone calls in October 2019 due to their limited postal accessibility.

Only two pregnant women and one medical assistant accepted the invitation, while two gynecologists and one medical assistant declined. No response was received from the remaining invitees. Because of this, all of the remaining participants already invited were contacted successively again by phone to ask if they were interested in an interview. While all contacted pregnant women were willing to be interviewed, 18 of the eligible gynecologists and 4 of the eligible midwives either rejected participation due to a lack of time or could not been reached. An appointment was scheduled with all of those who were interested. Once the interview was over, all of the interviewees received a gift (voucher) worth 15–20 euros as a thank you for their participation. After 12 interviews had been conducted with pregnant women, data saturation was discussed by the research team as no new themes emerged in the interviews. This was not possible in the same way for the HCP interviews, as no more HCPs could be recruited for an interview. The final sample consisted of 25 interviewees, of whom 12 were pregnant women and 13 were multi-professional HCPs (five gynecologists, five medical assistants, and three midwives). The sample characteristics are displayed in Tables 1 and 2. The participating women were about 33 years old on average, had an average body mass index (BMI) of 25.6, and half of them were first-time mothers. All of the interviews were conducted in the last trimester of pregnancy. The interviewed HCPs were mostly female, and their level of professional experience varied greatly between 4 and 42 years. They all had between 8 and 12 months of experience in implementing the GeMuKi intervention.

Table 1. Sample description of pregnant women; mean values (minimum; maximum).

	Participants ($n = 12$)
Interview duration (minutes)	21:16 (15:00; 26:44)
Age (years)	32.5 (30; 37)
Week of pregnancy	32 (28; 36)
BMI before pregnancy	25.64 (21.64; 33.06)
Parity	No children: 50.0% ($n = 6$) One child: 33.3% ($n = 4$) Two or more children: 16.7% ($n = 2$)

Table 2. Sample description of HCPs; mean values (minimum; maximum).

	Gynecologists (n = 5)	Assistants (n = 5)	Midwives (n = 3)
Interview duration (minutes)	40:00 (25:00; 60:00)	17:12 (7:00; 25:00)	28:20 (25:00; 30:00)
Gender	Male: 1/5 Female: 4/5	Male: 0/5 Female: 5/5	Male: 0/3 Female: 3/3
Professional experience (years)	8 (4; 16)	20,67 (5; 32)	22,67 (9; 42)
Office size	9 (3; 16)	9,8 (5; 20)	-
Employment relationship	-	-	Employed: 0/3 Self-employed: 3/3

2.4. Data Collection

The data collection for this study took place between July 2019 and March 2020 (in one of the five regions, the interviews were carried out in October and November 2020, as the implementation of the intervention in this region started one year later. This involved only the interviews with one pregnant woman and two medical assistants. These interviews were conducted during the COVID-19 pandemic. As the GeMuKi-intervention and the interviews for this study could be carried out in the same way as before the pandemic, there were no substantial differences). The first author (L.L.; female), who is a sociologist by training and an experienced qualitative researcher conducted 25 qualitative interviews. The interviewer was part of the evaluation team and had not met the interviewees before. The interviewees were informed in advance that the interviews would discuss their personal perspectives on and experiences of prevention and lifestyle counseling in prenatal care. They knew that their insights were needed to understand if the intervention fit their expectations and to improve the implementation process of the intervention in case of a national rollout. The interviews with the gynecologists were conducted in person in their offices. The interviews with the pregnant women, midwives, and medical assistants were conducted via telephone. All of the interviews were recorded digitally, anonymized, and transcribed verbatim according to the rules published by Dresing/Pehl (2011) [47]. The interviews with the pregnant women took an average of 21 min. The interviews with the medical assistants lasted a similar amount of time (17 min), whereas the interviews with the midwives and gynecologists took longer (Tables 1 and 2). A second researcher (F.K. or F.N.) was present during the interview and documented the atmosphere and specifics during the interview in a postscript. They also made sure that all of the aspects of the interview guide were covered.

2.5. Data Analysis

The transcribed interviews were analyzed by two researchers using 'thematic qualitative text analysis' as described by Kuckartz (2014), a particular form of qualitative content analysis [48,49]. An inductive–deductive category-based approach was used [48]. L.L. developed the category system. Initially, only deductive categories derived from the interview guides were applied. In an iterative process, two researchers coded the data and derived inductive categories from the text material. In a final pass, two researchers coded the interviews independently using the elaborate category system. Conflicts in coding were discussed among L.L., F.N., and F.K. until a consensualized version for all analyses was completed. All of the coding and analyzing processes were carried out with the aid of the MAXQDA 18 software (VERBI Software, Berlin, Germany) [50]. The interviews were conducted and analyzed in German. In order to make the results available to an international audience, two researchers translated the quotes independently into English. The names of the interviewees were pseudonymized. The thematic qualitative text analysis focused on categories relevant to the research questions, which could be grouped into five main themes (see Figure 1).

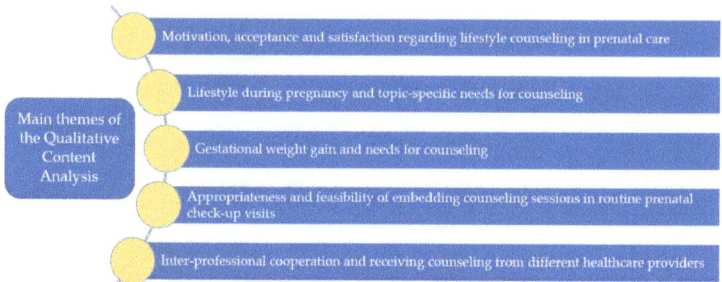

Figure 1. Main themes of the Qualitative Content Analysis.

3. Results

The results from the interviews are presented here for the five main themes (see Figure 1), each of which is discussed below from the perspectives of both the pregnant women and the HCPs. After both perspectives are presented in detail, they are each contrasted in a summary figure at the end of every section (see Figures 2–6).

3.1. Perspectives on Motivation, Acceptance, and Satisfaction Regarding Lifestyle Counseling in Prenatal Care

3.1.1. Pregnant Women's Perspective

The women were interested in the intervention, mainly because they expected to receive more extensive counseling for themselves and their babies. Several of the women stated that they believed obesity to be a socially important issue, and that they would like to help to improve care for pregnant women and infants. The first-time mothers were especially interested in receiving more detailed counseling sessions. They often felt uncertain about various issues and were pleased to be given the opportunity to receive extended counseling sessions with HCPs. Some of the women who had already given birth also reported that they were often overstrained, especially during the first pregnancy.

> "because when you don't have a clue at all and you're at the beginning and..: Hm, yes, what am I allowed to do now, what should I do, what can I NOT do, what would be better for me? At the beginning, you are a bit overwhelmed when you get your first [baby]" (Christine, paragraph 67)

The women who had already had children felt that their first pregnancies had already provided them with all of the information they needed. They stated several times that they felt less need to talk. In addition to this, due to their already busy childcare schedules, they had less time to implement the recommendations on lifestyle changes.

The pregnant women were of the opinion that the opportunity for lifestyle counseling should be available as part of routine care, but women should be able to decide for themselves whether and with whom they would like to address the topics, depending on their needs.

Pregnancy is rated as a good time for lifestyle counseling because it is a time when women report taking greater care of themselves. During check-up visits, almost all of the women wanted to discuss what they were allowed to do and what they should avoid. For example, they expected instructions on what foods or sports they should avoid during pregnancy.

The women were mainly satisfied with their participation in the intervention, as it gave them more time to spend with HCPs.

> "I am very pleased. In particular, the additional counseling from the gynecologist was of the main reasons why I participated in this intervention" (Kerstin, paragraph 86)

Nevertheless, some of the women reported that they already knew everything the HCPs had told them during their counseling sessions. Some of the interviewees pointed out that the counseling should always be adapted to each woman's individual needs, and that maintaining a healthy lifestyle was already important to them before they became pregnant.

Some of the participants found it difficult to assess whether they had changed any aspects of their lifestyle as a result of the counseling sessions. Nevertheless, they noted that a recommendation from a physician had more impact than when an attempted change was driven by self-commitment alone. For example, one participant identified her unhealthy lifestyle patterns, and now wants to pay more attention to them. She felt that a face-to-face conversation strengthened her focus more than simply reading up on recommendations would. Several of the women reported that jointly agreed goals helped them and provided motivation. They also considered it beneficial to discuss the progress of reaching their goals with their gynecologists.

"I have to say I really like that because that gives you a little bit of an extra motivation, because every time when checking the app after visiting the doctor, there is a summary of what we talked about and what we agreed upon. That is an additional reminder and then you simply want to accomplish that [goal]." (Kerstin, paragraph 26)

The pregnant women wanted their counseling goals to realistically fit their daily lives and be easy to implement. Only one of the participants reported that the sessions failed to motivate her at all, and that she already knew everything she was told prior to participating in the intervention.

In summary, minor changes, such as participants eating more fruit or getting up to exercise more, were attributed to counseling. Additionally, some of the women were repeatedly encouraged to exercise by their HCP, even though they had concerns at first.

3.1.2. Healthcare Providers' Perspective

All of the HCPs interviewed said that their patients generally responded positively to the offer of the intervention. In particular, they reported that the women who were going through their first pregnancies tended to be anxious, and were, therefore, grateful for receiving additional support. Furthermore, some of the women had weight problems during previous pregnancies, and therefore appreciated the counseling sessions.

The HCPs came away with the impression that most of the women were already very well informed prior to the intervention. They often needed reassurance that they were doing things right. When asked, some of the women would also always say that they were doing just fine and did not need the lifestyle advice.

All of the HCPs who were interviewed considered taking the time to provide additional counseling on lifestyle issues to be very worthwhile. They emphasized their intrinsic interest in participating, and noted that they had already dealt with the topics before. Some of the medical assistants stated that they had realized that additional counseling would be beneficial as a result of their own pregnancies. In addition to this, all of the HCPs agreed that there was a need for intervention with regard to overweightness and obesity issues.

Some of the HCPs felt that the counseling had helped the participants. In some cases, awareness was raised regarding the need for change. Sometimes, the help was nothing more than small tips for everyday routines that the patients had not come up with on their own. The HCPs also reported that the joint goal-setting process motivated their patients to give things a try. Some of the HCPs came away with the impression that the women preferred to have their hands held and be given a guideline.

According to one gynecologist, pregnant women are confronted by so many major changes in their life circumstances during pregnancy that they are not able to fundamentally change their diet and exercise if they have not already been eating/exercising adequately. Likewise, this gynecologist believed that women who were already overweight would fail to change their dietary habits, and said that the counseling intervention would thus be unable to help them.

"I think that during pregnancy, women are confronted with so many things, so many changes in life, that it is DIFFICULT for them to put everything into action, to have adequate physical activity, a healthy diet, when they didn't even manage to do that before. And that's what I've said right from the start: Those who do that ANYWAY, do not need the program, whereas those who weren't doing it before pregnancy, definitely won't manage it during pregnancy" (gynecologist 5, paragraph 66)

In addition to this, some of the HCPs believed that there were always some women who thought that they already knew everything. This particularly applied to women in their second or third pregnancy. Likewise, there were certain women who were described as resistant to counseling and who did not value additional counseling. Some of the HCPs noted that these were often overweight women who were unwilling to talk about their lifestyle.

One gynecologist had the impression that the counseling was particularly well received by women who were well-educated and physically active, and thus did not really need it. In contrast, another gynecologist explained that he sometimes had to phrase the information somewhat differently depending on the patient's socioeconomic status, though he would not necessarily say that the better-off knew a lot more. In his opinion, the counseling sessions always needed to be tailored to the patients' needs and background. In spite of this, some of the HCPs observed an information leak for women with little formal education.

There was consensus that an established relationship of trust between the woman and the HCP, e.g., due to treatment and consultation during previous pregnancies, improved the readiness of the women to accept the counseling.

3.1.3. Summary and Comparison of Perspectives

A summary of the findings and comparison of the perspectives on the motivation, acceptance and satisfaction regarding the lifestyle counselling in prenatal care is given in Figure 2.

Motivation, acceptance and satisfaction regarding lifestyle counseling in prenatal care	
Similar Perspectives	**Differing Perspectives & Further Impressions**
➢ first-time mothers were especially interested in receiving more detailed counseling sessions as they often felt uncertain; or anxious as HCPs described it ➢ women who had weight problems during previous pregnancies appreciated the counseling sessions ➢ jointly agreed goals (which realistically fit women's daily lives) had helped and provided motivation ➢ HCPs felt that counseling had helped women, i.e. by raising awareness regarding the need for change while women felt a face-to-face conversation strengthens their focus to identify unhealthy lifestyle patterns ➢ HCP and women stated that counseling sessions need to be tailored to the patients' needs and backgrounds ➢ pregnancy is rated as a good time for lifestyle counseling and it should be available as part of routine care	➢ minor changes, such as participants eating more fruit or getting up to exercise more, were attributed to the counseling by women ➢ women who had already had children felt less need to talk and had less time to implement recommendations on lifestyle changes ➢ HCPs stated that some women in their 2nd/3rd pregnancy think they already know everything and some are resistant to counseling ➢ some HCPs state that women who were already overweight fail to change their habits and that the intervention would thus be unable to help them. ➢ HCPs agreed on the need for intervention with regard to obesity issues and emphasized their intrinsic interest

Figure 2. Summary of the results in Section 3.1.

3.2. Perspectives on Lifestyle during Pregnancy and Topic-Specific Needs for Counseling

3.2.1. Pregnant Women's Perspective

All of the women reported that they took more care of themselves during pregnancy. Nearly all of the participants used various pregnancy apps, online searches, and books to obtain information on lifestyle topics. The unborn child motivated them to adopt a healthy lifestyle.

"[. . .]and I think, for the good of the child, I think every mom would like to contribute something[. . .]" (Elli, paragraph 97)

"Hm, how can I put it best? It's about doing my bit to ensure the development of our children" (Frida, paragraph 63)

Nutrition during pregnancy was considered a very important topic, and advice on it was desired by almost all of the participants. Some of the women expected to be educated on foods that were "forbidden" foods during pregnancy, and to receive a list of rules from HCPs.

> "Yes, so that she [the gynecologist] simply explains, what I can eat, and what's good for me and what's not." (Christine, paragraph 87)

Some of the participants exercised regularly, but their fitness declined during the course of their pregnancy. The participants were unsure of what activities they were still allowed to do.

During the counseling sessions, nutrition was the most frequently chosen discussion topic. One participant reported that she had more in-depth counseling sessions on nutrition due to her gestational diabetes. Another participant needed specific advice because she wanted to maintain her vegetarian diet. In addition to nutrition, the integration of physical activity into the women's day-to-day routines was also discussed, as well as sufficient water intake. Smoking and alcohol were not discussed in depth because they were of no concern to any of the women who were interviewed.

One interviewee stated that she knew enough about the topics herself and therefore did not want to waste time receiving counseling on lifestyle issues. She believed that people thought enough about healthy lifestyle choices without the need for further advice. She had gained more weight than she wanted, and considered this to be due to a lack of physical activity.

The women reported that they would also like something to take home after the counseling session, such as an information brochure on the lifestyle topics they had discussed. The participants reported that their minds were often very busy during the counseling sessions, and that it would be great to be able to remind themselves of the conversation using written information the next day.

The predefined topics corresponded to the participants' expectations. Most of the women felt that, in addition to these topics, they could also address any other issue as necessary. One participant said she would also be open to home visits for counseling sessions on breastfeeding.

3.2.2. Healthcare Providers' Perspective

The HCPs believed there was a tremendous need for lifestyle counseling, since they provide care to many overweight women. One gynecologist said that the needs of pregnant women varied greatly depending on their initial weight and level of education. One gynecologist said that many women had no idea what healthy food was, and that they stopped exercising the moment they discovered they were pregnant.

> "because they simply have no idea at all what is healthy food and what is not. They put themselves to bed: I'm not moving (laughs slightly), that could harm the child (laughs slightly). That's really blatant" (Gynecologist 3, paragraph 8)

One medical assistant came away with the impression that the women were mostly asking for confirmation on whether they were eating enough and whether their diets were healthy enough.

> "I would say that nutrition [is the most important topic for women]. Many are uncertain about this. Am I now eating sufficiently, am I now eating HEALTHY enough? So I always have this feeling, yes." (Medical Assistant 3, paragraph 44)

The HCPs confirmed that nutrition was the most popular counseling topic, followed by physical activity. They also stated that nutrition was usually particularly important to women during their first pregnancy. One gynecologist said that the participants often had problems with gaining weight or drinking water. Some physicians stated that alcohol and nicotine-related issues were a problem. Smokers often do not manage to quit completely, while alcohol consumption is very taboo and often kept secret. The gynecologists stated that many problems, such as substance abuse disorders, cannot be addressed in regular preventive care, and said that some women also needed psychological support.

One gynecologist reported that it was difficult for the participants to decide which lifestyle topic they wanted to discuss while still in the early phase of pregnancy. During this phase, worries and fears regarding the progress of the pregnancy are still highly prominent. In addition to this, the early stages of pregnancy involve a large number of medical tests and require the women in question to handle a multitude of information.

> "the pregnant woman COMES to the determination of the pregnancy, then one determines the pregnancy and then she is OVERCOME first with completely many information. Right? And there are really MANY, MANY, MANY things, so she must first come to terms with the fact that she is pregnant at all, is happy or not happy, is afraid whether the pregnancy will go well or not—you don't know at the beginning of the pregnancy. Then (clears throat) is the explanation, okay, now maternity care starts. What does prenatal care mean, what do all the examinations that are done in prenatal care mean?" (Gynecologist 4, paragraph 12)

As a result, they cannot remember everything. Due to this, some of their patients expressed disappointment that they did not receive any written information after the counseling sessions. They also noted that pregnant women needed to adjust to their new life circumstances, and did not consider lifestyle issues a priority for this reason.

3.2.3. Summary and Comparison of Perspectives

In Figure 3, the results on lifestyle during pregnancy and topic-specific needs for counselling are summarized and the perspectives on this main theme are compared.

Lifestyle during pregnancy and topic-specific needs for counseling	
Similar Perspectives	**Differing Perspectives & Further Impressions**
➢ predefined topics corresponded to the participants' expectations ➢ nutrition was the most popular counseling topic (some women had special needs, i.e. gestational diabetes, vegetarian diet), followed by physical activity ➢ some exercised regularly, but as their fitness declined, they were unsure what activities they were allowed to do ➢ women expressed the need for written information on the lifestyle topics they had discussed to remind themselves the next day; HCPs also considered this to be useful ➢ expected instructions on what foods or sports they should avoid during pregnancy; HCPs confirmed that women were mostly asking for confirmation	➢ HCPs stated that women's needs varied greatly depending on their initial weight and level of education ➢ HCPs reported that it was difficult for the participants to decide which lifestyle topic to choose, due to fears or the multitude of information in the early phase of pregnancy ➢ women stated that the unborn child motivated women to adopt a healthy lifestyle and all used pregnancy apps, books etc. to get information on lifestyle topics ➢ HCPs expressed the impression that some women have no idea what healthy food is and stop exercising when they discover they are pregnant ➢ smoking and alcohol were of no concern to any of the women ➢ HCPs explained that substance abuse disorders cannot be addressed in regular preventive care

Figure 3. Summary of the results in Section 3.2.

3.3. Perspectives on Gestational Weight Gain and Needs for Counseling

3.3.1. Pregnant Women's Perspective

For the women who participated in the study, weight gain was seen as a normal part of being pregnant. The participants gave the impression that they were not particularly concerned about weight gain, and did not think they could do anything about it anyway. None of the participants associated weight gain with consequences for their own health or that of their child.

> "I make sure that it's not so MUCH [weight], but I/Now if it's 15, 20 kilos, then that's just how it is [...] So it's just pregnancy (laughs lightly), so then you gain weight, right?" (Christine, paragraph 54)

> "Actually, it [weight gain] does not matter so much now. What is certain is that you gain weight. I am not exactly the skinniest of the participants. But I'm not worrying about it right now." (Elli, paragraph 26)

"Well, I mean, you can't really influence it [weight gain] much, or you shouldn't really influence it much, by saying: Oh dear, I'm putting on far too much weight, I want to cut back. So I wouldn't do that, also with regard to the health of the child, that the child would then, I don't know, suffer any disadvantages in its development." (Frida, paragraph 28)

Some of the interviewees seemed to be of the impression that they did not need to be counseled regarding weight gain, even if they had already gained a lot of weight or started their pregnancy at a high initial weight. One of the participants explicitly stated that she had gained very little weight, and, therefore, did not need to talk about weight. Some of the women reported that their weight was not discussed with a gynecologist or midwife at all. Others reported that sometimes, after weighing, they had been told that their weight gain was within limits, but that there was no further conversation on the topic afterwards.

Only one of the interviewees reported that her gynecologist had discussed and analyzed her weight gain with her. At the beginning of the pregnancy, she was afraid of gaining the same amount of weight as she had during her previous pregnancy. As a result, she was appreciative of the helpful advice on nutrition during the consultation.

One participant explained that she had gained a lot of weight, but said that she did not need to talk about it because she knew herself what had caused the gain. Her gynecologist advised her to write down her daily meals in spite of this, and she now reports that she is in better control of her weight.

In summary, it seems that none of the women were aware of weight gain recommendations or the risks associated with excessive weight gain.

3.3.2. Healthcare Providers' Perspective

The HCPs possessed differing views on the relevance of gestational weight gain. There were both midwives and gynecologists in the study who believed that it was not their job to talk about weight, and stated that they had many other important priorities.

"So I think as long as she feels good and does not have any side effects, so if blood pressure is okay, it's not important for me whether she gains 16 or 18 or 20 kg." (Gynecologist 1, paragraph 56)

Some midwives even said that they did not want to address weight gain because it felt uncomfortable.

"You just have to be a little bit careful, and when I don't see the women during the course of the pregnancy, and only at these counseling sessions, I'm just a little bit more cautious about bringing up the subject of weight if it would be extreme in any way." (Midwife 3, paragraph 24)

Moreover, some of the HCPs reported that they had had difficulty communicating recommendations regarding gestational weight gain to overweight women. One gynecologist believed that to do so would be in conflict with the MI technique, as consultants should not give instructions when using MI. In contrast, one medical assistant said that MI techniques were helpful because they provided a means of approaching the topic of weight gently and sensitively.

On the other hand, there were also gynecologists who said that they always addressed weight, and see regular weighing during check-ups in particular as an opportunity to repeatedly raise awareness. Their impression was that women were more sensitized to the issue of their weight when it was discussed frequently. In their opinion, a combination of regular weighing and information dissemination had the potential to change lifestyles. They, therefore, believed that pregnancy and the close accompanying monitoring can be particularly beneficial in this regard.

"So, of course, all you need is information, and also of course this/We weigh them every four weeks. They'll never have that again in their lives, right? So then they're like: (changes voice pitch) Oh, my God, I don't want to be asked about it again at the gynecologist." (Gynecologist 3, paragraph 56)

Another gynecologist said that his patients know how strict he is with regard to weight gain. Even outside of pregnancy, he discusses options with obese women or refers them to colleagues.

"and then pregnancy starts, and I say "Yes, you know, weight development, how high it SHOULD be" and then you can see how it develops and that's good [. . .] So it seems to help if you keep pointing it out." (Gynecologist 2, paragraph 26)

Another of the gynecologists said that, although she tries to address weight frequently, women have a very different focus and want to know if their child is healthy. Often, her patients are more concerned when they are perceived to not be gaining very much weight.

"The focus is on the child. After that, whether they've gained a lot of weight or not is only a minor concern. That's something that doesn't really interest them deeply. Funnily enough, it's more the NOT gaining weight. The significant weight gain shocks them rather less (laughs)." (Gynecologist 4, paragraph 26)

One of the gynecologists noted that, for obese women, body weight is without a doubt an issue before pregnancy and that it should ideally have been talked about beforehand. In contrast, another of the gynecologists explained that she would only discuss lifestyle issues in the context of prenatal care, because, in such scenarios, they also have a direct impact on the health of the child. Outside of pregnancy, she sees no obligation to address the issue, and considers it the responsibility of a general practitioner.

One of the gynecologists was convinced that pregnant women are concerned about their weight because they are constantly being asked about their appearance. Nevertheless, most of her patients were unaware of the recommendation. Practically all of the HCPs observed that the women were not familiar with the recommendations for adequate weight gain during pregnancy.

3.3.3. Summary and Comparison of Perspectives

Figure 4 summarizes the findings on gestational weight gain and needs for counselling and compares the perspectives of pregnant women and HCPs.

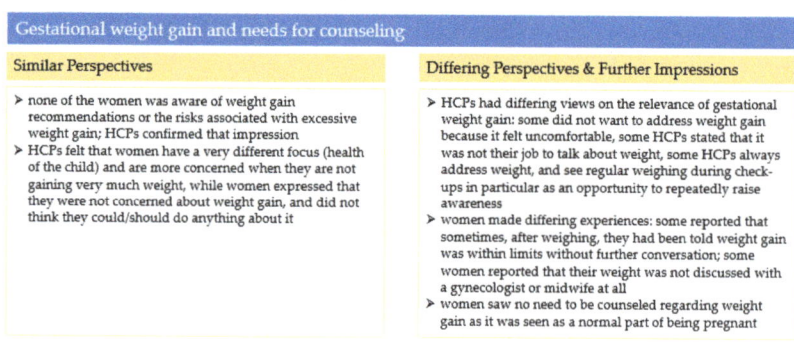

Figure 4. Summary of the results in Section 3.3.

3.4. Perspectives on the Appropriateness and Feasibility of Embedding Counseling Sessions into Routine Prenatal Check-Up Visits

3.4.1. Pregnant Women's Perspective

In all cases, the women appreciated the fact that the counseling sessions were carried out as part of their routine prenatal care.

"Yes, I think so. Because where else can you go/I think it makes sense when you're at the gynecologist's that you also talk about such topics." (Elli, paragraph 58)

The majority of the participants were opposed to additional appointments outside of their regular check-up visits. The pregnant woman also said they would also only consult other healthcare experts outside of their routine prenatal care setting if problems arose. For example, one participant said she could see herself contacting a lactation consultant if her breastfeeding was not going well.

The women provided highly differing descriptions of their counseling sessions. Some women felt that a lot of time was given to them. Others complained that there was little time for a conversation, and that things were rather hectic. One woman said that she stopped asking questions because everyone in the practice was so stressed. Some women reported that, despite being enrolled in the trial, they had not yet received counseling, nor had their lifestyle issues been addressed. However, the women also found it difficult to distinguish their standard care from the intervention.

Most of the interviewed women received lifestyle counseling at their gynecological practices. In half of the sample, there was no involvement at all from medical assistants in the intervention components. In some cases, they assisted with documentation or with preparing topics for the counseling sessions. For example, some medical assistants attempted to identify the topic the patients wanted to discuss. Two women reported that they had received counseling from medical assistants. Only one of the women who were interviewed received counseling from a trained midwife. The other participants reported that they only saw their midwives at a later stage of their pregnancy.

About half of the women who received counseling sessions chose the counseling topic themselves. The topics for the other half of the sample were predetermined by the respective HCP. From the interviews with the women, it appears that the HCPs often asked questions regarding their behaviors, then offered recommendations in response.

> "For example, when it comes to eating behavior, she first asks me what I like to eat or what I eat in general, i.e., whether I eat healthily or not, or when it comes to drinking, what I drink all day, how much I drink and (clears throat) I answer all the questions. Then, if she has any other information that doesn't match my questions, then she informs me about it." (Doris, paragraph 12)

3.4.2. Healthcare Providers' Perspective

All of the HCPs considered prenatal care to be an appropriate setting for preventive counseling. The gynecologists stressed that a gynecological practice is a good setting for preventive counseling because they usually already have a long-standing relationship with their patients and see them regularly. Emphasis was also placed on the fact that prenatal check-up visits at a gynecological practice present a reliable opportunity to speak to women about their health, since all women attend these services. Medical assistants can usually schedule appointments in order to tie the consultations to regular check-up visits.

The gynecologists did not take patient accessibility via midwives as a given, as many women are not in contact with midwives during their pregnancy; in fact, some have no contact with midwives at all. The gynecologists also pointed out that a medical practice provides a safe space where these conversations can take place uninterrupted. The gynecologists usually incorporated their consultations into the regular check-up visits. Some took 5–10 min for the consultation, and others between 15 and 20 min.

On the other hand, all of the gynecologists reported a lack of time due to many other issues relating to regular screening during check-up visits. One gynecologist stressed that gynecologists are mainly responsible for curative matters, and that preventive medicine is not something they generally deal with.

> "Preventive medicine in general just basically isn't something we do, we are basically there for curative issues. But then that's a contradiction in itself, because there is no curative activity for us to carry out in maternity care. So we definitely need to talk about the extent to which such a practice procedure really offers room for it. But, yes, on the other hand, this is again contrary to the relationship work that one does as a caring doctor." (Gynecologist 4, paragraph 64)

One gynecologist explained that she needed to educate the women on numerous topics, and suggested that midwives should be made more aware of prevention topics. However, she also pointed out that midwives all have different levels of training. Despite this, the gynecologists stated that breastfeeding was a topic traditionally discussed in midwifery.

Several of the HCPs did not apply the conversational MI technique, deciding instead to stick to their usual conversational approach. One physician stated that he did not consider the technique applicable at all. One of the gynecologists considered MI inappropriate for topics such as breastfeeding.

All of the midwives stressed that they had always provided lifestyle counseling and saw themselves as suitable counselors, since they also assisted families after the birth. Nutrition and breastfeeding have always been topics on which midwives have provided detailed counseling.

Contrary to the study protocol, all of the midwives reported that they always made additional appointments for lifestyle counseling as part of the intervention, as they did not normally see their patients until shortly before birth. The midwives visited the women in their homes and spent about 20 min on counseling. They felt that going to the woman's home specifically for this purpose gave the consultation special relevance. The midwives also highlighted a number of other advantages to providing counseling in the home environment—there were no interruptions, they were able to take more time for the conversation, and they also gained an insight into the women's lifestyles in their homes. Nevertheless, they noted that the visits were time-consuming and not very profitable. In terms of scheduling, they said that the facts that they do not have practice offices and that it is difficult to coordinate on-site home visits were problematic. One of the midwives said that they would like a predefined guideline on how to incorporate the counseling sessions into her workflow. On the other hand, another of the midwives expressed concern that gynecologists' offices are too overburdened, and said that midwives can be more flexible and provide longer counseling sessions on an individual basis.

One gynecologist pointed out that the quality of counseling varied greatly among all colleagues. In addition, he emphasized that, in the gynecological practice, they can only cover the tip of the iceberg and highlight topics. He refers obese women to nutritional counseling and draws their attention to the services offered by health insurance companies.

Another of the gynecologists expressed concern that dedicated and well-educated women would follow the recommendation to see a nutritionist when they were actually the group that least needed to do so.

> "So I think that it [the gynecological practice] is the right place, because they will definitely be there. [...] So if we now say that they should all go to a nutrition consultation, then I'll tell you: All the working women won't go, they're happy when they've managed to get the appointment here, ok? All those who more or less let everything slide anyway, i.e., the unmotivated ones, they will NOT go either. Then the women you have in the nutritional counseling are the ones who actually don't really need it, because they're already quite good anyway." (Gynecologist 3, paragraph 124)

Some of the HCPs stressed that the program was unable to reach the women who needed to be addressed most urgently. All of the HCPs agreed that there was an urgent need to find a way of conducting good counseling sessions with non-German-speaking women. In addition to this, they said that all of the information materials needed be translated as standard.

Another of the gynecologists reported that most of her patients had a huge need for counseling on childbirth, and many fears and concerns that needed to be discussed. She said that sometimes there was more focus on this than on lifestyle issues. This gynecologist suggested using the counseling time to discuss all of the patient's fears first, otherwise, the women would not be able to concentrate on lifestyle issues.

One of the gynecologists said that she would like to see general changes in the health care system, and that it was not cost-effective for her to conduct in-depth consultations with her patients. She claimed that HCPs needed more time and adequate compensation. Likewise, the midwives said that they would like to be reimbursed for the consultation in a manner similar to a postpartum visit. In addition to this, it was agreed that regular training should be provided. Some of the gynecologists also suggested that medical assistants should be more closely involved in the consultation process. The medical assistants echoed this preference.

> "I have an additional qualification as a nutrition consultant and […] I find it especially interesting in pregnancy and that was my motivation for me. […] I would like to do more personally, but I'm kind of not allowed to. So I think that's a bit of a shame" (Medical Assistant 1, paragraph 54; 92)

3.4.3. Summary and Comparison of Perspectives

A summary of the findings and comparison of the perspectives on the appropriateness and feasibility of embedding counselling sessions in routine prenatal check-up visits is given in Figure 5.

Appropriateness and feasibility of embedding counseling sessions in routine prenatal check-up visits	
Similar Perspectives	**Differing Perspectives & Further Impressions**
➢ women appreciated that the counseling sessions were carried out as part of their routine prenatal care; gynecologist incorporated their consultations into the regular check-up visits ➢ women reported that they only see their midwives at a later stage of their pregnancy and only one interviewed women received counseling sessions from a midwife; midwives confirmed that they had to make additional appointments for lifestyle counseling as they do not see their patients until shortly before the birth ➢ all considered prenatal care to be an appropriate setting for preventive counseling ➢ an established relationship of trust between favored the readiness of the women to accept the counseling ➢ women reported that HCPs often asked questions regarding their behaviors, then offered recommendations in response, which gave the impression that the conversional technique MI was not applied; some HCPs confirmed that they did not apply MI ➢ about half of the women who received counseling sessions chose the counseling topic themselves, while topics for the other half of the sample were predetermined by the respective HCP; interviews with HCPs confirmed this impression	➢ gynecologist rate their practices as the best setting while midwives highlighted the relevance of on-site home visits ➢ HCPs claim that they need more time and adequate compensation ➢ some HCPs stated that quality of counseling varies greatly among all colleagues and regular training should be provided ➢ some HCPs wanted medical assistants to be more closely involved in the consultation process ➢ women state they would only consult other experts outside of routine care if problems arose while one gynecologist refers obese women to nutritional counseling/draws their attention to other offered services ➢ HCPs stated that the program was unable to reach the women who needed to be addressed most urgently ➢ HCPs see an urgent need to find a way of conducting good counseling sessions with non-German-speaking women; information materials need to be translated as standard ➢ women gave highly differing descriptions of their received counseling sessions: a lot time was given to them/little time for conversation/HCPs so stressed that women hesitated to ask questions/some had not yet received counseling on lifestyle topics

Figure 5. Summary of the results in Section 3.4.

3.5. Perspectives on Inter-Professional Cooperation and Receiving Counseling from Different Healthcare Providers

3.5.1. Pregnant Women's Perspective

Several of the women liked the idea of receiving lifestyle counseling from multiple HCPs. They felt that the more often they heard the key messages, the better. In addition to this, they believed that it would be a good idea for all of the professions involved to consult on lifestyle topics, as they hoped that this would give them a more comprehensive picture and the opportunity to explore different perspectives. In contrast, one of the women, who had already given birth to several children, said that she would have liked to choose who her counseling session was with, and did not want to have to discuss the topics with everyone.

> "I am not sure whether I would be annoyed by this, when visiting all three providers, […] I would say (sighs) one time would be enough. So I think it would be good if you could choose, so everyone offers it and you can decide who you trust the most. But hearing it from everyone, I think that is too much." (Helga, paragraph 36)

Some of the women said that they only saw their midwives shortly before/after giving birth, or only for a birth preparation class. As a result, they had no counseling sessions with their midwives. In some cases, the women already knew their midwives from previous pregnancies, and said that there was no need to see them early.

The women described a relationship of trust with their HCP as being particularly crucial for counseling. Which HCPs were trusted varied greatly from one woman to the next. Some participants reported that they already had a relationship of trust that had been established during a previous pregnancy. One of the participants felt that the gynecologist was the best person to provide the counseling, but said that she would still like the midwife to be more involved. One participant specifically said that she would prefer to confer with her gynecologist because, unlike the midwife, the gynecologist was someone who would continue to provide her with medical assistance for many years to come.

Some of the participants experienced a close relationship of trust with their midwives, and said that they would particularly like to receive advice from their midwives on breastfeeding. One participant said she would like to discuss all of the topics with her midwife, because she sees the midwife both during and after birth. Another of the women also placed considerable trust in her midwife, as she felt it was safe to assume that the midwife would have a particular interest in ensuring that the birth was free of complications. One of the participants reported that her midwife was available to her at all times and always responded promptly. In contrast, she hardly felt comfortable asking any questions at all at her gynecological practice.

The pregnant women expressed uncertainty regarding the relationship between gynecologists and midwives. Some of the women explicitly requested that the HCPs not contradict each other in counseling. The women were under the impression that midwives and gynecologists do not exchange information with one another and do not have access to the same data. In addition to this, the women assumed that HCPs do not maintain any contact with each other. Some of the participants were highly dissatisfied with the lack of collaboration, saying that there seemed to be a lack of mutual acceptance and respect.

The participants felt torn between their gynecologists their and midwives. They felt that some gynecologists seemed to believe that a midwife was not needed, while the midwife had offered to take over the preventive care.

"My midwife offered to do the usual prenatal care, just like the doctor would do it. That would be my choice, whether seeing the doctor or seeing her. They are both from this village, and she made the remark that my gynecologist is not convinced about letting the midwife do that and said I don't need a midwife anyway, and that's why I am thinking there is no cooperation between them." (Frida, paragraph 46)

"Yes, I would say it [cooperation] is quite bad. I have a midwife who I am visiting for every second prenatal care appointment, because I want to give birth in a birthing center. And it seems like my gynecologist does not accept that. Every time I visit her she keeps saying to me that I should make the next appointment for in about two weeks, and I am not familiar with the legal situation of what is my right, and every time I see my midwife she keeps saying that my gynecologist did too much, and she wasn't allowed to do that, because it was agreed that my midwife would do that. That is a difficult situation for me." (Brigitte, paragraph 49–50)

In addition to this, the midwives and the gynecologists offered differing advice on a number of topics. One participant reported a discrepancy between the information she had received from her gynecologist and that from her midwife. For example, the midwife might have recommended something, then the gynecologist would state that the proposed action would not be of any help, and, as a result, the participant would not know what to do. At the same time, some of the women described midwives as peculiar, and said that they were thus hesitant to follow their advice. In this context, the women described their physicians as the authority.

"Midwives are usually kind of a bit, let's call it 'special.' Every one of them has her direction where she's heading and she is super convinced of that, but I am not sure if they

are able to judge objectively. Every one of them has her own, let's call it 'style.' So I would maybe rather lean towards the doctors." (Frida, paragraph 56)

One participant said that she was more likely to listen to or act on something a doctor might say than a midwife. The women were not generally referred to other health care experts. Unless there was any particular need, they might not think of visiting other experts. Two of the participants were diagnosed with gestational diabetes, and were, therefore, referred to a diabetologist.

3.5.2. Healthcare Providers' Perspective

All of the HCPs said that there was a need to engage more with their colleagues regarding counseling on lifestyle topics. All of the HCPs also reported that the intervention had not led to any changes with regard to collaboration.

One of the gynecologists has always worked hand-in-hand with midwives in her practice; three midwives rent offices in her practice and the collaboration works very well. The gynecologist carries out the preventive care first, then the women usually go to see the midwife afterwards. The gynecologist in question strongly supports this approach. In her opinion, gynecologists and midwives have different areas of expertise, and, therefore, complement each other well. Nonetheless, she expressed concern that this is not the way things are done in most practices. She believed that legislation has hindered collaboration between midwives and gynecologists, and said that this was bad for all of the parties involved.

"It has also been hindered by the legislation. [. . .] This is not good for the pregnant women, for pregnancy counseling, for the midwife, and not for the doctors either, right? Nobody knows what that was all about. But (...) midwives can do different things to me. And I can do different things to the midwife. And of course I do my regular prenatal care, that's obvious, that's also obligatory, that's how it should be, that's what the women want. But they come HERE because they read on the Internet that I work with midwives, right? And then that's exactly how it is: they have their own consultation hours, and then the patients can just go there additionally." (Gynecologist 3, paragraph 156)

The other participating gynecologists reported that they had no contact with midwives. One gynecologist expressed regret at this, as she believes that messages are received better when they come from different HCPs. She would be open to gynecologists and midwives sharing prenatal care in a better way. For example, gynecologists could focus on more of the technically related matters and midwives could conduct more of the preventive work.

"in this room, the pregnant women are perhaps more receptive [. . .], because they are more focused on getting this information, and if one were to speak the same language and the pregnant women knew, okay, my midwife says this, and my doctor says the same thing, so in that imaginary scenario, okay, it's my job as a doctor to somehow record the technical points and perhaps then consult with the midwife. Maybe I would advise her to pay a little more attention with one patient, or discuss what could be done with another one, but then I would leave the intervention itself to the midwife." (Gynecologist 4, paragraph 72)

The remaining gynecologists expressed little interest in working with midwives. One gynecologist explained this by saying that they did not have time to network. Another of the doctors had had bad experiences in the past, and said that midwives had made questionable recommendations he did not agree with. Nevertheless, he recognized that midwives perform an important job and can offer women a closer level of care than a gynecological practice is often able to. Due to the shortage of midwives, the gynecologist in question said that he already advises all newly pregnant women to seek midwifery care as soon as possible.

One of the gynecologists said that he was not interested in networking and discussion because, firstly, he had no further use for other people's information, and secondly, he did not want to interfere with anyone else.

The medical assistants reported that discussion and collaboration in a large practice is difficult because it is not clear which midwife is in charge of which pregnant woman.

One of the midwives described the nature of the communication between physicians and midwives as old-fashioned: the midwife approaches the physician, but not vice versa.

> "We midwives have been thinking about this for a long time, but it's hard to get the doctors to do it. So we go to them, but they don't come to us (laughs slightly) [. . .]. I think that's just an old-fashioned attitude to collaboration in general, which is certainly almost historically conditioned." (Midwife 2, paragraph 122–124)

One midwife suggested that the lack of discussion was due to tight schedules and the overburdening of both physicians and midwives. In addition to this, competitive thinking could also play a major role. One midwife observed that women were more likely to follow advice from gynecologists than that from midwives.

The midwives in particular indicated that they would like to see an improvement in their collaboration with gynecologists. They all considered joint training to be beneficial, and emphasized the importance of understanding the respective skill sets of each professional group and the way in which each one consults. They saw knowing one another's faces as important in facilitating the exchange of patient information and further referrals. In addition to this, they advocated for a more holistic approach to counseling during pregnancy.

3.5.3. Summary and Comparison of Perspectives

The results and perspectives on inter-professional cooperation and receiving counseling from different healthcare providers are summarized and compared in Figure 6.

Inter-professional cooperation and receiving counseling from different healthcare providers	
Similar Perspectives	**Differing Perspectives & Further Impressions**
➤ women liked the idea of receiving lifestyle counseling from multiple HCPs: the more often they heard the key messages, the better/get a more comprehensive picture ➤ women particularly like to receive advice from their midwives on breastfeeding; HCPs also see midwives as most appropriate counselors for breastfeeding ➤ women requested that HCPs should not contradict each other in counseling; HCPs saw a need to engage more with their colleagues regarding counseling on lifestyle topics and considered joint training to be beneficial ➤ got the impression that midwives and gynecologists do not exchange information and do not have access to the same data; most HCPs reported that they had no contact with other professions and that the intervention had not led to any changes with regard to collaboration	➤ only one gynecologists has always worked with midwives in her practice and highlights different areas of expertise that complement each other well ➤ midwives in particular indicated that they would like to see an improvement in their collaboration with gynecologists; some gynecologist expressed little interest in collaboration ➤ medical assistants reported that collaboration is difficult for a large practice, because it is not clear which midwife in the region is in charge of which pregnant woman ➤ women described a relationship of trust with their HCP as being particularly crucial for the counseling, which HCPs were trusted varied greatly from one woman to the next ➤ some women felt torn between their gynecologists their and midwives or were uncertain regarding their relationship ➤ some women were highly dissatisfied with the lack of collaboration

Figure 6. Summary of the results in Section 3.5.

4. Discussion

The results of this study are valuable for tailoring preventive measures in prenatal care according to the needs and expectations of pregnant women and their HCPs. The findings illustrate the similarities and differences in the expectations and experiences of women and HCPs with regard to the preventive counseling in pregnancy provided in the GeMuKi intervention. This demonstrates the importance of including both patients' and HCPs' perspectives when planning and designing implementation.

The pregnant women expressed a need to talk about lifestyle issues, mainly in terms of nutrition and physical activity. The first-time mothers in particular felt a great need for counseling and welcomed the extra time with HCPs. This was reflected by the HCPs in their daily practice as well. Furthermore, the HCPs pointed out a tremendous need for lifestyle counseling, since they provided care to many overweight women.

All of the pregnant women who participated in the study stated that they wanted to strive for a healthy lifestyle in order to benefit themselves and their child. This behavior was not questioned and could represent a form of social desirability. Atkinson et al. (2016) found that women whose pregnancies were not characterized by a sense of vulnerability or anxiety made lifestyle decisions based upon a "combination of automatic judgements, physical sensations, and perceptions of what is normal or 'good' for pregnancy" [18]. Furthermore, Rockliffe et al. (2021) found that women wanted to adopt to the role of the 'good mother' by making healthy lifestyle changes, but, at the same time, a lack of understanding with regard to health consequences and low risk perception represented barriers to change [51].

The interviews emphasized that perspectives on gestational weight gain varied widely. Pregnant women assumed that they could not influence gestational weight gain and did not link it to the health of the child. Although the HCPs described the women as well informed, the HCPs believed that the women were not aware of recommendations for weight gain during pregnancy. Despite this, HCPs differed in how and whether they addressed weight gain, if they did so at all, and what relevance they attached to it. Moreover, some HCPs reported difficulties in communicating gestational weight gain recommendations to overweight women.

This is in line with findings that stated that pregnant women were not aware of the risks associated with gestational weight gain [37,52,53]. Pregnant women often base their behavior regarding diet and physical activity on their social and community environment and their peers' beliefs [54,55]. While risks, such as smoking during pregnancy, are discussed in these contexts, the risks relating to weight gain are often not known and are not talked about [55]. This further highlights the importance of sharing information on gestational weight gain through HCPs. There is evidence that women who have received information from their gynecologists have a higher level of knowledge with regard to lifestyle-related factors during pregnancy [56]. Liu et al. (2016) showed that weight gain recommendations made by HCPs are an important predictor of actual weight gain [57]. Furthermore, Deputy et al. (2018) found that both inadequate and excessive weight gains were more likely in women who had received no recommendation at all [58]. Research has also indicated that pregnant women assume that weight gain is not a relevant issue if it is never addressed by HCPs [59]. Additionally, findings illustrate a need for accurate advice from HCPs regarding gestational weight gain recommendations [60]. Research is needed on appropriate resources and materials to support HCPs in giving consistent weight gain advice [36].

All of the interviewees agreed that regular check-up visits in prenatal care were a good setting for lifestyle counseling. While the HCPs reported a lack of time due to many other issues related to regular screening, the women appreciated the fact that they did not have to attend additional appointments for lifestyle counseling outside of their normal check-up visits. Embedding additional counseling into routine care was not always feasible for midwives, while it was easy to organize in gynecological practices. While this was not a concern of the interviewed women, some HCPs pointed out that the intervention was unable to reach the women who needed to be addressed most urgently. More research is needed regarding methods to improve outreach to these women and to refer them to experts.

All of the interviewees agreed that joint goal setting and reminders may help pregnant women in making lifestyle changes. Aside from incorporating joint goal setting, the best approach for counseling on lifestyle-related topics remains unclear. The MI technique was not always used and some of the women tended to expect concrete instructions, rather than an open conversation. In contrast, the HCPs stressed that MI techniques had been particularly helpful in enabling them to address difficult and sensitive topics, such as weight. This is in line with other findings, which demonstrated that implementing MI techniques can facilitate openness and create trust, but pose challenges to medical practices due to a lack of time in their daily routine [61,62].

However, it is important to consider that HCPs should be trained in sensitive communication. There is a risk that HCPs who are not trained and not aware of obesity and lifestyle issues may provide discriminatory advice. HCPs, therefore, require additional training to ensure that they do not stigmatize their patients and inadvertently harm the relationship or health outcomes [63,64]. Continuing education on lifestyle counseling could also benefit patients in other stages of life, such as those undergoing hormonal changes during menopause or cancer and cardiovascular disease [32].

The pregnant women described a relationship of trust with their HCP as particularly crucial for counseling. They were dissatisfied with the collaboration between gynecologists and midwives. Conflicts between the professional groups were sometimes acted out at the patients' expense, resulting in insecurity. The midwives in particular expressed a desire for improved cooperation, while the gynecologists mostly believed that discussion was only needed if complications occurred. Many women do not receive care from a midwife until the last few weeks before birth. Some of the interviewed gynecologists proposed a better division and coordination of consultations so that each profession could focus on their respective field of expertise. Interdisciplinary stakeholders in health care relating to childbirth in Germany have also called for improved collaboration, for example, through joint education and training, and resolution of legal ambiguities [65]. Different authors point to the importance of commitment, interpersonal skills, effective communication, respect, and trust among HCPs for successful collaboration [66–68]. More research is needed to examine the deep-rooted reasons for the difficulties in collaboration between gynecologists and midwives in Germany. Van der Lee et al. (2016) described a combination of exploring contemporary inter-professional practice with a historical perspective on inter-professional collaboration as beneficial to understand problems, and to provide guidance for improving collaboration [69]. From this, implications for policy and practice could be derived and could enable practitioners to implement actions for improving collaboration.

Strengths and Limitations

One strength of the study was the open and explorative character of the interviews. At the beginning, the women were asked to tell the interviewer about their last counseling session with their gynecologist and/or midwife. This led to an open flow of conversation in which the women were able to decide for themselves what to focus on. Another strength was the study's ability to incorporate inter-professional perspectives, as it allowed gynecologists, midwives, and medical assistants to share their experiences. The fact that different researchers were involved in the iterative analysis process represents another advantage, as it meant that the results were discussed in depth at various stages and according to the text material.

As shown in an evaluation of the recruitment procedures during the GeMuKi trial, intrinsic motivation was one of the major factors that led to HCPs participating in the GeMuKi trial [70]. The HCPs who consented to be interviewed were most likely motivated. It was, therefore, reasonable to assume that they did not represent typical HCPs in terms of implementing the intervention. A larger sample of different healthcare providers would have been beneficial. Unfortunately, it was not possible to recruit more healthcare providers for an interview. The interviews did not provide the information required for a comprehensive evaluation of the use of MI techniques. This would have required recurring observations of the counseling sessions, which was unfortunately not possible in practice.

5. Conclusions

Pregnant women and HCPs rated regular check-up visits during pregnancy as a good setting in which to focus on lifestyle topics. In particular, both pregnant women and HCPs reported that the combination of joint goal setting, reminders via push notifications, and feedback sessions helped women to make minor lifestyle changes. Nevertheless, it became apparent that there was a lack of information among pregnant women with regard to the recommendations for adequate gestational weight gain, and that the counseling approaches adopted by HCPs varied greatly. A discussion should be held regarding using sensitive techniques to inform all pregnant women of the risks and consequences of excessive weight gain. In addition to this, strategies should be sought to improve inter-professional collaboration between all of the HCPs involved in regular prenatal care. The results of this study will help to improve health care in pregnancy by taking into account the perspectives of both pregnant women and their HCPs.

Supplementary Materials: The following supporting information can be downloaded at: https://www.mdpi.com/article/10.3390/ijerph19106122/s1, Figure S1: COREQ Checklist; Table S1: Interview guides. Table S2: Topics of the interview guide*: Interviews with healthcare providers.

Author Contributions: L.L. designed the study, collected and analyzed the data, and wrote the manuscript. F.K. and F.N. assisted in the recruitment of the interviewees and supported the iterative process of data coding. A.A., F.K., F.N., L.L. and S.S. were members of the research team for the host trial. A.A. and S.S. designed the evaluation of the host trial. All authors have read and agreed to the published version of the manuscript.

Funding: The Innovation Fund of the German Federal Joint Committee (G-BA), Module 3, funded the trial: Improving communication with patients and promoting health literacy (Project no. 01NVF17014).

Institutional Review Board Statement: The study was conducted according to the guidelines of the Declaration of Helsinki. Ethical approval was received from the University Hospital of Cologne Research Ethics committee on 22 June 2018 (ID: 18-163), and from the State Chamber of Physicians in Baden-Wuerttemberg on 28 November 2018 (ID: B-F-2018-100). The trial was registered in the German Clinical Trials Register (DRKS00013173; date of registration: 3 January 2019). The study data were processed exclusively in a pseudonymized form in accordance with the EU General Data Protection Regulation (GDPR).

Informed Consent Statement: Written informed consent for the interviews and to publish the study was obtained from all the participants.

Data Availability Statement: The datasets used and analyzed in this study are available from the corresponding author on reasonable request.

Acknowledgments: The GeMuKi project was supported by the Innovation Fund of the German Federal Joint Committee, the G-BA (Project no. 01NVF17014), and was carried out by a consortium of five partners: Plattform Ernährung und Bewegung, Institut für Gesundheitsökonomie und Klinische Epidemiologie Universitätsklinikum Köln, Fraunhofer Institut für Offene Kommunikationssysteme FOKUS, BARMER, and Kassenärztliche Vereinigung Baden-Wuerttemberg. First, we would like to thank all of the interviewees—both the pregnant women and the healthcare providers—for their participation in the study and their openness to sharing their experiences and perspectives with us. We would also like to thank Isabel Lück and the team of study coordinators for their assistance in recruiting the interview participants. Additionally, we would like to thank the whole project team for their efforts and fruitful discussions. In the context of the host trial, the authors would like to thank all participating practices, gynecologists, pediatricians, medical assistants, midwives, pregnant women, and their families for their involvement. We would like to extend our deep thanks to Isabel Lück, Judith Kuchenbecker, Andrea Moreira, Andrea Seifarth, Elena Tschiltschke, Denise Torricella, and Hilke Friesenborg, who coordinated the study in the study regions in Baden-Wuerttemberg and provided essential support for data management in the field, and Anne-Madeleine Bau, GeMuKi project leader, who coordinated the consortium. We would also like to thank Brigitte Neumann and Sonja Eichin for developing and conducting the training in all intervention regions. Furthermore, we acknowledge Stefan Klose, Christian Giertz, Benny Häusler, and Michael John for developing and operating all of the digital intervention components. In addition, we would like to extend our thanks to Karsten Menn, Tobias Weigel, Rüdiger Kucher, and Simone Deininger for their help with the legal and contractual aspects of the project. We also acknowledge the members of the scientific advisory committee: Hans Hauner, Joachim Dudenhausen, Liane Schenk, Julika Loss, and Andrea Lambeck. We also thank Arim Shukri for his assistance with the statistical analyses. Additionally, we would like to thank the following partners, who have had an essential role in the success of the GeMuKi project: Gesund ins Leben—Netzwerk Junge Familie, Berufsverband der Kinder—und Jugendärzte,

Berufsverband der Frauenärzte, Hebammenverband Baden-Wuerttemberg, Landesärztekammer Baden-Wuerttemberg, Universität Freiburg, AOK Baden-Wuerttemberg, Techniker Krankenkasse, and all other health insurers participating in the project through GWQ Service Plus. Further, we would like to thank Cornelia Wäscher for her contribution to the grant proposal. Finally, we gratefully acknowledge Thomas Kauth and Ulrike Korsten-Reck for contributing to the initial project idea and for their support during implementation.

Conflicts of Interest: The authors declare no conflict of interest.

References

1. Varnaccia, G.; Zeiher, J.; Lange, C.; Jordan, S. Adipositasrelevante Einflussfaktoren im Kindesalter—Aufbau eines Bevölkerungsweiten Monitorings in Deutschland. *J. Health Monit.* **2017**, *2*, 90–102. [CrossRef]
2. World Health Organization. *Obesity—Preventing and Managing the Global Epidemic: Report on a WHO Consultation*; World Health Organization: Geneva, Switzerland, 2000; ISBN 9789241208949.
3. Ensenauer, R.; Chmitorz, A.; Riedel, C.; Fenske, N.; Hauner, H.; Nennstiel-Ratzel, U.; von Kries, R. Effects of suboptimal or excessive gestational weight gain on childhood overweight and abdominal adiposity: Results from a retrospective cohort study. *Int. J. Obes.* **2013**, *37*, 505–512. [CrossRef] [PubMed]
4. Mourtakos, S.P.; Tambalis, K.D.; Panagiotakos, D.B.; Antonogeorgos, G.; Arnaoutis, G.; Karteroliotis, K.; Sidossis, L.S. Maternal lifestyle characteristics during pregnancy, and the risk of obesity in the offspring: A study of 5125 children. *BMC Pregnancy Childbirth* **2015**, *15*, 66. [CrossRef] [PubMed]
5. Hrolfsdottir, L.; Rytter, D.; Olsen, S.F.; Bech, B.H.; Maslova, E.; Henriksen, T.B.; Halldorsson, T.I. Gestational weight gain in normal weight women and offspring cardio-metabolic risk factors at 20 years of age. *Int. J. Obes.* **2015**, *39*, 671–676. [CrossRef]
6. Goldstein, R.F.; Abell, S.K.; Ranasinha, S.; Misso, M.; Boyle, J.A.; Black, M.H.; Li, N.; Hu, G.; Corrado, F.; Rode, L.; et al. Association of Gestational Weight Gain with Maternal and Infant Outcomes: A systematic review and meta-analysis. *JAMA* **2017**, *317*, 2207–2225. [CrossRef]
7. Goldstein, R.F.; Abell, S.K.; Ranasinha, S.; Misso, M.L.; Boyle, J.A.; Harrison, C.L.; Black, M.H.; Li, N.; Hu, G.; Corrado, F.; et al. Gestational weight gain across continents and ethnicity: Systematic review and meta-analysis of maternal and infant outcomes in more than one million women. *BMC Med.* **2018**, *16*, 153. [CrossRef]
8. Rong, K.; Yu, K.; Han, X.; Szeto, I.M.Y.; Qin, X.; Wang, J.; Ning, Y.; Wang, P.; Ma, D. Pre-pregnancy BMI, gestational weight gain and postpartum weight retention: A meta-analysis of observational studies. *Public Health Nutr.* **2015**, *18*, 2172–2182. [CrossRef]
9. Guo, L.; Liu, J.; Ye, R.; Liu, J.; Zhuang, Z.; Ren, A. Gestational weight gain and overweight in children aged 3–6 years. *J. Epidemiol.* **2015**, *25*, 536–543. [CrossRef]
10. Kominiarek, M.A.; Saade, G.; Mele, L.; Bailit, J.; Reddy, U.M.; Wapner, R.J.; Varner, M.W.; Thorp, J.M.; Caritis, S.N.; Prasad, M.; et al. Association between gestational weight gain and perinatal outcomes. *Obstet. Gynecol.* **2018**, *132*, 875–881. [CrossRef]
11. Wu, Y.; Wan, S.; Gu, S.; Mou, Z.; Dong, L.; Luo, Z.; Zhang, J.; Hua, X. Gestational weight gain and adverse pregnancy outcomes: A prospective cohort study. *BMJ Open* **2020**, *10*, e038187. [CrossRef]
12. Brunner, S.; Stecher, L.; Ziebarth, S.; Nehring, I.; Rifas-Shiman, S.L.; Sommer, C.; Hauner, H.; von Kries, R. Excessive gestational weight gain prior to glucose screening and the risk of gestational diabetes: A meta-analysis. *Diabetologia* **2015**, *58*, 2229–2237. [CrossRef] [PubMed]
13. Arabin, B.; Baschat, A.A. Pregnancy: An underutilized window of opportunity to improve long-term maternal and infant health-an appeal for continuous family care and interdisciplinary communication. *Front. Pediatr.* **2017**, *5*, 69. [CrossRef] [PubMed]
14. Hayes, L.; McParlin, C.; Azevedo, L.B.; Jones, D.; Newham, J.; Olajide, J.; McCleman, L.; Heslehurst, N. The effectiveness of smoking cessation, alcohol reduction, diet and physical activity interventions in improving maternal and infant health outcomes: A systematic review of meta-analyses. *Nutrients* **2021**, *13*, 1036. [CrossRef] [PubMed]
15. Hussein, N.; Kai, J.; Qureshi, N. The effects of preconception interventions on improving reproductive health and pregnancy outcomes in primary care: A systematic review. *Eur. J. Gen. Pract.* **2016**, *22*, 42–52. [CrossRef] [PubMed]
16. Andreasen, K.R.; Andersen, M.L.; Schantz, A.L. Obesity and pregnancy. *Acta Obstet. Gynecol. Scand.* **2004**, *83*, 1022–1029. [CrossRef] [PubMed]
17. Bohrer, J.; Ehrenthal, D.B. Other adverse pregnancy outcomes and future chronic disease. *Semin. Perinatol.* **2015**, *39*, 259–263. [CrossRef]
18. Atkinson, L.; Shaw, R.L.; French, D.P. Is pregnancy a teachable moment for diet and physical activity behaviour change? An interpretative phenomenological analysis of the experiences of women during their first pregnancy. *Br. J. Health Psychol.* **2016**, *21*, 842–858. [CrossRef]
19. Streuling, I.; Beyerlein, A.; von Kries, R. Can gestational weight gain be modified by increasing physical activity and diet counseling? A meta-analysis of interventional trials. *Am. J. Clin. Nutr.* **2010**, *92*, 678–687. [CrossRef]
20. Heslehurst, N.; Hayes, L.; Jones, D.; Newham, J.; Olajide, J.; McLeman, L.; McParlin, C.; de Brun, C.; Azevedo, L. The effectiveness of smoking cessation, alcohol reduction, diet and physical activity interventions in changing behaviours during pregnancy: A systematic review of systematic reviews. *PLoS ONE* **2020**, *15*, e0232774. [CrossRef]

21. Thangaratinam, S.; Rogozinska, E.; Jolly, K.; Glinkowski, S.; Roseboom, T.; Tomlinson, J.W.; Kunz, R.; Mol, B.W.; Coomarasamy, A.; Khan, K.S. Effects of interventions in pregnancy on maternal weight and obstetric outcomes: Meta-analysis of randomised evidence. *BMJ* **2012**, *344*, e2088. [CrossRef]
22. Muktabhant, B.; Lawrie, T.A.; Lumbiganon, P.; Laopaiboon, M. Diet or exercise, or both, for preventing excessive weight gain in pregnancy. *Cochrane Database Syst. Rev.* **2015**, *6*, CD007145. [CrossRef] [PubMed]
23. Craemer, K.A.; Sampene, E.; Safdar, N.; Antony, K.M.; Wautlet, C.K. Nutrition and Exercise Strategies to Prevent Excessive Pregnancy Weight Gain: A Meta-analysis. *AJP Rep.* **2019**, *9*, e92–e120. [CrossRef] [PubMed]
24. Institute of Medicine (IOM); National Research Council. *Weight Gain during Pregnancy: Reexamining the Guidelines*; National Academies Press: Washington, DC, USA, 2009.
25. Deputy, N.P.; Sharma, A.J.; Kim, S.Y.; Hinkle, S.N. Prevalence and characteristics associated with gestational weight gain adequacy. *Obstet. Gynecol.* **2015**, *125*, 773–781. [CrossRef] [PubMed]
26. Chen, H.-Y.; Chauhan, S.P. Association between gestational weight gain adequacy and adverse maternal and neonatal outcomes. *Am. J. Perinatol.* **2018**, *36*, 615–623. [CrossRef] [PubMed]
27. Huang, A.; Ji, Z.; Zhao, W.; Hu, H.; Yang, Q.; Chen, D. Rate of gestational weight gain and preterm birth in relation to prepregnancy body mass indices and trimester: A follow-up study in China. *Reprod. Health* **2016**, *13*, 93. [CrossRef] [PubMed]
28. Noever, K.; Schubert, J.; Reuschel, E.; Timmesfeld, N.; Arabin, B. Changes in maternal body mass index, weight gain and outcome of singleton pregnancies from 2000 to 2015: A population-based retrospective cohort study in Hesse/Germany. *Geburtshilfe Frauenheilkd.* **2020**, *80*, 508–517. [CrossRef] [PubMed]
29. Dodd, J.; Thangaratinam, S. Researchers' position statement on tackling obesity in pregnancy: The International Weight Management in Pregnancy (i-WIP) collaboration pleads for public health intervention. *BJOG* **2016**, *123*, 163–164. [CrossRef]
30. Gemeinsamer Bundesausschuss. Richtlinien des Gemeinsamen Bundesausschusses über die Ärztliche Betreuung Während der Schwangerschaft und nach der Entbindung (Mutterschafts-Richtlinien). Available online: https://www.g-ba.de/richtlinien/19/ (accessed on 18 March 2021).
31. Goeckenjan, M.; Brückner, A.; Vetter, K. Schwangerenvorsorge. *Gynäkologe* **2021**, *54*, 579–589. [CrossRef]
32. Schaudig, K.; Schwenkhagen, A. Prävention—ein Thema für Gynäkologen? *Gynäkologe* **2016**, *49*, 224–225. [CrossRef]
33. Alayli, A.; Krebs, F.; Lorenz, L.; Nawabi, F.; Bau, A.-M.; Lück, I.; Moreira, A.; Kuchenbecker, J.; Tschiltschke, E.; John, M.; et al. Evaluation of a computer-assisted multi-professional intervention to address lifestyle-related risk factors for overweight and obesity in expecting mothers and their infants: Protocol for an effectiveness-implementation hybrid study. *BMC Public Health* **2020**, *20*, 482. [CrossRef]
34. Lück, I.; Kuchenbecker, J.; Moreira, A.; Friesenborg, H.; Torricella, D.; Neumann, B. Development and implementation of the GeMuKi lifestyle intervention: Motivating parents-to-be and young parents with brief interventions. *Ernährungsumschau* **2020**, *67*, e37–43. [CrossRef]
35. OECD; World Bank Group; World Health Organization. *Delivering Quality Health Services: A Global Imperative for Universal Health Coverage*; World Health Organization: Geneva, Switzerland, 2018; ISBN 9789241513906.
36. Whitaker, K.M.; Wilcox, S.; Liu, J.; Blair, S.N.; Pate, R.R. Patient and provider perceptions of weight gain, physical activity, and nutrition counseling during pregnancy: A qualitative study. *Women's Health Issues* **2016**, *26*, 116–122. [CrossRef] [PubMed]
37. Nehring, I.; Feurig, S.; Roebl-Matthieu, M.; Schiessl, B.; von Kries, R. Sichtweisen schwangerer Frauen zu ihrem Ernährungs- und Bewegungsverhalten: Eine Beratungsgrundlage zur Vermeidung exzessiver Gewichtszunahme. *Gesundheitswesen* **2017**, *79*, 461–467. [CrossRef] [PubMed]
38. Novick, G. Women's experience of prenatal care: An integrative review. *J. Midwifery Women's Health* **2009**, *54*, 226–237. [CrossRef] [PubMed]
39. Rollnick, S.; Miller, W.R. What is motivational interviewing? *Behav. Cognit. Psychother.* **1995**, *23*, 325–334. [CrossRef]
40. Miller, W.R.; Rollnick, S. *Motivational Interviewing: Helping People Change*, 3rd ed.; Guilford Publications: New York, NY, USA, 2013; ISBN 9781609182274.
41. Koletzko, B.; Cremer, M.; Flothkötter, M.; Graf, C.; Hauner, H.; Hellmers, C.; Kersting, M.; Krawinkel, M.; Przyrembel, H.; Röbl-Mathieu, M.; et al. Diet and lifestyle before and during pregnancy—Practical recommendations of the germany-wide healthy start—Young family network. *Geburtshilfe Frauenheilkd.* **2018**, *78*, 1262–1282. [CrossRef] [PubMed]
42. Nawabi, F.; Alayli, A.; Krebs, F.; Lorenz, L.; Shukri, A.; Bau, A.-M.; Stock, S. Health literacy among pregnant women in a lifestyle intervention trial: Protocol for an explorative study on the role of health literacy in the perinatal health service setting. *BMJ Open* **2021**, *11*, e047377. [CrossRef]
43. Curran, G.M.; Bauer, M.; Mittman, B.; Pyne, J.M.; Stetler, C. Effectiveness-implementation hybrid designs: Combining elements of clinical effectiveness and implementation research to enhance public health impact. *Med. Care* **2012**, *50*, 217–226. [CrossRef]
44. Tong, A.; Sainsbury, P.; Craig, J. Consolidated criteria for reporting qualitative research (COREQ): A 32-item checklist for interviews and focus groups. *Int. J. Qual. Health Care* **2007**, *19*, 349–357. [CrossRef]
45. Proctor, E.; Silmere, H.; Raghavan, R.; Hovmand, P.; Aarons, G.; Bunger, A.; Griffey, R.; Hensley, M. Outcomes for implementation research: Conceptual distinctions, measurement challenges, and research agenda. *Adm. Policy Ment. Health* **2011**, *38*, 65–76. [CrossRef]

46. Flottorp, S.A.; Oxman, A.D.; Krause, J.; Musila, N.R.; Wensing, M.; Godycki-Cwirko, M.; Baker, R.; Eccles, M.P. A checklist for identifying determinants of practice: A systematic review and synthesis of frameworks and taxonomies of factors that prevent or enable improvements in healthcare professional practice. *Implement. Sci.* **2013**, *8*, 35. [CrossRef] [PubMed]
47. Dresing, T.; Pehl, T. (Eds.) *Praxisbuch Transkription: Regelsysteme, Software und Praktische Anleitungen für Qualitative ForscherInnen*, 2nd ed.; Dr. Dresing und Pehl GmbH: Marburg, Germany, 2011; ISBN 9783818504892.
48. Kuckartz, U. *Qualitative Inhaltsanalyse: Methoden, Praxis, Computerunterstützung*, 3rd ed.; Beltz Juventa: Weinheim, Germany, 2016; ISBN 9783779933441.
49. Kuckartz, U. *Qualitative Text Analysis: A Guide to Methods, Practice & Using Software*; SAGE Publications Ltd.: London, UK, 2014; ISBN 9781446267745.
50. Rädiker, S.; Kuckartz, U. *Analyse Qualitativer Daten mit MAXQDA*; Springer: Wiesbaden, Germany, 2019; ISBN 9783658220945.
51. Rockliffe, L.; Peters, S.; Heazell, A.E.P.; Smith, D.M. Factors influencing health behaviour change during pregnancy: A systematic review and meta-synthesis. *Health Psychology Rev.* **2021**, *15*, 1–20. [CrossRef] [PubMed]
52. Vanstone, M.; Kandasamy, S.; Giacomini, M.; DeJean, D.; McDonald, S.D. Pregnant women's perceptions of gestational weight gain: A systematic review and meta-synthesis of qualitative research. *Matern. Child Nutr.* **2017**, *13*, e12607. [CrossRef] [PubMed]
53. Phelan, S.; Phipps, M.G.; Abrams, B.; Darroch, F.; Schaffner, A.; Wing, R.R. Practitioner advice and gestational weight gain. *J. Women's Health* **2011**, *20*, 585–591. [CrossRef]
54. Grenier, L.N.; Atkinson, S.A.; Mottola, M.F.; Wahoush, O.; Thabane, L.; Xie, F.; Vickers-Manzin, J.; Moore, C.; Hutton, E.K.; Murray-Davis, B. Be healthy in pregnancy: Exploring factors that impact pregnant women's nutrition and exercise behaviours. *Matern. Child Nutr.* **2021**, *17*, e13068. [CrossRef]
55. Verma, B.A.; Nichols, L.P.; Plegue, M.A.; Moniz, M.H.; Rai, M.; Chang, T. Advice given by community members to pregnant women: A mixed methods study. *BMC Pregnancy Childbirth* **2016**, *16*, 349. [CrossRef]
56. Oechsle, A.; Wensing, M.; Ullrich, C.; Bombana, M. Health knowledge of lifestyle-related risks during pregnancy: A cross-sectional study of pregnant women in Germany. *Int. J. Environ. Res. Public Health* **2020**, *17*, 8626. [CrossRef]
57. Liu, J.; Whitaker, K.M.; Yu, S.M.; Chao, S.M.; Lu, M.C. Association of provider advice and pregnancy weight gain in a predominantly Hispanic population. *Women's Health Issues* **2016**, *26*, 321–328. [CrossRef]
58. Deputy, N.P.; Sharma, A.J.; Kim, S.Y.; Olson, C.K. Achieving appropriate gestational weight gain: The role of healthcare provider advice. *J. Women's Health* **2018**, *27*, 552–560. [CrossRef]
59. Piccinini-Vallis, H.; Brown, J.B.; Ryan, B.L.; McDonald, S.D.; Stewart, M. Women's views on advice about weight gain in pregnancy: A grounded theory study. *Matern. Child Health J.* **2021**, *25*, 1717–1724. [CrossRef]
60. Emery, R.L.; Benno, M.T.; Salk, R.H.; Kolko, R.P.; Levine, M.D. Healthcare provider advice on gestational weight gain: Uncovering a need for more effective weight counselling. *J. Obstet. Gynaecol.* **2018**, *38*, 916–921. [CrossRef] [PubMed]
61. Lindhardt, C.L.; Rubak, S.; Mogensen, O.; Hansen, H.P.; Goldstein, H.; Lamont, R.F.; Joergensen, J.S. Healthcare professionals experience with motivational interviewing in their encounter with obese pregnant women. *Midwifery* **2015**, *31*, 678–684. [CrossRef] [PubMed]
62. Brobeck, E.; Bergh, H.; Odencrants, S.; Hildingh, C. Primary healthcare nurses' experiences with motivational interviewing in health promotion practice. *J. Clin. Nurs.* **2011**, *20*, 3322–3330. [CrossRef] [PubMed]
63. Incollingo Rodriguez, A.C.; Smieszek, S.M.; Nippert, K.E.; Tomiyama, A.J. Pregnant and postpartum women's experiences of weight stigma in healthcare. *BMC Pregnancy Childbirth* **2020**, *20*, 499. [CrossRef]
64. Hill, B.; Incollingo Rodriguez, A.C. Weight Stigma across the preconception, pregnancy, and postpartum periods: A narrative review and conceptual model. *Semin. Reprod. Med.* **2020**, *38*, 414–422. [CrossRef]
65. Abdallah, L.; Desery, K.; Eichenauer, J.; Fressle, R.; Oberle, A.; Soldner, G.; Stammer, G. Schwangerschaft und geburt als grundlage der gesundheit. *Geburtshilfe Frauenheilkd.* **2020**, *80*, 228–231. [CrossRef]
66. Gibiino, G.; Rugo, M.; Maffoni, M.; Giardini, A. Back to the future: Five forgotten lessons for the healthcare managers of today. *Int. J. Qual. Health Care* **2020**, *32*, 275–277. [CrossRef]
67. Smith, D.C. Interprofessional collaboration in perinatal care: The future of midwifery. *J. Perinat. Neonatal Nurs.* **2016**, *30*, 167–173. [CrossRef]
68. Waldman, R.; Kennedy, H.P.; Kendig, S. Collaboration in maternity care: Possibilities and challenges. *Obstet. Gynecol. Clin. N. Am.* **2012**, *39*, 435–444. [CrossRef]
69. Van der Lee, N.; Driessen, E.W.; Scheele, F. How the past influences interprofessional collaboration between obstetricians and midwives in the Netherlands: Findings from a secondary analysis. *J. Interprof. Care* **2016**, *30*, 71–76. [CrossRef]
70. Krebs, F.; Lorenz, L.; Nawabi, F.; Lück, I.; Bau, A.-M.; Alayli, A.; Stock, S. Recruitment in health services research—A study on facilitators and barriers for the recruitment of community-based healthcare providers. *Int. J. Environ. Res. Public Health* **2021**, *18*, 10521. [CrossRef] [PubMed]

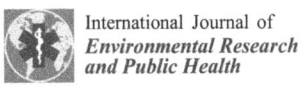

Article

"What Do You Need? What Are You Experiencing?" Relationship Building and Power Dynamics in Participatory Research Projects: Critical Self-Reflections of Researchers

Doris Arnold [1,*], Andrea Glässel [2,3], Tabea Böttger [4], Navina Sarma [5], Andreas Bethmann [6] and Petra Narimani [7]

1. Department of Social Work and Health Care, Ludwigshafen University of Business and Society, 67059 Ludwigshafen, Germany
2. Institute of Biomedical Ethics and History of Medicine, University of Zurich, 8006 Zurich, Switzerland; andrea.glaessel@ibme.uzh.ch
3. Institute of Public Health (IPH), Zurich University of Applied Sciences (ZHAW), 8400 Winterthur, Switzerland; andrea.glaessel@zhaw.ch
4. Institute of Health Science, Faculty of Medicine, University of Lübeck, 23562 Lübeck, Germany; tabea.boettger@uni-luebeck.de
5. Department of Infectious Disease Epidemiology, Robert Koch Institute, 13353 Berlin, Germany; sarman@rki.de
6. Centre for International Health Protection (ZIG), Robert Koch Institute, 13353 Berlin, Germany; bethmanna@rki.de
7. Protestant University of Applied Sciences Berlin (EHB), 14167 Berlin, Germany; petra.narimani@aol.de
* Correspondence: doris.arnold@hwg-lu.de; Tel.: +49-621-5203-570

Citation: Arnold, D.; Glässel, A.; Böttger, T.; Sarma, N.; Bethmann, A.; Narimani, P. "What Do You Need? What Are You Experiencing?" Relationship Building and Power Dynamics in Participatory Research Projects: Critical Self-Reflections of Researchers. *Int. J. Environ. Res. Public Health* **2022**, *19*, 9336. https://doi.org/10.3390/ijerph19159336

Academic Editor: Paul B. Tchounwou

Received: 29 June 2022
Accepted: 27 July 2022
Published: 30 July 2022

Publisher's Note: MDPI stays neutral with regard to jurisdictional claims in published maps and institutional affiliations.

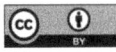

Copyright: © 2022 by the authors. Licensee MDPI, Basel, Switzerland. This article is an open access article distributed under the terms and conditions of the Creative Commons Attribution (CC BY) license (https://creativecommons.org/licenses/by/4.0/).

Abstract: Participatory approaches create opportunities for cooperation, building relationships, gaining knowledge, rethinking, and eventually changing power structures. From an international perspective, the article looks at the historical development of different participatory approaches in which building relationships and managing the balance of power between persons engaged in participatory research are central. The authors present and critically reflect on four research projects to show how they understood and implemented participatory research in different ways and what they have learned from their respective experiences. The "PaSuMi" project worked in the context of addiction prevention with migrants and provides a glimpse into different contexts of participatory research. The initiator of the study "Back into life—with a power wheelchair" works with post-stroke individuals who use the assistive device in community mobility and reflects on the shifting and intertwining roles of participants. In the research project "Workshops for implementation of expanded community nursing", new professional roles for nurses in community nursing were developed; here limitations to participation and ways to deal with them are illustrated. Finally, the "DIPEx" project deals with challenges of enabling participation of persons with multiple sclerosis via narrative interviews on the experience of health and illness. All examples underline the necessity of a permanent reflection on relationships and power dynamics in participatory research processes.

Keywords: participatory research; participation; health; power; reflection; research relationships; understanding of roles in research; error culture; DIPEx

1. Introduction

The concept of participation in practice and research is ambiguous and multifaceted and must therefore largely adapt to the respective living environments with their different socializations, experiences, emergencies, and needs. Participatory approaches are, therefore, not only dependent on different conditions, but they also have to be designed differently at different levels [1] (pp. 445–453) [2]. Involvement and participation in social decision-making processes always have been and still are a matter of course in many nations and cultures. As an example, some Latin American countries such as Ecuador or Chile—and recently Colombia—are mentioned here, in which quite a few of the numerous nations and ethnic groups want to maintain their ways of life based on very different forms of participation. At the same time, they are striving for a plurinational superordinate state whose tasks they would like to co-determine.

Participatory research approaches are rooted in social movements that stand up for a democratic and inclusive society. Among others, these include Participatory Rural Appraisal (CHAMBERS), Emancipatory Research Approaches (FREIRE), Action Research in Organizational Development (LEWIN), Action Research in Education (KEMMIS), Human Inquiry and Cooperative Inquiry (REASON), Appreciative Inquiry (COOPERRIDER), Community-Based Participatory Research (WALLERSTEIN), Action Science (ARGYRIS), Constructivist Research (LINCOLN), Feminist Research (LATHER), Empowerment Evaluation (FETTERMAN), and Democratic Dialogue (GUSTAVSEN) [3].

Participatory research in Germany draws on many different sources and traditions [4]. Its common denominator might be that the people and/or groups involved shape the research process as independent and equal actors. Their concerns, inequalities, and lives are at the core of the joint research processes as well as the intention to bring about change. The design of the relationship of all actors involved is of central importance for participatory research. At this point, different interests, roles, and power dynamics are inevitably at stake, as well as structural obstacles within and outside the research community. Thus, the issue of relationships in the research process represents a challenge as well as an opportunity to critically reflect on, improve and enhance participatory research.

Building on North American and South American approaches in the mid-20th century, "action research" flourished in the wake of the student movement of the late 1960s in Germany, Austria, and Switzerland. In 1993, Altrichter and Gstettner critically examined the booming publications on action research in the German-speaking world between 1972 and 1982 [5,6]. According to findings from a survey in 1990 action research had nearly disappeared from the German social science debate at that time, mostly due to its decreased attractiveness [5]. It came back as participatory research in the middle of the first decennial in the new millennium. Recently, we even saw an increased financial support of participatory research projects in Germany. Nevertheless, the definition of participatory research often seems to be unclear, both for researchers and for funders [4]. Currently, there are increasing discussions about suitable criteria and forms of funding for participatory research projects, which could lead to clearer regulations for funding participatory research in the near future [7,8]. On the other hand, Green and Johns [9] warned against "token" participation and pointed to recent pressure from ministries to make projects participatory.

Looking at the issues compiled by Altrichter and Gstettner on alleged and actual weaknesses of the action research approach today (in 2022), we find that many are still relevant and unanswered in Germany and worldwide. This article will focus on the issue of "relations between researchers and researched" [5] (p. 69) raised by Altrichter and Gstettner. In the English discourse on participatory health research, challenges connected with power and positionality of researchers in working with co-researchers are addressed in different contexts. Drawing on data from workshops with an international sample of participatory health researchers, Egid et al. [10] shed light on these issues and the need for reflexivity as a means for researchers to address power inequities in participatory research practice. Smith et al. [11] reflected on different positionalities of class, gender, race, sexual orientation and the status of insider or outsider of communities, using episodes taken from the experiences of novice participatory action researchers. In the context of CBPR, Muhammad et al. [12] discussed issues of identity, intersectional positionality and power dynamics by means of autoethnographic self-reflections of experienced researchers in working with partners from marginalized communities. In a slightly different vein, Jagosh et al. [13] showed the crucial importance of trust, power-sharing and co-governance for CBPR projects to be successful, employing a qualitative analysis of interviews with community members and researchers.

In this article, we discuss individual experiences in four research projects in the German context. We look at relationships and power dynamics between persons engaged in a participatory research process. By reflecting challenges and by showing how we understood and reacted to them, on one hand special features and the high value of participatory health research are emphasized. On the other hand, limitations to these endeavors are made transparent.

2. The Importance of Research Relationship and Power Dynamics from a Methodological Perspective

Facilitating participation in research processes has implications for the structure of relationships in the context of existing power dynamics among persons engaged in a participatory research process. With this essential characteristic the participatory research approach [14] differs from other approaches in social and health research. In this article, we refer mostly to the approach of Participatory Health Research (PHR).

The international Collaboration for Participatory Health Research (ICPHR) states the goal of PHR and the demands on participation in the research relationship within PHR as follows:

"The goal of PHR is to maximize the participation of those whose life or work is the subject of the research in all stages of the research process, including the formulation of the research question and goal, the development of a research design, the selection of appropriate methods for data collection and analysis, the implementation of the research, the interpretation of the results, and the dissemination of the findings. (...)" [15] (p. 6).

Participation refers to the co-operation in decision-making and research activities of those persons who are directly affected by the problems that are the subject of the respective research projects. Participatory Health Research understands participation as co-learning, co-operation or partnership in decision-making within research processes [16]. This requirement reaches beyond mere participation in the sense of consultation and involvement in data collection or analysis, as is also included, for example, in feminist, ethnographic, and other qualitative research designs (see, for example, [17] pp. 142–146). In participatory research and qualitative research designs, initiators of research projects should establish relationships based on trust with persons directly addressed by the research and with other stakeholders involved. In addition, common features of participatory research and other qualitative research designs, such as ethnography, might include creating spaces for hearing voices of persons in marginalized positions [18] (p. 435) and including their perspectives.

Thus, participation in research always addresses the relationship and power dynamics between researchers and the persons who are at the center of research processes, with and through whom knowledge on specific issues is generated [9–12,19]. At the same time, participatory research has the potential to enable the persons involved to bring about change within their communities and/or their individual situations through their co-operation in the research [20]. Epistemologically, the question here is how and in which social processes knowledge can emerge. Participation in research therefore has implications for epistemological aspects as well as for the design of the collaboration between researchers and other persons engaged in participatory research projects.

Issues concerning the design of research relationships and the epistemological aspects mentioned pertain to approaches of participatory research as well as to other qualitative research approaches and differentiate them from the prevailing positivist/post-positivist concept of science in quantitative research [21]. Thus, in quantitative research, the research relationship is supposed to be distant and characterized by objectivity, whereas in participatory research, as mentioned above, this issue is understood in a fundamentally different way due to the need to build a collaborative and trusting research relationship. For this reason, among others, participatory research or action research approaches had to grapple with criticism from established social research communities regarding the lack of "objectivity" and the scientific credibility of its results since their inception [5].

If participatory research is closely oriented towards the persons about whom it generates knowledge, and researchers work closely with these persons, researchers are at the same time consciously taking sides with persons who often belong to groups that are marginalized or disadvantaged in society. With reference to the history of action research in the German-speaking countries, one of the controversial issues discussed is the role of "admitted partiality" advocated by some action researchers [5] (p. 71). Hereby, the positivist/post-positivist claim to objectivity of conventional quantitative research was deliberately questioned in favor of a critical, politically motivated positioning of researchers on the side of those affected by the exercise of power and discrimination. Thus, in the early 1980s, Maria Mies assigned "partiality" a central place for feminist research in her "Methodological Postulates for Women's Studies" [22]. Mies's conception of feminist research included a clear commitment to politically motivated action research (with reference to Paolo Freire, among others) and understood "partiality" in favor of discrimination against women as a critique of the claim to absence of bias in the prevailing positivist/post-positivist understanding of science.

However, these epistemological and methodological implications of participation not only apply to participatory research, but also to other research styles of qualitative research, which, according to Yvonna Lincoln and colleagues, are oriented towards alternative inquiry paradigms [21,23]. One of the common characteristics of qualitative research approaches is the concept of research as a "situated activity" [24] that locates researchers and research activities in the social worlds of and thus in social interactions with the persons at the focus of research processes [23] (p. 10).

With reference to the German-language discourse, Hella Von Unger [20] mentioned three distinguishing features between participatory research and other interpretative, qualitative research styles:

(a) Co-operation of co-researchers in the research process on an equal basis.
(b) Initiation of " ... learning process[es] that enable individual and collective strengthening and development processes ... " among the persons involved in the research [20] (p. 162; translation by the authors).
(c) The "dual objective" of participatory research: firstly, to generate knowledge that contributes to a better understanding of the respective underlying problem, and, secondly, to bring about processes of change (ibid.).

According to Lincoln and colleagues [21], key differences between positivist/postpositivist research and qualitative research are, among others, tied up to the following questions about control over and participation in the research process:

"Who initiates? Who determines salient questions? Who determines what constitutes findings? Who determines how data will be collected? Who determines in what form the findings will be made public, if at all? Who determines what representations will be made of participants in the research?" [21] (p. 134).

This is particularly evident when compared with experimental studies (e.g., randomized controlled trials; [25]), which have played an increasingly powerful role in decision-making pertaining to policies in health care since the beginning of this century in the pursuit of evidence-based health care. Key characteristics of these studies are that control and decision-making power during the entire research process rest solely with the researchers. Any relinquishment of control over any of the aspects addressed in terms of participation in research would run the risk of creating bias, and thus would have a major detrimental impact on the quality of the study results (ibid.).

The questions mentioned above are answered in a decidedly different way in participatory research and at the same time address the significance of power in the research relationship between researchers and persons in the focus of the research. The importance of participation in terms of influence and co-design in the research process will be exemplified in the following examples from our research practice.

3. Four Examples of Designs of Research Relationships and Participation

3.1. Approach to Critical Self-Reflection on Research Experiences

The following examples are based on discussions and critical reflections on participation and participatory research that took place during an ICPHR Training in Participatory Health Research program in 2018 at the Catholic University of Applied Sciences, Berlin. We present four of the projects that were accompanied by all participants during the training in the form of collegial consultation. All projects were independent of each other in terms of time, content and aims. We chose an approach of critical self-reflection that in a similar way has been used by other researchers for sharing experiences and enhancing knowledge about the practice of participatory research [11,12]. First, we briefly introduce the aims, design and context of each project and describe their role as researchers or initiators of the projects. In a second step, we critically reflect our personal experiences as well as challenges during the research process that relate to issues of power dynamics and relationships. Finally, we point out aspects that facilitated or limited participation in research processes.

3.2. "Nothing about Us, without Us"—Participation in Addiction Prevention among Migrants—Reflections on Power Sharing and Roles within the PaSuMi Project by the Author Navina Sarma

3.2.1. Introduction

The PaSuMi (Participation, Addiction Prevention and Migration) project, duration 2017–2019, was a nationwide participatory model project of the German AIDS Service Organization (DAH) in the context of addiction prevention among migrants (https://pasumi.info/, (accessed on 26 July 2022)). Persons from and around eight addiction support and primary addiction prevention facilities in five German cities were involved. The common goal was to improve access to the help system with and for migrants. Clients, activists and community partners developed model approaches in a co-operative manner as research partners alongside employees of addiction support facilities (hereinafter referred to as practitioners) and academic researchers of the DAH [26].

In the first project phase, the project coordinators of the eight facilities formed local project teams. While one team consisted exclusively of activists from a self-organized initiative of Russian-speaking persons who use drugs (BerLUN) and persons from their community, other teams included staff (e.g., social workers, counselors, language mediators), (former) clients (e.g., from counseling or consumption rooms) and persons from specific communities (e.g., refugees, sex workers). Researcher partners called themselves peers or community partners (hereafter community partners). The size and composition of the project teams varied and was dynamic depending on the upcoming activities.

In the PaSuMi project, persons who previously acted in fixed hierarchical roles (community partners/practitioners/academics) developed model approaches for better access to migrant communities jointly, and if possible, with shared decision-making power. From the perspective of the PaSuMi project coordinator at DAH, I (D.S.) reflect on the changes in relationships and power dynamics, as well as on my own role in the project. From different contexts, I was familiar with both, addiction, and grassroots work with and for communities. Questions and reflections accompanied me throughout the course of the project: "Right now, I am very unsure whether I am at all suited for this task. I need a lot of structure, clear lines, goals, concrete measures. But that doesn't fit with the participatory approach. I don't know if I can accompany the projects competently." (Note from my research diary on 14 August 2017).

3.2.2. Formation of Research Teams: Relationship Building and Change of Perspective

A first challenge was the formation of the local project teams because of the positionality of the participants, who were situated in different levels of hierarchically structured power dynamics. Some of the community partners involved were clients of the facilities while others were key persons of specific communities, independent of the facilities. Many of the participants had a history of migration some were drug users, sex workers or persons with experience of poverty. These characteristics often led to discrimination and exclusion. Central and continuous components of the team building process were therefore the development of trust and forming of relationships. Other important factors were sufficient time and resources, sensitivity, knowledge about and openness to different realities of life, and already established trusting relationships among the practitioners in the facilities. In some cases, contacts to community partners were established through other institutions or peer recruitment which, according to international literature, is a useful approach in participatory processes [27].

From my perspective, participation is fundamentally based on the assumption that nobody knows everything. The Canadian HIV/AIDS Legal Network for instance states, that persons who use drugs know best what works in their community. Furthermore, all persons should have the right to be involved in decisions affecting their lives [28]. Accordingly, I understand expert knowledge from lived experience as equal to the professional expertise of practitioners and the methodological expertise of academic researchers. Communities are thus equal contributors to the knowledge production process [29]. This challenged familiar roles in the PaSuMi project and required a change in the attitude towards collaboration with research partners. Through the interaction of different bodies of knowledge, the PaSuMi project tried to influence structures, to create new knowledge among all participants, to produce results relevant for communities that could be applied in programs and practice directly, and to build networks [30]. To what extent this has succeeded is probably assessed differently by each person involved. "How can we create free spaces within the given framework and to what extent is what we do really participation?" (Quote from a staff member of a facility, WSII on 17 June 2017) was a question that accompanied us throughout the process. I observed individual moments of change enabled by participation in the PaSuMi project, which are described below.

3.2.3. Everything Is Different in Participatory Processes

Some of the eight local project coordinators not only faced the challenge of taking the PaSuMi project forward despite their own skepticism or insecurities concerning the participatory approach and in addition to their routine tasks in the facilities, but sometimes also had to work against resistance from within their organizations. For example, a coordinator had a tough time explaining travel and accommodation costs for participation of community partners at the regular joint workshops to the management. The management was not used to practitioners and clients in the role of community partners working as partners in a project. Another new aspect of the PaSuMi project compared to previous projects was that it was not only a matter of implementing specific prevention measures, but that the joint path that led to achieving this implementation, for example the formation of project teams and intervention planning, was an equally important part of the process. Some processes took longer in the PaSuMi project than in other projects and at first glance had little to do with the field of activity of the participating institutions or with direct addiction prevention. New methods were used and actions such as parties, a visit to an exhibition or a film shoot were implemented. Often, the initial focus was on confidence building, team building and skills acquisition, without addressing the issue of addiction prevention. In the first year of the project, participants increasingly allowed processes in PaSuMi to proceed differently than usual. It became apparent that participants discovered participation in the sense of a collaborative process as something that, due to changed relationships, opened new spaces for encounter and provided a previously unavailable insight into the lived experience of the community partners (and, perhaps that of the practitioners, too). "I need a lot of patience, but I'm really into the project", remarked a local project coordinator (project visit on 10 October 2017) after his project team was established and ready to act.

Familiar ways of working and hierarchies changed. As a result, community partners began to use their decision-making power to help shaping the research process and determine what benefits they would derive for themselves from the project. This required a high degree of flexibility and openness on the part of practitioners and researchers regarding their usual ways of working and claims to power.

The moment when community partners approached me, took the research process into their hands, and assigned tasks to me, such as arranging a translator or organizing a meeting, was a key moment for me as project coordinator. I interpret this as a sign of successful participation. The relationships and trust that emerged within the project provided the appropriate space for this. To this day, some of the community and practice partners from the PaSuMi project are friends, contacts in my practical work and research partners in other research projects. Relationships established in the PaSuMi project, also among the community partners, continue to exist in various forms after the end of the project.

I was also confronted with my own claim to power, which I illustrate with the following example. One of the local projects included me in most of the steps of project planning and implementation at the beginning of the PaSuMi project. As the network on the part of the community grew larger and larger, certain activities, such as workshops or a meeting with members of the German parliament, took place without my knowledge. For me, this initially appeared to be at odds with the close relationship we had established, and certainly with my role as coordinator, who always wanted to be informed about everything. I had to learn that my discomfort had to do with control and power. The fact that the community partners did not let me participate in everything had nothing to do with me personally, but with the fact that my participation in some areas was not required. In retrospect, I feel that this was exactly my contribution to participation: to support the community partners where they needed it, and at the same time to accept that our collaboration was shaped together and that they decided what they shared with me and what not.

Similar experiences were also reported from the local projects. For example, in some project teams, the community partners requested various trainings because they wanted to learn how to give presentations and front events with confidence. Local PaSuMi project meetings often took place in the evenings and on weekends and thus outside the practitioners' usual working hours. Without this flexibility and consideration of the community partners' commitments in language courses, school and jobs, the meetings could not have taken place. Flexibility was also required in communication: in several local projects, communication took place mainly via WhatsApp at the request of the community partners, a channel not previously used in the counseling practice of the corresponding institutions.

3.2.4. Complex Needs

Local PaSuMi project coordinators supported their community partners in writing job applications, finding functional clothes for internships and accompanied them on official visits. This was also part of the participatory research process, even if these activities had nothing to do with the content of the PaSuMi project and sometimes took place outside of regular working hours. Persons who do not have a secure residence status, whose rights are restricted by migration and asylum policies, and who are stigmatized and discriminated by society's normative ideas and racism have complex needs that, even if they lie outside the research interest, must be taken into consideration in participatory research. The clear distinction between research, social work, and private engagement that exists in more conventional scientific approaches becomes blurred in participatory research. All this is an expression of a kind of relationship that does not exist in other forms of research.

Key challenges in the PaSuMi project were my own expectations of the participatory approach, the desire to involve the entire PaSuMi team in all steps equally, and the concern about making decisions without sufficient involvement of some stakeholders. This made some processes complicated and time-consuming. I had to understand that some persons exercised their right not to participate, had other priorities than answering an email, some might not even have an email address, I did not speak all the languages of the persons involved—in short, I learned that participation by everyone in decision-making could be aimed at, but it was not always possible. In conclusion, I think the PaSuMi project can contribute to the discussion of whether a lack of privilege is a barrier to participation in participatory research. I assumed that participation in the PaSuMi project was not impeded due to a lack of privileges, but due to specifically identifiable structural barriers, such as migration-related legislation, structures, and procedures in institutions and in research that had been established over many years, and due to established framework conditions in individual projects. However, through reflection and flexibility in their own approach, all institutions were able to find a way to win community partners for the project. What has become of the relationships that have grown over 2.5 years is known only to those involved individually. I know of three cases in two participating agencies where community partners have formally become colleagues. From some I know that they were looking for community support for the time after the PaSuMi project to continue PaSuMi contents independently. In addition, new networks were formed. As I write this, I wonder how all the persons involved are doing and how, in retrospect, they assessed the relationships, roles, power, and benefits (or harms?) of the PaSuMi project.

3.3. Shifting and Interweaving Perspectives in the Project "Back into Life-with a Power Wheelchair": From Occupational Therapist to Research Initiator and Companion, by Author Tabea Böttger

3.3.1. Introduction

The project presented here was conducted between 2017 and 2019 in the context of the author's working environment, a long-term rehabilitation center for adults with severe acquired brain injury in Berlin. At the same time, the author took part in a part-time occupational therapy master's degree program at the University of Applied Sciences and Arts (HAWK) in Hildesheim, Germany. The author's aim was to address a practice-oriented issue in her final thesis and to involve former rehabilitation participations as co-researchers with equal status in order to implement the participatory research approach she had become familiar with in practice [31].

Many stroke survivors experience permanent limitations in their activities of daily living, including mobility. Some lose their usual walking mobility or are only able to walk a few steps inside their home without assistance. To be able to carry out activities outside the home (e.g., shopping, visits to the doctor, visiting friends) as autonomously as possible and without assistance, some rehabilitation patients are advised and provided with a power wheelchair. While intensive training with this assistive device takes place in different contexts (such as in public spaces) during rehabilitation, it is unclear whether individuals use it after discharge for mobility outside their home and to what extent it supports them in their participation in social life. Based on these considerations, the following research question, which I formulated on my own at the beginning of the project, was at the center of the project: How do persons with a severe acquired brain injury experience their community mobility in a powered wheelchair in the metropolitan area of Berlin and what changes do they want to initiate?

The entire research team (author, a colleague from the occupational therapy department from the rehabilitation center and five former rehabilitation participants) met in five group meetings over a period of one year (May 2018 to May 2019). Photovoice was chosen as a method to answer the research question [32]: five persons after stroke took photos of their living environment alone or with the help of others, presented them to each other in the meetings, discussed and analyzed them together with the aim of publishing their results to draw attention to their concerns. The photos and stories were first exhibited in the long-term rehabilitation center at the request of the co-researchers (January 2019), then in other contexts (e.g., scientific conferences, Occupational Therapy School).

3.3.2. Relationship Building between Research Initiator and Co-Researchers

From the author's point of view, the issue of relationships played a central role in the research project. The following hypothesis serves as a starting point to the discussion: Without the pre-existing, trusting relationships between the author, her colleague and the five co-researchers, this project would retrospectively probably not have taken place in this form.

All co-researchers had cognitive, communication and sensory motor impairments due to severe stroke (up to 12 years ago). So far, this group of persons has been hardly or not at all considered in traditional medical und participatory research [33,34]. Especially the severity of their cognitive as well as communicative impairments are mostly only considered as exclusion criteria, as these persons are, among other issues, considered incapable of giving consent and/or uncertainty prevails as to how their views can be captured despite their manifold impairments. This required ethical considerations and decisions on the part of the author before the beginning as well as during the entire research process. A positive vote was obtained from the Commission for Research Ethics of the University of Applied Sciences and Arts (HAWK Hildesheim, 3 April 2018). By communication impairments, the author means acquired speech and language disorders like aphasia and dysarthria [35]. Cognitive impairments are understood here primarily as impairments in the areas of attention, memory and executive functions, including deficits in self-awareness [36].

But what conditions are needed to actively involve these persons in a participatory research team on an equal basis?

From the author's point of view, this first required researchers who, in addition to openness and flexibility for the research process, above all had specialist knowledge of the individual impairments and their relevance to everyday life. It also required experience in being able to adjust appropriately to these persons in communication in order to open up protected spaces for them in which they could express themselves verbally and nonverbally via gestures, visual material, electronic communication aids or written language despite their impairments. Internationally, initial participatory research with persons after stroke exists, but mostly involved persons with little or no cognitive and/or communication impairments [37–39].

3.3.3. Common Background of Experience

The author and initiator of this research project had, through her professional background as an occupational therapist, both contact with persons with complex support needs and, through years of working in partnership in therapy, had become acquainted with and tested ways and means of enabling communication with each other. Thus, she took over the function of gatekeeper and, with her previous professional experience and contacts, enabled access to a group of persons often described as "difficult to reach" or "marginalized persons and groups" [40] (p. 52 translation by the authors). The author selected specific persons and contacted them in different ways, with whom she had worked to varying degrees of intensity during inpatient long-term rehabilitation in the last eight years. First, two former rehabilitants were contacted with an information letter in easy language, with whom the author still had sporadic personal contact. In a second step, these persons were able to name other former rehabilitants who were asked to participate in the project. In this way, the relationship is consciously considered in the recruitment of participatory co-researchers and thus in the composition of the research team. At the last group meeting, which was dedicated to the evaluation, two co-researchers confirmed that this aspect was quite decisive for their "participation": "I participated [...] because I also wanted to meet persons again" (Steven, 18 May 2019) "[...] and I was interested in (...) research (...). Daniel, Petra, (...) and Ines (counts with fingers and points to persons present). And then I say yes. Because I know them" (Berta, 18 May 2019).

At the time of invitation or cooperation in the research project, a therapeutic relationship no longer existed. But they received an invitation from a person known to them to participate as active co-researchers. The pre-existing therapeutic relationship established a basis of trust for further joint cooperation, as it was oriented towards the principles of client-centered practice [41]. Client-centered practice is characterized by a relationship based on partnership, which requires an active and equal involvement of the clients in decisions about goals and interventions of therapy, recognizing the individual wishes and needs as well as autonomy of each person (ibid.). Despite this demand for therapeutic collaboration, in the author's view, a relationship of dependency remains, defined among other aspects by the traditional roles of therapist and patient/client. The desired cooperation in the research project should depart from these familiar role patterns and allow for a more liberal cooperation, for example, without entering into a therapy contract.

Another central issue was the chosen research topic "community mobility with a power wheelchair" that connected author and co-researchers. Within occupational therapy, the possibilities of this assistive device for independent mobility outside the home were discussed and, above all, intensive training sessions were conducted in public spaces in the various settings. Thus, the author, her colleague as well as the co-researchers had numerous shared experiences regarding the everyday challenges in using the assistive device and were thus able to draw on a common content basis/experiential knowledge.

3.3.4. Experience in the New Role

Due to the pre-existing personal relationship mentioned above, there was a basic openness for the project idea among the people concerned, without knowing precisely what a participatory research project was and what their cooperation could look like. Taking into account the risk of exercising power and influence involved, the persons approached were given extensive and appropriate information (at several points in time and through various media and communication channels) about the nature of the research style and their associated active role. This initially included a personal conversation in their familiar home environment using written educational material in easy language and was carried out continuously at the beginning of the meetings in the sense of an ongoing assent [42].

The description of collaboration, joint research, and the attempt to initiate change spontaneously led to uncertainty and rejection among all persons asked. Fears were expressed of not being able to live up to the attributed competence of being active as equal co-researchers, as well as a feeling of powerlessness, of not being able to influence the prevailing social conditions. Further, very practical concerns mentioned for the planned group meetings included not having enough time due to busy daily schedules or not being able to reach the meeting place alone without assistance and much effort. The author finally succeeded in convincing the persons for a first joint meeting. The following factors were probably essential for this, which the author took into account in the organization: a centrally located and barrier-free room (and toilets) in Berlin, that was easily accessible by public transport, assistance in organizing the time window and the route, the use of various communication channels and, in part, appointment reminders. In addition, the author was clear in the discussions that this project was a joint effort that could also fail. Even before the first meeting, it became clear that the "researcher's" area of responsibility encompassed much more than the preparation and design of the content of the meetings and what significance the aspect of accessibility also had in the specific research context.

The author constantly expressed her ideas of equal cooperation and at the same time had to get involved in a process that could only be controlled to a limited extent. The participating co-researchers repeatedly decided for themselves to what extent they would contribute to the project-or not.

This project focused on mutual encounters and learning as Altrichter and Gstettner [5] (cited in Heinze 1986, p. 8) stated. Co-researchers were integrated into the research process on an equal basis to jointly explore their experiences and to initiate change. This meant that the author had to leave familiar paths and slip into the role of a researcher, which was new to her, and fill it with life, especially in contact with persons she had already supported as a therapist in another setting. In the process, it became apparent to her that it could profitably apply many competencies and ways of acting from her professional practice. At the same time, it became clear again and again in the research process that the initially ambitious goals of "equal inclusion" in the "joint" project needed gradation. Thus, in the first two meetings, the co-researchers understandably did not speak of their or our project; after all, they had not initiated it, but had been invited to "participate". Accepting this was difficult at first. Patience and an open discussion during the meetings about the own claim of the "joint project" beyond the writing of a qualification paper, however, made clear to the persons concerned their status in the project. At the same time, their tasks and responsibilities increased. For example, in the later course of the project, a lengthy discussion arose in the research team about where the first exhibition and thus presentation of the results should take place. The co-researchers stated their different opinions, and the author and her colleague supported the decision-making process, especially through facilitation.

Nevertheless, it was important to accept that each person could and wanted to participate with different intensity and that therefore there were differences in participation that should not be negated or concealed. Disclosing the unequal preconditions, such as different cognitive and communication abilities, and demands prevented egalitarianism. In this participatory research project, it was important to allow for different scopes of co-design, situated in an area of tension between enabling influence and avoiding excessive demands.

Many things were new for the author: she learned to reflect more consciously on the characteristics of her role as a therapist and to take a step back when, for example, behavior was shown that was classified normatively as negative (such as excessive consumption of stimulants such as sweets, nicotine and alcohol), and to address this only when, in her view, it influenced the group work process negatively or when other co-researchers, including herself, felt disturbed by the behavior. However, this confrontation was not only about her professional role as a therapist but involved a conscious reflection on her own personal attitudes towards socially prevailing norms and values. It became clear once again that persons with disabilities are still primarily seen as weak and in need of help and less as experts in their own lives. This was also reflected very clearly in the goals the participating co-researchers stated for the project: on the one hand, they wanted to inform their personal environment, friends, and family, about their own lives–especially the challenges and discrimination they experience every day. Furthermore, they wanted to show a different image of persons with disabilities in general and contribute to the reduction of prejudices, fear of contact and discrimination.

Nevertheless, the behavior and action on the author's part were shaped by my previous experience in the therapeutic context, which was ultimately helpful in many situations, such as the spontaneous assistance with a toilet transfer, which was proactively requested by the person concerned. To develop a better understanding of the living environment of the co-researcher, it was necessary to allow unexpected situations to occur spontaneously that did not primarily contribute to the goal of the project but were in the interest of the co-researcher. This approach was perceived as enriching for the joint process. For example, the author twice went out to dinner with individual co-researchers in a restaurant at their request after a joint excursion of photographing. Thereby she gained very vivid impressions of their perspectives and thus gained more knowledge as a researcher and practicing occupational therapist as well as an individual person outside these contexts and used this knowledge for critical reflection. During the entire research process, it became clear that there was space for both roles of the author, as they were relevant depending on the situation and at the same time, there was an increase in knowledge for both activity profiles.

3.3.5. Enabling New Spaces

Even though the project was initiated and led by the author, no new dependencies were created [5] (p. 69). Instead, a temporary space for exchange, getting to know each other and mutual appreciation was created, which had not existed before. The co-researchers lived in various districts of Berlin, in their own apartments or shared apartments, usually with little or no social contact outside their regular help or family system. During the group meetings, they were able to experience that they were not alone with their everyday problems. They supported each other at the meetings when, for example, a person with aphasia and/or apraxia of speech could not find the words. At the beginning of the meetings, they greeted each other warmly and inquired about each other's well-being. Some exchanged contact addresses. The sense of belonging to the project and the feeling of "we" among each other increased significantly during the meetings. To what extent the exchange among each other was continued after the end of the research project is not clear. Some co-researchers meet irregularly in other contexts (regulars' tables, parties at the former rehabilitation facility). The author has kept loose contact to the co-researchers, in case of requests for project presentation she forwards them to all co-researchers.

Each co-researcher decided for him/herself how long he/she would participate in the research project: for example, one co-researcher decided after the first exhibition that this was the end of the project for her and that she did not want to participate in further events. The author received further offers to make the results available to a wider audience in the form of exhibitions. She decided to do this only with the consent of the co-researchers and their participation (at least one person), so that it would remain a joint project also in the presentation and not become a pure end in itself.

The personal experiences presented here intend to illustrate that a participatory research project with persons with diverse impairments (cognitive, communication and mobility) rests on many preconditions and that pre-existing personal relationships and specific professional competencies play an important role in the implementation of such a project. At the same time, persons interested in participatory research are invited to engage in the critical reflection of their own competences in the preparation and during the research process. Furthermore, prospective scientists from the therapeutic and social professions are encouraged to consciously use their professional background for this research approach.

3.4. Towards Participation for Nurses in the Realization of New Professional Roles in Community Care: Workshops with Stakeholders as a Pilot Project by the author Doris Arnold

3.4.1. Introduction

The realization of participatory research projects in which participants take an active part in the research process as co-researchers depends on many conditions. This sums up my experiences in a research project on the development of expanded professional roles for nurses in community care for persons with dementia, which was carried out in the final phase of the project "E to the power of B—Nursing and Health", funded by the German Ministry of Education and Research. The original plan was to conduct a participatory project with participation of research participants as co-researchers [43]. However, we found that participation in research requires time and resources that were not available at that point. Thus, we carried out a pilot project to create the conditions necessary for the realization of meaningful participation in a subsequent participatory research project.

I acted as primary researcher in the pilot project, who planned the research process, conducted workshops employing focus groups together with colleagues from the project "E to the power of B—Nursing and Health" and interpreted the findings. The workshops aimed, firstly, at the design of a new professional role for experienced nurses who are qualified through a certificate program on extended community nursing practice for persons with dementia, and secondly, the identification of ways for financing these extended nursing tasks. Participants of the workshops were experienced nurses, who had attended the certificate program and other stakeholders in community care and health insurance.

In the following, the context of the project "E to the power of B—Nursing and Health" is initially described. The limiting circumstances that led to the decision to abandon the plan to use a participative approach and to implement the pilot project instead, consisting of three focus groups and its differences to participatory research are explained. Finally, the intended subsequent participatory project is briefly introduced.

3.4.2. The Background: The Project "E to the Power of B—Nursing and Health"

The certificate program "Care Strategies and Psychosocial Support for Living with Dementia at Home" [44] is as a scientific continuing education program developed and tested in the project "E to the power of B—Nursing and Health", which was funded as part of a government initiative aimed at the development of continuing academic education in German Universities. Academic education in German nursing still is very poor in all sectors, with only about one percent of nurses working in direct patient care in German teaching hospitals holding academic degrees [45].

The focus of the project was to develop, test and sustainably establish scientific continuous education for experienced nurses, who represent a non-traditional target group for academic education in Germany. An important argument for the approval of the funding for the originally planned participatory project was that the implementation of a new professional role for graduates in community nursing may contribute substantially to the sustainability of the certificate program. The development of the certificate program was based on the results of a comprehensive assessment of needs in community care and in further education for nurses [46,47]. It qualifies professionally experienced nurses to systematically evaluate, understand and answer the needs of persons with dementia who show so-called challenging behavior, as well as the needs of their family caregivers, based on a person-centered approach [44]. Thus, on one hand, the results of the needs assessment point to the need for extended tasks in caring for persons with dementia living at home, that should be carried out by appropriately trained nurses. On the other hand, these tasks had not yet been realized in the practice of community care and had not been financed accordingly. Given this background, the aim of the research was to identify and overcome challenges for implementing expanded nursing care for persons with dementia by drawing on the knowledge of nurses experienced in community nursing, who attended the certificate program, and that of other relevant stakeholders in community nursing and financing of health care. However, even though initially a participatory research project aiming at the implementation of expanded community care for persons with dementia appeared to be the most suitable approach, it quickly became clear that the tight time span of the overall project as a third-party funded project severely limited the possibilities for more extensive participation in a joint research process. For example, due to the limited time for appropriate advertising, relatively few nurses working in community nursing services could be recruited to participate in the piloting of the certificate program on dementia in community care. Therefore, it was not possible to involve the community nursing services in which the participants were employed as care professionals in the project to a sufficient extend. The original plan intended the establishment of local working groups, in which participation of nurses who had attended the certificate program and other local stakeholders as co-researchers in focus groups should be facilitated [43].

In the ultimately realized pilot project, only an involvement of participants was achieved, and its goals were limited to gaining more knowledge about what new, expanded professional roles and tasks for scientifically trained nursing professionals in community nursing services could look like in the context of dementia care and how this can be financed as a first step. This should be followed in a second step by a participatory project aimed at the implementation and evaluation of this expanded nursing role in community care, which is planned as a separate project.

3.4.3. The Pilot Project: Opportunities for Participation and Barriers to Participation in the Research Process

The pilot project finally comprised three workshops with focus group discussions with different groups of relevant stakeholders: (1) graduates of the piloting of the certificate program, (2) nursing service managers (PDLs) and managing directors of community nursing services, and (3) experts on the financing of community nursing care [48].

The project used qualitative research methods that allowed participants to be involved in some research activities but remained in the realm of involvement and did not allow for active co-operation in research activities and decision-making as co-researchers. Thus, the method of data collection in focus groups [49,50] offered the participants the opportunity to set their own priorities. As results of the individual focus groups, summary protocols were prepared, oriented on the procedure of qualitative content analysis [51]. Protocols were sent to participants with an invitation for feedback, so that they had the opportunity both to check on their contributions represented in the data and to make additions. In the second and third workshops, the available findings from each of the previous workshops were presented at the beginning. In this way, the cyclical process of participatory research was to some extend included in the procedure [40,52,53].

As mentioned, active participation of participants as co-researchers or shared decision-making in the research process could not be implemented in the workshops [14]. Participants did not participate actively as co-researchers in data collection and analysis and were not involved to any significant extent in the publication of the results. Most participants of all three workshops contributed with their respective valuable expert knowledge to the research process, as is usual in the context of qualitative research, and only a few persons participated in feedback. This gave them the opportunity to read and check their own contributions to the discussion in the form of "member checks".

However, some participants did mention a direct interest in the planned implementation project: for example, one nurse who had attended the certificate program was interested in implementing such a project in her community nursing service, and individual nursing managers expressed a special interest in the project. In this way, important contacts in the field were made, which can be followed up in the implementation project. In the workshop on financing, further specific considerations on the subsequent research project were discussed with the representatives of a nursing care insurance company and of a provider of community nursing services. At their suggestion, the planned model project will include two subprojects: The participatory implementation project and evaluation project that should provide evidence for the efficiency of the new nursing role. Thus, this also created substantial contributions that provide a sound basis for the future second step.

3.4.4. Evaluation, Outlook, and Thoughts on Participatory Research

In retrospect, the implementation of the workshops with focus groups within the limited conditions of a third-party funded project seems justified. On the one hand, it was necessary to forego the creation of additional possibilities for the participation of participatory researchers. On the other hand, meaningful first drafts for an extended professional role of a "dementia consultant in community care" and its activities were developed with comparatively little effort. Most significantly, a first proposal for financing these extended nursing tasks was drafted together with the representatives of a nursing care insurance company. It was particularly important that the cooperation with the respective participants at the workshops was as transparent and respectful as possible. We asked the respective actors to provide their expert knowledge for a specific goal and offered them opportunities for feedback and thus also for control over their data.

I have continued to maintain contact with three participants, who have expressed a special interest in further cooperation: one nurse who attended the certificate program, one contact person in a nursing care insurance company and one representative of a provider of community nursing services. To these persons, I have sent publications that I wrote about the project, and hope that the plans for the envisaged future participatory implementation project can be realized, in which I would then like to work more intensively with them.

The results of the workshops as a pilot project represent nothing more, but also nothing less than important prerequisites for the planned participatory implementation project –provided suitable funding can be obtained. Then, the research team would work in close cooperation with individual community nursing services. Nurses working in teams of community nursing services would be trained in the next certificate program offered and subsequently work together with the researchers as central actors and co-researchers. In doing so, they would lead the research and development process in implementing this new nursing role in their community nursing services in collaboration with other key stakeholders. Most importantly, among these stakeholders should be persons with dementia and their caregivers acting as co-researchers, as their health and wellbeing is in the focus of the expanded nursing tasks of the future consultants for dementia in community care. In this future project context, active participation of all co-researchers in all parts of the research process on an equal basis is not only plausible but is also indispensable.

However, there are still some hurdles to overcome before that project can be realized. The biggest of these is the acquisition of funding, for which it is helpful to be able to refer to the results of the pilot study. On the other hand, community nursing services whose managers support this project must be recruited. Most importantly, individual nurses who work in these facilities, and who are interested in participating in the certificate program and in becoming co-researchers in the participatory research project must be found.

In the planned participatory project, empowerment as an emancipatory moment of participatory research is not intended for clients of health care in the first place, even though their wellbeing is the aim of the nursing care in question. Rather, that project is an example of participatory practitioner research, and nurses as professionals and employees of community nursing services are central actors and therefore, they are the persons who are to be empowered to change their professional role as nurses. As mentioned above, persons with dementia and their family caregivers, should also be encouraged to participate actively as co-researchers. This means that their voices should also be heard and their perspectives on problems should be made visible, but they are not the in the focus of the project. Rather, the implementation of a new professional role for scientifically trained nurses is closely linked to an organizational development process [3] within community nursing services as service providers.

3.5. Approaches to Participation in the DIPEx Project on Illness Experiences Based on Narratives from the Patient's Perspective by Author Andrea Glässel

3.5.1. Introduction

On the one hand, the implementation and success of participatory approaches in research projects holds great potential in terms of joint development and learning from and with each other and shaping the research process. On the other hand, these participatory elements that hold promising potential pose difficulties to implement in research practice and can sometimes be demanding for researchers and participants involved. The participants in the project are in this case, patients. For them, as well as for the researchers, the research process, and the building of the relationship between researchers and participants, are characterized by different challenges and expectations. Based on a current research project, which focuses on experiences of and perspectives on the experience of health and illness by means of narrative interviews, this example would like to show experiences from the perspective of the researchers on participatory elements within the shared process experience and relationship design. In this context, individual elements of participatory research are integrated at various points within the research process. This contrasts with an approach to participatory health research, as described by the ICPHR with the goal "to maximize the participation of those whose life or work is the subject of the research in all stages of the research process" [15] (p. 6).

3.5.2. Presentation and Introduction to the "DIPEx" Project

The Swiss project DIPEx.ch is short for Database of Individual Patients' Experiences and is a national database for individual patient experiences based on narratives from the patient's or affected person's perspectives on health and illness (www.DIPEx.ch, (accessed on 26 July 2022)). This approach of building a national database was developed at Oxford University in 2000 as a pioneering project with direct patient participation, in which patients and their experiences were at the center as experts and thus given a public voice for the first time. Since then, international, and German-language participatory research and the possibilities of empowerment, participatory co-design, on the one hand, and the reception habits of users, on the other hand, have developed further due to digitalization (Web 2.0/social media), as shown by approaches to experienced-based co-design procedures and integrating a participatory approach [54].

The database contains a systematic and methodological collection of narratives on the subjective experience of illness and health from the perspective of those affected, as patients and/or as relatives. The guiding questions of the project are: "What do persons experience when they suffer from a serious illness or health condition? What experiences do they have as patients in doctors' and health professionals' offices, or hospitals? How do they cope with their everyday life with the restrictions caused by their illness, new functioning and changed health situation? What kind of support do they find helpful and where would they like to see more services? What problems, questions or answers do patients have that doctors, therapists, nurses or researchers may not yet have in mind?" and other questions.

The DIPEx project was designed to present excerpts of real patient narratives on the topic of multiple sclerosis (MS) as an example, on the website in the form of video, audio, or text excerpts. This includes a systematic collection and analysis of interviews about the individual experiences, descriptions of the emotional experience, allows insights into the biography, as well as into the everyday experience, or to different forms of treatment and more. In addition, information on self-help groups and other materials, including links to answers to participants' questions, are provided.

At this point, according to Bergold and Thomas [55], the association to participatory research becomes apparent. Without participation in research, "DIPEx" cannot be implemented. It takes place "together with the persons directly affected and aims at reconstructing their knowledge and skills in a process of self-understanding and empowerment. The majority of these are vulnerable groups of the population whose perspectives and voices are otherwise rarely included and who themselves hardly have the opportunity to justifiably introduce and assert their interests" [49] (pp. 7–8, translation by the authors). To be vulnerable because of the disease process, which demands its very own attention, which requires different or new daily structures, under which one's own participation and involvement raises the question: As a patient and/or family member, do I want to belong to this group at all and/or actively confront this difficult topic?

DIPEx Switzerland (www.dipex.ch, (accessed on 26 July 2022)) is an interdisciplinary group of researchers at the Institute of Biomedical Ethics and Medical History (IBME) of the University of Zurich and its partner the Zurich University of Applied Sciences (ZHAW) at the Department of Health Sciences. It is both integrated into a Swiss-wide network of partners in health care and a member of the international umbrella organization DIPEx International (www.dipexinternational.org, (accessed on 26 July 2022)). The network currently includes 14 countries with national websites for the UK (www.healthtalk.org, (accessed on 26 July 2022)), Germany (www.krankheitserfahrungen.de, (accessed on 26 July 2022)), or www.healthexperiencesusa.org, (accessed on 26 July 2022) in the US and others. These national databases follow the long-established qualitative research methodology set out in the Handbook of the Health Experience Research Group (HERG), Department of Primary Health Care, University of Oxford. The publication of real patient narratives in DIPEx follows the HON criteria (Health on the Net Code) and as a freely accessible resource, it forms an important support for patients, relatives, clinicians in training as well as teachers in the health professions and for research. Studies could show that patient narratives can have an impact on the individual experience of illness, but also on health policy, and on affected individuals reconsidering their own approach to illness, as when reading the German DIPEx website [25,56–58]. Drewniak, Glässel, Hodel, and Biller-Andorno [59] were able to show that access to individual experience is perceived as relevant support and can positively influence the empowerment of patients regarding disease management. The findings of Fadlallah et al. [60] suggest that, in addition to individual inspirational and empowerment effects, illness narratives can also serve as educational and awareness-raising tools of the political discourse on illnesses or health. The strength of individual patient narratives is also invoked by the 2018 European Report for Health, entitled "More than Numbers" (WHO). It calls for individual patient narratives to serve as illustrations alongside statistical information and facts, to strengthen the understanding of health, and to be specifically included in the formation of health literacy in the population [57].

3.5.3. Experiences on the Implementation of Participatory Elements within the DIPEx Project

The DIPEx project follows a qualitative study design according to the HERG manual, which DIPEx members are taught during mandatory training. This training is a prerequisite for the research groups to obtain a national DIPEx license. The DIPEx Switzerland project is conducted according to the principles of the Declaration of Helsinki [61] and received Swiss-wide approval from the cantonal ethics committee with the number BASEC Req-Nr. 2018-00050.

The procedure for the survey of lived experiences of patients with MS was methodologically based on a phenomenological approach using narrative and semi-structured interviews, which are based on the sampling strategy of maximum variation. Possibilities for limited participation or involvement of the patients in the research process become apparent in this approach, such as the fact that the participants are given a lot of space to set their own priorities within the narrative interviews. Some of the interviewees saw this as an opportunity to stimulate conversation and to be able to recount their experiences in depth from their own perspective. At the same time, it was precisely this open form of narration and of setting one's own focus that was experienced as challenging by other interviewees. These persons found the guiding questions by the researchers to be relieving and helpful. They helped to structure the narrative of their experience and their thoughts along the questions so that they could communicate more easily. In this interactive event of the first personal contact and encounter, the researcher is challenged to establish a relationship level conducive to conversation as a basis for the interview immediately and to convey an open and approachable attitude.

To create an atmosphere that was as natural as possible and that stimulated the conversation, the interviews were conducted in everyday language and recorded with video and audio. Verbatim transcripts were prepared using established rules for transcription as a basis for evaluating the interviews. Transcripts were sent to the participants by mail with the request for feedback, so that they had the opportunity for transparency about their data and statements as well as for additions. From the researcher's perspective, this type of participation or involvement in the research process revealed a great deal of ambivalence among respondents regarding (a) reading their own story and experience of illness and (b) reading their own linguistic expression. Reliving one's own story again and yet anew via the written discussion requires a deeper engagement with oneself. The personal state of mind and feeling in this situation of narration is due to the moment and to the atmosphere of the conversation with the interviewer. It thus also acquires a temporal and very personal, emotionally individual, even partly intimate dimension. Reading one's own transcript is not only about reading and correcting a statement or coherence of content. It is also a moment of reflection and awareness of emotional vulnerability and deep illness reflection [56].

Reading one's own language, formulation, and expression in everyday language or in a modified form of one's own dialect partly triggered a great discomfort, a defense, a confrontation with the statements produced in spontaneous speech, the text. Despite assurances by the interviewer that it was normal for spontaneous speech to be grammatically incorrect, that a spoken word did not correspond to a written word, this discomfort arose in some of the participants. The same applies to the unfamiliar text format of a transcript with special characters, although the researchers announced in advance the rather special text format, which does not conform to everyday speech, compared to linguistically polished texts in journals or books. As shown by Lucius-Hoene et al. [56]: the transcript aroused astonishment to the point of horror in the patients about the unfamiliar confrontation with what was said in the text's own language. The statement of one patient: "When I received the first written excerpt from what I had said, I was first of all shocked at myself and said, 'Is that how I present myself? What did I say? The way it was written, that's how I speak? That is terrible and that is not possible" [56] (p.199).

The feedback of the data to the interviewees is intended as a participatory element in this process and is perceived as a balancing act from the researcher's point of view. It requires an examination of one's own research contribution and a balanced relationship of closeness and distance between the researcher and the participants. Participation addresses the relationship between the researchers and the participants, including the researched objects about which they generate knowledge, and that new knowledge already emerges in relation to the discussion of this relationship within the research process. The design of this relationship level influences the handling of the data and information and thus in turn the participation and further development in the project.

As already described in Altrichter and Gstettner [5] (p. 68), the claim of participation with a symmetrical dialogue situation and cooperative research of researchers and participants in practice is presuppositional and is only conditionally achievable due to limited framework conditions in research to invest in this relational work. This form of relational work also often does not meet the expectations of research from the perspective of both researchers and participants. In our experience, participants in DIPEx do not expect researchers continuing in the role to maintain contact after the interview until the transcripts are received or the experiential posts and narratives are unlocked on the website. In the run-up to the interview, detailed information about the project was provided and the subsequent steps described were outlined. Nevertheless, according to previous experience, it was only partially possible to sufficiently convey the feedback of the data to the interviewees or to alleviate or even dispel concerns about it. This means for the research practice that cooperation and a form of co-production is in principle intended. In the design of the roles, however, this co-production in the sense of a participatory procedure usually succeeds only inadequately with rather one-sided role differentiation. The imbalance consists in the fact that the researchers have more experience about research-related circumstances and do not question the unusual format of a transcript further but regard it as part of the methodological procedure. At the same time, researchers themselves have usually never or rarely been in the situation where their own statements were written down in everyday language and had to be proofread by them with the knowledge that parts of them would be published. This creates an imbalance that does not promote true participation in the sense of sharing. In principle, mutual learning is possible, but the gain in knowledge is not visible to the participants in the same form or elaborated accordingly within this rule-governed research process [5].

3.5.4. Thoughts on Participatory Research and Outlook

With a self-critical view of the participatory element described in this project, the "intended level of participation" of the participants was rather limited. Sharing the experience: Yes, and gladly! But more participation is not needed. In this case, the intended project design with the goal of a high level of participation demanded more from the persons involved than they were willing or able to contribute, and thus also made limits clear.

In the further research process of the DIPEx project, other participatory elements can be identified, such as the advisory group, which is composed of different persons including patients. Based on this abbreviated insight into the DIPEx project, this approach cannot be further demonstrated. With reference to the chance of improving participation within the DIPEx project, the possibilities for an improved participatory and co-creative co-design of the personal contributions on the website are currently being investigated within the framework of a participatory project, to prospectively strengthen the project through participation in the form of participation and to work out its potential in a co-creative process.

4. Discussion

Based on the four examples presented, our central concern is to identify, name and reflect on the numerous factors that influenced the course of the concrete projects in their respective contexts in order to further the development of participatory research. In the following, we discuss these factors in relation to the shaping of relationships and the level of participation achieved and highlight both the various success factors and the challenges in participatory research processes.

4.1. Building Trusting Relationships in Participatory Research Processes

The experiences and reflections from the four projects described here show that the establishment of trusting relationships between academics as researchers and other research participants is a central element and a foundation for the success of a participatory project, as is shown in other research about CBPR [13]. At the same time, it is evident that this process has taken up different amounts of space, time, and weight in the four projects. While in the projects PaSuMi (Navina Sarma) and "Back into Life" (Tabea Böttger), trusting relationships between and among the research participants and the research initiator or the project coordinators existed in part already before the start of the project, these were initiated in the "Workshops" (Doris Arnold) and DIPEx (Andrea Glässel) only during the project. In the descriptions of the PaSuMi and "Back to Life" projects it becomes clear how access to the desired target group, the persons, and institutions relevant to the research in each case was facilitated by already established trusting relationships. Thus, various migrant individuals and groups and persons with severe stroke could be successfully involved, while in the "Workshops" the lack of existing relationships and networking also limited access to nurses in community nursing services and thus their recruitment for participation in the research project. Building these relationships would have required significantly more time and effort than was feasible under the conditions of the externally funded project. This observation applies to DIPEx, where in-depth work on building relationship with participants was only possible to a limited extent given the external condition of a one-off interview. This underlines limitations posed by deadlines of funded projects that cause too little time and resources to facilitate more than tokenistic participation in applied health research mentioned by Green and Johns [9].

In the context of CBPR, the need to work and reflect on the positionality of researchers when building trust with members of marginalized communities has been shown [12,19]. Similarly, despite partly pre-existing relationships in the PaSuMi and "Back into Life" projects, the new kind of cooperation as partners had to be negotiated to overcome problems with positionality in previously existing hierarchically structured power relationships in the respective work contexts. This grew gradually during the project, primarily through sufficient sensitivity, knowledge, and openness to the different realities of life and experiences made, as well as in encounters outside the joint working meetings. Both authors describe how opportunities were created for activities desired by the research participants outside the originally planned joint working meetings repeatedly. Thus, also concerns of the persons involved, which at first glance had nothing to do with the goal of the research project, were considered. According to Navina Sarma and Tabea Böttger, formulating and dealing with (personal) needs of research partners was part of the participatory process and supported trust building.

To what extent are these activities to be understood as a necessary part of participatory research? Or, to what extent do they reveal to us, the "primary researchers", in which everyday issues individuals have perhaps received too little support so far and/or that they do not know where they should turn, for example, to look for work clothes for internships? Do existing grievances show up more clearly, or at all, in participatory research projects due to the existing trusting relationship? And how do the project initiators deal with this?

Our experiences have led us to enter into participatory projects with the knowledge that, precisely because relationships and trust are there, situations will arise in which we will act as individual persons and not as scientists. To which extent and how much private time is invested for this purpose is a matter for discussion and individual decision.

The PaSuMi and "Back to Life" projects make it clear that, in addition to pre-existing relationships, the number of joint working meetings over a longer period contributed significantly to relationship building. Neither was the case in the other two projects: in the "workshops" there were one-time meetings with the respective group to conduct the focus groups; in DIPEx there was also only one meeting each to establish contact and conduct interviews—partly initiated while planning and arranging the interviews—by e-mail or telephone or through mediating contact persons. Based on the projects described above and their progress, it becomes clear that a person initiating the research with already existing long-standing, close contacts to a group of co-researchers has much more far-reaching possibilities to establish sustainable relationships in the research process. The form in which relationships are established also has to do, among other things, with the question of the form in which the methods used are (or can be) designed to be participatory.

Another influencing factor is our own understanding of our roles as researchers or project initiators, which we bring with us and live out in the projects. Some of us see ourselves as impulse givers, activists, or perhaps see themselves as practice partners, or move back and forth in double roles between therapy and science. The experiences in the PaSuMi and "Back to Life" projects show that the collaboration with the respective research participants can result in a sustainable relationship if we as academics disclose the different preconditions in the research team and at the same time focus on the necessity of the different backgrounds of experience for the common interest of creating knowledge. The disclosure of different preconditions and interests can result in the consequence of distributing tasks and responsibilities differently in the project team depending on the research step and allowing non-participation. For example, Tabea Böttger in "Back into Life" wrote down the results of the group discussion alone in a text form based on the jointly determined categories from the evaluation meetings and submitted these to the persons involved for proofreading before publication in her qualification thesis. Just like Doris Arnold in the "Workshops" and Andrea Glässel in DIPEx, she did not receive feedback from all persons involved in the desired Member Check. This also became apparent in the DIPEx project based on the question: May, or should or even must the standardized procedure of the Member Check by counter-reading the interview transcripts, as required in the method manual, be deviated from, if it does not correspond to the individual needs of the individual persons, as suggested in the contribution by Andrea Glässel? The method manual is seen as a helpful, quality-assuring basis for a common approach, especially for a cross-national research project. At the same time, it should open space for project-related experiences, so that on both sides, the researchers as well as the participants, positive or at least satisfactory experiences are not subsequently overlaid by negative experiences, which the researchers can only influence to a limited extent, as they cannot satisfactorily accompany the process of reading and dealing with the transcript in certain situations. It becomes clear that a standardized approach without allowing for individual nuances cannot meet or even contradicts the demands of participatory research.

4.2. Participation in the Area of Tension between Time and Dosage

At the end of the project, the question arose for all four projects about to how to deal with relationships that had arisen in the context of the research project.

With whom do I maintain contact and with what intensity? What criteria do I use to decide this matter? Does it play a central role whether, at the time of termination, I have already planned a future research project involving the persons involved (Doris Arnold)? Or do I continue the established relationships because of a personal bond ("friends"/Navina Sarma) has developed? What responsibility do I carry as project initiator or researcher? Was I able to initiate positive developments and avoid the emergence of new dependencies by creating a common space of exchange and support?

It is clear from the PaSuMi and "Back to Life" projects that new networks for mutual support had formed among the persons involved—independently of the academic coordinators. It remains to be seen to what extent these new networks will become permanent in the long term or to what extent research participants may feel abandoned if there is no further regular contact after completion.

From the point of view of the "workshops" and the DIPEx project, on the other hand, it is important to bear in mind that participants in these research projects only wanted to be contacted with queries to a certain extent, as the persons in these projects were able and wanted to make an individually limited commitment for their participation. On the one hand, concerning the design of the research relationship, the question arises here of the individual "dosage" of involvement or participation or of closeness and distance in this relationship. Participants and researchers have different perceptions and needs in this regard. These needs must be made transparent and must be reflected upon individually in participatory research. This was done, for example, in the "Back to Life" project. However, unlike in conventional, positivist/post-positivist research, participatory researchers cannot retreat to their scientific distance.

On the other hand, it should be borne in mind that the research participants' involvement in all four of the research projects presented required a different amount of time and effort. In the PaSuMi project, for example, community partners were also paid an expense allowance. Thus, in the participatory follow-up project to the "workshops", it will be necessary to finance payment for the time spent on research activities as working time for the participating nurses in outpatient services or finance compensation for expenses for family caregivers (for persons to stand in for their care responsibilities) to enable their reliable participation in the research process. This is because these persons make a very similar and important contribution to data collection and analysis or to development processes as the researchers and can therefore also expect a payment in return that seems appropriate to them [27].

4.3. Understand Participation as a Two-Way Process That Requires Adjustments

An important potential of participatory research is to make voices audible or to make realities visible from the perspective of actors of groups that are often not heard clearly enough in public and scientific discourse [18]. In the DIPEx project, the researchers' intention was to present the lifeworld and reality of persons affected by chronic illnesses from their own perspective and to give them the opportunity to have their say. However, the counter-reading of transcripts in the form of "Member Checks" was sometimes perceived by the participants as excessive and the reading of these texts, which arise from spoken language and cannot be compared with texts that are grammatically well formulated word for word in writing [62], caused discomfort for some respondents. Even the presented explanation and preparation for the unusual format of transcripts could only absorb this impression to a limited extent. An intensive examination of one's own illness experience, sometimes written over 30 to 60 pages, can be emotionally and cognitively demanding, or even overwhelming for respondents [63]. From a research ethics perspective, there is also the question of the researcher's responsibility to critically examine the procedure recommended in the methods manual for reasonableness [64]. Thus, the fact that those involved in the research did not want their voices heard and read in the way suggested to them became a problem in the DIPEx project, contrary to the intentions of the researchers.

The researchers in the DIPEx project would also like to avoid irritations of this kind among the participants in the future, so that the moment of the interview, which was experienced as positive, is not overshadowed negatively afterwards. Therefore, alternative approaches are currently being investigated in a participatory project with DIPEx participants. In this context, an "experienced-based co-design" [54] was used, which provided for participatory action and would give the participants options to determine the personally feasible level of participation. A possible suggestion for this could be to discuss selected text passages from the transcripts with the participants, which could be considered for publication on the website.

In contrast, the co-researchers in the project "Back into Life" presented their view of their reality by not only taking and discussing the photos, but also as independent actors and thus participated actively in the dissemination of the research findings. In the PaSuMi project, community partners took the space that was provided by the participatory approach to participate and shape the common project goal, but also to develop their personal skills and to manage their everyday life. Empowerment took place through the participants themselves and participatory research can help to recognize, activate, and use one's own resources.

In the "workshops", the participating actors contributed their respective expert knowledge to the research process. However, their involvement was limited to checking and, to a limited extend, to deciding whether their voices were heard and represented adequately. However, this did not enable them to participate in the research actively as co-researchers. The original plan for this project envisioned an approach more closely aligned with participatory research, which ultimately could not be implemented. More to the point, the initially intended involvement of participants in data analysis would ultimately have entailed the risk of mere tokenistic participation [9]. Because of the very limited time available, the participation would have had more the character of "assistance with research activities" without, however, opening sufficient possibilities for shared decision making in the research process, which was not possible under these circumstances.

5. Conclusions

The four research projects presented in this article provide a critical examination of the construction of relationships and of power dynamics in research processes that facilitated or limited possibilities for participation. These opportunities rested on different preconditions and resulted in different evaluations and experiences of researchers.

Relationships may take very different forms but remain the essential element of participatory research processes, where those persons who are at the center of research must have the opportunity to contribute their own experiences and perspectives to the research process on an equal basis. Thus, the distinctive features of participatory approaches are not only the democratic design of the research process itself but also their contribution for empowering the persons involved to overcome discriminating living conditions or hierarchically structured power dynamics in their lives.

The prerequisite for this is that persons representing science and practice see themselves equally as learners in the research process to be able to share their questions and uncertainties as well as to engage in joint reflection. Different expectations on both sides, different levels, and kinds of knowledge as well as issues of power or individual interests and goals can thus be taken up and dealt with.

In this article, scientists from different health professions acting in different research contexts shared, discussed, and reflected on their respective experiences with participative research to provide opportunities for other researchers to reflect on their own past and future research.

The practical implication of the article lies above all in the recognition that the critical self-reflection of participatory research processes prevents misinterpretations, provides deeper insights, and facilitates processes of change for everyone involved.

Author Contributions: The manuscript was developed in a collaborative process with all authors commenting mutually on each other's contribution up to the finalization of the manuscript. P.N. and A.B. initiated the process and shared the idea for the first conception of the text. Both wrote the introductory chapter on participatory research that represents the foundation for the article. Within the initial writing phase, facilitation for the collective writing process passed to D.A. and A.G. Within a collaborative writing and reflection process by all authors, they coordinated the collective revision of the article with thematic focus on power and research relationships during several commenting loops. D.A. wrote the methods chapter. A.G. integrated the introduction to the project contributions, and the text components framing the manuscript. D.A., T.B., A.G. and N.S. (in alphabetical order) contributed the project examples to the manuscript. The project examples went through multiple feedback loops by all authors. T.B. wrote the draft for the discussion chapter and integrated the arguments of the respective authors with reference to their project examples. P.N. rounded off the manuscript with concluding thoughts. All authors contributed with substantial comments to the final version of the overall manuscript. All authors have read and agreed to the published version of the manuscript.

Funding: The project of writing this manuscript received no external funding.

Institutional Review Board Statement: Not applicable. This article reflects on researcher experiences and does not report research results.

Informed Consent Statement: Not applicable. This article reflects on researcher experiences and does not report research results.

Data Availability Statement: Not applicable.

Acknowledgments: We would like to thank our colleagues Tanja Gangarova, Maike Grube, Inka Kleinecke and Stefan Paulus from the ICPHR Training in Participatory Health Research program in 2018 at the Catholic University of Applied Sciences, Berlin, who have supported us significantly with their critical feedback and comments on the manuscript.

Conflicts of Interest: The authors declare no conflict of interest. The project of writing this manuscript was not funded by third parties.

References

1. Narimani, P.; Wright, M.T. Partizipation in der Gesundheitsförderung und Prävention mit Migrant*innen. In *Handbuch Migration und Gesundheit.Grundlagen, Perspektiven und Strategien*; Spallek, J., Zeeb, H., Eds.; Hogrefe: Bern, Switzerland, 2021; pp. 445–453. ISBN 9783456859958.
2. Narimani, P. Dilemmas in the (anti-discriminatory) communication of migration-related research results. Consideration from the point of view of the practice researcher with participatory claim. In Proceedings of the Lecture at the Congress Poverty & Health, Berlin, Germany, 14–15 March 2019.
3. Bethmann, A.; Hilgenböcker, E.; Wright, M.T. Partizipative Qualitätsentwicklung in der Prävention und Gesundheitsförderung. In *Prävention und Gesundheitsförderung*; Tiemann, M., Mohokum, M., Eds.; Springer: Berlin/Heidelberg, Germany, 2021; pp. 1083–1095. ISBN 978-3-662-62425-8.
4. Wright, M.T.; Burtscher, R.; Wihofszky, P. PartKommPlus: German Research Consortium for Health Communities-New Developments and Challenges for Participatroy Health Research in Germany. In *Participatory Health Research: Voices from around the World*; Wright, M.T., Kongats, K., Eds.; Springer: Berlin/Heidelberg, Germany, 2018; pp. 117–126.
5. Altrichter, H.; Gstettner, P. Aktionsforschung-ein abgeschlossenes Kapitel in der Geschichte der deutschen Sozialwissenschaft? *Soz. Lit.-Rundsch.* **1993**, *16*, 67–83.
6. Altrichter, H.; Gstettner, P. Action Research: A closed chapter in the history of German social science? *Educ. Action Res.* **1993**, *1*, 329–360. [CrossRef]
7. Bethmann, A.; Behrisch, B.; Peter, S. Förder-und Rahmenbedingungen für Partizipative Gesundheitsforschung aus Projektsicht. *Bundesgesundh. Gesundh. Gesundh.* **2021**, *64*, 223–229. [CrossRef] [PubMed]
8. Von Peter, S.; Bär, G.; Behrisch, B.; Bethmann, A.; Hartung, S.; Kasberg, A.; Wulff, I.; Wright, M. Partizipative Gesundheitsforschung in Deutschland—Quo vadis? *Das Gesundh.* **2020**, *82*, 328–332. [CrossRef] [PubMed]
9. Green, G.; Johns, T. Exploring the Relationship (and Power Dynamic) Between Researchers and Public Partners Working Together in Applied Health Research Teams. *Front. Sociol.* **2019**, *4*, 20. [CrossRef] [PubMed]
10. Egid, B.R.; Roura, M.; Aktar, B.; Quach, J.A.; Chumo, I.; Dias, S.; Hegel, G.; Jones, L.; Karuga, R.; Lar, L.; et al. 'You want to deal with power while riding on power': Global perspectives on power in participatory health research and co-production approaches. *BMJ Glob. Health* **2021**, *6*, e006978. [CrossRef] [PubMed]
11. Smith, L.; Bratini, L.; Chambers, D.-A.; Jensen, R.V.; Romero, L. Between idealism and reality: Meeting the challenges of participatory action research. *Action Res.* **2010**, *8*, 407–425. [CrossRef]
12. Muhammad, M.; Wallerstein, N.; Sussman, A.L.; Avila, M.; Belone, L.; Duran, B. Reflections on Researcher Identity and Power: The Impact of Positionality on Community Based Participatory Research (CBPR) Processes and Outcomes. *Crit. Sociol.* **2015**, *41*, 1045–1063. [CrossRef]
13. Jagosh, J.; Bush, P.L.; Salsberg, J.; Macaulay, A.C.; Greenhalgh, T.; Wong, G.; Cargo, M.; Green, L.W.; Herbert, C.P.; Pluye, P. A realist evaluation of community-based participatory research: Partnership synergy, trust building and related ripple effects. *BMC Public Health* **2015**, *15*, 725. [CrossRef]
14. PartNet. PartNet-Diskussionspapier: Beteiligte an Partizipativer Gesundheitsforschung. Available online: https://opus4.kobv.de/opus4-ash/frontdoor/index/index/searchtype/latest/docId/475/start/0/rows/10 (accessed on 26 July 2022).
15. International Collaboration for Participatory Health Research. Position Paper 1: What is Participatory Health Research? *Version: Mai 2013*. 2013. Available online: https://www.academia.edu/6895905/What_is_Participatory_Health_Research? (accessed on 26 July 2022).
16. Unger, H. Partizipative Gesundheitsforschung: Wer partizipiert woran? *Particip. Qual. Res.* **2012**, *13*, 1. [CrossRef]
17. Arnold, D. *"Aber Ich Muss ja Meine Arbeit Schaffen!": Ein Ethnografischer Blick auf den Alltag im Frauenberuf Pflege*; Mabuse: Frankfurt am Main, Germany, 2008; ISBN 9783940529343.
18. Fine, M.; Torre, M.E. Critical Participatory Action Research: A Feminist Project for Validity and Solidarity. *Psychol. Women Q.* **2019**, *43*, 433–444. [CrossRef]

19. Wallerstein, N.; Muhammad, M.; Sanchez-Youngman, S.; Rodriguez Espinosa, P.; Avila, M.; Baker, E.A.; Barnett, S.; Belone, L.; Golub, M.; Lucero, J.; et al. Power Dynamics in Community-Based Participatory Research: A Multiple-Case Study Analysis of Partnering Contexts, Histories, and Practices. *Health Educ. Behav.* **2019**, *46*, 19S–32S. [CrossRef]
20. Von Unger, H. Partizipative Forschung. In *Handbuch Interpretativ Forschen*; Akremi, L., Baur, N., Knoblauch, H., Traue, B., Eds.; Beltz Juventa: Weinheim, Germany, 2018; pp. 161–182. ISBN 3779931265.
21. Lincoln, Y.S.; Lynham, S.A.; Guba, E.G. Paradigmatic Controversies, Contradictions, and Emerging Confluences, Revisited. In *The SAGE Handbook of Qualitative Research*, 5th ed.; Denzin, N.K., Lincoln, Y.S., Eds.; Sage: Los Angeles, CA, USA, 2018; pp. 108–150. ISBN 978-1-4833-4980-0.
22. Mies, M. Methodische Postulate zur Frauenforschung. *Beiträge Zur Fem. Theor. Und Prax.* **1984**, *7*, 7–25.
23. Denzin, N.K.; Lincoln, Y.S. Introduction: The Discipline and Practice of Qualitative Research. In *The SAGE Handbook of Qualitative Research*, 5th ed.; Denzin, N.K., Lincoln, Y.S., Eds.; Sage: Los Angeles, CA, USA, 2018; pp. 1–26.
24. Haraway, D. Situated knowledges: The science question in feminism and the priviledge of partial perspective. *Fem. Stud.* **1988**, *14*, 575–599. [CrossRef]
25. Greenhalgh, T. *Einführung in Die Evidenzbasierte Medizin*, 3; Vollständig Überarbeitete Auflage; Verlag Hans Huber: Bern, Switzerland, 2015; ISBN 978-3-456-95473-8.
26. Coupland, H.; Maher, L. Clients or Colleagues? Reflections on the Process of Participatory Action Research with Young Injecting Drug Users. *Int. J. Drug Policy* **2005**, *16*, 191–198. [CrossRef]
27. Souleymanov, R.; Kuzmanović, D.; Marshall, Z.; Scheim, A.I.; Mikiki, M.; Worthington, C.; Millson, M.P. The ethics of community-based research with people who use drugs: Results of a scoping review. *BMC Med. Ethics* **2016**, *17*, 25. [CrossRef]
28. Canadian HIV/AIDS Legal Network. "Nothing about Us without Us". Greater, Meaningful Involvement of People Who Use Illegal Drugs: A Public Health, Ethical, and Human Rights Imperative; Canadian HIV/AIDS Legal Network: Montreal, QC, Canada, 2006. Available online: http://www.hivlegalnetwork.ca/site/wp-content/uploads/2013/04/Greater+Involvement+-+Bklt+-+Drug+Policy+-+ENG.pdf?lang=en (accessed on 3 June 2022).
29. Wallerstein, N.; Duran, B. Community-based participatory research contributions to intervention research: The intersection of science and practice to improve health equity. *Am. J. Public Health* **2010**, *100* (Suppl. 1), S40–S46. [CrossRef]
30. Wallerstein, N.; Duran, B. Theoretical, historical, and pratice roots of CBPR. In *Community-Based Participatory Research for Health: Advancing Social and Health Equity*, Third ed.; Wallerstein, N., Duran, B., Oetzel, J.G., Minkler, M., Eds.; Jossey-Bass a Wiley Brand: San Francisco, CA, USA, 2018; pp. 17–29. ISBN 9781119258872.
31. Böttger, T.; Dennhardt, S.; Knape, J.; Marotzki, U. "Back into life—With a power wheelchair": Learning from people with severe stroke through a participatory photovoice study in a metropolitan area in Germany. in press.
32. Wang, C.; Burris, M.A. Photovoice: Concept, methodology, and use for participatory needs assessment. *Health Educ. Behav.* **1997**, *24*, 369–387. [CrossRef]
33. Keeley, C.; Munde, V.; Schowalter, R.; Seifert, M.; Tillmann, V.; Wiegering, R. Partizipativ forschen mit Menschen mit komplexem Unterstützungsbedarf. *Teilhabe* **2019**, *58*, 96–102.
34. Bernasconi, T.; Keeley, C. Empirische Forschung mit Menschen mit schwerer und mehrfacher Behinderung. *Teilhabe* **2016**, *55*, 10–15. [CrossRef]
35. American Stroke Association. Communication Effects of Stroke. Available online: https://www.stroke.org/en/about-stroke/effects-of-stroke/cognitive-and-communication-effects-of-stroke (accessed on 26 July 2022).
36. Gillen, G.; Nilsen, D.M.; Attridge, J.; Banakos, E.; Morgan, M.; Winterbottom, L.; York, W. Effectiveness of interventions to improve occupational performance of people with cognitive impairments after stroke: An evidence-based review. *Am. J. Occup. Ther.* **2015**, *69*, 6901180040p1–6901180040p9. [CrossRef] [PubMed]
37. Balakrishnan, R.; Kaplan, B.; Negron, R.; Fei, K.; Goldfinger, J.Z.; Horowitz, C.R. Life after Stroke in an Urban Minority Population: A Photovoice Project. *Int. J. Environ. Res. Public Health* **2017**, *14*, 293. [CrossRef] [PubMed]
38. Maratos, M.; Huynh, L.; Tan, J.; Lui, J.; Jarus, T. Picture This: Exploring the Lived Experience of High-Functioning Stroke Survivors Using Photovoice. *Qual. Health Res.* **2016**, *26*, 1055–1066. [CrossRef]
39. Barclay-Goddard, R.; Ripat, J.; Mayo, N.E. Developing a model of participation post-stroke: A mixed-methods approach. *Qual. Life Res.* **2012**, *21*, 417–426. [CrossRef]
40. Unger, H. *Partizipative Forschung: Einführung in Die Forschungspraxis*; Springer: Wiesbaden, Germany, 2014; ISBN 9783658012892.
41. Sumsion, T. *Client-Centred Practice in Occupational Therapy*, 2nd ed.; Churchill Livingstone: Edinburgh, Scotland; Elsevier: New York, NY, USA, 2006; ISBN 9780443101717.
42. Slaughter, S.; Cole, D.; Jennings, E.; Reimer, M.A. Consent and assent to participate in research from people with dementia. *Nurs. Ethics* **2007**, *14*, 27–40. [CrossRef]
43. Arnold, D.; Gold, A.W. *Partizipative Forschung für die Umsetzung Erweiterter Gemeindenaher Pflegepraxis: Konzeption eines Partizipativen Forschungs-und Entwicklungsprojekts*; Arbeits-und Forschungsberichte aus dem Projekt E-hoch-B (32); Technische Universität Kaiserslautern: Kaiserslautern, Germany, 2018. Available online: https://nbn-resolving.org/urn:nbn:de:hbz:386-kluedo-58616 (accessed on 26 July 2022).
44. Gold, A.W.; Helbig, A.K.; Römer, C.; Arnold, D. Der Zertifikatskurs "Versorgungsstrategien und Psychosoziale Unterstützung für ein Leben mit Demenz zu Hause": Evidenzbasierte und Bedarfsorientierte Entwicklung des Bildungsangebots. Arbeits- und Forschungsberichte aus dem Projekt E Hoch B-Bildung als Exponent Individueller und Regionaler Entwicklung (29).

45. Tannen, A.; Feuchtinger, J.; Strohbücker, B.; Kocks, A. Survey zur Einbindung von Pflegefachpersonen mit Hochschulabschlüssen an deutschen Universitätskliniken-Stand 2015. *Z. Fur Evidenz Fortbild. Und Qual. Im Gesundh.* **2017**, *120*, 39–46. [CrossRef]
46. Helbig, A.K.; Poppe, S.; Gold, A.W.; Steuerwald, T.; Arnold, D. *Hochschulische Bildungsangebote zu erweiterter Pflege im ambulanten Bereich: Ergebnisse quantitativer Studien unter Pflegefachpersonen, Pflegedienstleitungen und Hausärzt_innen aus der Region Westpfalz*; Arbeits-und Forschungsberichte aus dem Projekt E-hoch-B (28); Technische Universität Kaiserslautern: Kaiserslautern, Germany, 2018. Available online: https://nbn-resolving.org/urn:nbn:de:hbz:386-kluedo-58577 (accessed on 26 July 2022).
47. Scheipers, M.; Arnold, D. *Rekonstruktion von Bedarfslagen zur Erweiterung Gemeindenaher Pflegepraxis anhand von Expert*Inneninterviews mit Geschäftsführungen, Pflegedienstleitungen und Pflegefachkräften Ambulanter Pflegedienste*; Arbeits-und Forschungsberichte aus dem Projekt E-hoch-B (15); Technische Universität Kaiserslautern: Kaiserslautern, Germany, 2017. Available online: https://nbn-resolving.org/urn:nbn:de:hbz:386-kluedo-58438 (accessed on 26 July 2022).
48. Arnold, D.; Gold, A.W. Der Beitrag wissenschaftlicher Bildungsangebote als Antwort auf Versorgungsbedarfe in der ambulanten Pflege. In *Wissenschaftliche Weiterbildung und Region.Bedarfsorientierte Angebotsentwicklung für neue Zielgruppen*; Rohs, M., Dallmann, H.-U., Schmidt, H.-J., Eds.; wbv: Bielefeld, Germany, 2020; pp. 193–208. ISBN 978-3-7639-6108-5.
49. Lamnek, S. *Gruppendiskussion: Theorie und Praxis*, 2nd ed.; Beltz: Weinheim, Germany; Basel, Switzerland, 2005; ISBN 3-621-27417-0.
50. Wilkinson, S. Focus Group Research. In *Qualitative Research, Theory, Method and Practice*, 2nd ed.; Silverman, D., Ed.; Sage: London, UK, 2004; pp. 177–199.
51. Kuckartz, U. *Qualitative Inhaltsanalyse. Methoden, Praxis, Computerunterstützung*, 3rd ed.; Beltz Juventa: Weinheim, Germany; Basel, Switzerland, 2016; ISBN 3-7799-3344-6.
52. Kemmis, S.; McTaggart, R. Participatory Action Research. In *Handbook of Qualitative Research*, 2nd ed.; Denzin, N.K., Lincoln, Y.S., Eds.; SAGE Publications: Thousand Oaks, CA, USA, 2000; pp. 567–605. ISBN 0-8039-4679-1.
53. Breda, K.L. Participatory Action Research. In *Nursing Research Using Participatory Action Research. Qualitative Designs and Methods in Nursing*; Chesnay, M., Ed.; Springer Publishing Company: New York, NY, USA; Boston, MA, USA, 2016; pp. 1–12. ISBN 978-0-8261-2613-9.
54. Mulvale, A.; Miatello, A.; Hackett, C.; Mulvale, G. Applying experience-based co-design with vulnerable populations: Lessons from a systematic review of methods to involve patients, families and service providers in child and youth mental health service improvement. *Patient Exp. J.* **2016**, *3*, 117–129. [CrossRef]
55. Bergold, J.; Thomas, S. Partizipative Forschungsmethoden: Ein methodischer Ansatz in Bewegung. *Forum Qual. Soz./Forum Qual. Soc. Res.* **2012**, *13*, 13.
56. Lucius-Hoene, G.; Groth, S.; Becker, A.-K.; Dvorak, F.; Breuning, M.; Himmel, W. Wie erleben Patienten die Veröffentlichung ihrer Krankheitserfahrungen im Internet? *Die Rehabil.* **2013**, *52*, 196–201. [CrossRef]
57. World Health Organization-Europe. *European Health Report 2018: More than Numbers-Evidence for All*; World Health Organization: Geneva, Switzerland; Regional Office for Europe: Copenhagen, Denmark, 2018.
58. Breuning, M.; Schäfer-Fauth, L.; Lucius-Hoene, G.; Holmberg, C. Connecting one's own illness story to the illness experiences of others on a website-An evaluation study using the think aloud method. *Patient Educ. Couns.* **2020**, *103*, 199–207. [CrossRef]
59. Drewniak, D.; Glässel, A.; Hodel, M.; Biller-Andorno, N. Risks and benefits of web-based patient narratives: Systematic review. *J. Med. Internet Res.* **2020**, *22*, e15772. [CrossRef]
60. Fadlallah, R.; El-Jardali, F.; Nomier, M.; Hemadi, N.; Arif, K.; Langlois, E.V.; Akl, E.A. Using narratives to impact health policy-making: A systematic review. *Health Res. Policy Syst.* **2019**, *17*, 26. [CrossRef]
61. World Medial Association. Declaration of Helsinki. Available online: https://www.wma.net/policies-post/wma-declaration-of-helsinki-ethical-principles-for-medical-research-involving-human-subjects/ (accessed on 26 July 2022).
62. Carlson, J.A. Avoiding traps in member checking. *Qual. Rep.* **2010**, *15*, 1102–1113. [CrossRef]
63. Birt, L.; Scott, S.; Cavers, D.; Campbell, C.; Walter, F. Member Checking: A Tool to Enhance Trustworthiness or Merely a Nod to Validation? *Qual. Health Res.* **2016**, *26*, 1802–1811. [CrossRef]
64. Forbat, L.; Henderson, J. Theoretical and practical reflections on sharing transcripts with participants. *Qual. Health Res.* **2005**, *15*, 1114–1128. [CrossRef]

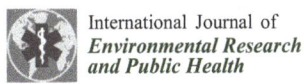

Article

"Back into Life—With a Power Wheelchair": Learning from People with Severe Stroke through a Participatory Photovoice Study in a Metropolitan Area in Germany

Tabea Böttger [1,2,*], Silke Dennhardt [3], Julia Knape [4] and Ulrike Marotzki [2]

1. Institute of Health Science, Faculty of Medicine, University of Lübeck, 23562 Lübeck, Germany
2. Faculty of Social Work and Health, University of Applied Sciences and Arts Hildesheim, Holzminden, Göttingen (HAWK), 31134 Hildesheim, Germany
3. Physio- and Occupational Therapy Program, Faculty of Health, Alice Salomon Hochschule Berlin (ASH), University of Applied Sciences, 12627 Berlin, Germany
4. Independent Researcher, 10439 Berlin, Germany
* Correspondence: tabea.boettger@uni-luebeck.de

Abstract: Severe stroke leads to permanent changes in everyday life. Many stroke survivors depend on support in community mobility (CM). This leads to restrictions and limited social participation. A power wheelchair (PWC) can enable independent CM and reduce such restrictions. This participatory study focused on how people with severe stroke experience their CM in a PWC in Berlin/Germany and what changes they want to initiate. A research team of five severe stroke survivors and two occupational therapists examined the question using photovoice. Stroke survivors took photos of their environment, presented, discussed, and analyzed them at group meetings to identify themes, and disseminated their findings at exhibitions and congresses. The photos emphasize the significance of and unique relationship to the PWC for the self-determined expression of personal freedom. As a complex, individualized construct, CM requires an accessible environment and diverse planning strategies by PWC users to arrive at their destination and overcome suddenly occurring obstacles. Desired changes stress CM independent of external help, increased social esteem, and active involvement in the provision of assistive devices. Voices of severe stroke survivors need to be heard more in healthcare and research to ensure the possibility of equal social participation.

Keywords: participatory research; photovoice; power wheelchair; community mobility; social participation; stroke; rehabilitation

1. Introduction

For people who suffer a brain injury, life changes suddenly and unexpectedly. Stroke, as a form of acquired brain injury, is a major cause of disability in adults worldwide [1,2], and due to demographic changes, the absolute number of people affected is continuously increasing [3]. Experiencing a stroke also affects one's mobility; for about two-thirds of stroke patients, mobility is initially limited [4,5]. Three months after the acute event, about 20% of those affected are still dependent on a wheelchair, and in about 70%, gait speed and endurance are reduced to an extent relevant to everyday life [5]. Around 14–31% of stroke survivors are severely affected because they have multiple functional impairments and remain dependent on assistance in activities of daily living (ADLs) and mobility, regardless of rehabilitation efforts [6].

After a stroke or traumatic brain injury, many people are able to move independently again within their own home, but relating to community mobility (CM), they are dependent on support [7–11]. A recent review [7] about CM after stroke concludes that moderate to severe limitations in CM persist up to and beyond four years after stroke. It showed that all domains of the International Classification of Functioning, Disability, and Health

(ICF) [12] affected the ability to reach CM, "including body structures and function, activity performance, as well as personal and environmental factors" [7] (p. 12). Even though CM encompasses all modes of functional mobility, including mobility in a (power) wheelchair [13], studies rarely take this into account [7]. Thus, the current review could not include any study in which stroke survivors used alternative means of transport (e.g., wheelchair) or had communicative and cognitive impairments, as this was an exclusion criterion in all studies (ibid.). This example shows that there is little evidence to date that addresses CM in stroke survivors who use other means of transportation, such as a PWC, and/or have severe impairments.

As a central connecting function in everyday life, CM takes on and facilitates social participation. It enables us to leave our homes to go grocery shopping or to work, meet friends, travel—and much more [8]. Experiencing limitations in social participation and choice of activities that were taken for granted before the stroke has a huge negative impact on health and life satisfaction [14,15]. The loss of activities and occupations, specifically outside the house, often leads to a sense of dependence [16,17], social isolation, and being bound to one's home [9,18,19].

The use of a mobility assistive device, especially a wheelchair, can be an important "enabler of community participation" [20] (p. 18) for stroke survivors. A power wheelchair (PWC) or a scooter may have various positive effects, such as being able to transport oneself independently to places that enable participation in leisure and social activities and, thus, role enablement [21–24]. Studies point out the high satisfaction of users with their PWC, mainly due to the created independent mobility outside the home [22,23,25,26]. These positive results are also evident in small initial studies with people after acquired brain injury [20,21,24]. First studies show that limitations in activities and participation reported by stroke survivors can be reduced in most cases by the provision of a PWC [20,24]. However, stroke survivors experience many environmental barriers when using a PWC, such as the nature and layout of buildings as well as personal attitudes towards assistive devices (ibid.). Most of the studies involved people with an average age of 67 years or older and who had no or only few communication and cognitive impairments. Less is known about younger stroke survivors ($\leq$55 years) with communication and cognitive impairments, how they use their PWC in CM, and how satisfied they are.

In Germany, the provision process of assistive devices is an integral part of the German healthcare system and neurological rehabilitation [27,28]. Nevertheless, there is little data about provision processes, frequency of use, and satisfaction with assistive devices available [28–30], and various problems in the provisioning process are discussed, such as by the German Society for Rehabilitation (Deutsche Vereinigung für Rehabilitation e.V., DVfR) [31,32]. The very few existing studies reveal that PWCs are seldom or not at all prescribed for neurological rehabilitation in Germany [28,33,34]. The possibilities for successful social participation, which can be especially facilitated by a PWC, are not yet sufficiently considered by decision-makers and health care professionals involved in the care process [32]. This shows the need for further research that focuses on this issue.

According to the International Classification of Functioning, Disability and Health (ICF) [12] and the UN Convention on the Rights of Persons with Disabilities (UN CRPD) [35], effective and equal participation of people with disabilities in social life is an aim of the rehabilitation process that has to be ensured [29,36]. This reorientation also requires a practice-relevant, applied, and participatory research landscape in which stroke survivors are involved in research beyond therapeutic rehabilitation practice [36,37]. Participatory health research (PHR), which involves people whose living conditions are the topic of the research as equal research partners in the research process, is becoming increasingly important in Germany [38]. At the same time, the use of this research approach to people with disabilities is still in its infancy in German health research [39].

Photovoice [40] is a visual methodology that is frequently used in qualitative and, above all, participatory health research (PHR) [41–44]. The number of international photovoice studies involving people after brain injury and especially after stroke has increased in the last 10 years [18,45–50]. Although the produced personal photos represent a form of communication that does not require reading or writing [40] and thus provide an alternative to language-based methods in research for people with post-stroke aphasia that shows promising results [45], researchers often exclude stroke survivors with aphasia from photovoice research [51]. The authors of this recent scoping review, therefore, concluded that further studies on the adaptation of photovoice for these groups are needed to facilitate their inclusion in future participatory action research "in ensuring that all post-stroke stakeholders are involved in projects related to social justice and policy for stroke survivors" (ibid., p. 219). Furthermore, the authors do not describe the participation of severe stroke survivors in these studies. Likewise, no photovoice study focuses on the experiences of CM using a PWC in a metropolitan area.

Therefore, the purpose of this study was to involve persons with severe acquired brain injury as research partners in a participatory research process to learn about their everyday life with a PWC in Berlin. This study specifically explored CM with a PWC in a metropolitan area using Berlin as an example to understand community mobility, identify needs for change, and draw attention to persons with severe acquired brain injury using a PWC. Based on these considerations, the preliminary research question for this participatory photovoice study, drafted prior to the start of the participatory project, was: How do people with severe acquired brain injury experience their community mobility in a power wheelchair in the metropolitan area of Berlin, and what changes do they want to initiate?

2. Materials and Methods

This study is situated within the context of participatory health research (PHR) [52,53]. In PHR, participation is the guiding intention throughout the research process. Maximum participation should be achieved in the sense of the decision-making power of all people who are actively involved in the research. Collaboration among all participants in the research team is organized in a spirit of partnership, and power relations are continuously reflected. The involvement of stroke survivors as co-researchers aimed to facilitate shared learning and empowerment processes, gain new local knowledge, and initiate change (ibid.). The term "co-researcher" instead of "participants" is used throughout this paper to emphasize the particularly active role of stroke survivors in this research process, beyond the usual form of participation [54,55]. The form and extent of participation in participatory research often represent a continuum; while full participation can sometimes not be achieved, the highest level of quality in community participation in the research process is sought [55]. This means that researchers try to "develop egalitarian partnerships with community members that equalize the decision-making power between researchers and community members ... and will make joint decisions that reflect our shared goals and interest in the research project" (ibid, p. 2131). This study was initiated by the first author (TB) as part of her final master's thesis in the master's program in Occupational Therapy at the University of Applied Sciences and Arts (HAWK) in Hildesheim, Germany (2016–2018) and was continued after she graduated.

2.1. Ethics

The study was approved by the University of Applied Sciences and Arts Commission for Research Ethics (HAWK Hildesheim/Germany, 3 April 2018). In participatory research, research ethics issues have a high priority, as the research often takes place with marginalized or vulnerable groups, and a trusting, equal collaboration takes place over a longer period of time [54,56]. Using photovoice requires reflection on specific ethical concerns, such as the possible violation of privacy by making individuals identifiable and public, the researcher's influence on the photo's topics, the photo selection for exhibitions and publications, and questions of photo ownership [44,57,58]. A key critical question is "whose voice" is made visible through the presentation of the photos and titles or captions [44,58]. In this study, the recommendations of the International Collaboration for Participatory

Health Research (ICHPR) [52,59] were considered, which demand, among other things, that the ownership of Participatory Health Research Projects "lies in the hands of the group conducting the study" [52] (p. 10). Therefore, the research team collectively decides how best to report and publish the research findings to achieve the group's stated goals. This refers to all publications (e.g., exhibitions, congresses, articles). The rights to photos and narratives generated in the study belong to the individual co-researchers and are obtained separately for each publication. For this publication, all co-researchers were involved in the selection of the photos, gave their written consent about the use of the photos, and wanted to be mentioned by their first or full names in the acknowledgments.

All participating co-researchers were able to provide written informed consent. Some have legal guardianship for certain areas of life but still have full legal capacity. To account for the co-researchers cognitive and communication impairments, consent was understood as a process, and alternative consent procedures were considered [60,61]. All information about the study (e.g., invitation letter, consent form) was written in easy language [62,63], checked by two stroke survivor peers beforehand, given multimodal, and explained at multiple points in time.

In addition to discussing research ethics with co-researchers during the project, the first author (TB) and her colleague (JK) completed a postscript separately after each meeting for ongoing reflection on research ethics and exchanged ideas regularly. In addition, the first author kept a research journal and used peer discussion with other participatory researchers through an ICHPR training course at the Catholic University of Applied Sciences in Berlin (2018). The critical self-reflections about relationship building and power dynamics in participatory research projects of four research projects from this course, including this study, resulted in a collaborative article [64].

2.2. Recruitment of Co-Researchers

People who had undergone specialized, long-term rehabilitation for adults with an acquired brain injury in the past five years and lived in Berlin were invited to be co-researchers in this study. At the time of the study, the first author (TB) and her colleague (JK) were working as occupational therapists in the rehabilitation center and thus had the opportunity to involve these "seldom heard" [65] (p. 163) individuals in the research project.

Recruitment took place in several steps and through different access ways. Invitations were sent to persons who fulfilled the following inclusion criteria:

- stroke or traumatic brain injury (acquired after the age of 18);
- acute event at least 1 year ago;
- motor, cognitive, and/or communication impairments as a result of the acute event;
- living in an outpatient living arrangement in Berlin for at least 6 months (with or without assistance);
- provided with a power wheelchair (PWC) during rehabilitation and using a PWC outside the home;
- interest and willingness to actively participate in a research project that includes several group meetings;
- enjoyment of photography.

The number of participants was limited to a maximum of five in order to ensure that all co-researchers would have sufficient opportunities to participate in the group meetings [45,50]. People with whom the research initiator already had a relationship of trust were deliberately invited. TB considers herself a gatekeeper to this marginalized group of people [54] because she regularly worked with individuals in this group in a therapeutic context over a longer period of time and was, thus, a part of their lives for a certain period of time (from 1 to 4 years).

When individuals expressed interest in participating in the research project as co-researchers (via email or text message), an appointment was made for a home visit. TB explained her project idea and answered questions and concerns that potential participants might have had. Custom-made information sheets on participatory research and photovoice were used to clarify potential concerns, inspired by a photovoice study with people with intellectual disabilities [66]. Upon written informed consent, a brief questionnaire on demographic data (e.g., living and working situation) and mobility (e.g., assistive device use inside and outside the home) was filled out together. Furthermore, individual time capacities were noted to be able to plan the meetings of the final research team. Likewise, support needs for meeting attendance and desired communication pathways were discussed and recorded. The home visits took place in April 2018 and lasted between 90 and 120 min.

2.3. Photovoice Process

The study used the participatory visual research methodology photovoice [44] based on the principles of Wang and Burris [40] "by which people can identify, represent, and enhance their community through a specific photographic technique" (p. 369). People from an often marginalized group are invited to take photos of their living environment under one or more questions, share and discuss them with each other in the group, and make them available to others. The three main goals of using photovoice in participatory research are to empower people to document and reflect on their community's strengths and concerns, to foster critical dialogue and knowledge about important issues through group discussions about the photos, and to reach decision-makers, such as policymakers and important stakeholders, in the process [40,54].

The photovoice process was guided by von Unger's seven phases [54] and occurred between June 2017 and May 2019 (Scheme 1). The first steps of Phase 1 (Planning and Preparation) were carried out by the first author alone due to the pre-determined time of her master's thesis. Further preparatory steps of Phase 1 were carried out together with the co-researchers in the first group meeting: getting to know each other, introducing and discussing the participatory research approach, and setting the research question and common goals (Table 1). The following phases involved the co-researchers as equal partners. The research topic CM in a PWC evolved from a literature review and TB's professional experience as an occupational therapist. A focus group preceding the study with different participants (except one person) who also had a severe acquired brain injury (October 2017) confirmed the importance of the research topic and provided initial foci and questions. Based on this, the first author decided to use a photovoice methodology to provide an appropriate opportunity for stroke survivors to give a visible voice to their concerns in a participatory research approach. TB and JK pre-planned and facilitated the five group meetings.

Phases	Date	Form
1 Planning and Preparation	June 2017–April 2018	Primarily TB
2 Training of Co-Researchers	April–May 2018	1. Meeting
3 Photo Shooting Phase	May–July 2018	Individually
4 Discussion	June–July 2018	2. Meeting
5 Analysis and Findings	June–August 2018	3. Meeting
6 Presentation and Use	As of September 2018	4. Meeting
7 Evaluation	May 2019	5. Meeting

Scheme 1. Photovoice Research Process (following von Unger, 2014 [54], pp. 71–76).

Table 1. Collective Research Goals.

> - Inform friends and family about my life
> - Inform other affected people about the possibilities of a power wheelchair
> - To point out and reduce discrimination
> - To reduce fear of contact and prejudice
> - To show a different image of people with disabilities

Based on the co-researchers' request, the meetings took place in a centrally located, accessible neighborhood center as well as in the former rehabilitation center. Each meeting lasted between 3 and 3.5 h and was recorded with audio and video. Ongoing process consent for recording was obtained in accordance with a dialogic process about research participation at the beginning of each meeting. The video recordings were used to support the transcription since the audio recordings were not always understandable or comprehensible due to the impairments in speech production and manner of speaking. Due to limited resources, a partial transcription of all meetings took place, whereby the verbatim transcription was limited to central statements and dialogues according to the research question of the project.

Co-researchers' training (Phase 2) included an introduction to photovoice (formulating a storytelling prompt, training on legal and ethical issues, sharing about photos, and desired need for help) using the graphic "A Photovoice Path" by Lorenz [67,68]. The research team decided against restricting the subject of the study (only limitations or possibilities), as it was initially planned by the first author. Instead, a storytelling prompt, "What would you like to tell other people about your life in a power wheelchair?" was formulated to guide the process of photo taking. Co-researchers expressed skepticism about the degree to which change could be initiated, as the original research question suggested. The setting of collective research goals clarified this point; at the same time, it was stated that the first goal of the project was to inform other people (Table 1). The group jointly decided that each person would bring 5 to 10 photos to the second group meeting.

For photo shooting (Phase 3), the co-researchers mainly used their smartphones, and one person was lent a camera as hers broke down in the process of the study. Four of the five co-researchers asked for and received support from the first author in taking photos. They felt uncertain about what they could photograph, were unsure about handling their smartphones due to hemiparesis, or could only leave their homes in power wheelchairs with help from others due to the lack of a grab bar for the transfer (one person). Requested support was given at one to three appointments, during which photos were only taken at the suggestion of the co-researchers. The first author expressed her own opinions only when asked. She then explained the research question and the storytelling prompt again and reported what the co-researchers had already mentioned in previous conversations.

The discussion (Phase 4) and participatory analysis (Phase 5) of the photos occurred in the second and third group meetings. Here, all photos were presented, discussed, and analyzed according to Wang and Burris' three-stage process: (1) selection of the most relevant photos, (2) contextualization, and (3) codification [40,54]. For stage 1 and 2, the co-researchers presented and described each of their photos. The first author (TB) moderated and facilitated the discussion, and her colleague (JK) noted keywords on moderation cards. In the next step, noted keywords and topics were validated by communication. The research group searched for commonalities, patterns, and differences as well as for "umbrella terms" that grouped ideas and themes together. With verbal direction from the co-researcher, the moderation cards were ordered on a flipchart (stage 3). The resulting categories were discussed, and everyone was invited to assign their photos to the themes or to create new categories. During the discussion, the co-researchers gave working titles to each of their photos. In the fourth group meeting and in subsequent individual meetings, the co-researchers were assisted in formulating their stories to clarify the content of the photos. Wang and Burris describe this under the acronym "VOICE—*voicing our individual* and *collective experience*" [40] (p. 381). The results of these discussion and analysis meetings were written up and sent to everyone to review in order to prevent possible misunderstandings that could arise, for example, due to memory deficits.

In the third and fourth group meetings, dissemination of the research results were discussed (Phase 6, Presentation and Use). The planning of a first exhibition and further possible publications took place (see Section 2.1 Ethics). The co-researchers discussed the advantages and disadvantages of different exhibition places. Finally, a decision was made that the first exhibition would occur in the former rehabilitation center. This was to meet the co-researchers' collective goal that, above all, other persons with disabilities need to be informed about the possibilities of a power wheelchair to give courage and hope to those in rehabilitation. The group searched for a title that best expressed their results and could be used for their presentation. One co-researcher's suggestion met agreement from all: "Back into life—with a power wheelchair".

In the last group meeting, the project was evaluated by the research group (Phase 7, Evaluation). The following questions were used for reflection: "How did I feel about the project?", "What did I like?", "What did I not like?", "How can it continue?". All co-researchers received a photo book with their photos and photos from the first exhibition's opening.

3. Results

3.1. Co-Researcher Characteristics

Five stroke survivors participated in the research group. They were aged 36–54 years and had undergone long-term inpatient rehabilitation as a result of a first stroke between 2011 and 2017. All five have severe acquired brain injury with a degree of disability (GdB) varying between 90–100% (max. 100%) based on hemiparesis and cognitive and communication impairments. While communication impairments are cited in their medical reports, specific references to cognitive impairments are lacking (Table 2). According to the evaluation of TB and her colleague, JK, as occupational therapists, cognitive impairments in individually varying degrees exist in the areas of attention, memory, and executive functions, including deficits in self-awareness. During the long-term inpatient rehabilitation, all co-researchers were provided with a power wheelchair (PWC). They live in their own apartments and receive support from assisted independent living (Betreutes Einzelwohnen, BEW) or in an assisted living community; one of them is living with intensive support (Wohnen mit Intensivbetreuung, WMI).

The five co-researchers accomplish getting around in their homes differently. The majority use a wheelchair or PWC for independent mobility, one of these persons uses a rollator (walking frame), but rarely, and one person walks independently without an assistive device. All five use their PWC in community mobility, but not in all situations. Four of the five also temporarily use their manual wheelchair. Reasons for this are primarily space constraints, for example, in medical offices, stores, restaurants, event spaces, public toilets, or their workplace. Other reasons include the absence of the PWC due to repairs, as well as issues in the use of the special transportation service (Sonderfahrdienst, SFD). One person describes anxiety in safely managing the ramp when entering/exiting SFD with their PWC. Backing out causes the person anxiety, so all trips are made only with the manual wheelchair. Another co-researcher already walks short distances in her living environment and at work without an assistive device. Thus, for work, the PWC deliberately stays at home, but also because the commute to work is guaranteed with door-to-door special transport service. For all co-researchers, the frequency of leaving the apartment is related to the occupational status and the need for help. The three persons who are employed leave their homes daily. The other two leave their homes one to two days or three to five days/week. The first one is dependent on assistance from other persons for activities outside the home because she needs help to transfer to the PWC due to a missing grab bar in the apartment. The grab bar was prescribed before leaving the rehabilitation facility, but after 6 months, it has still not been installed. As she lives alone, she can only leave her home with her PWC when care services or family visit and help her.

Table 2. Characteristics of the Co-Researchers.

	Alex [1]	Charlie	Chris	Mika	Lukas
Age (years)	49	52	37	54	36
Sex (female/male)	f	f	m	f	m
Living condition	Alone, Apt.	Alone, Apt.	Alone, Apt.	Ass. LC	Ass. LC
Job status	SW	Retired	SW	Retired	SW
Year of stroke	2010	2013	2012	2010	2005
Symptoms [2]	Hemiplegia right, Aphasia, Apraxia of speech	Hemiplegia right	Hemiplegia left, Dysarthria	Hemiplegia right, Aphasia, Apraxia of speech	Hemiplegia left, Dysarthria
At home since (months)	50	13	12	64	57
Power wheelchair since (months)	79	55	69	85	100
Use of mobility device at home	No	WC	WC	WC, RR	PWC
GdB [3] (Degree of disability	90	100	100	90	100

[1] The names used are pseudonyms. [2] Based on self-assessment of the co-researchers and offered medical reports. Apt.: apartment, Ass. LC: assisted living community, SW: sheltered workshop, WC: wheelchair, PWC: power wheelchair, RR: rollator (walking frame). [3] Degree of disability (GdB) in Germany: "The effects on the participation in community life are assessed as degree of disability in increments of 10 (20 to 100)." [69], "as severely handicapped persons are regarded, who are not only temporarily physically, mentally or emotionally handicapped with a degree of disability of at least 50" [70].

3.2. Back into Life—With a Power Wheelchair—Themes from Photos

Six central themes were identified and named by the co-researchers in the group discussion meetings: 1. Built environment, 2. Personal freedom, 3. Me and my power wheelchair, 4. Demands on users of a power wheelchair, 5. Demands on other persons, and 6. Desires for change. The wording of the categories presented is the result of participatory analysis by the entire research team. Discussions with the five stroke survivors made it evident that foreign words and specialized terminology would reduce comprehensibility. Therefore, formulations in easy language were deliberately chosen. Photos and quotes from the co-researchers are included using pseudonyms and referring to the meetings (M1, M2, etc.).

3.2.1. Theme 1: Built Environment

In their photos, the co-researchers depicted different conditions in public spaces or buildings that constrict or, sometimes, enable mobility in a PWC. Uneven boardwalks or streets (such as cobbled streets, see Figure 1), high or steep curbs, and cars parked on boardwalks or crosswalks hinder group members' community mobility. As a result, they cannot always cross the streets where they would like to, or they swerve their PWC into the street to drive (Figure 2. On the road with the PWC):

"Yes, ... there are pedestrian paths. But they are relatively narrow, everything is relatively green. That means you always have to circle back and forth. And in between there are always these (.) "Huckelpflaster" (cobblestones). When there are driveways." (Charlie, M2).

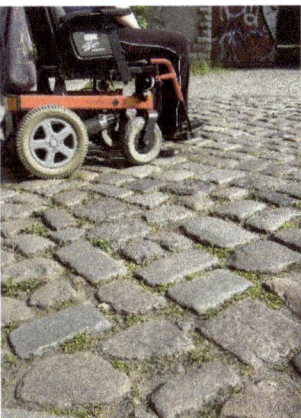

Figure 1. Cobblestones.

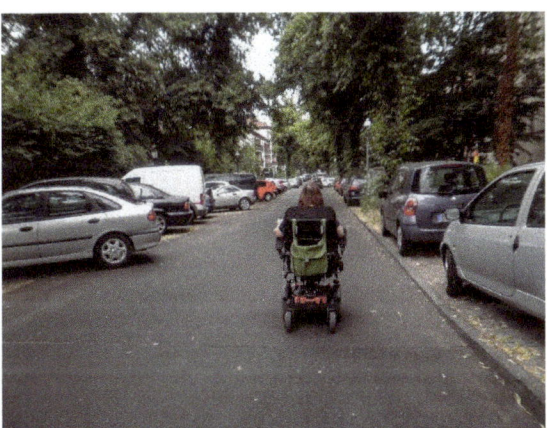

Figure 2. On the road with the PWC.

To board or deboard public transport such as the bus, tramway, underground, and metropolitan railway with a wheelchair in Berlin mostly requires the assistance of the drivers. Wheelchair users must stand at specific assigned places and make their ride requests visible when the train or bus arrives, which feels annoying to the co-researchers. On the other hand, the use of public transport enables various meaningful occupations (Figure 3. Bus stop):

> "I usually go (.) when I (.) visit friends or (.) go for a walk. Or logo (.) [speech and language therapy] do. Yes." (Mika, M2).

Some photos showed elevators. Elevators are principally considered useful by the co-researchers, but there is seldom any information about alternatives if they are out of order, and not every station in Berlin has an elevator yet. Restricted accessibility and deficient space for power wheelchairs in buildings are also seen as a barrier to doing what one needs or wants, especially in medical practices. Stairs often prevent people from choosing a family doctor close to home—unless one can walk a few steps again, as visible in the photos from one co-researcher (Figure 4. Medical practice).

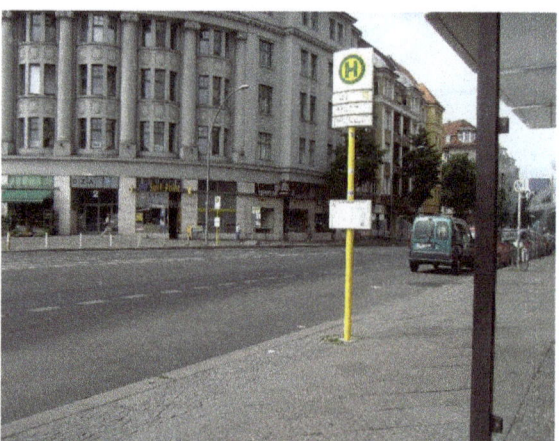

Figure 3. Bus stop.

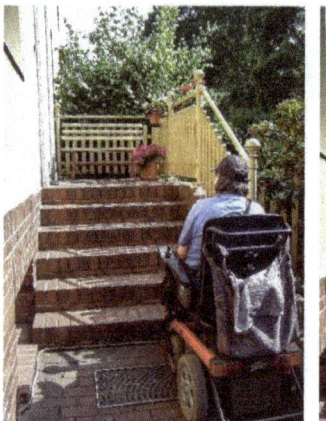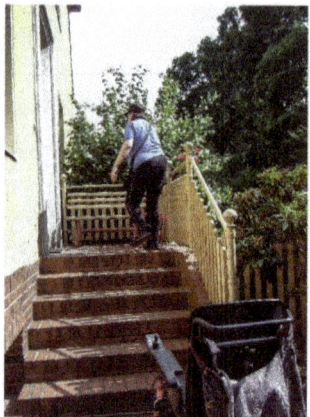

Figure 4. Medical practice.

3.2.2. Theme 2: Personal Freedom

Four of the five co-researchers narrate the possibility of independently doing various meaningful occupations outside their homes, such as going to the cinema, cafés, parks, or for a walk in the neighborhood using their PWC. The PWC provides an important resource in community mobility (CM), for example, by facilitating leisure activities. Lukas reports on his visits to the cinema with a friend who also took the photo of him (Figure 5. Cinema):

> "You can see the cinema there. Alexanderplatz. And I did that because I'm there quite often. (.) ... Because all the cinemas there are barrier-free. ... In the PWC or wheelchair you sit in the back. And you have a good view of the screen. That's why I think it's so good." (Lukas, M3).

For another person, it is important to simply be in a public space, to be among and part of other people:

> "I enjoy that (.) when I (.) go to market hall. And (.) then (.) people arrive. And watch (moves her head to do so). And (.) people approach me. "What did you do" and dedede (.) ... But (.) this is (..) my home (gestures with her hand). (.) Yes. (.) Like this." (Mika, M2).

With the support of the first author, Alex took a photo in a public park near her home, which she likes to visit regularly. She describes how the PWC compensates for her limited walking mobility, enabling her to resume individual interests and routines, thus supporting her self-determination and well-being. Alex formulated for her photo (Figure 6. Schlosspark):

> "I like to be outside with my PWC. I like to go to the Schlosspark. I love the trees—always have. I like to be in nature. I can't get there on foot. With my PWC, I can go there by myself when I want. My wish: Despite my physical limitations, I would like to do the things I like to do. And that do me good. The PWC helps me to do that."

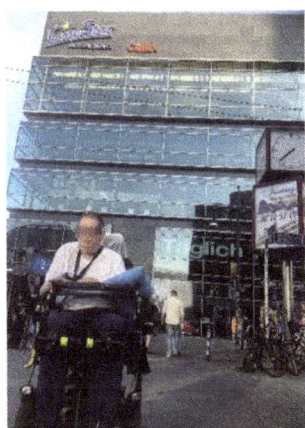

Figure 5. Cinema.

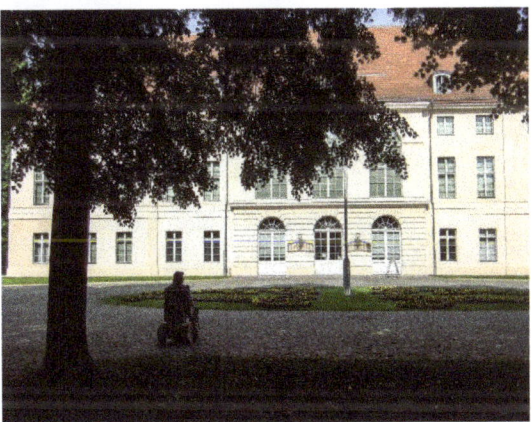

Figure 6. Schlosspark.

3.2.3. Theme 3: Me and My Power Wheelchair (PWC)

The central role of the PWC in enabling meaningful occupations and choice causes a high identification with the assistive device. One member of the research group named their PWC with her second surname (Figure 7. Bonita):

> "Uh (runs her hand over the armrest of her PWC and considers) (. . .) Bonita. And (..) I love (..) (taps hand on armrest in time to speaking) PWC." (Mika, M2).

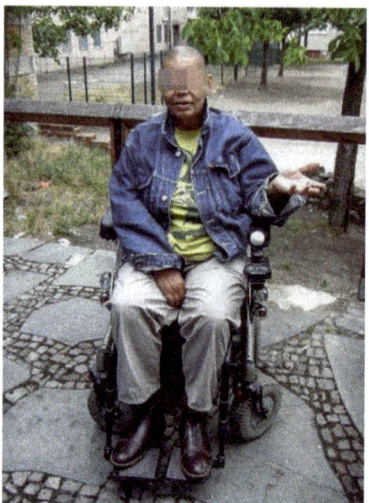

Figure 7. Bonita.

In the meetings, she used this name repeatedly when she spoke praisingly of her PWC. She is very satisfied with her aid because it enables her to do a lot: *"My wheelchair is (.) Bonita. (.) And (.) love freedom. (..). Yes."* (Mika, M3).

These very personal descriptions led to a joint discussion in the group on how this could be represented in a photo. One co-researcher expressed the suggestion that Mika should take a picture of herself with her PWC. When asked where this photo could be created, she responded, "now, here". For the making of the photo, the environment was not important because the photo should primarily depict a satisfied Mika with her assistive device.

Another co-researcher even got a license plate with the words *"se-xy 50"* for her birthday and is thinking about attaching it to her PWC as she did with her former car. She has not attached the self-made license plate to her PWC yet, but can imagine doing so in the future if her relationship with her PWC evolves:

"I ... have always given my car a name. So, I think I would then also, if I can identify with that, somehow. ... If I can then say that it is mine. (.) Then I would also give it a name." (Charlie, M2).

Another co-researcher associates his PWC with a tank (Figure 8. T34/Tank). This association refers to both the size and the driving characteristics, which are either helpful or a barrier, depending on the context. The PWC is *"(.) also designed to (.) simply take the terrain"* (Chris, M3). In confined spaces, such as a café, this could lead to unwanted situations:

"If I ... drive into the café (.) too briskly (.) ... then I drive into the tables. (.) A path of destruction in" (Chris, M2).

Despite the off-road capability of his PWC, there are also *"insurmountable obstacles"* for him, such as curbs that were too high: *"Well. And (.) sometime is also times closing time. No?"* (Chris, M2).

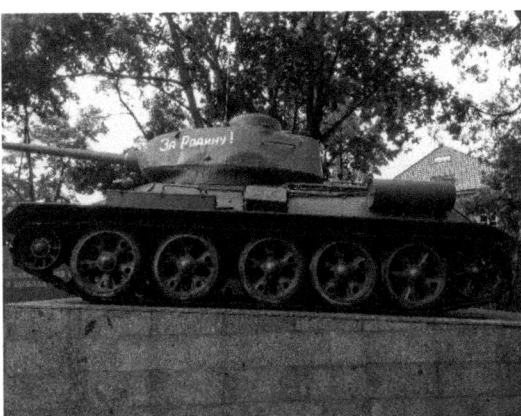

Figure 8. T34/Tank.

3.2.4. Theme 4: Demands on Users of a Power Wheelchair (PWC)

Independent mobility with a PWC needs planning and preparation. Co-researchers describe that they have to be informed beforehand about the accessibility of, for example, a cinema and how it is necessary to check if there are elevators at the transport station when going to the cinema. If they want to use a special transportation service, they also have to book in advance. Before longer rides with a PWC, the battery needs to be checked. PWC users have to know alternatives if plans need to be adapted, they have to be able to ask for assistance, and they have to have knowledge of how to get assistance. A co-researcher describes that it is not always known where one can find or receive appropriate help, for example, who could accompany one on a voluntary basis, or where to find reliable information about accessible places: *"Yes, but it's not always (.) clear. So, barrier-free restaurants. That is totally difficult to find!"* (Charlie, M3).

In addition to planning and preparation, it is also important to know alternatives, have knowledge about the PCW, as well as to be able to ask for help. Broken elevators sometimes cause a change in the original route. If the PWC is broken, one has to know how to unblock it and ask people to push. It is also necessary to know a service or emergency number as well as one's rights. A co-researcher described that while his PWC was being repaired, he was not provided with a replacement PWC despite being entitled to one. Upon inquiry, he was told that no PWC was available in his size. As a result, he was unable to do his grocery shopping and lived on his supplies, as he reported after a meeting. From this account, it is clear that knowing one's rights and being able to advocate for them to others is also a requirement—and to ask for help if one's rights are not met. A co-researcher concludes: *"And then I think you really have to be well-structured."* (Charlie, M3).

3.2.5. Theme 5: Demands on Other Persons

The co-researchers described many situations where they missed appropriate assistance and support from other persons. A shop assistant coming out of a small shop with stairs by his initiative and asking what one needs is welcome. In another situation, one person was offered help by the waitress at a café because the toilet was not barrier-free. She describes very impressively how this was perceived as 'crossing the line':

"Sure, with my brother I would manage that. (.) Well, I would also be able to walk 2, 3 steps (.) to the toilet. That would not be a problem. (.) But I wouldn't do that with a complete stranger. ... (laughs). I don't say to the waitress: "Yes, go with me to the toilet!" (Charlie, M3).

The co-researchers also describe exclusions and prejudices they experience in everyday life. Lukas described how, when visiting a restaurant with family or friends, he was the only person not offered a menu on several occasions. His conclusion is: *"Well, if you're in a wheelchair, you're automatically stupid."* (Lukas, M3).

The bus drivers of public transport were often described as verbally or non-verbally unkind for reasons that are not clear. *"Uh (.) grumble"*. (Mika, M2) *"One can see it in the face."* (Charlie, M2).

A co-researcher described an experience: *"I had that last time, too. (.) I was on the road with . . . . And we were trying to catch the M . . . [number of the bus] in the direction of . . . . She ran ahead. Because she already saw that he was coming. (..) And then I ran after him. And then he was in a really bad mood and threw his gloves and everything he had (..) onto this shelf in front. And then (.) asked in all seriousness why we were going with him and not taking the later bus. (.) The next one is coming soon. . . . Because then they don't have the will/they don't have the will to make the ramp out."* (Charlie, M2).

The research group thought about how this could be expressed in a photo. One co-researcher spontaneously stuck out her middle finger and received approval from the other co-researchers. As a result, Figure 9 was created as a joint photomontage (Figure 9. Stinky finger at a bus stop).

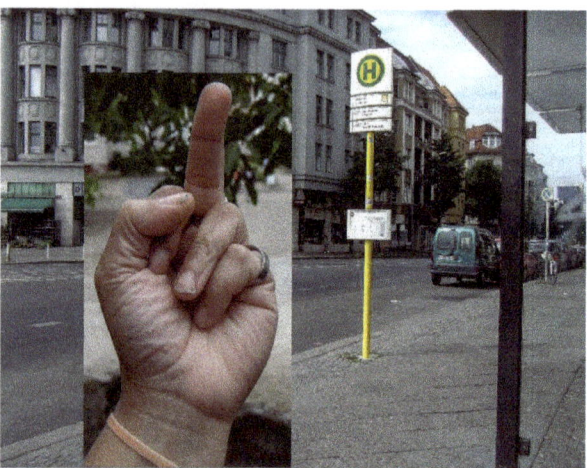

Figure 9. Stinky finger at a bus stop.

Another important theme was the adequate individual provision of assistive devices in relation to the context. One group member was able to go shopping independently with her PWC while in rehabilitation. Independent transfer to her PWC is not possible in her own flat because for nearly one year, the supplier of medical equipment did not deliver a grip bar and other adaptations for her PWC (Figure 10. Power wheelchair).

> *"That it is not enough (.) to have such an expensive part [PWC] there. But that you also have to get it adequately adapted. . . . Yes. And now I just sit in the shack. (.) It's really like that."* (Charlie, M2).

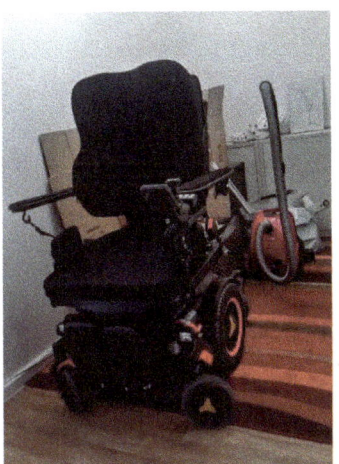

Figure 10. Power wheelchair.

3.2.6. Theme 6: Desires for Change

The co-researchers constantly—in all group meetings—expressed their wishes for change, such as more accessible medical practices or stores. *"Well, I think that (.) not accessible stores (.) too few for us. . . . where you can drive in and look. (.) Like a normal customer. (.) Customer is king."* (Charlie, M3).

Basically, they all wish to be independently mobile in buildings and public transport with their PWC—without the assistance of other people, such as being dependent on someone who handles a ramp. The co-researchers expressed their wish for recognition and appreciation of their knowledge and experience and to be treated with an attitude of equality. They assume that people are not aware that the co-researchers had a "normal" life some time ago.

"I was healthy until five years ago, too. And jumped around. And now I am sitting in one of these. I imagined it differently, too. And tomorrow you could be hit by a stroke!" (Charlie, M3).

In the provisioning process of assistive devices, stroke survivors want to be heard more so that the assistive devices meet their individual wants and needs. Likewise, they would like more support in advocating for their rights with payers, such as insurance. One co-researcher reported that she spent a lot of time making phone calls inquiring about approval or delivery. She expressed during the first home visit, *"I could spend my free time in other ways!"*

A central concern of the research group was and is to communicate courage and the possibilities of assistive devices like PWCs to other persons with disabilities.

"This is the place [rehabilitation center] where you are made fit again . . . for life (.) And (.) . . . I'm sure some people have already resigned. (..) There's no progress at all. And (..) And yes, everything sucks. And so on. (.) But (.) the people should also see that it (.) goes up. That there are assistive devices." (Chris, M3).

3.3. Dissemination of Findings

In January 2019, the findings of the study were exhibited for the first time in the cafeteria of the long-term rehabilitation center over four weeks. The place was decided upon the majority request of the co-researchers. Current rehabilitants were present, in addition to staff and management of the institution. After introductory, appreciative words from the head physician, the co-researchers and the first author presented the project, the results, and their concerns (see Figure 11). The representative for seniors and passengers with disabilities of the Berlin transport company (BVG) was invited to the exhibition opening and showed interest in the results. However, as often, the initial contact that was established at the exhibition was not followed up.

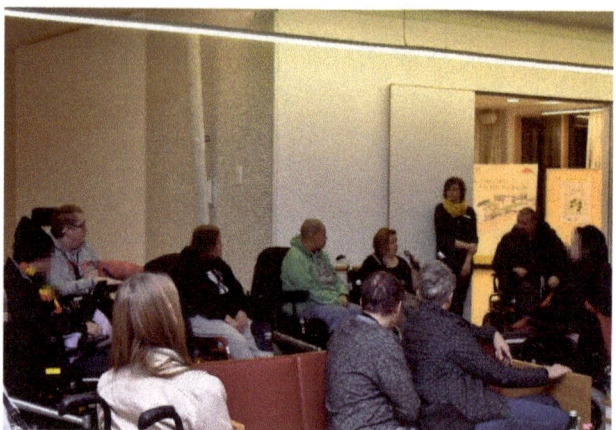

Figure 11. Exhibition opening.

Afterward, three co-researchers expressed a general interest in accompanying the authors to congresses and reporting on the project—at least if these were to take place in Berlin. One co-researcher went to the opening of the exhibition at the Catholic University of Applied Sciences Berlin (conference of the Berlin Workshop for Participatory Research, March 2019), and one co-researcher and another rehabilitant reported about the project at the opening of the exhibition at an occupational therapy school in Berlin (December 2019). Furthermore, the results were presented at four scientific conferences in the form of verbal presentations, at two of which the first author was accompanied by a co-researcher.

3.4. Evaluation

The planned evaluation after the first exhibition in early 2019 had to be canceled due to illness and was postponed by three months. All co-researchers spoke positively about the project that had been carried out. At the same time, most of them found it difficult to make an evaluation and thus a conscious reflection. Two smileys cards (sad and laughing facial expressions) supported the process: the two cards were attached to the flipchart to visualize the questions, "What did I like?" and "What did I not like?". Two co-researchers emphasized the importance of the exhibition in the rehabilitation center, and one co-researcher proposed the idea of meeting other, former, and familiar rehabilitants again and doing something together. All emphasized sharing with each other and how they experienced the associated feeling of not being alone with the problems they experienced. One co-researcher expressed the amount of time and organizational effort associated with the meetings as negative. Above all, the long journey of one hour by SFD was perceived as burdensome. In order to share their own motivation for the project and to communicate it to others, e.g., at congress presentations, the authors suggested that short statements by the co-researchers should be recorded on video. Four agreed to this idea, and the fifth person did not want to do this.

4. Discussion

The aim of the presented participatory study was to find out how people with a severe stroke experience their community mobility (CM) using a power wheelchair (PWC) in the metropolitan area of Berlin and what changes they want to initiate. Our results show that all co-researchers regularly use their PWC outside the home despite numerous existing barriers and challenges experienced on a daily basis. Thus, the assistive device prescribed during rehabilitation occupies a central, if not irreplaceable, part in the independent lifestyle of the co-researchers. The impressive descriptions and discussions of the co-researchers reveal that successful CM with a PWC is a very complex construct; it depends on several factors and has an individual level of meaning. In the following section, we want to discuss the most important results and methodological considerations for future research before we finally mention the limitations of the study.

4.1. Complexity of Community Mobility Using a Power Wheelchair

4.1.1. Accessible Environment and Transport Possibilities

The results of the presented study support the statement that CM is a complex construct for social participation that depends on many factors [8,71,72], especially for people after acquired brain injury who are mobile in a wheelchair [20,24,73,74]. The most common physical barriers in the environment described by our co-researchers and previous studies were access to buildings and the surface condition of footpaths (potholes, curbs). This shows that public space still does not provide equal access to all people and that wheelchair users are still not considered enough in inclusive urban planning in Germany. A recent statement by the German Institute for Human Rights (Deutsches Institut für Menschenrechte, DIMR), which was commissioned as an independent national human rights institution for the implementation of the UN CRPD, confirms that the strategic planning of the administrations in Berlin hardly or not at all take the special mobility needs of people with disabilities into account [75]. This statement has wide-ranging, public health-relevant consequences for the persons concerned. For example, due to only limited barrier-free public transport, lack of barrier-free cabs, and complicated billing modalities for the special transport service (SFD), many people had great difficulties attending their SARS-CoV-2 vaccination appointments in the established vaccination centers in Berlin in 2021 (ibid.). Our co-researchers also describe the limited accessibility and accessible equipment of medical practices: only one in three medical practices in Germany is barrier-free to date [76]. Our results reinforce previous research from other countries that people with disabilities often experience health disparities resulting from the inaccessibility of healthcare services, see, e.g., [77]. To promote the social participation of wheelchair users in Berlin, there is a need for the coordinated overall planning of public space, including footpaths, roads, buildings, and means of transport, as well as a general national legal obligation for accessibility in all areas of life, as has been implemented in other countries, such as Austria or the U.S., for decades. It is important to systematically involve the people concerned in these decisions. It should also be discussed and investigated to what extent the SFD can be reduced by expanding generally accessible transport services, such as barrier-free call cabs [75]. This could not only contribute to a reduction in costs but, above all, realize full and equal participation in the sense of the UN-CRPD and minimize the dependence on others, such as family members.

Previous international studies show that people after stroke are more likely to use special transport services or be passengers in cars with family members [15,26,78], but partly without their PWC because transporting it is not possible in most cars, so the PWC then remains at home. The experiences of the co-researchers in our study do not coincide with these previous findings: only one person used SFD regularly, although all were eligible. The low use of special transportation services like the SFD in Berlin was explained by the co-researchers as a lack of flexibility and unreliability of the service, as shown in a previous study from Iceland [79]. Desired trips have to be planned and booked with a lot of advance time and organization, the SFD can only be used at certain times of the day, and sometimes there are significant delays. Their descriptions illustrate that SFD does not automatically increase CM since it does often not support spontaneous CM and that other transport options should.

4.1.2. Invisible and Unexpected Challenging Experiences

The explanations on the use of the SFD and further descriptions of the co-researchers reveal, in addition to an accessible environment and transport possibilities, that it requires much more to be independently and self-determinedly mobile with a PWC in the community. First, it requires a massive amount of planning, which is not visible to other people and, thus, often not known. This highlights that CM does not start when leaving home, but much earlier. PWC users must obtain a lot of information before making their daily trips to reach their destinations on time and use the services provided there. Thus, they need comprehensive strategies of where to look for this information and access to the skills to use information sources, such as the internet. A recent scoping review highlights that by elaborating the different cognitive functions required for safe use of powered mobility devices [80]. Similarly, such planning efforts require an enormous amount of time. These barriers to access became highly "visible" to the non-PWC-using researchers as they attempted the collective dissemination of the research findings. The participation of two co-researchers in a scientific congress in a city 500 km away required numerous planning steps as early as 6 months before the event, including booking and reserving train travel with as few changes as possible and requesting assistance (by a lift) to get on and off the train, researching and booking accessible accommodation that met the co-researchers' individual needs, and booking an assistant for dressing and undressing. Because of this elaborate planning and the fear that something might go wrong, only a few co-researchers were willing to go on this "adventure". It took a lot of positive reinforcement for two co-researchers to get involved. The joint trip almost failed at the starting point because the scheduled bus to the train station did not run that morning, and the co-researchers could not change to any other barrier-free public transportation (subway or cab). Fortunately, a wheelchair space was still available on a later train service that day, so the congress visit could be made together. These experiences and findings have practical implications for rehabilitative practice, developers of digital assistance systems, as well as the planning of participatory research projects. In rehabilitation, in addition to training with the PWC in the desired environment in the community, the focus must be on counseling stroke survivors and their caregivers on what planning steps are necessary and where to find relevant information. Peer support groups or peer counseling may be an appropriate intervention. Previous research has shown that these can help stroke survivors cope with their lives [81,82]. Likewise, it is important to educate about the fact that spontaneous, unexpected challenges can occur and to prepare possible solutions together. This includes, for example, always carrying a cell phone and knowing which person to call in a difficult situation, or alternatively, which app can generate alternative barrier-free travel routes using public transportation. This requires digital assistance systems such as apps that can be used without assistance by people with cognitive impairments. When planning participatory research projects, sufficient time and financial resources must be available, as well as the willingness to engage in the adventure of the experiences of the researchers concerned to establish the required equality in the collaboration. In order to achieve not only symbolic or sham participation, it is necessary to adapt the existing funding conditions for participatory health research in Germany [83].

4.1.3. Individually Meaning of Community Mobility

The photo narratives of our co-researchers reinforce the diversified meaning of CM. First, being mobile outside the home enables a variety of activities of daily living, especially for shopping and numerous leisure activities, which is consistent with the findings of other international studies [20,21,24,73]. Second, to be mobile in the community means "'being a part of" and being "a respected, valued member of the community" [73] (p. 55). The co-researchers describe how they can do things that are personally important to them when they want, for example, visiting a café or a park. CM thus contributes to maintaining their own identity. Alternatively, as Nanninga and colleagues formulated, "mobility is considered as a way to connect places that are meaningful to individuals rather than as movements from A to B" [8] (p. 2016). Third, the photos and narratives of the co-researchers also indicate that the statement "to be mobile" refers to a limited spatial area. This means that, above all, the possibility of being able to carry out everyday activities in one's own local living environment—in Berlin called "Kiez"—with the PWC without accompaniment. There seems to be an individual mobility radius that is essential for satisfaction, social participation, and belonging: *"That's enough. . . . Yes. In my "Kiez". . . . And still I am on the road in Berlin"* (Mika). This statement also has practical implications for rehabilitative practice; it reveals the high importance of a locally community-based, socially oriented rehabilitation for stroke survivors in order to enable independent and meaningful CM and social participation [84–86]. Further research can investigate how even a limited mobility radius contributes to this group's independence, self-confidence, and quality of life and to what extent this represents a special feature for the included target group of people with cognitive and communication impairments.

4.2. Identification with the Power Wheelchair

Despite the multiplicity of barriers to using a PWC in CM, the co-researchers highlighted the important role of the PWC. They show a high degree of identification with the PWC, which led to individually naming them in some cases. This expresses a kind of personal 'ownership' and even empowerment. The PWC seems to be much more than an assistive device object that compensates only a physical impairment. This could mean that the PWC has become part of their subjectivity because it gives back control over their lives and autonomy that they had lost due to the disease. With the PWC, they are once again able to decide for themselves when and where they go. Evans' findings support that the provision of a PWC can lead to overcoming the experienced occupational deprivation [21] (p. 551). Wilcock defines occupational deprivation as an occupational risk factor, an external circumstance that keeps individuals from performing meaningful occupations and that, if prolonged, poses a health risk [87]. Disability as a social construct is one such influencing factor and applies, for example, to people who are dependent on a wheelchair (ibid.). The relevance in relation to subjective health perception is shown in the statement of Charlie, who currently cannot use her PWC without assistance: *"If my wheelchair (laughs) would work, I would feel better. (.) That's just a bit on my stomach"* (Charlie).

The core value of the PWC for severe stroke survivors highlights the central importance of the provisioning process of assistive devices in rehabilitation. Indeed, a key finding of our study is that this high level of identification with the PWC was not present from the outset, which might be one reason why the co-researchers highlight the desire to inform peers. All co-researchers described that they were unsure to what extent they could "become friends" with the PWC when being introduced to and testing a PWC in the rehabilitative context. Only through the positive experiences during the use outside the home—in the community—did the high value increasingly become apparent to them. Their own experiences led the co-researchers to the objective of the project "to inform other affected people about the possibilities of a power wheelchair" (see Table 1). Future research should further investigate the aspect of peer support groups or counseling in the context of assistive device provision with a PWC. In addition, all actors (e.g., physicians, allied health professionals, as well as payers) involved in the provisioning process should be aware of the possibilities of PWCs so that they can point them out in counseling and during testing of driving while minimizing existing fears. In Germany, there seems to be limited recognition of these possibilities among payers to date, as evidenced by high rejection rates of around 19–36% for assistive devices such as wheelchairs, PWCs, and electric scooters in the few existing studies [88,89]. The provision of wheelchairs in German health care often focuses only on the close range ("Nahbereich" such as living space) and thus does not meet the participation requirements of persons with disabilities [32]. Especially people with multiple disabilities can achieve an effective improvement in their independently manageable radius of CM by being equipped with a PWC or with an auxiliary drive (ibid.).

4.3. Methodological Considerations

Regarding methodological considerations, our study shows that photovoice is an appropriate, accessible method for collaborative, participatory research with people with severe strokes. Even if reading and writing skills are not necessary, the importance of verbal expression skills was evident in describing, discussing, and analyzing the photos. It was helpful that the first author had accompanied some of the co-researchers in photo taking and could support the communication through her memories when needed. In addition, our experiences indicate the benefit of a "mixed group" of stroke survivors with and without communication impairments. The other co-researchers intuitively showed understanding and responded by describing what they saw in the photos and what it might mean. The communication-impaired person confirmed or denied the statements verbally or with head nodding/shaking. However, it remains to be seen whether Mika and Alex, the two persons with aphasia and apraxia of speech, were able to communicate all their concerns. It is also not clear to what extent the verbal statements of the other members of the research team influenced this, according to the key question, "whose voice" is made visible through the photos and narratives [44,58]. When selecting the photos for the exhibitions as well as for this article, the first author noted that she would have chosen different photos in some cases. For example, it was important for Alex to include Figure 1, Cobblestones, in the article. Even though the co-researchers were involved in this step of the publication, it should be noted that they were not involved in the writing of this manuscript and text selection. According to Evans-Agnew and Rosemberg, this reflects a widespread challenge in photovoice research designs [44]. Some selected photos show the individuals in portrait, thereby making them publicly identifiable. Although this aspect and possible associated dangers, such as stigmatization, were addressed with the co-researchers, the consequences of publication can only be predicted to a limited extent. Methodological considerations should also take into account the positioning and reflection of the two researchers (TB, JK) who prepared and conducted the research meetings. The pre-existing trusting relationships from the therapeutic rehabilitation setting were not seen as limiting but rather as a special resource [64,90]. Nevertheless, it required a constant reflection on their roles, expectations, possible influence, and open communication about them with the co-researchers. For example, at the beginning of the research project, it was important to acknowledge that the people included did not see themselves as "co-researchers" and thus did not speak of "our" project until the study was underway. Reflections of an inclusive research team on their working relationships support the experience that it takes shared time and situations before a "we" emerges throughout the team [90]. Future research should investigate further accessible methods that enable participatory research by people with severe communication impairments.

4.4. Limitations

There are also some study limitations. First, the co-researchers did not receive cameras, were not provided with special camera training, or assessed for camera adaptations, such as one-handed access, as in other studies [45,47]. This could have reduced the support and a possible influence by external persons when taking photos [51]. Joint "neighborhood walks" through a district of Berlin would probably have been helpful as a first step to take pictures and try out the cameras [66]. In this study, the co-researchers not only had hemiparesis, which made it difficult for them to handle the cameras or smartphones, but they were also on the road with a motorized assistive device, which is controlled by the active hand. In future studies, newer technical possibilities could be tested, such as cameras attached to the head (headwear), which can be used to take hands-free pictures from one's own perspective. Second, the participatory involvement of the co-researchers could have been higher under different circumstances, e.g., from the beginning of the planning phase. This research project was developed in the context of a master's thesis and thus had limited resources. Due to this, not all of the co-researchers' concerns could be implemented in the research process. The majority expressed a preference not to hold the joint meetings at the former rehabilitation center, which is located in the suburbs of the city and thus would have meant a long, exhausting journey for some. The search for a centrally located, barrier-free room that could be used free of charge due to limited financial resources was successful. Since the co-researchers live in different districts of Berlin, travel times remained at 45–60 min for individuals. The length of the meetings was not reduced because of this, although most of the co-researchers showed signs of fatigue despite breaks, which can be discussed as overload due to disregard of the reduced capacity. Third, the co-researchers' cognitive impairments were neither directly named by them nor cited in their medical reports. Not all co-researchers provided medical reports; this was a voluntary option. Even though the evaluations of cognitive impairments are based on the first author's and her colleague's (JK) years of professional experience with this clientele, these evaluations may be liable to bias and might not be relevant to one's voice being heard, but for searching for alternative methods. Fourth, more public exhibitions in the different districts of Berlin could have increased the impact of the project. Finally, in terms of sustainability of the results and the associated initiation of change, it would have been useful to involve political decision-makers from Berlin transport companies, representatives of health insurance companies, service providers of assistive devices, and medical and therapeutic staff involved in the provision of assistive devices in a follow-up project.

5. Conclusions

This participatory photovoice study demonstrates that the active inclusion of severely affected stroke survivors as equal co-researchers in the research process is possible and provides important insights and findings. The power wheelchair plays a crucial role in the lives of stroke survivors involved in this study, as it decisively supports their desire for a self-determined and independent lifestyle by enabling community mobility in Berlin and social participation for them. However, community mobility should be understood as a complex, individualized construct that requires both an accessible environment and multiple planning strategies by PWC users. According to their own statements, after a long period of rehabilitation, these people have "*managed to jump back . . . into life*" (Chris, M3).

The practical implications of this study lie in the need for increased involvement of the target group in rehabilitation, research, and public planning processes. In rehabilitation, interested individuals should be involved as peer experts in the various stages of the provision process of assistive devices, and access to a power mobility device should be supported by the interdisciplinary rehabilitation team as well as by payers. The special challenges in community mobility should be extended by peer support services. Further research on this issue is needed.

Author Contributions: T.B. designed the study, T.B. and J.K. collected and analyzed the data with the co-researchers in the group meetings and wrote a first draft of the manuscript. U.M. and S.D. supervised the project. All authors have read and agreed to the published version of the manuscript.

Funding: The P.A.N. Zentrum for Post-Akute Neurorehabilitation, Berlin, Germany, funded the printing of the photos and promotional materials for the first exhibition in January 2019. This research received no further funding.

Institutional Review Board Statement: The study was conducted in accordance with the Declaration of Helsinki, and approved by Ethics Committee of University of Applied Sciences and Arts Hildesheim, Holzminden, Göttingen (HAWK), Germany (3 April 2018).

Informed Consent Statement: Informed consent was obtained from all subjects involved in the study. Written informed consent has been obtained from the co-researchers to publish this paper.

Data Availability Statement: The datasets used and analyzed in this study are available from the corresponding author on reasonable request.

Acknowledgments: Participatory research is the work of many participants who often remain invisible in scientific publications. We would like to express our sincere thanks to all those who made this contribution possible, but especially to the five co-researchers who have given their consent to be named here: Andrea Hergt, Aurelia Topyürek, Daniel Cornelius, Kevin Kraaß, and Sabine. Without you, this project would not exist. These people have taken the time to share their experiences and views with us openly and confidently, to exchange and to document them in photos. In doing so, they have given us a very personal and previously blocked insight into their respective living environments, which has had a sustainable effect. The first author (T.B.) would like to thank her supervising professors, Ulrike Marotzki and Silke Dennhardt, for their trust in her project idea and for their constructive advice and support. The first author would also like to thank her colleague Julia Knape for her wide-ranging support of the project. The authors thank the P.A.N. Zentrum for Post-Akute Neurorehabilitation, Berlin, and the neighborhood house Prinzenallee 58, Berlin, for the use of their premises for the meetings. We also would like to thank the P.A.N. Zentrum for Post-Akute Neurorehabilitation, Berlin, for supporting and facilitating the first exhibition on their facilities, especially for funding the printing of the photos and the promotional material. The University of Applied Sciences and Arts Hildesheim, Holzminden, Göttingen (HAWK) funded the cost of open access publication of this manuscript in this journal.

Conflicts of Interest: The authors declare no conflict of interest.

References

1. Krishnamurthi, R.V.; Ikeda, T.; Feigin, V.L. Global, Regional and Country-Specific Burden of Ischaemic Stroke, Intracerebral Haemorrhage and Subarachnoid Haemorrhage: A Systematic Analysis of the Global Burden of Disease Study 2017. *Neuroepidemiology* **2020**, *54*, 171–179. [CrossRef] [PubMed]
2. Hay, S.I.; Abajobir, A.A.; Abate, K.H.; Abbafati, C.; Abbas, K.M.; Abd-Allah, F.; Abdulkader, R.S.; Abdulle, A.M.; Abebo, T.A.; Abera, S.F.; et al. Global, regional, and national disability-adjusted life-years (DALYs) for 333 diseases and injuries and healthy life expectancy (HALE) for 195 countries and territories, 1990–2016: A systematic analysis for the Global Burden of Disease Study 2016. *Lancet* **2017**, *390*, 1260–1344. [CrossRef]
3. Busch, M.A.; Kuhnert, R. 12-Monats-Prävalenz von Schlaganfall oder chronischen Beschwerden infolge eines Schlaganfalls in Deutschland: Robert Koch-Institut. *J. Health Monit.* **2017**, *2*, 70–76. [CrossRef]
4. Shaughnessy, M.; Michael, K.M.; Sorkin, J.D.; Macko, R.F. Steps after stroke: Capturing ambulatory recovery. *Stroke* **2005**, *36*, 1305–1307. [CrossRef] [PubMed]
5. Jørgensen, H.S.; Nakayama, H.; Raaschou, H.O.; Vive-Larsen, J.; Støier, M.; Olsen, T.S. Outcome and time course of recovery in stroke. Part II: Time course of recovery. The copenhagen stroke study. *Arch. Phys. Med. Rehabil.* **1995**, *76*, 406–412. [CrossRef]
6. McGlinchey, M.P.; James, J.; McKevitt, C.; Douiri, A.; Sackley, C. The effect of rehabilitation interventions on physical function and immobility-related complications in severe stroke: A systematic review. *BMJ Open* **2020**, *10*, e033642. [CrossRef]
7. Wesselhoff, S.; Hanke, T.A.; Evans, C.C. Community mobility after stroke: A systematic review. *Top. Stroke Rehabil.* **2018**, *25*, 224–238. [CrossRef]
8. Nanninga, C.S.; Meijering, L.; Postema, K.; Schönherr, M.C.; Lettinga, A.T. Unpacking community mobility: A preliminary study into the embodied experiences of stroke survivors. *Disabil. Rehabil.* **2018**, *40*, 2015–2024. [CrossRef]
9. Hesse, S.; Staats, M.; Werner, C.; Bestmann, A.; Lingnau, M.L. Ambulante Krankengymnastik von Schlaganfallpatienten zu Hause. *Nervenarzt* **2001**, *72*, 950–954. [CrossRef]
10. Logan, P.A.; Dyas, J.; Gladman, J.R.F. Using an interview study of transport use by people who have had a stroke to inform rehabilitation. *Clin. Rehabil.* **2004**, *18*, 703–708. [CrossRef]
11. Logan, P.A.; Armstrong, S.; Avery, T.J.; Barer, D.; Barton, G.R.; Darby, J.; Gladman, J.R.F.; Horne, J.; Leach, S.; Lincoln, N.B.; et al. Rehabilitation aimed at improving outdoor mobility for people after stroke: A multicentre randomised controlled study (the Getting out of the House Study). *Health Technol. Assess.* **2014**, *18*, 1–113. [CrossRef] [PubMed]
12. World Health Organization. International Classification of Functioning, Disability and Health: ICF. Available online: https://apps.who.int/iris/handle/10665/42407 (accessed on 18 July 2022).
13. AOTA. Occupational Therapy Practice Framework: Domain and Process—Fourth Edition. *Am. J. Occup. Ther.* **2020**, *74*, 7412410010p1–7412410010p87. [CrossRef]
14. Eriksson, G.; Kottorp, A.; Borg, J.; Tham, K. Relationship between occupational gaps in everyday life, depressive mood and life satisfaction after acquired brain injury. *J. Rehabil. Med.* **2009**, *41*, 187–194. [CrossRef] [PubMed]
15. Wendel, K.; Ståhl, A.; Risberg, J.; Pessah-Rasmussen, H.; Iwarsson, S. Post-stroke functional limitations and changes in use of mode of transport. *Scand. J. Occup. Ther.* **2010**, *17*, 162–174. [CrossRef] [PubMed]
16. O'Sullivan, C.; Chard, G. An exploration of participation in leisure activities post-stroke. *Aust. Occup. Ther. J.* **2010**, *57*, 159–166. [CrossRef]
17. Burton, C.R. Living with stroke: A phenomenological study. *J. Adv. Nurs.* **2000**, *32*, 301–309. [CrossRef]
18. Balakrishnan, R.; Kaplan, B.; Negron, R.; Fei, K.; Goldfinger, J.Z.; Horowitz, C.R. Life after Stroke in an Urban Minority Population: A Photovoice Project. *Int. J. Environ. Res. Public Health* **2017**, *14*, 293. [CrossRef]
19. Salter, K.; Hellings, C.; Foley, N.; Teasell, R. The experience of living with stroke: A qualitative meta-synthesis. *J. Rehabil. Med.* **2008**, *40*, 595–602. [CrossRef]

20. Barker, D.J.; Reid, D.; Cott, C. The Experience of Senior Stroke Survivors: Factors in Community Participation among Wheelchair Users. *Can. J. Occup. Ther.* **2006**, *73*, 18–25. [CrossRef]
21. Evans, R. The Effect of Electrically Powered Indoor/Outdoor Wheelchairs on Occupation: A Study of Users' Views. *Br. J. Occup. Ther.* **2000**, *63*, 547–553. [CrossRef]
22. Edwards, K.; McCluskey, A. A survey of adult power wheelchair and scooter users. *Disabil. Rehabil. Assist. Technol.* **2010**, *5*, 411–419. [CrossRef] [PubMed]
23. Wressle, E.; Samuelsson, K. User Satisfaction with Mobility Assistive Devices. *Scand. J. Occup. Ther.* **2004**, *11*, 143–150. [CrossRef]
24. Pettersson, I.; Törnquist, K.; Ahlström, G. The effect of an outdoor powered wheelchair on activity and participation in users with stroke. *Disabil. Rehabil. Assist. Technol.* **2006**, *1*, 235–243. [CrossRef] [PubMed]
25. Buning, M.E.; Angelo, J.A.; Schmeler, M.R. Occupational Performance and the Transition to Powered Mobility: A Pilot Study. *Am. J. Occup. Ther.* **2001**, *55*, 339–344. [CrossRef] [PubMed]
26. Brandt, A.; Iwarsson, S.; Ståhle, A. Older people's use of powered wheelchairs for activity and participation. *J. Rehabil. Med.* **2004**, *36*, 70–77. [CrossRef]
27. Deutsche Gesellschaft für Allgemeinmedizin und Familienmedizin. Schlaganfall S3-Leitlinie: DEGAM-Leitlinie Nr. 8. Available online: https://www.awmf.org/uploads/tx_szleitlinien/053-011l_S3_Schlaganfall_2021-03.pdf (accessed on 25 June 2022).
28. Bestmann, A.; Lingnau, M.L.; Staats, M.; Hesse, S. Phasenspezifische Hilfsmittelverordnungen in der neurologischen Rehabilitation. *Rehabilitation* **2001**, *6*, 346–351. [CrossRef]
29. Reuther, P.; Wallesch, C.-W. Teilhabesicherung nach Schlaganfall. *Gesundheitswesen* **2015**, *77*, 513–523. [CrossRef]
30. Perotti, L.; Klebbe, R.; Maier, A.; Eicher, C. Evaluation of the quality and the provision process of wheelchairs in Germany. Results from an online survey. *Disabil. Rehabil. Assist. Technol.* **2020**, 1–10. [CrossRef]
31. Deutsche Vereinigung für Rehabilitation. Für eine optimierte Versorgung mit Hilfsmitteln: Eine Expertise der Deutschen Vereinigung für Rehabilitation zu aktuellen Problemen bei der Versorgung mit Hilfsmitteln. 2006. Available online: https://www.dvfr.de/fileadmin/user_upload/DVfR/Downloads/Stellungnahmen/DVfR-Hilfsmittel-Expertise_061017.pdf (accessed on 18 June 2022).
32. Deutsche Vereinigung für Rehabilitation. Empfehlungen zur Verbesserung des Teilhabeorientierten Versorgungsprozesses Mobilitätseingeschränkter Menschen mit Rollstühlen. 2018. Available online: https://www.dvfr.de/fileadmin/user_upload/DVfR/Downloads/Stellungnahmen/DVfR-Stellungnahme_Rollstuhlversorgung_-_Juni_2018_bf.pdf (accessed on 18 June 2022).
33. Hesse, S.; Gahein-Sama, A.L.; Mauritz, K.-H. Technical aids in hemiparetic patients: Prescription, costs and usage. *Clin. Rehabil.* **1996**, *10*, 328–333. [CrossRef]
34. Hoeß, U.; Schupp, W.; Schmidt, R.; Gräßel, E. Versorgung von Schlaganfallpatienten mit ambulanten Heil- und Hilfsmitteln im Langzeitverlauf nach stationärer neurologischer Rehabilitation. *Phys. Med. Rehabil. Kurortmed.* **2008**, *18*, 115–121. [CrossRef]
35. UN General Assembly. Convention on the Rights of Persons with Disabilities: Resolution/Adopted by the General Assembly, 24 January 2007, A/RES/61/106. Available online: https://www.refworld.org/docid/45f973632.html (accessed on 18 July 2022).
36. Bundesministerium für Arbeit und Soziales. "Unser Weg in eine Inklusive Gesellschaft": Nationaler Aktionsplan 2.0 der Bundesregierung zur UN-Behindertenrechtskonvention (UN-BRK). 2016. Available online: https://www.bmas.de/DE/Soziales/Teilhabe-und-Inklusion/Nationaler-Aktionsplan/nationaler-aktionsplan-2-0.html (accessed on 25 June 2022).
37. Deutsche Vereinigung für Rehabilitation. Stellungnahme: Partizipation an der Forschung–Eine Matrix zur Orientierung. Available online: https://www.dvfr.de/arbeitsschwerpunkte/stellungnahmen-der-dvfr/detail/artikel/dvfr-stellungnahme-partizipation-an-der-forschung-eine-matrix-zur-orientierung/ (accessed on 25 June 2022).
38. Wright, M.T. Partizipative Gesundheitsforschung: Ursprünge und heutiger Stand. *Bundesgesundheitsblatt-Gesundh.-Gesundh.* **2021**, *64*, 140–145. [CrossRef] [PubMed]
39. Munde, V.; Tillmann, V. Partizipative Forschung: Umsetzungsbeispiele und Zukunftsperspektiven. *Teilhabe* **2022**, *61*, 74–80.
40. Wang, C.; Burris, M.A. Photovoice: Concept, methodology, and use for participatory needs assessment. *Health Educ. Behav.* **1997**, *24*, 369–387. [CrossRef]
41. Catalani, C.; Minkler, M. Photovoice: A review of the literature in health and public health. *Health Educ. Behav.* **2010**, *37*, 424–451. [CrossRef] [PubMed]
42. Dassah, E.; Aldersey, H.M.; Norman, K.E. Photovoice and Persons With Physical Disabilities: A Scoping Review of the Literature. *Qual. Health Res.* **2017**, *27*, 1412–1422. [CrossRef] [PubMed]
43. Lal, S.; Jarus, T.; Suto, M.J. A Scoping Review of the Photovoice Method: Implications for Occupational Therapy Research. *Can. J. Occup. Ther.* **2012**, *79*, 181–190. [CrossRef]
44. Evans-Agnew, R.A.; Rosemberg, M.-A.S. Questioning Photovoice Research: Whose Voice? *Qual. Health Res.* **2016**, *26*, 1019–1030. [CrossRef]
45. Levin, T.; Scott, B.M.; Borders, B.; Hart, K.; Lee, J.; Decanini, A. Aphasia Talks: Photography as a means of communication, self-expression, and empowerment in persons with aphasia. *Top. Stroke Rehabil.* **2007**, *14*, 72–84. [CrossRef]
46. Lorenz, L.S. Visual metaphors of living with brain injury: Exploring and communicating lived experience with an invisible injury. *Vis. Stud.* **2010**, *25*, 210–223. [CrossRef]
47. Barclay-Goddard, R.; Ripat, J.; Mayo, N.E. Developing a model of participation post-stroke: A mixed-methods approach. *Qual. Life Res.* **2012**, *21*, 417–426. [CrossRef]

48. Hebblethwaite, S.; Curley, L. Exploring the role of community recreation in stroke recovery using participatory action research and photovoice. *Ther. Recreat. J.* **2015**, *49*, 1–17.
49. Maratos, M.; Huynh, L.; Tan, J.; Lui, J.; Jarus, T. Picture This: Exploring the Lived Experience of High-Functioning Stroke Survivors Using Photovoice. *Qual. Health Res.* **2016**, *26*, 1055–1066. [CrossRef] [PubMed]
50. Törnbom, K.; Lundälv, J.; Palstam, A.; Sunnerhagen, K.S. "My life after stroke through a camera lens"—A photovoice study on participation in Sweden. *PLoS ONE* **2019**, *14*, e0222099. [CrossRef] [PubMed]
51. Dietz, A.; Mamlekar, C.R.; Bakas, K.L.; McCarthy, M.J.; Harley, D.; Bakas, T. A scoping review of PhotoVoice for people with post-stroke aphasia. *Top. Stroke Rehabil.* **2021**, *28*, 219–235. [CrossRef]
52. International Collaboration for Participatory Health Research. *Position Paper 1: What Is Participatory Health Research?* International Collaboration for Participatory Health Research: Berlin, Germany, 2013. Available online: http://www.icphr.org/uploads/2/0/3/9/20399575/ichpr_position_paper_1_defintion_-_version_may_2013.pdf (accessed on 5 June 2022).
53. German Network for Participatory Health Research. PartNet Definition–Partizipative Gesundheitsforschung. Available online: http://partnet-gesundheit.de/ueber-uns/partnet-definition/ (accessed on 24 June 2022).
54. Von Unger, H. *Partizipative Forschung: Einführung in die Forschungspraxis*; Springer: Wiesbaden, Germany, 2014; ISBN 9783658012892.
55. Chung, K.; Lounsbury, D.W. The role of power, process, and relationships in participatory research for statewide HIV/AIDS programming. *Soc. Sci. Med.* **2006**, *63*, 2129–2140. [CrossRef]
56. Von Unger, H.; Narimani, P. *Ethische Reflexivität im Forschungsprozess: Herausforderungen in der Partizipativen Forschung*; WZB Discussion Paper SP I 2012-304; Wissenschaftszentrum Berlin für Sozialforschung (WZB): Berlin, Germany, 2012.
57. Wang, C.C.; Redwood-Jones, Y.A. Photovoice ethics: Perspectives from Flint Photovoice. *Health Educ. Behav.* **2001**, *28*, 560–572. [CrossRef]
58. Abma, T.; Breed, M.; Lips, S.; Schrijver, J. Whose Voice is It Really? Ethics of Photovoice with Children in Health Promotion. *Int. J. Qual. Methods* **2022**, *21*, 160940692110724. [CrossRef]
59. International Collaboration for Participatory Health Research. *Position Paper 2: Participatory Health Research: A Guide to Ethical Principals and Practice*; International Collaboration for Participatory Health Research: Berlin, Germany, 2013. Available online: http://www.icphr.org/uploads/2/0/3/9/20399575/ichpr_position_paper_2_ethics_-_version_october_2013.pdf (accessed on 5 June 2022).
60. Fields, L.M.; Calvert, J.D. Informed consent procedures with cognitively impaired patients: A review of ethics and best practices. *Psychiatry Clin. Neurosci.* **2015**, *69*, 462–471. [CrossRef]
61. Pearl, G.; Cruice, M. Facilitating the Involvement of People with Aphasia in Stroke Research by Developing Communicatively Accessible Research Resources. *Top. Lang. Disord.* **2017**, *37*, 67–84. [CrossRef]
62. Hansen-Schirra, S.; Maaß, C. Easy Language, Plain Language, Easy Language Plus: Perspectives on Comprehensibility and Stigmatisation. In *Easy Language Research: Text and User Perspectives*, 2nd ed.; Hansen-Schirra, S., Maaß, C., Eds.; Frank & Timme: Berlin, Germany, 2020; pp. 17–38.
63. Bundesministerium für Arbeit und Soziales. Leichte Sprache. Ein Rat ge ber. Available online: https://www.bmas.de/DE/Service/Publikationen/Broschueren/a752-leichte-sprache-ratgeber.html (accessed on 27 June 2022).
64. Arnold, D.; Glässel, A.; Böttger, T.; Sarma, N.; Bethmann, A.; Narimani, P. "What do you need? What are you experiencing?" Relationship building and power dynamics in participatory research projects: Critical self-reflections of researchers. *Int. J. Environ. Res. Public Health* **2022**, *19*, 9336. [CrossRef]
65. Schaefer, I.; Kümpers, S.; Cook, T. "Selten Gehörte" für partizipative Gesundheitsforschung gewinnen: Herausforderungen und Strategien. *Bundesgesundheitsblatt-Gesundh. -Gesundh.* **2021**, *64*, 163–170. [CrossRef] [PubMed]
66. Allweiss, T.; Perowanowitsch, M.; Burtscher, R.; Wright, M.T. Participatory Exploration of Factors Influencing the Health of People with Intellectual Disabilities in an Urban District: A photovoice study. In Proceedings of the 3rd International Conference on Public Health, Kuala Lumpur, Malaysia, 27–29 July 2017; pp. 237–245. [CrossRef]
67. Lorenz, L.S. *Brain Injury Survivors: Narratives of Rehabilitation and Healing*; Lynne Rienner Publishers: Boulder, CO, USA, 2010; ISBN 1588267288.
68. Lorenz, L.S. What Is Photovoice? A Photovoice Path. Available online: https://www.photovoiceworldwide.com/what-is-photovoice/ (accessed on 26 June 2022).
69. The Federal Health Monitoring System. Definition: Degree of Disability. Available online: https://www.gbe-bund.de/gbe/ergebnisse.prc_tab?fid=8296&suchstring=&query_id=&sprache=E&fund_typ=DEF&methode=&vt=&verwandte=1&page_ret=0&seite=1&p_lfd_nr=13&p_news=&p_sprachkz=E&p_uid=gast&p_aid=18602946&hlp_nr=2&p_janein=J (accessed on 25 June 2022).
70. The Federal Health Monitoring System. Definition: Severely Handicapped Persons. Available online: https://www.gbe-bund.de/gbe/ergebnisse.prc_tab?fid=2108&suchstring=&query_id=&sprache=E&fund_typ=DEF&methode=&vt=&verwandte=1&page_ret=0&seite=1&p_lfd_nr=15&p_news=&p_sprachkz=E&p_uid=gast&p_aid=18602946&hlp_nr=2&p_janein=J (accessed on 25 June 2022).
71. Nieß, M.; Aichele, V. Selbstbestimmt Unterwegs in Berlin? Mobilität von Menschen mit Behinderungen aus Menschenrechtlicher Perspektive. Available online: http://www.institut-fuer-menschenrechte.de/fileadmin/user_upload/Publikationen/BERICHT/Bericht_Selbstbestimmt_unterwegs_in_Berlin.pdf (accessed on 25 June 2022).

72. Römisch, K.; Tillmann, V. Mobilität als Voraussetzung für selbstbestimmte Mobilität im Sinnne der UN-BRK. *Teilhabe* **2017**, *56*, 100–1006.
73. Hammel, J.; Jones, R.; Gossett, A.; Morgan, E. Examining barriers and supports to community living and participation after a stroke from a participatory action research approach. *Top. Stroke Rehabil.* **2006**, *13*, 43–58. [CrossRef] [PubMed]
74. Smith, E.M.; Sakakibara, B.M.; Miller, W.C. A review of factors influencing participation in social and community activities for wheelchair users. *Disabil. Rehabil. Assist. Technol.* **2016**, *11*, 361–374. [CrossRef]
75. Deutsches Institut für Menschenrechte. Mobilität von Menschen mit Behinderungen in Berlin Verbessern: Empfehlungen für Eine an der UN-Behindertenrechtskonvention Ausgerichtete Mobilitätsplanung. Available online: https://www.institut-fuer-menschenrechte.de/fileadmin/Redaktion/Publikationen/Position/Position_Mobilitaet_von_Menschen_mit_Behinderungen_in_Berlin_verbessern.pdf (accessed on 4 June 2022).
76. Deutsche Presse-Agentur. Ist nur Jede Dritte Arztpraxis Behindertengerecht Ausgestattet? Available online: https://www.aerztezeitung.de/Wirtschaft/Ist-nur-jede-dritte-Arztpraxis-behindertengerecht-ausgestattet-409719.html (accessed on 4 June 2022).
77. Pharr, J.R.; James, T.; Yeung, Y.-L. Accessibility and accommodations for patients with mobility disabilities in a large healthcare system: How are we doing? *Disabil. Health J.* **2019**, *12*, 679–684. [CrossRef]
78. Ståhl, A.; Månsson Lexell, E. Facilitators for travelling with local public transport among people with mild cognitive limitations after stroke. *Scand. J. Occup. Ther.* **2018**, *25*, 108–118. [CrossRef]
79. Jónasdóttir, S.K.; Egilson, S.Þ.; Polgar, J. Services, systems, and policies affecting community mobility for people with mobility impairments in Northern Iceland: An occupational perspective. *J. Occup. Sci.* **2018**, *25*, 309–321. [CrossRef]
80. Pellichero, A.; Kenyon, L.K.; Best, K.L.; Lamontagne, M.-E.; Lavoie, M.D.; Sorita, É.; Routhier, F. Relationships between Cognitive Functioning and Powered Mobility Device Use: A Scoping Review. *Int. J. Environ. Res. Public Health* **2021**, *18*, 12467. [CrossRef]
81. Christensen, E.R.; Golden, S.L.; Gesell, S.B. Perceived Benefits of Peer Support Groups for Stroke Survivors and Caregivers in Rural North Carolina. *North Carol. Med. J.* **2019**, *80*, 143–148. [CrossRef]
82. Wijekoon, S.; Wilson, W.; Gowan, N.; Ferreira, L.; Phadke, C.; Udler, E.; Bontempo, T. Experiences of Occupational Performance in Survivors of Stroke Attending Peer Support Groups. *Can. J. Occup. Ther.* **2020**, *87*, 173–181. [CrossRef]
83. von Peter, S.; Bär, G.; Behrisch, B.; Bethmann, A.; Hartung, S.; Kasberg, A.; Wulff, I.; Wright, M. Partizipative Gesundheitsforschung in Deutschland–quo vadis? *Gesundheitswesen* **2020**, *82*, 328–332. [CrossRef] [PubMed]
84. Reuther, P. Teilhabe für Schwerbetroffene: Ambulante und mobile neurologische Rehabilitation im Wohn- und Lebensraum. In *Teilhaben!!: NeuroRehabilitation und Nachsorge zu Teilhabe und Inklusion*, 2nd ed.; Fries, W., Reuther, P., Lössl, H., Eds.; Aktualisierte und Erweiterte Auflage; Hippocampus: Bad Honnef, Germany, 2017; pp. 37–48.
85. Doig, E.; Fleming, J.; Kuipers, P. Achieving Optimal Functional Outcomes in Community-Based Rehabilitation following Acquired Brain Injury: A Qualitative Investigation of Therapists' Perspectives. *Br. J. Occup. Ther.* **2008**, *71*, 360–370. [CrossRef]
86. Hillier, S.; Inglis-Jassiem, G. Rehabilitation for community-dwelling people with stroke: Home or centre based? A systematic review. *Int. J. Stroke* **2010**, *5*, 178–186. [CrossRef]
87. Wilcock, A.A. *An Occupational Perspective of Health*, 2nd ed.; Slack: London, UK, 2006.
88. Funke, A.; Grehl, T.; Großkreutz, J.; Münch, C.; Walter, B.; Kettemann, D.; Karnapp, C.; Gajewski, N.; Meyer, R.; Maier, A.; et al. Hilfsmittelversorgung bei der amyotrophen Lateralsklerose. Analyse aus 3 Jahren Fallmanagement in einem internetunterstützten Versorgungsnetzwerk. *Nervenarzt* **2015**, *86*, 1007–1017. [CrossRef] [PubMed]
89. Sander, M.; Albrecht, M.; Loos, S.; Möllenkamp, M.; Stengel, V.; Igl, G. *Leistungsbewilligungen und -Ablehnungen durch Krankenkassen; Studie für den Beauftragten der Bundesregierung für die Belange der Patientinnen und Patienten Sowie Bevollmächtigten für Pflege*; IGES Institut: Berlin, Germany, 2017. Available online: https://www.iges.com/sites/igesgroup/iges.de/myzms/content/e6/e1621/e10211/e15829/e20499/e20500/e20502/attr_objs20506/StudiezuLeistungsbewilligungenund-ablehnungen_ger.pdf (accessed on 13 June 2022).
90. Sergeant, S.; Peels, H.; Sandvoort, H.; Pseudonym, B.; Schelfhout, P.; de Schauwer, E. A collective biography on working relationships in inclusive research teams. *Disabil. Soc.* **2022**, 1–18. [CrossRef]

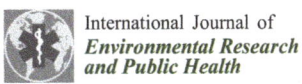

Protocol

Promoting Health and Behavior Change through Evidence-Based Landscape Interventions in Rural Communities: A Pilot Protocol

Shan Jiang [1,*], Udday Datta [2] and Christine Jones [3]

1 GBBN Architects, Pittsburgh, PA 15206, USA
2 School of Design and Community Development, West Virginia University, Morgantown, WV 26506, USA
3 Community Care of West Virginia at Big Otter (Big Otter Clinic), Ivydale, WV 25113, USA
* Correspondence: sjiang@gbbn.com

Abstract: Rural communities in the United States have many public health issues, including a high prevalence of physical inactivity, obesity, and higher risks for major non-communicable diseases. A lack of safe and convenient places to exercise could intensify healthy lifestyle disparities. Individually adapted physical activity prescriptions at the primary level of healthcare could play a role in behavior change for rural residents. Healthcare professionals and designers created the rural wellness hub concept, which integrates walking trails and therapeutic landscape features on the clinic site, to support patient physician-prescribed activities and treatments. This research protocol reports the design and implementation of the rural wellness hub at a clinic in Clay County, West Virginia. Following a participatory, evidence-based landscape intervention (EBLI) protocol, 58 user representatives (patient = 49; clinic employee = 9) participated in the four-phase protocol: (1) pre-design survey, (2) design and development, (3) post-design interview, and (4) post-occupancy evaluation. Survey and interview data from all phases were collected and analyzed. The preliminary results indicate that the redesigned clinic campus could promote several health programs among local communities, with the benefits of walking trails, in particular, highlighted. The rigorous EBLI protocol could serve as a template for rural communities that seek to develop similar healthcare intervention programs.

Keywords: evidence-based design; therapeutic landscapes; physical activity; rural community; health promotion

1. Introduction

Sedentary lifestyles and physical inactivity have been associated with many chronic diseases and a significant portion of death in the United States [1]. Physical inactivity prevalence among rural populations is much higher than their non-rural counterparts [2]. Public health professionals have been advocating behavior interventions that focus on physical activity promotion, in which the core intervention programs should match the unique attributes and preferences of the target population [3]. Individually adapted physical activity prescriptions at the primary level of healthcare have emerged as a new method to engage people and deliver positive outcomes; however, physicians are facing multiple obstacles, including a lack of access to resources and facilities, and inadequate coordination of the health intervention programs [4]. Therapeutic landscapes in clinical environments as a health intervention have started to gain attention in contemporary research. This article reports an evidence-based landscape intervention (EBLI) protocol that designs and develops a rural wellness hub in support of physical activity prescriptions and healthy lifestyle promotion.

1.1. Physical Inactivity Prevalence in Rural Communities

Physical inactivity for adults is defined as not participating in any regular leisure-time physical activities such as running, walking for exercise, or gardening [5]. According to a

series of studies conducted by the Centers for Disease Control and Prevention (CDC) [6], seven states in the U.S. (i.e., West Virginia, Oklahoma, Louisiana, Alabama, Kentucky, Arkansas, and Mississippi) and Puerto Rico have a physical inactivity prevalence of 30% or more. A lack of safe and convenient places to exercise in those areas could intensify disparities in leading a healthy lifestyle [6]. The World Health Organization (WHO) [7] has warned that physically inactive lifestyles are a leading cause of major non-communicable diseases and can seriously impact people's health status. Strong evidence has shown significant correlations between physical inactivity and the increased risk of obesity, coronary heart disease, diabetes, cancer, and shorter life expectancy [8].

West Virginia is categorized as one of the most rural states in the U.S., with more than 50% of its population living in rural communities [9]. The state has been ranked as the 11th state with high physical inactivity prevalence—more than 28.5% of West Virginian adults did not routinely participate in leisure-time physical activity or exercise [10]. Despite the highly ranked forest coverage and abundant natural resources, the West Virginian rural population—particularly seniors, the disabled, and the medically underserved—have limited daily access to public open spaces and physical activity opportunities [11,12]. According to a cross-sectional study on more than 400 participants who participated in primary care, the most common barrier to physical activity was lack of resources (80.5%), which was particularly significant among people of lower income socioeconomic status [13]. Gilbert et al. [14] made similar conclusions that the physical activity participation rate among rural populations is significantly lower than urban and suburban counterparts, and environmental barriers were significant obstacles to physical activities, including the lack of desired amenities and design characteristics, location, accessibility, and safety.

In the context of emerging needs for safe, accessible, and convenient sites to host various health intervention programs, the rural wellness hub concept was coined collectively by healthcare professionals and designers, and first piloted in southern West Virginia. The hub integrates walking trails and therapeutic landscape features to support physician-prescribed physical activities and treatments on the clinic site. The design and development of the hub followed a rigorous protocol, namely that of evidence-based landscape intervention (EBLI), which involves stakeholder participation and research components to ensure the hub's usability and wellness outcomes.

1.2. Behavior Change through Community Building

Several behavioral change models contribute to the theoretical framework for the EBLI protocol. The Health Belief Model (HBM) was originally developed by a group of social psychologists in the U.S. Public Health Service who aimed to detangle a series of applied research problems that had emerged since the 1950s, and has been expanded and updated to serve as a dominant model in health behavior change [15–17]. Among the six key constructs of HBM, the "perceived barriers" were negative aspects of a particular health action that may act as obstacles for individuals undertaking recommended behaviors [18]. The "cues to action" suggest that cues such as bodily events and media publicity could help trigger the actions to perform the recommended behavior [18]. The theory of planned behavior (TPB) focuses on explaining individual motivation as a decisive factor in performing a specific behavior—a person's strong beliefs that positive outcomes are associated with the behavior (i.e., behavioral belief) determines the individual's willingness to perform the behavior [19]. A person's perceived control over behavioral performance, including the perceived ease or challenge, is expected to have a direct effect on executing the behavior [20].

Rural communities hold unique cultures that vary in their approach to physical activities and health behaviors [14,21]. "Important determinants of health-related behavior are embedded in relationships that tie individuals to organizations, neighborhoods, families, and friends in their community" [22]. Therefore, building rural community organizations with accessible resources and collective goals could be effective models for facilitating health behavior change among rural populations [23]. Recreational and fitness programming in indoor facilities have been suggested to promote physical activity and healthy lifestyles for rural communities [24]. Rural communities in regions that have heavy industries such as coal mining and steel industry face serious challenges regarding environmental health [25]. Green public open spaces in rural communities in West Virginia will promote residents' exposure to healthy environments and lead to positive health outcomes [26]. Considering the numerous benefits of green exercise (i.e., participating in physical activities in a natural setting) on people's physical and mental health [27], implementing therapeutic landscapes and outdoor features in rural wellness centers as interventions to promote physical activities and wellbeing deserves further exploration.

1.3. Evidence-Based Design Approach

Evidence-based design (EBD) is a process of planning, designing, and constructing healthcare environments that makes decisions according to credible research to achieve the best possible outcomes [28]. The EBD has proven its effectiveness in promoting patient and user experiences and medical outcomes in the healthcare context, which has become a leading trend and effective tool in the healthcare design realm [29]. Eight key steps in EBD span the entire cycle of the healthcare project: (1) defining the EBD goals and objectives, (2) identifying sources of information, (3) critical interpretation of relevant research evidence, (4) the generation of innovative EBD concepts, (5) hypothesis development and testing, (6) collecting baseline performance measures, (7) monitoring design implementation and construction, and finally (8) conducting post-occupancy evaluations [28]. Along the different phases of an EBD project, sources of reliable information should cover relevant research evidence in the knowledge field as well as key stakeholders' and end-users' opinions to ensure that the information can be appropriately interpreted in line with the cultural norms of local communities [30]. The essence of EBD is user-centered, which maximizes the usability of the design for optimal outcomes. In situations where gaps exist between research evidence and practices, ad hoc studies with research questions and hypotheses arising from the project could be strategically embedded in the EBD process. Using community-based, non-empirical samples to address those questions and hypotheses could aid decision-making by providing loops of feedback quickly in a well-situated context [31,32].

1.4. Research Objectives

This study aimed at the development and implementation of an EBLI protocol that converts a traditional rural clinic to a wellness hub that facilitates several physical activity intervention programs directly on the clinic site. Primary research objectives addressed in the study include: (1) to explore suitable physical activities and design features that fulfill users' needs on the clinic site. (2) to implement the EBLI protocol to support the rural wellness hub concept on a pilot clinic site.

2. Materials and Methods

2.1. The Pilot Site and Context

The Community Care of West Virginia (CCWV) Big Otter Clinic in Clay County is the pilot site for this study. The CCWV organization is a federally qualifying health clinic network that serves low-income and underinsured patients in West Virginia. The CCWV Big Otter Clinic (henceforth referred to as the clinic) sought to renovate its outdoor environments by introducing a series of landscape features to support treatments and physical activities and to host educational programs for local communities in the county. The need to renew the existing clinic grounds arose in response to two emergent healthcare approaches: (1) the clinic physicians intended to prescribe exercises and walking time for their primary care patients and coordinate physical activity programs directly on the clinic site to improve participation [3]; and (2) the clinic therapists intended to offer walk-and-talk therapy sessions to facilitate patients' psychological processing [33]. Therefore, the rural wellness hub concept was introduced to the clinic site not just to deliver sickness treatment but to support disease prevention and wellness care. The wellness hub will provide safe and accessible opportunities for people to walk, exercise, and meditate in nature; the hub includes paths for walking and exercise, seating areas with different levels of privacy, and gathering spaces for community events and educational programs. The clinic physicians and staff members can also use the outdoor space to take breaks from work-related stress [34,35]. The ultimate project goal is to transition a traditional clinic site to a wellness center to serve as a node in an extensive network of trails and parks in the region.

2.2. The Four-Phased EBLI Protocol

The project follows a mixed-method, four-phase EBLI protocol that integrates key components of evidence-based design and community-based participatory design, as discussed, including (1) pre-design survey, (2) site design and development, (3) post-design interview, and (4) post-occupancy evaluation (POE). The pre-design survey was designed to explore user's preferred outdoor activities, desired landscape features, behavior patterns, and overall usage situations of the clinic site. Patients and clinic staff members were randomly recruited to form a representative sample of users. Two versions of the survey questionnaires were administrated, including a hard copy survey for the patients and an online version for the employees. Each version of the survey had some tailored questions for the user group; for instance, the patient participants were asked questions such as "how often do you visit the clinic?" and "how do you spend your waiting time before seeing the doctor?" Comparatively, employee participants were asked questions such as "how much break time do you have per day?" and "how do you spend your break time?" Both surveys asked the same questions about the participant's preferred physical and leisure activities, and their preferred landscape design features using 5-point Likert scales.

The site design and development phase were conducted by the project team consisting of faculty and graduate students in landscape architecture from West Virginia University. The design team conducted a thorough site analysis and a literature review of relevant research evidence, then utilized the pre-design survey to inform the initial site design. After completing the first round of site design, a post-design interview (Phase 3) was conducted to collect user representatives' feedback on the initial design ideas. The initial site design plan, together with a series of reference images depicting different design elements, were presented to the interviewees. Participants' preference for different programming elements and design styles was recorded, transcribed, and analyzed by the project team. The design suggestions were looped back to reshape the site design and development and finalize the Phase 2 efforts (Figure 1). There could be multiple rounds of post-design interviews with different emphases depending on the scope of the project and the level of details. Frequent feedback and quick assessments during design implementation and site construction are also desirable from the knowledge-sharing perspective [36]. The pre-design surveys and post-design interview questions can be accessed as supplementary materials through the open access data deposit [37].

Due to funding constraints, the clinic prioritized the implementation of walking trails and phased development of other features over future years. As reported in February 2022, the outside border trail and benches along the trail were completed and some minimal landscaping along the site border was under construction. The next round of funding will be used to install additional seating, signage, and to develop the meditation garden near the behavioral health office. The trails have been used by patients and physicians and the clinic doctor has provided some written feedback as preliminary POE data (Phase 4). The project team plans to conduct a full POE after the site construction is completed and has been experienced by the users.

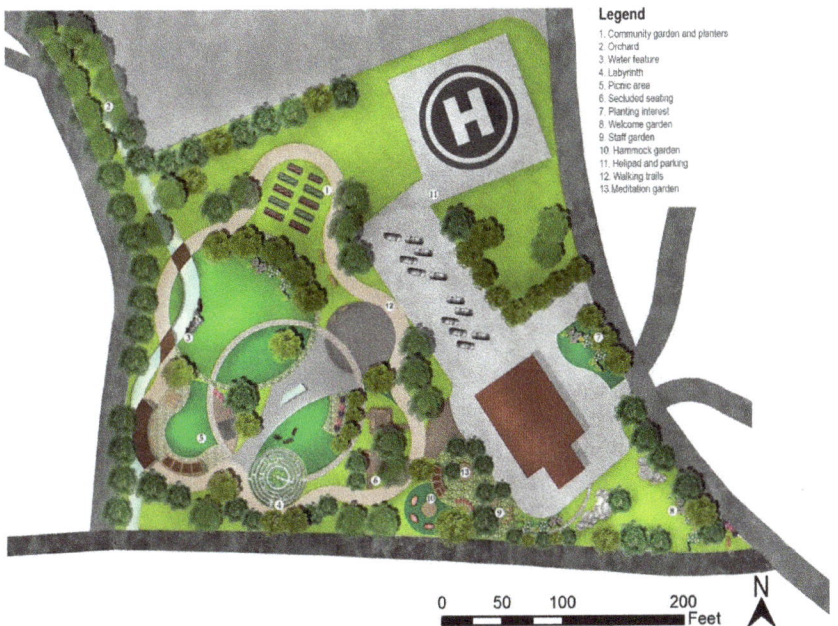

Figure 1. Finalized site plan for the clinic after Phase 2 and 3 following the EBLI protocol.

2.3. Methods and Participants

A total of 58 user representatives (patient = 49; clinic employee = 9) participated in the four-phased EBLI protocol, including 48 patients and 6 clinic employees during Phase 1 pre-design survey, 1 patient representative and 1 employee representative during Phase 3 post-design interview, and 2 employees who provided preliminary POE feedback during Phase 4. Participants in the project were protected by the Office of Research Integrity and Compliance at West Virginia University.

2.3.1. Pre-Design Survey

Patient Survey. The project was conducted during the COVID-19 pandemic with restricted in-person visiting policies. Therefore, the clinic doctor helped coordinate the pre-design survey. Considering the potential of the digital divide among rural and senior populations, a paper-pencil survey questionnaire was administrated to patient participants onsite [38]. Patients who visited the clinic between September 2020 and February 2021 were recruited by the front desk receptionist and asked to fill out the questionnaire onsite if the patient agreed to participate in the survey. The survey period followed the project funding period and the site design and construction timeline. The number of survey invitations and the response rate was not traceable.

A convenience sample of 48 adult patients participated in the pre-design survey and the demographic information of the sample is provided in Table 1. Participants in the sample belong to diverse age groups but were skewed to the seniors, with 4.2% from 18–24 years old, 6.3% from 25–34 years old, 18.8% from 35–44 years old, 8.3% from 45–54 years old, 25% from 55–64 years old, and 37.5% who were 65 years of age or older. The sample was dominated by white (97.9%) and female (83.3%) participants. The majority, 72.9% of the participants, were regular patients of the clinic, and 20.8% were occasional clinic visitors when they need to see a doctor. The sample's age distribution was representative as the clinic doctor described the clinic as serving mostly senior patients. Looking at the broad picture, the Big Otter clinic serves Clay County in West Virginia. According to the census data estimation as of July 2021, the county's population estimates was 7892, with 22.3% senior residents (65 years and above) and 49.1% female residents; about 97.6% of the county's residents were white alone, and 23.3% of the county residents were in poverty [39].

Table 1. Survey participants demographic information.

Demographic Information		Patient Survey Participants	
		Count	Valid Percent
Age	18–24 years old	2	4.2
	25–34 years old	3	6.3
	35–44 years old	9	18.8
	45–54 years old	4	8.3
	55–64 years old	12	25
	65–74 years old	12	25
	75+ years old	6	12.5
Gender	Male	8	16.7
	Female	40	83.3
Ethnicity	White	47	97.9
	Native American/American Indian	1	2.1
Clinic Visit	Regular patient	35	72.9
	Occasionally as needed	10	20.8
	Emergency	2	4.2
	Missing data	1	2.1
Demographic Information		Staff Survey Participants	
		Count	Valid Percent
Age	25–34 years old	1	16.7
	35–44 years old	3	50
	45–54 years old	2	33.3
Gender	Female	6	100
Ethnicity	White	6	100

Employee Survey. The web-version of the pre-design survey was distributed to all clinic employees through the internal email system, including three behavioral health specialists and nine general clinic staff. Six clinic employees participated in the pre-design survey and the demographic information of the sample is shown in Table 1. The employee survey response rate was about 66.7%. Employee participants in the sample belong to three age groups, with 16.7% from 25–34 years old, 50% from 35–44 years old, and 33.3% from 45–54 years old. All employee participants were white females (Table 1).

2.3.2. Post-Design Interview and Content Analysis

All participants in the survey phase were asked if they agreed to be contacted for Phase 3 of the study. Among those who indicated willingness to participate, a total of two user representatives (1 patient and 1 nurse) showed up for post-design interviews (Phase 3) through one-on-one Zoom meetings on 26 March 2021. Transcribed interviews were analyzed using content analysis techniques aided by QDA Miner Lite software [40]. Transcribed interviews were coded in four main categories: (1) Design Favored, (2) Design Unfavored, (3) Functionality, and (4) Interaction. Under each category, multiple themes emerged. These themes were used to analyze each interview to understand the participants' responses to the proposed designs.

2.3.3. Preliminary POE Feedback

The site construction was not fully completed when the protocol was documented, and only one doctor provided preliminary POE feedback through conventional email communications. A diagnostic POE study will be conducted after the site is fully constructed [41].

2.4. Statistical Analyses

Descriptive statistics (mean [M], standard deviation [SD]) and one-way between-group analysis of variance (ANOVA) with Tukey's HSD Test for multiple comparisons were conducted to compare the differences between age groups regarding the preferred physical activities and site design features. All statistical analyses were conducted using the IBM SPSS (Version 28.0) software (IBM, Armonk, NY, USA) [42].

3. Results
3.1. Pre-Design Survey
3.1.1. Patient Survey

The pre-design survey results served as guidelines to indicate design decisions. Patient participants were asked to rate their level of preference for a series of recreational activities on 5-point Likert scales (1 = "Dislike very much", 5 = "Like very much"). One response was excluded due to missing values and eventually, 47 responses were analyzed. Referring to Sullivan and Artino [43], "parametric tests are sufficiently robust to yield largely unbiased answers that are acceptably close to 'the truth' when analyzing Likert scale responses," therefore, the mean preference scores of the survey items are reported below.

The top five preferred activities were reading (M = 4.49, SD = 0.93), roaming in the woods (M = 4.4, SD = 1.1), gardening (M = 4.38, SD = 1.05), hiking (M = 4.26, SD = 1.21), and music/instruments (M = 4.06, SD = 1.21), and the bottom five preferred activities were climbing (M = 2.6, SD = 1.33), jogging/running (M = 2.79, SD = 1.37), yoga (M = 2.98, SD = 1.28), art (M = 3.21, SD = 1.35), and cycling (M = 3.28, SD = 1.31). Because age was a major variable in the study sample, the participants' preferred recreational activities were analyzed and compared across different age groups. Figure 2 demonstrates that as the age increases, participants' general interest in intensive physical activities decreased. A one-way between-group ANOVA was conducted to explore the impact of age on preference scores for recreational activities. The results indicated statistically significant differences for jogging/running, climbing, and reading among different age groups, with jogging $F(6, 40) = 6.28$, $p < 0.001$; climbing $F(6, 40) = 4.49$, $p = 0.001$; and reading $F(6, 40) = 3.54$, $p = 0.007$. Tukey's HSD Test for multiple comparisons found that the mean preference scores for participants in age groups above 65 years old were significantly lower than participants under 45 years old for jogging and climbing, and the mean preference scores for reading among participants older than 65 years were significantly higher than participants in younger age groups (Table 2).

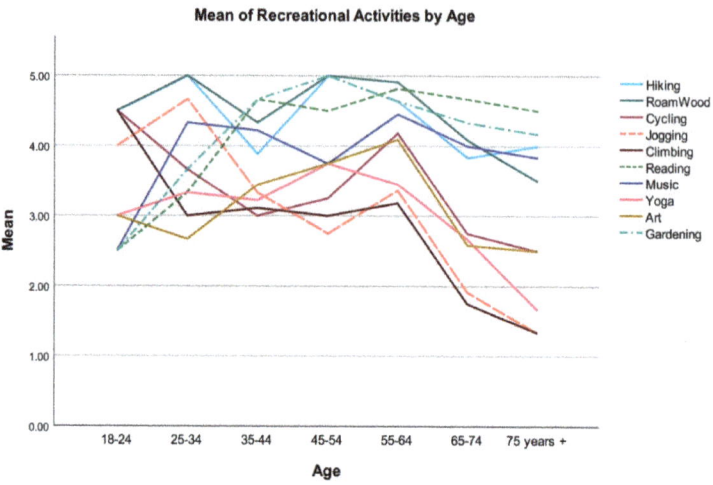

Figure 2. Preference of recreational activities by age.

Table 2. Tukey's HSD Test for Multiple Comparisons by Recreational Activities. This table reports only the statistically significant results because of the great number of variables and categories.

Dependent Variable	(I) Age	(J) Age	Difference (I–J)	Std. Error	Sig.	95% Confidence Interval	
						Lower Bound	Upper Bound
Jogging or Running	18–24	75+	2.67	0.86	0.05	0.00	5.33
	25–34	65–74	2.75	0.68	0.00	0.64	4.86
		75+	3.33	0.74	0.00	1.03	5.64
	35–44	75+	2.00	0.55	0.01	0.28	3.72
		65–74	1.45	0.44	0.03	0.09	2.81
	55–64	65–74	1.45	0.44	0.03	0.09	2.81
		75+	2.03	0.53	0.01	0.37	3.69
Climbing	18–24	65–74	2.75	0.84	0.03	0.14	5.36
		75+	3.17	0.90	0.02	0.37	5.96
	55–64	65–74	1.43	0.46	0.05	0.00	2.86
		75+	1.85	0.56	0.03	0.11	3.58
Reading	18–24	35–44	−2.17	0.63	0.02	−4.12	−0.21
		55–64	−2.32	0.62	0.01	−4.24	−0.40
		65–74	−2.17	0.62	0.02	−4.08	−0.26

Participants were asked to rate their level of preference for five landscape programming elements for the site on 5-point Likert scales (1 = "Dislike very much", 5 = "Like very much"). The average scores for the programming elements, ranked from the most to least preferred were: trails (M = 4.91, SD = 0.35), picnic areas (M = 4.68, SD = 0.73), community garden (M = 4.49, SD = 0.95), gathering space (M = 4.06, SD = 1.19), water feature (M = 3.87, SD = 1.21), and playground (M = 3.72, SD = 1.31). Figure 3 demonstrates that trails were ranked as the most preferred programming element by all age group participants, and the playground was ranked the least preferred by participants under 25 or older than 55 years old. A one-way between-group ANOVA indicated a statistically significant difference for playground among participants from different age groups, $F(6, 40) = 2.76$, $p = 0.024$, and post hoc tests did not identify statistical significance between different age groups.

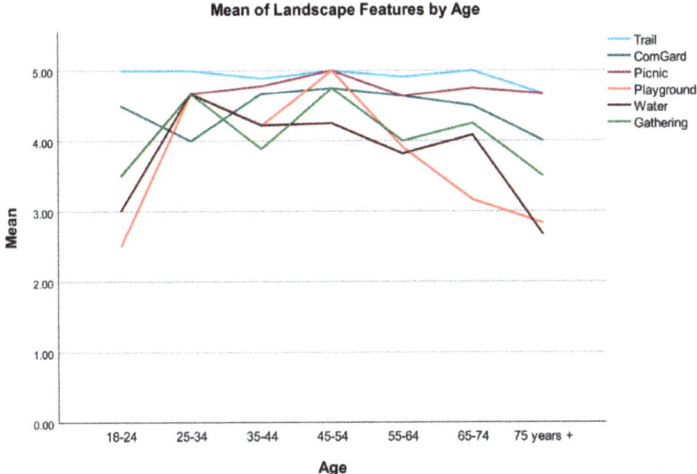

Figure 3. Preference of landscape features by age.

3.1.2. Employee Survey

Participants were asked to rate their level of preference for a series of recreational activities on 5-point Likert scales (1 = "Dislike very much", 5 = "Like very much"). Due to the small sample size, only descriptive statistics were conducted on their preferred recreational activities and landscape programming. The top five preferred activities were cycling ($M = 4.83$, $SD = 0.41$), music or instruments ($M = 4.83$, $SD = 0.41$), roaming in the woods ($M = 4.67$, $SD = 0.52$), hiking ($M = 4.17$, $SD = 0.75$), and yoga ($M = 4$, $SD = 1.55$), and the bottom five referred activities were art ($M = 3.5$, $SD = 0.84$), gardening ($M = 3.5$, $SD = 1.05$), jogging or running ($M = 3.5$, $SD = 1.23$), reading ($M = 3.5$, $SD = 1.05$), and climbing ($M = 3.67$, $SD = 1.03$). Employee participants were also asked to rate their level of preference for five landscape programming elements. The average scores for the programming elements, ranked from the most to least preference were: playground ($M = 5$, $SD = 0$), community garden ($M = 4.67$, $SD = 0.82$), trails ($M = 4.5$, $SD = 0.55$), gathering space ($M = 4.5$, $SD = 0.55$), and water feature ($M = 3.33$, $SD = 1.51$).

3.1.3. Summary and Additional Feedback

To summarize the pre-design survey results from all user groups, the site design should emphasize trails that support walking and roaming in the woods, places to sit or read, gardening in community gardens, and multifunctional spaces for music or similar community events. Additionally, the patient participants reported their feedback about the quality of the clinic's built environment through open-ended questions. Nineteen participants contributed their suggestions regarding the features they wish to improve for the clinic. The top-ranked items were all relevant to the outside environments, including landscapes/landscaping (6 times/31.6%), adding trails on the clinic ground (3 times/15.8%), and more outside lighting (2 times/10.5%). Other minor suggestions included interior paint and flooring, parking lot, waiting room layout, and modernizing the overall architectural style (1 time/5.3% for each). Employees reported having 15–30 min of break time during a typical workday in the clinic with moderate stress level. Their average satisfaction score with the overall physical environment of the clinic was neutral ($M = 3.4$, $SD = 0.89$), and their desired landscape programming elements included: places to sit outside for lunch, trails to walk before or after work, a more naturalistic design, and more lighting outside.

3.2. Post-Design Interview

The patient representative had an overall positive response to the initial site design proposal. Handicap accessibility and ease for wheelchair users were the primary concerns. The overall mood of the place was very important. The participant preferred designs that helped create a warm, welcoming, joyous environment. In terms of functionality, the participant welcomed the inclusion of outdoor lighting, wayfinding signage, an outdoor bathroom, and a healing garden. A colorful planting palette with a naturalistic style was preferred over designs with geometrical shapes and hardscape elements. The participant thought a dense, shaded, and secluded type of trail looked lonely and preferred an open parkland style to encourage socialization. Water features were also preferred because of their calming effect. Design elements such as firepits were not considered fitting as they can be hazardous for small children accompanying the elderly. The participant welcomed the idea of a hammock garden and thought it could be a good place to read. Design elements such as a greenhouse and a yoga or meditation area were welcomed. Noise from the adjacent road was identified as a major problem, and a noise buffer was suggested.

The employee representative also had a positive response to the initial preliminary site design plan. The safety of the elderly occupants and ease of maintenance were priorities for selecting detailed design style and elements. The naturalistic landscaping was preferred over high-maintenance geometric styles. The participant welcomed the inclusion of water features due to their soothing impact on the users and the seasonal wet conditions of the site were identified as a potential design opportunity to create an immersive landscape. A mixture of socializing spaces and spaces that allow users to relax and contemplate might be ideal for this project. Low maintenance traditional planter boxes at a raised height were favored. Naturalistic landscaping and a vivid color palette were preferred over manicured lawns. The public park style outdoor furniture was preferred over homey style patio-type furniture. Design elements such as fire pits and hammock gardens were considered unfitting for an older generation target population. The presence of a power line going across the proposed helipad location was identified as a significant limitation.

3.3. Preliminary Post Occupancy Evaluation (POE)

Two clinic doctors reported their observations of the site usage as preliminary POE data through email communications from February to September 2022. The behavior health doctor reported that they have started using the therapeutic landscape features and walking trails for the walk-and-talk therapy: "Our counselor sees a lot of benefit with the school-age children when she takes them outside. We also have had positive feedback from the adult patients as well."

One family medicine doctor provided some feedback about the trail usage situation by different patient groups (Figure 4A–C):

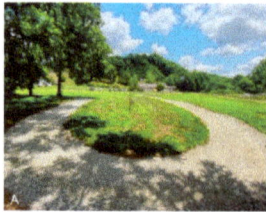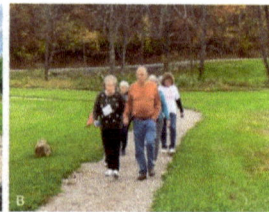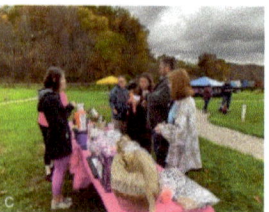

Figure 4. (**A**) The first loop of trails installed on the clinic site; (**B**) trails supporting the patient walking club organized by the clinic doctor; and (**C**) the fundraising event for breast cancer hosted on the site in October 2021.

"The park, even in the beginning stages, is being used already. Our behavioral health team find the walking appt options very useful for ADHD children. They feel they can get 10–15 min of solid time with them in a much more relaxed atmosphere. We hosted a fundraiser for breast cancer on the site in October. The staff is using it for walking at lunch ... I have begun a walking club on Tuesday afternoon with patients, although this is weather dependent in the winter. We have had some feedback already that everyone wants the outside trail to be paved so they can take wheelchairs."—Big Otter Clinic Doctor Feedback

4. Discussion

The rural population in the U.S. is facing increased rates of physical inactivity, obesity, and the associated health risks for major non-communicable diseases [44]. Infrastructure interventions, such as trails and parks where outdoor exercises and healthful events are hosted, could play an important role in promoting physical activity and raising health awareness among local communities [45]. For rural communities that are isolated or lack safe and convenient places to exercise and host those healthful events, it becomes imperative to establish a network of rural wellness centers that consolidate the resources and extend public health support. This study documented the process that transformed a traditional rural clinic to a wellness hub from ideation to design and implementation following the EBLI protocol. The protocol emphasized design decision-making and iteration informed by research evidence and direct input by the community users. Pre-design survey, post-design interview, and preliminary post-occupancy evaluation was conducted to collect representative users' opinions on different landscape programming and design features.

When offering outdoor recreational opportunities, sites should be chosen carefully considering users' preferences and attitudes. The pre-design survey revealed that participants' preferred recreational activities and landscape design features vary significantly by age group, which corresponds with previous research that found a reduction in physical activity intensity and functional fitness was associated with the aging process [46]. Generally, major site users favored activities and design features such as trails and roaming in the woods, places to sit or read, and gardening in community gardens.

The post-design interview results indicated that different user groups have different design concerns: the clinic employee prioritized the daily maintenance of the site, and the patient was concerned with wheelchair users' ability to access and use the design features. Different opinions about water features emerged from the pre-design survey and the post-design interview. Because the sample size was small for the post-design interview, users' attitudes about water features on a clinic site requires further exploration in future studies.

Preliminary POE feedback demonstrated additional functions of the site beyond the initial intent. The walking trail could offer a relaxed atmosphere in facilitating treatments during walk-and-talk therapy sessions. Existing studies have indicated that ongoing professional guidance in a face-to-face format may improve the effectiveness of physical activity programs [47,48]. The individually adapted physical activity prescriptions guided by the clinic doctor, such as the patient walking club, could be an effective behavioral intervention.

The small sample size using a convenience sampling technique was a limitation of the study. There have been similar studies that used smaller sample sizes and gained reliable research insights [49,50]. Considering the EBLI protocol was still in the pilot testing stage, the sample of patients and employees recruited directly from the clinic site provided meaningful insight to guide the design and implementation of the wellness hub [51]. The protocol will need to be validated using a larger sample size in various rural locations.

The wellness hub concept is not new to rural communities; some hubs were piloted on school sites [52], and others were centered on parks and recreation opportunities [53]. This protocol intended to fill the gap between therapeutic landscapes, physical activity intervention programs, and a physician-led wellness hub on a rural clinic site, with an emphasis on the evidence-based design and evaluation of the site features from user-centered perspectives. The implementation of the EBLI protocol was completely a bottom-up process that involved multiple stakeholders, including the core design-research team, community participants, public university extension programs, and numerous nonprofit funding agencies. Gathering community input and feedback during all phases of the project was important to the successful construction of the physical environment of the hub. Recognizing that each user group has its own unique culture and needs sheds light on the equitable access and inclusiveness of the rural wellness hub.

5. Conclusions

The EBLI protocol emphasized participatory design, community building, and cultural uniqueness when implementing behavioral intervention programs for rural communities. It suggested walking trails and other age-appropriate programs that converted a traditional clinic site into a wellness hub in a rural county of West Virginia. The protocol could serve as a template for the design and development of a rural wellness hub that integrates therapeutic landscape features to support physical activities through doctor prescriptions and community-level health intervention programs. The effectiveness of various intervention programs hosted by the wellness hub, such as the patient walking club and walk-and-talk therapy programs, need systematic measurements and documentation in the next step of the study.

Author Contributions: A multi-disciplinary team led the research and design phase of the project, including a healthcare designer (S.J.), a graduate researcher (U.D.), and a doctor (C.J.) who served as the key contact person from the clinic. Detailed author responsibilities were: conceptualization, methodology, data analysis, and manuscript writing, S.J.; data analysis, tables and graphics, and manuscript writing, U.D.; survey, interview and preliminary POE coordination and site construction coordination, C.J. All authors have read and agreed to the published version of the manuscript.

Funding: This research phase of the project was jointly funded by (1) West Virginia University Faculty Grants for Community Engagement; Funder: West Virginia University. (2) Hatch/ Multistate NE1962 Grant. Project No. WVA00729. Funder: National Institute of Food and Agriculture (NIFA), United States Department of Agriculture (USDA).

Institutional Review Board Statement: The study was approved by the Institutional Review Board of West Virginia University (protocol ID #2009127770); the initial date of approval: 10 November 2020.

Informed Consent Statement: Informed consent was obtained from all subjects involved in the study.

Data Availability Statement: The study's supplementary materials are available online with open access: https://github.com/UddayDatta/Pilot_Protocol_supplementary_materials/tree/main.

Acknowledgments: We would like to thank the West Virginia University Community Engagement Lab and the School of Design and Community Development for providing research facilitation. We would also like to thank Pooja Pawar, Graduate Research Assistant from West Virginia University who helped with the design and graphics of the project.

Conflicts of Interest: The authors declare no conflict of interest.

References

1. Carlson, S.A.; Adams, E.K.; Yang, Z.; Fulton, J.E. Percentage of Deaths Associated with Inadequate Physical Activity in the United States. *Prev. Chronic Dis.* **2018**, *15*, 170354. [CrossRef] [PubMed]
2. Patterson, P.D.; Moore, C.G.; Probst, J.C.; Shinogle, J.A. Obesity and Physical Inactivity in Rural America. *J. Rural Health* **2004**, *20*, 151–159. [CrossRef] [PubMed]
3. Morgan, P.J.; Young, M.D.; Smith, J.J.; Lubans, D.R. Targeted Health Behavior Interventions Promoting Physical Activity: A Conceptual Model. *Exerc. Sport Sci. Rev.* **2016**, *44*, 71–80. [CrossRef] [PubMed]
4. Seth, A. Exercise Prescription: What Does It Mean for Primary Care? *Br. J. Gen. Pract.* **2014**, *64*, 12–13. [CrossRef]
5. CDC. CDC Maps America's High Levels of Inactivity. Available online: https://www.cdc.gov/media/releases/2020/0116-americas-inactivity.html (accessed on 11 September 2022).
6. CDC. Adult Physical Inactivity Prevalence Maps by Race/Ethnicity. Centers for Disease Control and Prevention. Available online: https://www.cdc.gov/physicalactivity/data/inactivity-prevalence-maps/index.html (accessed on 11 September 2022).
7. Physical Inactivity a Leading Cause of Disease and Disability, Warns WHO. Available online: https://www.who.int/news/item/04-04-2002-physical-inactivity-a-leading-cause-of-disease-and-disability-warns-who (accessed on 11 September 2022).
8. Lee, I.-M.; Shiroma, E.J.; Lobelo, F.; Puska, P.; Blair, S.N.; Katzmarzyk, P.T. Effect of Physical Inactivity on Major Non-Communicable Diseases Worldwide: An Analysis of Burden of Disease and Life Expectancy. *Lancet* **2012**, *380*, 219–229. [CrossRef]

9. Vanderboom, C.P.; Madigan, E.A. Federal Definitions of Rurality and the Impact on Nursing Research. *Res. Nurs. Health* **2007**, *30*, 175–184. [CrossRef]
10. Statistics about the Population of West Virginia. Available online: https://dhhr.wv.gov/hpcd/data_reports/pages/fast-facts.aspx (accessed on 11 September 2022).
11. Vogt, J.T.; Smith, B.W.; United States Forest Service. Forest Inventory and Analysis Program (U.S.). In *Forest Inventory and Analysis: Fiscal Year 2016 Business Report*; USDA: Washington, DC, USA, 2017; p. 74.
12. Crouch, B.J.; Gupta, R.; Williams, A.; Christy, D.M. *West Virginia Behavioral Risk Factor Surveillance System Report 2016*; Health Statistic Center: Charleston, WV, USA, 2017; p. 211.
13. AlQuaiz, A.M.; Tayel, S.A. Barriers to a Healthy Lifestyle among Patients Attending Primary Care Clinics at a University Hospital in Riyadh. *Ann. Saudi Med.* **2009**, *29*, 30–35. [CrossRef]
14. Gilbert, A.S.; Duncan, D.D.; Beck, A.M.; Eyler, A.A.; Brownson, R.C. A Qualitative Study Identifying Barriers and Facilitators of Physical Activity in Rural Communities. *J. Environ. Public Health* **2019**, *2019*, 1–7. [CrossRef]
15. Janz, N.K.; Becker, M.H. The Health Belief Model: A Decade Later. *Health Educ. Quar.* **1984**, *11*, 1–47. [CrossRef]
16. Rosenstock, I.M. Historical Origins of the Health Belief Model. *Health Educ. Monogr.* **1974**, *2*, 328–335. [CrossRef]
17. Glanz, K.; Rimer, B.K.; Viswanath, K. (Eds.) *Health Behavior and Health Education: Theory, Research, and Practice*, 4th ed.; Jossey-Bass: San Francisco, CA, USA, 2008.
18. Champion, V.; Skinner, C. The Health Belief Model. In *Health Behavior and Health Education: Theory, Research, and Practice*, 4th ed.; Glanz, K., Rimer, B.K., Viswanath, K., Eds.; Jossey-Bass: San Francisco, CA, USA, 2008; pp. 45–65.
19. Montano, D.E.; Kasprzyk, D. Theory of Reasoned Action, Theory of Planned Behavior, and the Integrated Behavioral Model. In *Health Behavior and Health Education: Theory, Research, and Practice*, 4th ed.; Glanz, K., Rimer, B.K., Viswanath, K., Eds.; Jossey-Bass: San Francisco, CA, USA, 2008; pp. 67–92.
20. Ajzen, I. Perceived Behavioral Control, Self-Efficacy, Locus of Control, and the Theory of Planned Behavior 1. *J. Appl. Soc. Psychol.* **2002**, *32*, 665–683. [CrossRef]
21. Hartley, D. Rural Health Disparities, Population Health, and Rural Culture. *Am. J. Public Health* **2004**, *94*, 1675–1678. [CrossRef] [PubMed]
22. Eng, E.; Salmon, M.E.; Mullan, F. Community Empowerment: The Critical Base for Primary Health Care. *Family Commun. Health* **1992**, *15*, 1–12. [CrossRef]
23. Minkler, M.; Wallerstein, N.; Wilson, N. Improving Health through Community Organization and Community Building. In *Health Behavior and Health Education: Theory, Research, and Practice*, 4th ed.; Glanz, K., Rimer, B.K., Viswanath, K., Eds.; Jossey-Bass: San Francisco, CA, USA, 2008; pp. 287–351.
24. Salonen, T. Promoting Wellness to a Rural Area through Recreation Facility and Programming. In *Culminating Projects in Kinesiology*; St. Cloud State University: St. Cloud, MN, USA, 2017.
25. Johnston, J.; Cushing, L. Chemical Exposures, Health, and Environmental Justice in Communities Living on the Fenceline of Industry. *Curr. Environ. Health Rep.* **2020**, *7*, 48–57. [CrossRef] [PubMed]
26. Song, Y.; Huang, B.; Cai, J.; Chen, B. Dynamic Assessments of Population Exposure to Urban Greenspace Using Multi-Source Big Data. *Sci. Total Environ.* **2018**, *634*, 1315–1325. [CrossRef] [PubMed]
27. Pretty, J.; Peacock, J.; Sellens, M.; Griffin, M. The Mental and Physical Health Outcomes of Green Exercise. *Int. J. Environ. Health Res.* **2005**, *15*, 319–337. [CrossRef]
28. What Is Evidence-Based Design (EBD)? *The Center for Health Design*. Available online: https://www.healthdesign.org/certification-outreach/edac/about-ebd (accessed on 11 September 2022).
29. McCullough, C.S. (Ed.) *Evidence-Based Design for Healthcare Facilities*; Sigma Theta Tau International: Indianapolis, IN, USA, 2010.
30. Carr, V.L.; Sangiorgi, D.; Büscher, M.; Junginger, S.; Cooper, R. Integrating Evidence-Based Design and Experience-Based Approaches in Healthcare Service Design. *HERD* **2011**, *4*, 12–33. [CrossRef]
31. Carr, E.C.; Babione, J.N.; Marshall, D. Translating Research into Practice through User-Centered Design: An Application for Osteoarthritis Healthcare Planning. *Int. J. Med. Inform.* **2017**, *104*, 31–37. [CrossRef]
32. Rashid, M. The Question of Knowledge in Evidence-Based Design for Healthcare Facilities: Limitations and Suggestions. *HERD* **2013**, *6*, 101–126. [CrossRef]
33. Revell, S.; McLeod, J. Experiences of Therapists Who Integrate Walk and Talk into Their Professional Practice. *Couns. Psychother. Res.* **2016**, *16*, 35–43. [CrossRef]
34. Cordoza, M.; Ulrich, R.S.; Manulik, B.J.; Gardiner, S.K.; Fitzpatrick, P.S.; Hazen, T.M.; Mirka, A.; Perkins, R.S. Impact of Nurses Taking Daily Work Breaks in a Hospital Garden on Burnout. *Am. J. Crit. Care* **2018**, *27*, 508–512. [CrossRef] [PubMed]
35. Naderi, J.R.; Shin, W.-H. Humane Design for Hospital Landscapes: A Case Study in Landscape Architecture of a Healing Garden for Nurses. *HERD* **2008**, *2*, 82–119. [CrossRef] [PubMed]
36. Henderson, J.R.; Ruikar, K.D.; Dainty, A.R.J. The Need to Improve Double-loop Learning and Design-construction Feedback Loops: A Survey of Industry Practice. *Eng. Constr. Archit. Manag.* **2013**, *20*, 290–306. [CrossRef]
37. Datta, U.; Jiang, S. Pilot_Protocol_Supplementary_Materials. 2022. Available online: https://github.com/UddayDatta/Pilot_Protocol_supplementary_materials/tree/main (accessed on 1 October 2022).

38. Vogels, E. Some digital divides persist between rural, urban and suburban America. Pew Research Center. USA. 2021. Available online: https://policycommons.net/artifacts/1808201/some-digital-divides-persist-between-rural-urban-and-suburban-america/2543052/ (accessed on 1 October 2022).
39. United States Census Bureau. Quick Facts Clay County, West Virginia. n.d. Available online: https://www.census.gov/quickfacts/fact/table/claycountywestvirginia/IPE120221#IPE120221 (accessed on 1 October 2022).
40. Provalis Research. *QDA Miner: Qualitative and Mixed-Method Software (Version 4.1) [Software]*; Provalis Research: Montreal, QC, Canada, 2004.
41. Jiang, S.; Staloch, K.; Kaljevic, S. Diagnostic Post Occupancy Evaluation of the Landscape Environments in a Primary Care Clinic: The Environmental and Social Performances. Available online: https://www.semanticscholar.org/paper/DIAGNOSTIC-POST-OCCUPANCY-EVALUATION-OF-THE-IN-A-Jiang-Shan/9e5944c5293e34788d621d6ad2bd2fb4b7a0df2a (accessed on 11 September 2022).
42. IBM Corp. *IBM SPSS Statistics for Windows, Version 28.0*; IBM Corp.: Armonk, NY, USA, 2021.
43. Sullivan, G.M.; Artino, A.R. Analyzing and Interpreting Data from Likert-Type Scales. *J. Grad. Med. Educ.* **2013**, *5*, 541–542. [CrossRef]
44. Bhuiyan, N.; Singh, P.; Harden, S.M.; Mama, S.K. Rural Physical Activity Interventions in the United States: A Systematic Review and RE-AIM Evaluation. *Int. J. Behav. Nutr. Phys. Act.* **2019**, *16*, 140. [CrossRef]
45. Physical Activity: Park, Trail, and Greenway Infrastructure Interventions when Combined with Additional Interventions. The Guide to Community Preventive Services (The Community Guide). Available online: https://www.thecommunityguide.org/content/one-pager-physical-activity-park-trail-and-greenway-infrastructure-interventions-when-combined-with-additional-interventions (accessed on 12 September 2022).
46. Milanovic, Z.; Jorgić, B.; Trajković, N.; Sporis, G.; Pantelić, S.; James, N. Age-Related Decrease in Physical Activity and Functional Fitness among Elderly Men and Women. *CIA* **2013**, *2013*, 549–556. [CrossRef]
47. Foster, C.; Hillsdon, M.; Thorogood, M.; Kaur, A.; Wedatilake, T. Interventions for Promoting Physical Activity. In *Cochrane Database Systematic Reviews*; John Wiley & Sons, Ltd.: Chichester, UK, 2005. [CrossRef]
48. Richards, J.; Foster, C.; Thorogood, M.; Hillsdon, M.; Kaur, A.; Wickramasinghe, K.K.; Wedatilake, T. Face-to-Face Interventions for Promoting Physical Activity. In *Cochrane Database of Systematic Reviews*; The Cochrane Collaboration, Ed.; John Wiley & Sons, Ltd.: Chichester, UK, 2013; p. CD010392. [CrossRef]
49. Pasha, S.; Shepley, M.M. Research Note: Physical Activity in Pediatric Healing Gardens. *Landsc. Urban Plan.* **2013**, *118*, 53–58. [CrossRef]
50. Finkel, J.; Printz, B.; Gallagher, L.M.; Au, A.; Shibuya, K.; Bethoux, F. Patient Perceptions of Landscape and Abstract Art in Inpatient Cardiac Units: A Cross-Sectional Survey. *HERD* **2021**, *14*, 66–83. [CrossRef]
51. Etchegaray, J.M.; Fischer, W.G. Understanding Evidence-Based Research Methods: Pilot Testing Surveys. *HERD* **2011**, *4*, 143–147. [CrossRef]
52. DeBolt, M.; Southwick, A. Wellness Hub Approach to School Health in Rural Oregon. [Conference Poster]. Available online: https://www.oregon.gov/oha/HPA/dsi-tc/Documents/Summit-Poster-Wellness-Hub.pdf (accessed on 2 October 2022).
53. National Recreation and Park Association. Community Wellness Hubs: A Toolkit for Advancing Community Health and Well-Being through Parks and Recreation. ArcGIS StoryMaps. Available online: https://storymaps.arcgis.com/stories/53045b41ea204719a6aace92481f99ee (accessed on 12 September 2022).

Review

Reframing Patient Experience Approaches and Methods to Achieve Patient-Centeredness in Healthcare: Scoping Review

Eun-Jeong Kim [1], Inn-Chul Nam [2,*] and Yoo-Ri Koo [3,*]

1. Department of Otorhinolaryngology-Head and Neck Surgery, The Catholic Medical Center, The Catholic University of Korea, Seoul 06591, Korea; dodam.design.research@gmail.com
2. Department of Otorhinolaryngology-Head and Neck Surgery, Incheon St. Mary's Hospital, The Catholic University of Korea, Seoul 21431, Korea
3. Department of Service Design, Graduate School of Industrial Arts, Hongik University, Seoul 04066, Korea
* Correspondence: entnam@catholic.ac.kr (I.-C.N.); yrkoo@hongik.ac.kr (Y.-R.K.)

Abstract: (1) There has been growing attention among healthcare researchers on new and innovative methodologies for improving patient experience. This study reviewed the approaches and methods used in current patient experience research by applying the perspective of design thinking to discuss practical methodologies for a patient-centered approach and creative problem-solving. (2) A scoping review was performed to identify research trends in healthcare. A four-stage design thinking process ("Discover", "Define", "Develop", and "Deliver") and five themes ("User focus", "Problem-framing", "Visualization", "Experimentation", and "Diversity"), characterizing the concept, were used for the analysis framework. (3) After reviewing 67 studies, the current studies show that the iterative process of divergent and convergent thinking is lacking, which is a core concept of design thinking, and it is necessary to employ an integrative methodology to actively apply collaborative, multidisciplinary, and creative attributes for a specific and tangible solution. (4) For creative problem-solving to improve patient experience, we should explore the possibilities of various solutions by an iterative process of divergent and convergent thinking. A concrete and visualized solution should be sought through active user interactions from various fields. For this, a specific methodology that allows users to collaborate by applying the integrative viewpoint of design thinking should be introduced.

Keywords: patient experience; patient-centered care; design thinking; holistic approach; creative problem-solving; multidisciplinary perspective

1. Introduction

1.1. Patient Experience (PE) Approaches and Design Thinking (DT) as a Creative Problem-Solving Method

Recently, PE for quality improvement (QI) has increasingly evoked interest among researchers [1]. To achieve high-quality care in medical services, patient-centeredness should be considered a key attribute of healthcare [2,3]. Patient-centered care is defined as (1) being responsive to patients' needs, values, and preferences; and (2) involving patients in decision-making [3–5]. Accordingly, efforts to improve PE through patient engagement in healthcare are intensified. PE involves several stakeholders, such as patients, caregivers, medical staff, and administrators, dealing with complex and diverse problem situations. However, the existing traditional healthcare method for patient engagement has limited the patient's role in the problem-solving process by putting healthcare experts and researchers in the center of PE improvement [1], which resulted in the patient's passive attitude toward their quality of care.

As a new way to engage patients, participatory design, experience-based co-design (EBCD), and co-design were introduced by employing service design methods such as service blueprints, user journeys, and stakeholder maps. These methodologies are relatively unfamiliar design approaches derived from the concept of DT and were originally meant as a holistic and integrative process and methods for problem-solving by using research, prototyping (visualized evidence), and co-creating values for relevant stakeholders [1,6,7]. DT is also an approach that iteratively repeats the process of diverging and converging ideas by engaging all relevant users in a human-centered and collaborative manner [6,8]. The converging process corresponds to the concept of narrowing down choices to find a solution to a specific problem. In contrast, the diverging process considers the problem space from a new perspective and reviews the situation in various creative ways that were not previously thought of. Since DT holistically and iteratively deals with the overall process for problem-solving, from problem recognition and definition, from a new perspective to problem identification and ideation, and for solutions to a concrete presentation of visualized results, it can serve as a useful viewpoint and methodology in solving complex and diverse problems from a patient perspective in healthcare. Stakeholders' views are actively reflected in the solution by conducting collaborative work among users to deeply understand interrelated human activities.

Therefore, it provides a holistic and integrative view of exploring the complex problems of healthcare [6,9–11]. This approach is very different from the attitude in evidence-based, analytical medicine. A patient's perspective in a problem-solving process can be strongly influenced by diverging and converging ideas and by effectively visualizing a solution into tangible artifacts [6]. For example, identifying patient's unmet needs for the improvement of person-centered care [7], identifying the causes of problems in the patient engagement process [12], visualizing future services by presenting scenarios and prototypes through workshops [13], or offering strategies by performing persona-scenario sessions [14] could be explained as divergent processes. However, identifying the preferences of patients or clinicians for specific factors [1], analyzing barriers to a particular topic [15], assessing the usefulness of a questionnaire [16], or refining a tool and evaluating the tool's feasibility [17] correspond to a convergence process.

1.2. DT Process

The DT process deals with the overall problem-solving process holistically and integratively by diverging and converging ideas iteratively. This process helps to solve complex and mutually conflicting PE issues flexibly. Applying a patient-centered approach to the problem-solving process is a useful deviation from the system-focused thinking approach.

The DT process was originally introduced by the Design Council (2015) [18] and consisted of four stages: "Discover"; "Define"; "Develop"; "Deliver". Each stage requires collaboration with stakeholders, reflecting multidisciplinary perspectives [19]. "Discover" corresponds to the divergent stage of DT by considering the problematic situation and by searching for new insights to explore potential ideas for a solution by conducting user research. "Define" is the stage of converging the ideas to narrow insights for potential opportunities. "Develop" is the stage of diverging the ideas again to turn abstract concepts or ideas into visual structures as tangible result forms. "Deliver", as a re-converged stage of ideas, suggests a specific solution to a problematic issue and tests its feasibility (Figure 1).

The DT process can be understood as a framework for viewing problems from an integrated point of view. Therefore, designing the study by including the four stages, rather than focusing on a specific stage in the DT process, can be an effective methodology for PE improvement in healthcare.

1.3. DT Themes

DT themes introduced by Carlgren et al. (2016) deal with five important concepts for creative problem-solving: "User focus", "Problem-framing", "Visualization", "Experimentation", and "Diversity". They emphasize that creative problem-solving is possible through (1) the deep understanding or involvement of users in identifying their pain points or latent needs by using design ethnography such as user journeys, empathy map, and persona; (2) reframing the initial problem space to catch an unexpected potential solution with the techniques of how-might-we-questions, the five whys technique, and the problem statement; (3) transforming ideas into visual structures to effectively communicate ideas among users by using physical prototypes, sketching, and storyboarding; (4) iterative working for the refinement and testing feasibility of the solution for evaluation by conducting brainstorming; (5) involving multiple teams and the collaborative approach to reflect diverse perspectives in the decision-making process by using study visits, analogies, and demographics [20].

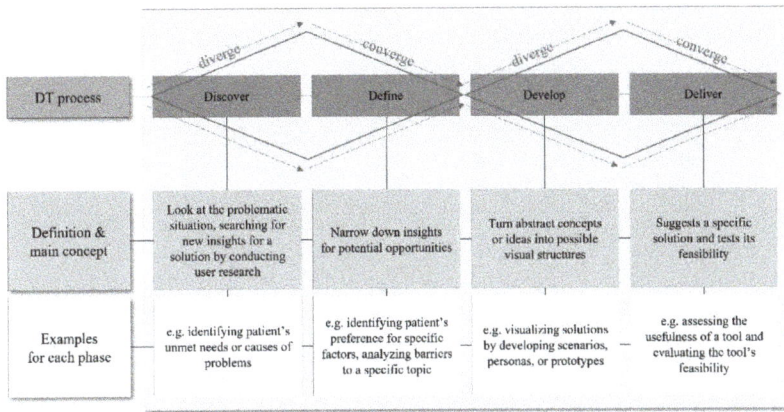

Figure 1. The DT process as a framework for creative problem-solving.

These themes are closely related to the DT process and emphasize holistic, integrative, iterative, and user-centered attitudes by actively engaging users.

Among these themes, "User focus" looked at its contents focusing on user engagement and type. Anderson et al. (2021) classified user engagement approaches for PE improvement into three types according to the degree of intervention. They include (1) "Consultation" by gathering feedback from users through surveys, interviews, and focus groups; (2) "Collaboration" by participating in the discussion, brainstorming, developing solutions, and evaluating results with diverse stakeholders; (3) "Blended approach" that combines "Consultation" and "Collaboration" (co-creation of the solution by working with diverse stakeholders based on the consultation data identified in the early phase) [21]. This classification helps the understanding of how active user engagement was induced to obtain patient-centeredness and how it can guide the design of user engagement methods.

"Problem-framing" involves gathering insights for a potential solution by identifying the specific needs of users. "Visualization" deals with exploring solutions to the problems identified in the previous step by employing divergent thinking and developing them as a tangible prototype. "Experimentation" deals with evaluating and testing the prototypes developed for problem-solving in the last stage by using convergent thinking to focus on the feasibility of the solution. "Diversity" is related to the involvement of diverse members from different backgrounds and the consideration of different user perspectives (Figure 2).

Figure 3 explains the relationships of five DT themes with the DT process. "User focus" is related to the whole stages of the DT process, mainly focusing on the stage of "Discover". It helps to set the level of user engagement and decide the type and the scope of participants for employing different perspectives in the overall process. "Problem-framing" is related to the stage of "Discover" and "Define" in the DT process, focusing on the stage of "Define". It tries to reframe the problem from a new or different perspective and tries to identify user needs. This theme includes divergent and convergent aspects to expand the research scope and narrow down the study purpose to set up a more specific problem-solving goal. In this case, both divergent and convergent thinking must be included, and when only one of them is dealt with, the research scope can become too broad and vague, making it difficult to apply a new perspective; therefore, it cannot be differentiated from the existing traditional problem-solving methods. "Visualization" mainly corresponds to the "Develop" stage, involving "Define" and "Deliver" stages for the iterative work process. It explores the solution in a specific and tangible manner by expanding the search area for possible solutions. "Experimentation" deals with iterative work for the refinement and feasibility test, which corresponds to the "Deliver" stage by narrowing down the solution to a specific result. It also involves the "Develop" stage in the process of complementing the prototype iteratively. "Diversity" involves the whole DT process by affecting the perspectives of users engaged. These five themes are helpful when determining specific methods for each step of the DT process or deciding the comprehensive nature of the research or the characteristics of participants.

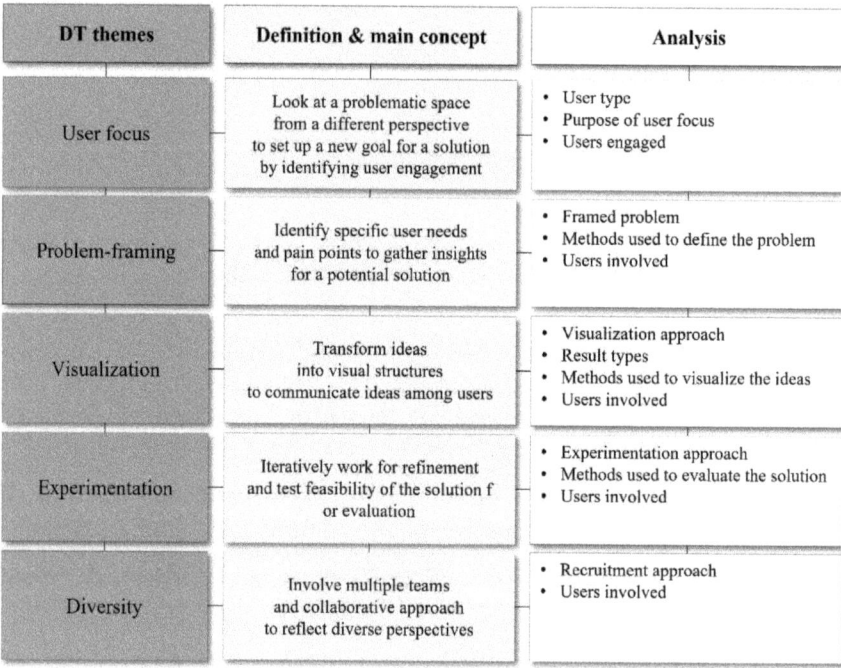

Figure 2. The DT themes representing methodological concepts.

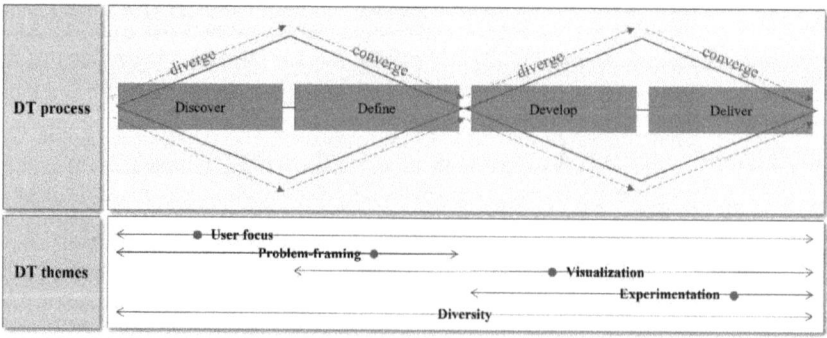

Figure 3. The relationship of DT themes with the DT process.

The above frameworks, as shown in Figures 1–3, suggest essential concepts to understand how holistic and integrative the current studies approached problem situations and how they designed the methods from a patient-centered point of view.

With this background, this study aimed to review how current studies on PEs have approached problem-solving from the DT perspective, and it explored the possibility that the integrative DT approach can be applied as an effective, powerful method to improve the quality of care from the patient perspective.

A scoping review was conducted to examine the approaches and methods used in the current PE-related studies. It was a systematic approach to reviewing the literature on a given topic, providing an overview of the case [22–25]. To actively achieve patient-centeredness in healthcare, we attempted to draw meaningful insights for applying a holistic, integrative, and practical DT methodology to the medical field. In addition, we aimed to help related researchers increase their understanding of DT to provide insights for dynamically engaging patients in the PE improvement process. The specific research questions were as follows:

RQ 1. What are the characteristics of current studies (study countries, study subjects, and study focus)?

RQ 2. How holistic is the approach and how iterative the process of each study when applied to the DT process?

RQ 3. What approaches and methods were employed, and what user types were involved in the reviewed studies?

RQ 4. How did these studies achieve patient-centeredness in terms of collaboration?

2. Materials and Methods

Arksey and O'Malley's (2005) model [22], a commonly used scoping review method [25], was employed to develop the research framework. It comprises five phases, and the practices described by Tricco et al. (2016) [26] were referred to for each phase. The data were analyzed by detailed coding items corresponding to the research question in each cell using Excel. Based on the method introduced by Levac et al. (2010) [24,27], we performed statistical and thematic analyses based on DT themes and attributes drawn from the literature.

For search strategy, "healthcare", "QI", "PE", "service design" (since service design is more commonly used than DT, it was used in the search condition), "communication", and "barriers" were used as primary search keywords. For barriers, various terms with similar meanings were used, and terms such as "needs", "insights", "protocols", "evidence", and "improvements" were additionally used for article search.

Four electronic databases (Google Scholar, PubMed, Web of Science, and Taylor & Francis journal) were used for the study search and selection, and a total of 7008 papers were collected after the primary search. After screening the title and abstract of 6183 papers (excluding duplicates) for relevance to the subject, 131 papers were selected. A total of 67 articles [1,7,12–17,21,28–85] were selected for the final analysis, excluding unfinished work with no results ($n = 21$), review articles ($n = 13$), case studies ($n = 28$), and theses ($n = 2$) (Figure 4).

For the 67 papers selected for the scoping review, study characteristics were examined, focusing on the country where the study was conducted, study subjects, and study focus. The study subjects were classified through a content analysis based on the similarity of the subject range. The study focus was analyzed to determine whether the purpose of the study was to collect user needs or to improve the efficiency of the system or tool.

As the main framework for review, the approaches and methods of the selected studies were examined in two aspects of DT: the process and themes. Each selected study was examined to see how much holistic and iterative work was achieved by identifying which of the four stages of the DT process was applicable. Thereafter, for each of the five DT themes, what specific methods and approaches were applied to each study, what type of participants were involved, and to what extent the DT perspective for creative problem-solving was reflected and used for each analysis were examined.

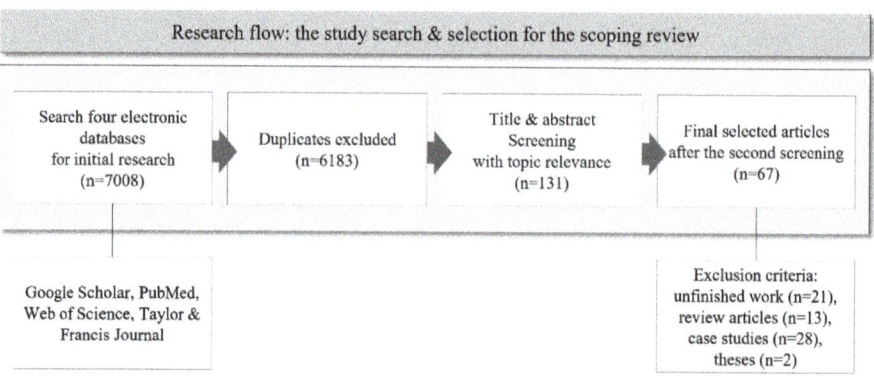

Figure 4. The flow of the research for the scoping review.

3. Results

3.1. Study Characteristics

The distribution of countries where the studies were conducted, by continent, was as follows: 32 studies in North America, showing the highest frequency, followed by 25 studies in Europe. Of the 67 studies, 57 were conducted in North America and Europe, indicating that research to improve PE is the most active in these countries. In Europe, studies for improving PE were conducted mainly in the UK (n = 11). Six studies were conducted in Australia and one in Spain in South America. In Africa, two studies were conducted, one in Ghana and one in Nigeria. Joint research between countries was identified in two cases, Denmark and the Netherlands, and 34 countries distributed on various continents. Remarkably, we found no studies based in Asia (Table 1).

From the above results, it is evident that research on PE in healthcare is being intensively conducted in Europe and North America. Contrarily, active research is not being conducted in Africa and Asia, although the importance of a service design for PE is recognized.

Table 1. Summary of the study countries and continents.

Continent	Countries	Count	Total (%)
Africa	Ghana	1 [15]	2 (2.99%)
	Nigeria	1 [28]	
Europe	Belgium	1 [29]	25 (37.31%)
	Denmark	1 [30]	
	France	1 [16]	
	Germany	1 [17]	
	Netherlands	3 [12,31,32]	
	Norway	1 [7]	
	Sweden	4 [13,33–35]	
	Switzerland	1 [36]	
	UK	11 [37–47]	
	Denmark/Netherlands	1 [48]	
North America	Canada	8 [14,21,49–54]	32 (47.76%)
	USA	24 [55–78]	
South America	Spain	1 [79]	1 (1.49%)
Australia	Australia	6 [1,80–84]	6 (8.96%)
Multiple continents	34 countries	1 [85]	1 (1.49%)
Total	-	67	67 (100%)

The study aims were analyzed in terms of study subjects and study focus. From the content analysis based on the similarity of the subject range covered by each study, the study subjects were classified into five types: data collection and use, user involvement, user needs, care services/intervention, and patient education (Table 2). The issues with the highest frequency were user involvement and user needs ($n = 24$ each), followed by PE data ($n = 9$), care services/intervention ($n = 8$) and patient education ($n = 2$). These results indicate that the recent PE research for QI focused on the unmet needs and involvement of the user-centeredness on the patient rather than on systems such as care service, education, or intervention.

Table 2. Summary of study subjects.

Study Subjects			Count (%)
Focusing on patient data collection and use	The use of PE data	5	9 (13.43%)
	Capturing feedback/gathering data from patients	4	
User involvement	User engagement for QI	14	24 (35.82%)
	Reciprocity/communication among users	10	
Identifying user needs	User perception/satisfaction to care	10	24 (35.82%)
	Unmet needs among users	14	
Care services/intervention	Care services to be improved	5	8 (11.94%)
	Intervention for improvement	3	
Patient education	Patient education	2	2 (2.99%)
Total		67	67 (100%)

In user involvement, the active engagement ($n = 14$) and communication ($n = 10$) of users were identified as sub-topics, and for user needs, the topics of unmet needs ($n = 14$), user perception, or satisfaction ($n = 10$) were covered. This indicates that the service provider realizes the importance of understanding the users' needs and direct user participation and interaction in improving the PE. In the data collection and use, the topics of data usage ($n = 5$) and data gathering ($n = 4$) were treated with similar frequencies, indicating that collecting problems and barriers to healthcare experience from the patient's perspective and processing and managing the collected data for the improvement of PE had the same importance.

The study's focus was to identify whether the focus of research was on collecting and reflecting users' opinions and needs or on improving the efficiency of tools or systems. Tool focus includes the improvement of medical decision aids, mobile apps, questionnaires, toolkits, and communication cards. System focus had blood test system, patient engagement hospital plan, primary care system, and outpatient palliative care system. Only two studies focused on both the active understanding of user needs and tool development. A representative case was a study that identified the needs of young asthma patients and developed a mobile app through direct patient participation. Focusing on improving tools and systems was limited to achieving patient-centeredness because its primary purpose was to effectively solve existing structural problems rather than viewing the problematic situation from a whole new point of view for developing a unique solution. As seen in Table 3, several studies still focused on improving tools and systems, and few studies lead to the presentation of new solutions based on profound user needs.

Table 3. Summary of study focus.

Study Focus	User-Focused	Tool-Focused	System-Focused	User/Tool-Focused
Count (%)	32 (47.76%) [1,7,15,28,30–35,37,40,43,45,47–49,51,52,56,65,67,68,71–74,78–80,82,84]	21 (31.34%) [12–14,16,17,29,36,39,44,46,50,53,55,57–59,62,66,70,75,77]	12 (17.91%) [21,38,41,42,54,60,61,63,64,76,83,85]	2 (2.99%) [69,81]
Total		67 (100%)		

3.2. Process for a Holistic and Iterative Approach

The results of examining which stage of the DT process each study included, as presented in Table 4, show that 49 studies dealt with only one stage, followed by two studies that dealt with 14 studies that dealt with two stages and three studies with three stages. No studies were found that dealt with all the stages of the DT process. This clearly shows that the existing research focuses only on a specific stage without iteratively going through divergent and convergent thinking. Since such segmental research design cannot go through the four stages of a flexible thinking process, it is difficult to adopt an approach with an integrated point of view and creative problem-solving.

Among the papers that focused on only one stage of the DT process, four papers corresponded to the "Discover" stage. Rather than an intensive analysis of specific problem situations, these were studies that listened to comprehensive opinions for the improvement of overall care services or systems from the perspective of patients or medical staff. For example, Schäfer et al. (2015) [85] investigated patients' perceptions of improvement potential in primary care in 34 countries. Rather than limiting the scope to a specific country to find improvement points, it provided insights to compare differences in the patients' perspectives by country and set a differentiated improvement direction for each country in the future.

Most of the papers (n = 31) were found in the "Define" stage. They focused on discovering pain points for immediate improvement by identifying users' preferences or needs for a series of interventions or initiatives in detail. For example, Song et al. (2020) [83] identified specific barriers when implementing PE surveys and discussed using their findings for service improvement. This was to find ways to improve and utilize a particular survey tool. It corresponds to a deep dive into a problem space to specifically solve the previously identified problem situation rather than discovering the problem from a new perspective.

There are two papers in the "Develop" stage. Revenäs et al. (2015) [13] developed scenarios and prototypes through a co-design workshop to improve the system requirements and specifications for the mobile Internet service. This study transformed the solution for a specific problem situation into a visible form, enabling it to present results at a more realistic level.

There were 12 studies corresponding to "Deliver". Lyes et al. (2020) [39] evaluated the extent to which the questionnaire for assessing patient satisfaction in the intensive care unit reflects the patient's opinion. Miatello et al. (2018) [50] examined the effectiveness of smartphone and web apps for PE data collection. This is to evaluate how effective a particular tool is, and it is necessary for the continuous development and update of the device or system.

In studies involving only one stage of the DT process, the convergent thinking stage of "Define" and "Deliver" appeared the most. This has limitations in creative problem-solving because it is difficult to expand the problem space allowing for flexible thinking due to the absence of divergent thinking stages. Each stage of the DT process has integrity and value as substantial research. However, each stage has different functions and objectives. It is possible to present more detailed and in-depth results when research is designed with continuity rather than proceeding in an independent form. The holistic approach of (1) raising a problem from a new perspective (Discover), (2) analyzing the cause of a specific problem (Define), (3) approaching a possible solution visually and structurally (Develop), and (4) evaluating its usefulness and developing it into a more successful result (Deliver) corresponds to a creative research process that recognizes and solves more real problem situations in patient-centered communication.

In studies involving two stages, 14 cases appeared in the "Define" and "Develop" stages. Since this is an approach of searching for solutions based on problems that have been directly exposed, it is difficult to understand the patient's latent needs. Moreover, it is hard to reflect a patient-centered perspective in the problem-solving process because the healthcare experts usually hold strong opinions. For example, Fitch et al. (2021) [49]

reviewed the main challenges of adolescent and young adult cancer survivors and discussed their suggestions regarding care improvements. However, the needs data collected from patients were not actively utilized. They did not lead to a practical solution because a specific prototype was not developed, and the delivery stage was not progressed to evaluate its usefulness.

Research involving three stages showed integrative thinking and iterative problem-solving processes, but the "Discover" stage was still missing. For example, identifying barriers to the current healthcare system helps researchers focus on the specific problematic situation, but understanding the system's mechanism from a patient's perspective can help healthcare researchers set up a new goal for problem-solving.

As such, studies in which the stages of the DT process are not continuously applied hold significant values in themselves. However, from a macro perspective, to creatively solve complex and difficult-to-solve problems in the medical field by adding a different and new perspective, it is necessary to apply each DT stage responsible for other functions continuously.

Table 4. Summary of the study stage in the DT process.

DT Stage	Discover	Define	Develop	Deliver	Count (%)
Involve one stage	[7,12,41,85]				4 (5.97%)
		[1,15,28–34,40,42,45, 48,54,60,65–68,70–76,78,79,82–84]			31 (46.27%)
			[13,14]		2 (2.99%)
				[16,17,36,39,46,50,53, 55,58,61–63]	12 (17.91%)
Involve two stages		[21,35,37,43,44,49,51,52,56,57,64,69,80,81]			14 (20.89%)
Involve three stages			[38,47,77]		3 (4.48%)
Total					67 (100%)

3.3. DT Themes for a User-Centered Approach

3.3.1. User Focus Aspect

Concerning the user types who participated in each study, 23 studies included patients and/or families, and 18 showed the highest frequency of patient participation compared to other users. The involvement of medical staff and/or caregivers and professionals was identified in 12 studies, and the participation of professionals, healthcare leaders, and society members was identified in four cases. Patients and medical staff participated together in 26 cases, which accounted for the most significant proportion among user types, and the mixed participation of patients and professionals was reported in two cases (Table 5).

Table 5. Summary of user types.

User Types		Count (%)	
Involving patients/families	Patients	18	23 (34.33%)
	Patients/caregivers	4	
	Caregivers (families)	1	
Involving medical staff	Medical staff	7	12 (17.91%)
	Medical staff/caregivers	2	
	Medical staff/professionals/researchers	3	
Involving professionals	Professionals/leaders/society members	4	4 (5.97%)
Involving patients/medical staff	Patients/medical staff	12	26 (38.81%)
	Patients/caregivers/medical staff	8	
	Patients/medical staff/professionals	4	
	Patients/medical staff/development team (designers)	2	
Involving Patients/professionals	Patients/professionals	1	2 (2.98%)
	Patients/caregivers/professionals	1	
Total	-		67 (100%)

When examining the significance of user participation, user involvement was the most frequent topic, with 34 cases, followed by user understanding, with 26 cases. Thus, it is evident that, for PE improvement, users' direct participation is crucial to understand their needs rather than just contacting users. Seven studies combined user understanding and participation, indicating a significant attempt to involve users in deriving improvement directions directly and understanding user needs to improve the PE (Table 6).

However, it is interesting to note that 48 cases of consultation, 12 cases of a blended approach, and seven cases of collaboration were reported in user engagement. This implies that the users' participation activity is more of a passive and one-way opinion gathering rather than an active reflection of the users' opinion and interaction with other stakeholders. When users include patients, user engagement at the consultation level is higher. These results suggest that researchers recognize the importance of direct patient participation and are trying to engage them for patient-centered care. However, they are still accustomed to methods focused on simple data collection from the users rather than managing active interaction.

Table 6. Purpose of user focus and engagement aspects.

Category		Result	Count (%)	
Purpose of user focus	User understanding	[1,7,15,28,30–35,40,45,48,49,65,67–69,71–74,78,79,82,84]	26 (38.80%)	67 (100%)
	User involvement	[12–14,16,17,21,29,36,38,39,41,42,44,46,50,51,53–55,57–64,66,70,75–77,83,85]	34 (50.75%)	
	User understanding and involvement	[37,43,47,52,56,80,81]	7 (10.45%)	
User engagement	Consultation	[1,12,15–17,21,29–35,40,41,45,46,48–50,53–56,58,60–76,78,79,82–85]	48 (71.64%)	67 (100%)
	Collaboration	[7,13,14,28,36,42,59]	7 (10.45%)	
	Blended (co-creation)	[37–39,43,44,47,51,52,57,77,80,81]	12 (17.91%)	

3.3.2. Problem-Framing Aspect

For the problems framed at this stage, identifying users' needs/barriers/preferences/satisfaction had the highest number of cases, with 33 cases, followed by understanding the current tool or system, with 19 cases. The most common methods used for 'Problem-framing' were interviews ($n = 34$), surveys ($n = 21$), and focus groups ($n = 11$). The focus was on identifying insights on specific issues directly from stakeholders, which means that the current studies lack the efforts to reframe the initial problem by reflecting the viewpoints of various users. It is difficult to achieve a creative problem-solving approach when the focus is on identifying the user's needs within the range of a problem that has already been established rather than reframing the initial problem.

In addition, for the framed problems, while identifying users' needs and analyzing issues with existing systems and tools that were mainly used, access to intangible problems such as users' emotions, attitudes, and perceptions was relatively lacking. However, since these factors are critical in understanding the patient's potential needs, a balance of research to understand the emotions and attitudes of patients is needed, along with simple satisfaction or preference-based needs analysis. As for the method of defining the problem, the questionnaire was frequently used following the interview, clearly showing that there is a limit to understanding the patient's inner voice. The scope of users related to the problem-framing aspect involved mainly direct stakeholders such as patients, medical staff, and caregivers. To understand the patient's unmet needs, the participation of experts in different fields such as cognition and psychology can help for an in-depth problem-framing approach (Table 7).

Table 7. Summary of study's problem-framing.

Perspective	Description	Count (n)	
Framed problem	Users' needs/barriers/pain points/preferences/satisfactions	33	
	Current/existing tool or system	19	62
	Users' perception/knowledge/attitudes/emotions	6	
	Potential improvement of the current system	4	
Methods used to define the problem	Interviews	34	
	Focus group	11	
	Workshop	4	73
	Survey (Delphi)	21	
	Checklist	1	
	Observation	2	
Users involved	Patients	21	
	Patients/caregivers	4	
	Caregivers	3	
	Patients/medical staff	10	
	Patients/caregivers/medical staff	3	58
	Medical staff	9	
	Professionals	2	
	Medical staff/professionals	6	
	Patients/caregivers/medical staff/professionals	3	

3.3.3. Visualization Aspect

As for the "Visualization" approach, visualization of suggestions/strategies accounted for the most with seven cases (e.g., creating personas and scenarios to suggest strategies or building a visual structure of suggestions), followed by storyboarding ideas for tool/system development (e.g., developing a film to share and collect feedback from users) with four cases and mapping needs for priority setting with four cases. In three cases, the detailed specifications of a prototype (e.g., refining the existing decision aid tool) and the development of new prototypes (e.g., a mobile app or screening tool as a checklist) were found in three cases. This approach has been introduced in various formats. However, most of them have remained at the level of suggesting conceptual ideas for improvement rather than developing a tangible prototype, thus failing to actively explore the opportunity of creating a solution.

Most result types ($n = 18$) corresponded to visible software such as a mobile app, tool/program, film, or more abstract suggestions, strategies, processes, models, and interventions. Only one whiteboard design was identified as the hardware. The results were verified only in five studies, and a user test, focus group, audit, and interview were used for prototype evaluation. These results showed that an abstract conceptual discussion prevails over tangible results in this process.

As a visualization method, it was found that workshops involving various stakeholders were the most used. The active participation of users and the reflection of opinions were achieved to some extent in the visualization stage.

Most of the users involved in the visualization method were direct stakeholders such as patients, medical staff, and caregivers, but what stands out is that some experts, such as the design team, were included in the visualization process. It was interpreted that the designer's role is necessary for developing a high-fidelity prototype. The number of designer-participating cases was still as few as four, indicating that workshops made up of professionals in various fields are needed for the active exploration of tangible prototypes as solutions to healthcare problems (Table 8).

3.3.4. Experimentation Aspect

For the "Experimentation" approach, five approaches were identified: (1) providing feedback for improvement ($n = 4$); (2) testing the feasibility of the tool/program ($n = 5$); (3) discussing the prototypes for improvement ($n = 5$); (4) evaluating the values of the prototypes ($n = 5$); and (5) prioritizing the recommendations ($n = 1$). A survey, focus group, interview, and trial test were used as methods, and users involved in the "Experimentation" showed various configurations (Table 9).

Table 8. Summary of the study's visualization.

Perspective	Description	Count (n)	
Visualization approach	Visualization of suggestions/strategies	7	21
	Storyboarding ideas for tool/system development	4	
	Mapping the needs for priority setting	4	
	Provide/develop detailed specifications	3	
	Develop prototypes	3	
Result types — Software	Mobile app	4	19
	Visual structure of suggestions/strategies	7	
	Film	1	
	Tool/program	4	
	Process/model	1	
	Intervention	1	
Result types — Hardware	Whiteboard	1	1
Methods used to visualize the ideas	Interviews	4	22
	Focus group	6	
	Workshop	10	
	Survey	2	
Users involved	Patients	3	21
	Patients/caregivers	1	
	Patients/medical staff	1	
	Patients/professionals	1	
	Patients/caregivers/medical staff	5	
	Patients/medical staff/professionals	1	
	Medical staff	3	
	Professionals (design team)	4	
	Medical staff/professionals	1	

The "Experimentation" aspect is related to verifying feasibility through testing different solutions, and various users must participate and work iteratively to explore the answers. However, since many studies use questionnaires to receive user feedback, there is a limit to interrelated collaborative work between users by employing personal meetings or surveys. For users to actively present their opinions, test various solutions, and converge their thoughts to a specific result, it is necessary to apply an interactive method for brainstorming, such as a workshop.

Table 9. Summary of the study's experimentation.

Perspective	Description	Count (n)	
Experimentation approach	Provide feedback for improvement of the existing tool	4	20
	Test the feasibility of the program/tool	5	
	Discuss the prototypes for improvement	5	
	Evaluate the values of the results (prototypes)	5	
	Rate and prioritize the recommendations	1	
Method used to evaluate the solution	In-person meeting	1	26
	Focus group	5	
	Feedback session	1	
	Survey (Delphi)	8	
	Checklist	1	
	Audit	1	
	Interview	5	
	Workshop	1	
	Prototype test as a trial	3	
Users involved	Patients	5	19
	Patients/caregivers/medical staff	3	
	Patients/medical staff	2	
	Patients/professionals	1	
	Patients/medical staff/professionals	2	
	Medical staff	2	
	Medical staff/caregivers	2	
	Caregivers	1	
	Professionals	1	

3.3.5. Diversity Aspect

Regarding the "Diversity" aspect of DT themes, the recruitment approach was classified as internal/external to identify team composition and diversity of viewpoints. For 52 out of the 67 studies, there was external recruitment of the team members, and for studies focused on specific healthcare settings, team members were recruited internally ($n = 15$).

User involvement was analyzed by categorizing the user groups into direct and indirect stakeholders. Of the selected studies, 51 involved only direct stakeholders, showing the highest frequency. A mixture of direct and indirect stakeholders was reported in eight studies, and four studies reflected diverse viewpoints by including non-medical staff and professionals such as a design team, a game researcher, a program development team, and a multidisciplinary team.

Nineteen studies directly mentioned EBCD, co-design, and participatory design as methods to reflect the perspectives of various users. Most of these researchers ($n = 14$) preferred involving direct stakeholders obtained through external recruitment ($n = 13$). The results showed that the EBCD studies were active in acquiring diversity in recruitment but were limited to specific users and viewpoints in applying user involvement and DT themes. Although collaboration with external factors has been sufficiently achieved in terms of the recruitment approach, it is insufficient to reflect a multidisciplinary perspective on user participation types (Table 10).

Table 10. Summary of the study's diversity aspects.

Perspective		Description	General Count		EBCD Count
Recruitment approach		Internal recruitment	15		6
		External recruitment	52		13
Users Involved	Direct stakeholders	Patients	20	51	14
		Patients/caregivers/medical staff	8		
		Patients/medical staff	10		
		Patients/caregivers	3		
		Caregivers/medical staff	2		
		Medical staff	7		
		Caregivers	1		
	Indirect stakeholders	Interprofessional team (non-clinical team)	1	4	1
		Professionals	3		
	Mixed stakeholders	Patients/caregivers/medical staff/professionals	2	8	1
		Medical staff/professionals	4		
		Patients/medical staff/professionals	2		
	Multidisciplinary perspectives	Multidisciplinary team (adolescents, health informaticians, medical anthropologist, psychiatrist, gaming and digital media researcher)	1	4	3
		Patients/medical staff/design team	1		
		Patients/professionals (digital game researcher)	1		
		Patients/medical staff/program development team	1		

4. Discussion

The following insights were derived when examining the approaches and methods of the research for PE improvement.

First, in the distribution of countries, most of the studies centered on North America and Europe, while South America, Africa, and Asia hardly appeared. Considering that the overall quality of life in countries has improved and the importance of PE and the level of patient expectations have increased, active research should also be introduced in these countries.

Second, the user's perspective was treated as necessary in the study subject, focusing on topics related to user participation, interaction, needs, and satisfaction. However, patient feedback, data utilization, patient education, and intervention showed relatively low proportions; therefore, it is necessary to expand the scope to more diverse research topics in the future.

Third, when selected studies were viewed in the DT process, rather than dealing with the iterative process of divergent and convergent thinking, the focus was on the stages of "Define" and "Deliver", which correspond to the convergent thinking for problem identification. Given that medicine is accustomed to the analytical approach corresponding to convergent thinking, a holistic approach through the iteration of divergent and convergent thinking should be introduced to enable flexible and creative problem-solving.

Fourth, in terms of the "User focus" aspect, which corresponds to understanding user needs and using qualitative user research methods through empathy, user involvement at the consult level was higher. It indicated that user participation was increased, but it was still at the level of simple one-way communication. As user participation is still at the level of passive and one-way opinion listening, it is necessary to deeply understand and empathize with the patient's needs by applying ethnographic design techniques, such as "persona", "scenario", and "user journey". This approach allows researchers to solve problems with the question of "why" rather than "what" by observing, experiencing, and interviewing users from a patient's perspective.

Fifth, in terms of the "Problem-framing" aspect relevant to reframing the problem space from a user perspective, the current study's scope was confined to the stage of "Define". It mainly focused on presenting the current problems rather than discovering the potential needs of patients and redefining previously unseen problems. For creative problem-solving to improve PE, it is essential to share and interpret problems discovered through site visits and user research with various members and reframe the problem to find potential opportunities. To define the problem from the user's perspective by understanding the behavior and emotions of the patient through "Persona", a strategic fictional person based on precise observation information and "Patient journey map", a user-centered analysis tool, can be used. Therefore, problems related to PE in healthcare require a unique perspective on the problem and restructuring based on user research from the patient's point of view.

Sixth, for "Visualization", which explores creative solutions by co-creating with various users through divergent thinking, the current studies showed relatively low weight compared to other aspects. "Visualization" provides a tangible communication platform through visual prototyping. Thus, it is helpful for users to exchange opinions more efficiently and to materialize solutions by using the specified artifacts. To obtain a tangible result, relevant experts must participate in each stage of the research and be able to communicate and share their opinions while presenting solutions. Therefore, this aspect, which enables divergent thinking for creative solutions through the participation and interaction of various users, should be actively employed as a methodology for improving the patient-centered healthcare experience. For this, active communication through multidisciplinary team formation and co-creative workshops are required to develop ideas into specific and tangible prototypes.

Seventh, "Experimentation" is a process of iteratively exploring feasibility through testing and verifying solutions that have been explored in the "Visualization" stage. This aspect presents practical and tangible results by narrowing the scope of the divergent thinking back to a concrete solution. However, it is challenging to derive various and creative solutions from current studies because they directly extract keys from the problems identified analytically in the "Define" stage while skipping the "Develop" stage, which explores diverse possibilities. Thus, for developing creative solutions to achieve patient-centeredness, the aspect of "Experimentation" relevant to the attributes of iterative, collaborative, and convergent attributes in DT should be employed. It would be more effective as a methodology for creative problem-solving when various users incorporate methods such as brainstorming.

Lastly, in terms of "Diversity" relevant to the various configurations and viewpoints of the participating users, the recruitment approach is still limited to a specific stakeholder group, thereby not fully reflecting a multidisciplinary perspective in terms of involving diverse professionals from a variety of fields. To fulfill the "Diversity" aspect, it is necessary to form a team with various users and stakeholders for the PE improvement by consciously recruiting team members from a variety of fields such as doctors, UX designers, programmers, and psychologists and by conducting broad research to enable open communication among participants. In this process, a holistic perspective and integrative thinking can be developed, which suggest meaningful insights for improving patient-centered experiences in healthcare.

5. Conclusions

This study systematically viewed current studies on PE in healthcare from the DT perspective to explore the future applicability of the DT methodology that can apply an integrative approach and derive creative solutions through the iterative process of divergent and convergent thinking. The viewpoint of DT was reviewed in this study by employing the four-staged DT process and the five DT themes. As a result, it was found that the DT process is helpful as an approach for designing or evaluating a holistic and iterative research process. Dt themes presented criteria for designing and evaluating specific methodologies for each process step. However, the DT process and themes presented in this study provide a conceptual framework as a new methodology for creative problem-solving in the future medical field. Therefore, for this new approach to be actually applied to healthcare practice, application cases and the evaluation of specific methods should be made.

A patient-centered approach is vital for improving PE. For this purpose, it is meaningful to apply the DT methodology that emphasizes the holistic approach and iterative process of diverging and converging an idea to a problem space for healthcare innovation. This study has the potential to provide significant insights for healthcare researchers to seek a practical methodology for patient-centered healthcare improvement by introducing the concept of DT.

Author Contributions: All the authors contributed to the study design and analysis. Material preparation, data collection, and analysis were performed by E.-J.K., I.-C.N. and Y.-R.K. The main idea underlying the study was proposed by Y.-R.K., and an initial concept was built up with I.-C.N. The first draft of the manuscript was written by E.-J.K., and all authors commented on previous versions of the manuscript. All authors have read and agreed to the published version of the manuscript.

Funding: This research received no external funding.

Institutional Review Board Statement: Not applicable.

Acknowledgments: This research was supported by Basic Science Research Program through the National Research Foundation of Korea (NRF) funded by the Ministry of Education (2021R1I1A4A01059504).

Conflicts of Interest: The authors declare no conflict of interest.

References

1. Fradgley, E.A.; Paul, C.L.; Bryant, J.; Collins, N.; Ackland, S.P.; Bellamy, D.; Levi, C.R. Collaborative Patient-Centered Quality Improvement: A Cross-Sectional Survey Comparing the Types and Numbers of Quality Initiatives Selected by Patients and Health Professionals: A Cross-Sectional Survey Comparing the Types and Numbers of Quality Initiatives Selected by Patients and Health Professionals. *Eval. Health Prof.* **2016**, *39*, 475–495. [CrossRef] [PubMed]
2. Institute of Medicine, Committee on Quality of Health Care in America, Iom, National Academy of Sciences. *Crossing the Quality Chasm: A New Health System for the 21st Century*; National Academies Press: Washington, DC, USA, 2014.
3. Wong, E.; Mavondo, F.; Fisher, J. Patient Feedback to Improve Quality of Patient-Centred Care in Public Hospitals: A Systematic Review of the Evidence. *BMC Health Serv. Res.* **2020**, *20*, 530. [CrossRef] [PubMed]
4. Constand, M.K.; MacDermid, J.C.; Dal Bello-Haas, V.; Law, M. Scoping Review of Patient-Centered Care Approaches in Healthcare. *BMC Health Serv. Res.* **2014**, *14*, 271. [CrossRef] [PubMed]
5. Shaller, D. *Patient-Centered Care: What Does it Take?* Commonwealth Fund: New York, NY, USA, 2007.
6. Stickdorn, M.; Hormess, M.E.; Lawrence, A.; Schneider, J. *This Is Service Design Doing: Applying Service Design Thinking in the Real World*; O'Reilly Media: Sebastopol, CA, USA, 2018.
7. Kværner, K.J.; Støme, L.N.; Romm, J.; Rygh, K.; Almquist, F.; Tornaas, S.; Berg, M.S. Coassessment Framework to Identify Person-Centred Unmet Needs in Stroke Rehabilitation: A Case Report in Norway. *BMJ Innov.* **2021**, *7*, 148–156. [CrossRef]
8. Thies, A. On the Value of Design Thinking for Innovation in Complex Contexts: A Case from Healthcare. *Interact. Des. Archit.* **2015**, *27*, 159–171.

9. Cross, N. *Design Thinking: Understanding How Designers Think and Work*; Bloomsbury Visual Arts: London, UK, 2019.
10. Roberts, J.P.; Fisher, T.R.; Trowbridge, M.J.; Bent, C. A Design Thinking Framework for Healthcare Management and Innovation. *Healthcare* **2016**, *4*, 11–14. [CrossRef]
11. Gottlieb, M.; Wagner, E.; Wagner, A.; Chan, T. Applying Design Thinking Principles to Curricular Development in Medical Education. *AEM Educ. Train.* **2017**, *1*, 21–26. [CrossRef]
12. Van de Bovenkamp, H.M.; Zuiderent-Jerak, T. An Empirical Study of Patient Participation in Guideline Development: Exploring the Potential for Articulating Patient Knowledge in Evidence-Based Epistemic Settings. *Health Expect.* **2015**, *18*, 942–955. [CrossRef]
13. Revenäs, Å.; Martin, C.; Opava, C.H.; Brusewitz, M.; Keller, C.; Åsenlöf, P. A Mobile Internet Service for Self-Management of Physical Activity in People with Rheumatoid Arthritis: Challenges in Advancing the Co-Design Process during the Requirements Specification Phase. *JMIR Res. Protoc.* **2015**, *4*, e111. [CrossRef]
14. Lokker, C.; Gentles, S.J.; Ganann, R.; Jezrawi, R.; Tahir, I.; Okelana, O.; Yousif, C.; Iorio, A.; Valaitis, R. Knowledge Translation Strategies for Sharing Evidence-Based Health Information with Older Adults and Their Caregivers: Findings from a Persona-Scenario Method. *BMC Geriatr.* **2021**, *21*, 665. [CrossRef]
15. Maame Kissiwaa Amoah, V.; Anokye, R.; Boakye, D.S.; Gyamfi, N. Perceived Barriers to Effective Therapeutic Communication among Nurses and Patients at Kumasi South Hospital. *Cogent Med.* **2018**, *5*, 1459341. [CrossRef]
16. Grimaldi, A.; Penfornis, A.; Consoli, S.; Falissard, B.; Eymard, E.; Williams, P.; Dejager, S. Breaking Barriers to Effective Type 2 Diabetes Management: Findings from the Use of the OPTIMA© Questionnaire in Clinical Practice. *Adv. Ther.* **2016**, *33*, 1033–1048. [CrossRef]
17. Lindberg-Scharf, P.; Steinger, B.; Koller, M.; Hofstädter, A.; Ortmann, O.; Kurz, J.; Sasse, J.; Klinkhammer-Schalke, M. Long-Term Improvement of Quality of Life in Patients with Breast Cancer: Supporting Patient-Physician Communication by an Electronic Tool for Inpatient and Outpatient Care. *Support. Care Cancer* **2021**, *29*, 7865–7875. [CrossRef] [PubMed]
18. What Is the Framework for Innovation? Design Council's Evolved Double Diamond. Available online: http://www.designcouncil.org.uk/news-opinion/design-process-what-double-diamond (accessed on 2 May 2022).
19. Badwan, B.; Bothara, R.; Latijnhouwers, M.; Smithies, A.; Sandars, J. The Importance of Design Thinking in Medical Education. *Med. Teach.* **2018**, *40*, 425–426. [CrossRef] [PubMed]
20. Carlgren, L.; Rauth, I.; Elmquist, M. Framing Design Thinking: The Concept in Idea and Enactment: Creativity and Innovation Management. *Creat. Innov. Manag.* **2016**, *25*, 38–57. [CrossRef]
21. Anderson, N.N.; Baker, G.R.; Moody, L.; Scane, K.; Urquhart, R.; Wodchis, W.P.; Gagliardi, A.R. Approaches to Optimize Patient and Family Engagement in Hospital Planning and Improvement: Qualitative Interviews. *Health Expect.* **2021**, *24*, 967–977. [CrossRef]
22. Arksey, H.; O'Malley, L. Scoping Studies: Towards a Methodological Framework. *Int. J. Soc. Res. Methodol.* **2005**, *8*, 19–32. [CrossRef]
23. Gough, D.; Thomas, J.; Oliver, S. Clarifying Differences between Review Designs and Methods. *Syst. Rev.* **2012**, *1*, 28. [CrossRef]
24. Levac, D.; Colquhoun, H.; O'Brien, K.K. Scoping Studies: Advancing the Methodology. *Implement. Sci.* **2010**, *5*, 69. [CrossRef]
25. Peterson, J.; Pearce, P.F.; Ferguson, L.A.; Langford, C.A. Understanding Scoping Reviews: Definition, Purpose, and Process: Definition, Purpose, and Process. *J. Am. Assoc. Nurse Pract.* **2017**, *29*, 12–16. [CrossRef]
26. Tricco, A.C.; Lillie, E.; Zarin, W.; O'Brien, K.; Colquhoun, H.; Kastner, M.; Levac, D.; Ng, C.; Sharpe, J.P.; Wilson, K.; et al. A Scoping Review on the Conduct and Reporting of Scoping Reviews. *BMC Med. Res. Methodol.* **2016**, *16*, 15. [CrossRef] [PubMed]
27. Cacchione, P.Z. The Evolving Methodology of Scoping Reviews. *Clin. Nurs. Res.* **2016**, *25*, 115–119. [CrossRef] [PubMed]
28. Oguntunde, O.; Nyenwa, J.; Kilani-Ahmadu, S.; Salihu, A.; Yusuf, I. Addressing Socio-Cultural Barriers to Family Planning and Co-Designing Services to Improve Utilization: Evidence from Northern Nigeria. *Res. Sq.* **2019**, 1–17. [CrossRef]
29. Theys, S.; Lust, E.; Heinen, M.; Verhaeghe, S.; Beeckman, D.; Eeckloo, K.; Malfait, S.; Van Hecke, A. Barriers and Enablers for the Implementation of a Hospital Communication Tool for Patient Participation: A Qualitative Study. *J. Clin. Nurs.* **2020**, *29*, 1945–1956. [CrossRef] [PubMed]
30. Thayssen, S.; Hansen, D.G.; Søndergaard, J.; Høybye, M.T.; Christensen, P.M.; Hansen, H.P. Completing a Questionnaire at Home Prior to Needs Assessment in General Practice: A Qualitative Study of Cancer Patients' Experience. *Patient* **2016**, *9*, 223–230. [CrossRef]
31. Roodbeen, R.; Vreke, A.; Boland, G.; Rademakers, J.; van den Muijsenbergh, M.; Noordman, J.; van Dulmen, S. Communication and Shared Decision-Making with Patients with Limited Health Literacy; Helpful Strategies, Barriers and Suggestions for Improvement Reported by Hospital-Based Palliative Care Providers. *PLoS ONE* **2020**, *15*, e0234926. [CrossRef]
32. Yılmaz, N.G.; Sungur, H.; van Weert, J.C.M.; van den Muijsenbergh, M.E.T.C.; Schouten, B.C. Enhancing Patient Participation of Older Migrant Cancer Patients: Needs, Barriers, and EHealth. *Ethn. Health* **2020**, *27*, 1123–1146. [CrossRef]
33. Hovén, E.; Lannering, B.; Gustafsson, G.; Boman, K.K. Information Needs of Survivors and Families after Childhood CNS Tumor Treatment: A Population-Based Study. *Acta Oncol.* **2018**, *57*, 649–657. [CrossRef]
34. Bergerum, C.; Engström, A.K.; Thor, J.; Wolmesjö, M. Patient Involvement in Quality Improvement-a "tug of War" or a Dialogue in a Learning Process to Improve Healthcare? *BMC Health Serv. Res.* **2020**, *20*, 1115. [CrossRef]
35. Grim, K.; Rosenberg, D.; Svedberg, P.; Schön, U.-K. Shared Decision-Making in Mental Health Care-A User Perspective on Decisional Needs in Community-Based Services. *Int. J. Qual. Stud. Health Well-Being* **2016**, *11*, 30563. [CrossRef]

36. Selby, K.; Cardinaux, R.; Metry, B.; de Rougemont, S.; Chabloz, J.; Meier-Herrmann, V.; Stoller, J.; Durand, M.-A.; Auer, R. Citizen Advisory Groups for the Creation and Improvement of Decision Aids: Experience from Two Swiss Centers for Primary Care. *Res. Involv. Engagem.* **2021**, *7*, 37. [CrossRef] [PubMed]
37. Coy, K.; Brock, P.; Pomeroy, S.; Cadogan, J.; Beckett, K. A Road Less Travelled: Using Experience Based Co-Design to Map Children's and Families' Emotional Journey Following Burn Injury and Identify Service Improvements. *Burns* **2019**, *45*, 1848–1855. [CrossRef]
38. Litchfield, I.J.; Bentham, L.M.; Lilford, R.J.; McManus, R.J.; Hill, A.; Greenfield, S. Adaption, Implementation and Evaluation of Collaborative Service Improvements in the Testing and Result Communication Process in Primary Care from Patient and Staff Perspectives: A Qualitative Study. *BMC Health Serv. Res.* **2017**, *17*, 615. [CrossRef]
39. Lyes, S.; Richards-Belle, A.; Connolly, B.; Rowan, K.M.; Hinton, L.; Locock, L. Can the UK 24-Item Family Satisfaction in the Intensive Care Unit Questionnaire Be Used to Evaluate Quality Improvement Strategies Aimed at Improving Family Satisfaction with the ICU? A Qualitative Study. *J. Intensive Care Soc.* **2020**, *21*, 312–319. [CrossRef]
40. Renedo, A.; Marston, C. Developing Patient-Centred Care: An Ethnographic Study of Patient Perceptions and Influence on Quality Improvement. *BMC Health Serv. Res.* **2015**, *15*, 122. [CrossRef] [PubMed]
41. Ramos, M.; Bowen, S.; Wright, P.C.; Ferreira, M.G.G.; Forcellini, F.A. Experience Based Co-Design in Healthcare Services: An Analysis of Projects Barriers and Enablers. *Des. Health* **2020**, *4*, 276–295. [CrossRef]
42. Locock, L.; Montgomery, C.; Parkin, S.; Chisholm, A.; Bostock, J.; Dopson, S.; Gager, M.; Gibbons, E.; Graham, C.; King, J.; et al. How Do Frontline Staff Use Patient Experience Data for Service Improvement? Findings from an Ethnographic Case Study Evaluation. *J. Health Serv. Res. Policy* **2020**, *25*, 151–161. [CrossRef]
43. Haddow, J.B.; Walshe, M.; Aggarwal, D.; Thapar, A.; Hardman, J.; Wilson, J.; Oshowo, A.; Bhan, C.; Mukhtar, H. Improving the Diagnostic Stage of the Suspected Colorectal Cancer Pathway: A Quality Improvement Project. *Healthcare* **2016**, *4*, 225–234. [CrossRef] [PubMed]
44. Thomson, A.; Rivas, C.; Giovannoni, G. Multiple Sclerosis Outpatient Future Groups: Improving the Quality of Participant Interaction and Ideation Tools within Service Improvement Activities. *BMC Health Serv. Res.* **2015**, *15*, 105. [CrossRef] [PubMed]
45. Bowie, P.; McNab, D.; Ferguson, J.; de Wet, C.; Smith, G.; MacLeod, M.; McKay, J.; White, C. Quality Improvement and Person-Centredness: A Participatory Mixed Methods Study to Develop the "always Event" Concept for Primary Care. *BMJ Open* **2015**, *5*, e006667. [CrossRef]
46. Frith, L.; Hepworth, L.; Lowers, V.; Joseph, F.; Davies, E.; Gabbay, M. Role of Public Involvement in the Royal College of Physicians' Future Hospitals Healthcare Improvement Programme: An Evaluation. *BMJ Open* **2019**, *9*, e027680. [CrossRef] [PubMed]
47. Stevens, M.C.G.; Beynon, P.; Cameron, A.; Cargill, J.; Cheshire, J.; Dolby, S. Understanding and Utilizing the Unmet Needs of Teenagers and Young Adults with Cancer to Determine Priorities for Service Development: The Macmillan on Target Programme. *J. Adolesc. Young Adult Oncol.* **2018**, *7*, 652–659. [CrossRef]
48. Ågård, A.S.; Hofhuis, J.G.M.; Koopmans, M.; Gerritsen, R.T.; Spronk, P.E.; Engelberg, R.A.; Randall Curtis, J.; Zijlstra, J.G.; Jensen, H.I. Identifying Improvement Opportunities for Patient- and Family-Centered Care in the ICU: Using Qualitative Methods to Understand Family Perspectives. *J. Crit. Care* **2019**, *49*, 33–37. [CrossRef] [PubMed]
49. Fitch, M.I.; Nicoll, I.; Lockwood, G.; Chan, R.J.; Grundy, P. Adolescent and Young Adult Perspectives on Challenges and Improvements to Cancer Survivorship Care: How Are We Doing? *J. Adolesc. Young Adult Oncol.* **2021**, *10*, 432–442. [CrossRef] [PubMed]
50. Miatello, A.; Mulvale, G.; Hackett, C.; Mulvale, A.; Kutty, A.; Alshazly, F. Data Elicited through Apps for Health Systems Improvement: Lessons from Using the MyEXP Suite of Smartphone and Web Apps. *Int. J. Qual. Methods* **2018**, *17*, 160940691879843. [CrossRef]
51. Brosseau, M.; Gagnon, D.; Rohde, K.; Schellinck, J. Integrating Engagement and Improvement Work in a Pediatric Hospital. *Healthc. Q.* **2017**, *20*, 67–72. [CrossRef] [PubMed]
52. Fucile, B.; Bridge, E.; Duliban, C.; Law, M.P. Experience-Based Co-Design: A Method for Patient and Family Engagement in System-Level Quality Improvement. *Patient Exp. J.* **2017**, *4*, 53–60. [CrossRef]
53. Filler, T.; Foster, A.M.; Grace, S.L.; Stewart, D.E.; Straus, S.E.; Gagliardi, A.R. Patient-Centered Care for Women: Delphi Consensus on Evidence-Derived Recommendations. *Value Health* **2020**, *23*, 1012–1019. [CrossRef] [PubMed]
54. Liu, J.J.; Rotteau, L.; Bell, C.M.; Shojania, K.G. Putting out Fires: A Qualitative Study Exploring the Use of Patient Complaints to Drive Improvement at Three Academic Hospitals. *BMJ Qual. Saf.* **2019**, *28*, 894–900. [CrossRef]
55. St Clair Russell, J.; Southerland, S.; Huff, E.D.; Thomson, M.; Meyer, K.B.; Lynch, J.R. A Peer-to-Peer Mentoring Program for in-Center Hemodialysis: A Patient-Centered Quality Improvement Program. *Nephrol. Nurs. J.* **2017**, *44*, 481–496.
56. Powell, R.E.; Doty, A.; Casten, R.J.; Rovner, B.W.; Rising, K.L. A Qualitative Analysis of Interprofessional Healthcare Team Members' Perceptions of Patient Barriers to Healthcare Engagement. *BMC Health Serv. Res.* **2016**, *16*, 493. [CrossRef]
57. Haines, E.R.; Lux, L.; Smitherman, A.B.; Kessler, M.L.; Schonberg, J.; Dopp, A.; Stover, A.M.; Powell, B.J.; Birken, S.A. An Actionable Needs Assessment for Adolescents and Young Adults with Cancer: The AYA Needs Assessment & Service Bridge (NA-SB). *Support. Care Cancer* **2021**, *29*, 4693–4704. [CrossRef]
58. Duckworth, M.; Adelman, J.; Belategui, K.; Feliciano, Z.; Jackson, E.; Khasnabish, S.; Lehman, I.-F.S.; Lindros, M.E.; Mortimer, H.; Ryan, K.; et al. Assessing the Effectiveness of Engaging Patients and Their Families in the Three-Step Fall Prevention Process

across Modalities of an Evidence-Based Fall Prevention Toolkit: An Implementation Science Study. *J. Med. Internet Res.* **2019**, *21*, e10008. [CrossRef]
59. Sockolow, P.; Schug, S.; Zhu, J.; Smith, T.J.; Senathirajah, Y.; Bloom, S. At-Risk Adolescents as Experts in a New Requirements Elicitation Procedure for the Development of a Smart Phone Psychoeducational Trauma-Informed Care Application. *Inform. Health Soc. Care* **2017**, *42*, 77–96. [CrossRef]
60. Bekelman, D.B.; Rabin, B.A.; Nowels, C.T.; Sahay, A.; Heidenreich, P.A.; Fischer, S.M.; Main, D.S. Barriers and Facilitators to Scaling up Outpatient Palliative Care. *J. Palliat. Med.* **2016**, *19*, 456–459. [CrossRef] [PubMed]
61. Luna, A.; Price, A.; Srivastava, U.; Chu, L.F. Critical Patient Insights from the Same-Day Feedback Programme at Stanford Health Care. *BMJ Open Qual.* **2020**, *9*, e000793. [CrossRef]
62. Stoyell, J.F.; Jordan, M.; Derouin, A.; Thompson, J.; Gall, S.; Jooste, K.R.; Keskinyan, V.S.; Lakis, K.R.; Lee, Y.-L.A.; Docherty, S. Evaluation of a Quality Improvement Intervention to Improve Pediatric Palliative Care Consultation Processes. *Am. J. Hosp. Palliat. Care* **2021**, *38*, 1457–1465. [CrossRef]
63. Stockdale, S.E.; Zuchowski, J.; Rubenstein, L.V.; Sapir, N.; Yano, E.M.; Altman, L.; Fickel, J.J.; McDougall, S.; Dresselhaus, T.; Hamilton, A.B. Fostering Evidence-Based Quality Improvement for Patient-Centered Medical Homes: Initiating Local Quality Councils to Transform Primary Care. *Health Care Manag. Rev.* **2018**, *43*, 168–180. [CrossRef]
64. Li, J.; Du, G.; Clouser, J.M.; Stromberg, A.; Mays, G.; Sorra, J.; Brock, J.; Davis, T.; Mitchell, S.; Nguyen, H.Q.; et al. Improving Evidence-Based Grouping of Transitional Care Strategies in Hospital Implementation Using Statistical Tools and Expert Review. *BMC Health Serv. Res.* **2021**, *21*, 35. [CrossRef] [PubMed]
65. Agha, A.Z.; Werner, R.M.; Keddem, S.; Huseman, T.L.; Long, J.A.; Shea, J.A. Improving Patient-Centered Care: How Clinical Staff Overcome Barriers to Patient Engagement at the VHA. *Med. Care* **2018**, *56*, 1009–1017. [CrossRef]
66. Xin, H.; Kilgore, M.L.; Sen, B.P. Is Access to and Use of Primary Care Practices That Patients Perceive as Having Essential Qualities of a Patient-Centered Medical Home Associated with Positive Patient Experience? Empirical Evidence from a U.S. Nationally Representative Sample. *J. Healthc. Qual.* **2017**, *39*, 4–14. [CrossRef]
67. Hwang, A.; Warshaw, G. Joint AGS-CCEHI Survey Offers Insights into Patient Engagement in Geriatric Clinical Settings: Joint Ags-Ccehi Survey. *J. Am. Geriatr. Soc.* **2019**, *67*, 1791–1794. [CrossRef]
68. Alidina, S.; Martelli, P.F.; Singer, S.J.; Aveling, E.-L. Optimizing Patient Partnership in Primary Care Improvement: A Qualitative Study: A Qualitative Study. *Health Care Manag. Rev.* **2019**, *46*, 123–134. [CrossRef]
69. Creutzfeldt, C.J.; Engelberg, R.A.; Healey, L.; Cheever, C.S.; Becker, K.J.; Holloway, R.G.; Curtis, J.R. Palliative Care Needs in the Neuro-ICU. *Crit. Care Med.* **2015**, *43*, 1677–1684. [CrossRef]
70. Federman, A.D.; Sanchez-Munoz, A.; Jandorf, L.; Salmon, C.; Wolf, M.S.; Kannry, J. Patient and Clinician Perspectives on the Outpatient After-Visit Summary: A Qualitative Study to Inform Improvements in Visit Summary Design. *J. Am. Med. Inform. Assoc.* **2017**, *24*, e61–e68. [CrossRef]
71. Groller, K.D.; Teel, C.; Stegenga, K.H.; El Chaar, M. Patient Perspectives about Bariatric Surgery Unveil Experiences, Education, Satisfaction, and Recommendations for Improvement. *Surg. Obes. Relat. Dis.* **2018**, *14*, 785–796. [CrossRef]
72. Hsu, C.; Cruz, S.; Placzek, H.; Chapdelaine, M.; Levin, S.; Gutierrez, F.; Standish, S.; Maki, I.; Carl, M.; Orantes, M.R.; et al. Patient Perspectives on Addressing Social Needs in Primary Care Using a Screening and Resource Referral Intervention. *J. Gen. Intern. Med.* **2020**, *35*, 481–489. [CrossRef]
73. Palmer Kelly, E.; Agne, J.L.; Meara, A.; Pawlik, T.M. Reciprocity within Patient-Physician and Patient-Spouse/Caregiver Dyads: Insights into Patient-Centered Care. *Support. Care Cancer* **2019**, *27*, 1237–1244. [CrossRef]
74. Cardenas, V.; Rahman, A.; Zhu, Y.; Enguidanos, S. Reluctance to Accept Palliative Care and Recommendations for Improvement: Findings from Semi-Structured Interviews with Patients and Caregivers. *Am. J. Hosp. Palliat. Care* **2022**, *39*, 189–195. [CrossRef]
75. Clarke, M.A.; Moore, J.L.; Steege, L.M.; Koopman, R.J.; Belden, J.L.; Canfield, S.M.; Kim, M.S. Toward a Patient-Centered Ambulatory after-Visit Summary: Identifying Primary Care Patients' Information Needs. *Inform. Health Soc. Care* **2017**, *43*, 248–263. [CrossRef]
76. Scott, A.M.; Li, J.; Oyewole-Eletu, S.; Nguyen, H.Q.; Gass, B.; Hirschman, K.B.; Mitchell, S.; Hudson, S.M.; Williams, M.V.; Project ACHIEVE Team. Understanding Facilitators and Barriers to Care Transitions: Insights from Project ACHIEVE Site Visits. *Jt. Comm. J. Qual. Patient Saf.* **2017**, *43*, 433–447. [CrossRef] [PubMed]
77. Nowacki, K.; Gonzalez, T.; Mehnert, J.; Jacquemard, A.; Tyler, A. Using Patient Whiteboards to Engage Families in Harm Prevention and Care Planning: A Quality Improvement Study. *Hosp. Pediatr.* **2018**, *8*, 345–352. [CrossRef] [PubMed]
78. Grob, R.; Schlesinger, M.; Barre, L.R.; Bardach, N.; Lagu, T.; Shaller, D.; Parker, A.M.; Martino, S.C.; Finucane, M.L.; Cerully, J.L.; et al. What Words Convey: The Potential for Patient Narratives to Inform Quality Improvement. *Milbank Q.* **2019**, *97*, 176–227. [CrossRef] [PubMed]
79. Martínez-Guiu, J.; Arroyo-Fernández, I.; Rubio, R. Impact of Patients' Attitudes and Dynamics in Needs and Life Experiences during Their Journey in COPD: An Ethnographic Study. *Expert Rev. Respir. Med.* **2022**, *16*, 121–132. [CrossRef] [PubMed]
80. LaMonica, H.M.; Davenport, T.A.; Roberts, A.E.; Hickie, I.B. Understanding Technology Preferences and Requirements for Health Information Technologies Designed to Improve and Maintain the Mental Health and Well-Being of Older Adults: Participatory Design Study. *JMIR Aging* **2021**, *4*, e21461. [CrossRef] [PubMed]
81. Peters, D.; Davis, S.; Calvo, R.A.; Sawyer, S.M.; Smith, L.; Foster, J.M. Young People's Preferences for an Asthma Self-Management App Highlight Psychological Needs: A Participatory Study. *J. Med. Internet Res.* **2017**, *19*, e113. [CrossRef]

82. Fradgley, E.A.; Paul, C.L.; Bryant, J.; Oldmeadow, C. Getting Right to the Point: Identifying Australian Outpatients' Priorities and Preferences for Patient-Centred Quality Improvement in Chronic Disease Care. *Int. J. Qual. Health Care* **2016**, *28*, 470–477. [CrossRef]
83. Song, H.J.; Dennis, S.; Levesque, J.-F.; Harris, M. How to Implement Patient Experience Surveys and Use Their Findings for Service Improvement: A Qualitative Expert Consultation Study in Australian General Practice. *Integr. Health J.* **2020**, *2*, e000033. [CrossRef]
84. Hall, A.; Bryant, J.; Sanson-Fisher, R.; Grady, A.; Proietto, A.; Doran, C.M. Top Priorities for Health Service Improvements among Australian Oncology Patients. *Patient Relat. Outcome Meas.* **2021**, *12*, 83–95. [CrossRef]
85. Schäfer, W.L.A.; Boerma, W.G.W.; Murante, A.M.; Sixma, H.J.M.; Schellevis, F.G.; Groenewegen, P.P. Assessing the Potential for Improvement of Primary Care in 34 Countries: A Cross-Sectional Survey. *Bull. World Health Organ.* **2015**, *93*, 161–168. [CrossRef]

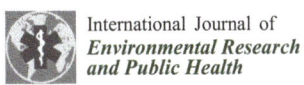

Article

Validation and Adjustment of the Patient Experience Questionnaire (PEQ): A Regional Hospital Study in Norway

Seth Ayisi Addo *, Reidar Johan Mykletun and Espen Olsen

Department of Innovation, Leadership and Marketing, University of Stavanger Business School, University of Stavanger, 4036 Stavanger, Norway; reidar.j.mykletun@uis.no (R.J.M.); espen.olsen@uis.no (E.O.)
* Correspondence: seth.a.addo@uis.no

Abstract: This paper assesses the psychometric qualities of the Patient Experience Questionnaire (PEQ), thereby validating a patient-oriented measurement model in a hospital environment, and modifies the model based on empirical results. This study employed survey data gathered by the Norwegian Institute of Public Health from adult inpatients at somatic hospitals in the Health South-East RHF in Norway. The survey engaged 4603 patients out of 8381 from five main hospitals in the region. The study found that an eight-factor model of the PEQ generally showed good fitness to the data, but assessment of discriminant validity showed that this was not the optimal factor solution among four of the eight dimensions. After comparing models, the study proposed a model with a second-order factor for four of the factors: "nurse services", "doctor services", "information", and "organization", collectively named "treatment services". The proposed model demonstrated good validity and reliability results. The results present theoretical and practical implications. The study recommends that inferential analyses on the PEQ should be done with the second-order factor. Furthermore, a revision of the PEQ is recommended subject to more confirmatory studies with larger samples in different regions. The study indicates a second-order factor structure for assessing and understanding patient experiences—a finding which has both theoretical and managerial implications.

Keywords: patient experiences; PREMs; psychometrics; CFA; hospital; second-order factor; Norway

1. Introduction

Healthcare professionals are facing heavy pressure to meet the growing needs of patients such as medical, physical, and psychological healthcare needs [1] as well as patients' expectations of quality services, products, and performance [2]. This is due to the increasing and alarming rate of morbidity and multi-morbidity in Western countries [3], together with aging populations and the healthcare needs of the aged. Pressure on healthcare professionals has increased in recent times with the outbreak of global pandemics such as COVID-19. Notwithstanding these morbidity rates and the growing needs of patients, healthcare providers and professionals are expected to ensure positive patient experiences. This study, focusing on hospitals and their professionals, seeks to examine patients' experiences with hospital service climates, focusing on the psychometric quality of a patient-reported experience measure (PREM).

The endeavour of gathering patients' experiences with healthcare has gained popularity, thus resulting in the development of PREMs that have been used in surveys in various countries [4–8]. In a bid to clarify the meaning of patient experiences, Wolf and Jason [9] synthesized various definitions of the concept and maintained that patient experiences comprise individual as well as collective events and occurrences that happen in the process of caregiving, and this has strong links with patients' expectations and how they were met. Wagland et al. [10] noted that significant progress has been made in understanding patient experience. The concept is viewed as interactions of patients with aspects of the healthcare delivery such as nurse services, doctor services, organization of the caregiving process in hospitals, and information delivery, where these aspects (dimensions) culminate in the entire continuum of experience that patients have with healthcare, as reported by the patients.

From patients' perspectives, interactions with dimensions of healthcare have been theoretically underpinned by the Donabedian framework for assessing healthcare quality [11], which is considered the most widely used in the healthcare sector to assess quality [12]. According to this framework, quality of healthcare can be assessed by making inferences under three categories: structure, process, and outcome. The structure deals with the setting in which care is given, for instance, facilities, equipment, and human resources. The process deals with what is done in giving and receiving care, for instance, nurse and doctor services as well as good communication and information sharing between patients and hospitals; and lastly, the outcome deals with the effects of care on health and well-being [11,13].

Increased understanding of patient experiences of hospital climate has similarly been aided by increased research and several studies on measuring the construct. Measurements in social science provide adequate guidelines for assessing phenomena and people's attributes that are not directly and easily observable [14]. Employing poor and inadequate measures in research can be very costly to practice, in terms of drawing invalid conclusions, making policy decisions based on false information, and wasting respondents' time and efforts [15]. DeVellis [15], however, indicated that a major challenge to developing adequate measures in social science is the immaterial nature of social science constructs supported by constantly changing theories. This makes measurements in social science susceptible to constant changes in performance and adequacy in assessing the constructs. Consequently, social science measures need to be constantly reviewed and reassessed to keep them abreast with changing theories and constructs and to uphold their validity and reliability. Therefore, reassessing PREMs to ensure adequate psychometric qualities is essential for theoretical and practical advancement of knowledge of patients' experiences, hence the focus and aim of this study.

Justification of the Study

The goal to accurately measure patient experiences has resulted in several PREMs for general and specialized healthcare [5]. The questions and dimensions that these PREMS have produced are indicative of patients' shared experiences. Most of these measures identified similar dimensions of experiences, such as those relating to nurse services, doctor services, information and communication, hospital organization and standards, and discharge from the hospital [5,6,16–18]. Although some of these studies differed with regard to the naming of the dimensions, the content of the items remained very similar among the PREMs. This study is underpinned by two main justifications: (i) psychometric statistical analyses have evolved over the years with more robust tools in validating scales; and (ii) due to the plethora of patient experience measures and unascertained psychometric qualities, existing PREMs should be re-examined to ascertain their validity and reliability, rather than developing new ones. These justifications are elaborated below.

The Norwegian Institute of Public Health (NIPH) conducted a survey in the east health region among a few hospitals, adapting an earlier validated PREM, the Patient Experience Questionnaire (PEQ) [8]. In the development and validation study, Pettersen, Veenstra (8) employed literature reviews, focus groups, pilot studies, and two cross-sectional surveys (1996 and 1998) across 14 hospitals in Norway. The study used exploratory factor analysis, a reliability test (Cronbach's alpha), and a construct validity test. The study found 10 factors and 20 final items out of an initial 35 items: "information on future complaints", "nursing services", "communication", "information examinations", "contact with next-of-kin", "doctor services", "hospital and equipment", "information medication", "organization", and "general satisfaction". All the factors recorded Cronbach's alpha scores between 0.61 and 0.83. Construct validity was also ascertained in the study by examining the relationship between the instrument and demographic factors such as age and gender. Stressing the lack of valid and reliable instruments, Pettersen et al. [8] concluded that it is imperative to re-examine existing patient experience measures so as to improve methodology. They further recommended employment of the PEQ for future in-patient experience surveys, hence the choice for the current study. Although this measure was adapted and modified for use by the NIPH, the performance of the measure should be called into question because this measure was developed and validated more than a decade ago. Psychometric analyses are evolving with more robust validating tools and methods, and this is evident in the study by Pettersen et al. [8] where issues such as discriminant validity and measurement invariance as well as other psychometric issues were absent in the analyses—a gap that the current study tackles.

Beattie et al. [19] also noted the problem of multiple patient experience measures with unascertained psychometric quality. This problem has hindered the use of data from patient experience surveys to adequately improve and sustain quality of care in hospitals. In the systematic review, Beattie et al. [19] developed a matrix to help choose PREMs for research and to identify research gaps in existing ones. This matrix showed that the PEQ study by Pettersen et al. [8] lacked analyses such as criterion-related validity. On this basis, the current study asserts that rather than developing more PREMs (which seem already saturated), existing ones should be re-examined, as recommended earlier by Pettersen et al. [8], in light of current analyses and conceptual underpinnings. This need for re-examination has also been recommended by other systematic reviews on patient experience [20,21].

Additionally, some PREMs have been developed in Norway to capture the phenomenon of patient experiences with general health practice as well as experiences with specific health issues and fields, with most of them asking questions on general patient satisfaction [8,18,22,23]. Haugum et al. [20] similarly recommended the need to repeat patient experience surveys and their outcomes in order to generate more validated instruments, as they are potentially affected by contextual factors. By inference, it can be said that the underlying psychometric rigors of a PREM can dwindle as they are employed over a long period. Although several surveys exist on patient experiences on various issues [2,24–27], a re-analysis of the psychometric performance of any particular measure is lacking. The quest to improve healthcare delivery and hospital service climate based on patients' experiences should begin with ascertaining the psychometric quality of PREMs. Based on these justifications, the purpose of this article is to test the psychometric qualities of the PEQ, thereby validating a measurement model in a hospital environment.

2. Materials and Methods

2.1. Sample and Data Collection

This study employed anonymous survey data from the Norwegian Institute of Public Health gathered from adult inpatients at somatic hospitals in the Health South-East RHF in Norway. These somatic hospitals dealt with issues generally affecting the bodies of patients and thus, were not specialized. The survey was started by the Norwegian Knowledge Centre for Health Services in the fall of 2015 and was continued at the Norwegian Institute of Public Health in the first quarter of 2016. It is worth noting that the last major reform and restructuring done in the Norwegian health sector was in 2002; where ownership of hospitals was transferred to the state. Thus, although changes have been made over the years since then, they are minor and incremental to the 2002 reform, focusing more on better standardization. These changes may therefore not affect this study in a major way. The survey engaged patients from 5 main hospitals in the region who were admitted for at least a day. The eligibility criteria were patients who were admitted between October and November in 2015 and who were admitted to the hospitals for at least one night. The study excluded outpatients. Patients who visited the 5 hospitals were identified through their contact information after they were discharged. Questionnaires were sent to their respective addresses via post mail with a return envelope. About 8381 patients were eligible and contacted. The total number of respondents who completed and returned their questionnaires was 4603, yielding a response rate of 54.92%. Patients were asked to consider various aspects of their experience being admitted. The questionnaire aimed at using feedback to identify which areas are working well and which areas the hospital should work to improve.

2.2. Instrument

The Patient Experience Questionnaire (PEQ) comprised 8 dimensions and 33 items as well as items on patient safety, patient satisfaction, and overall health benefits and health level. The NIPH adapted the questions for the survey from the PEQ developed and validated by Pettersen et al. [8]: "nurse services" (items N1–N7), "doctor services" (items D1–D7), "information" (items IF1–IF3), "organization" (items OR1–OR4), "next of kin" (items NK1 and NK2), "standard" (items S1–S6), "discharge" (items DC1 and DC2), and "interaction" (items IT1 and IT2). These items were measured on a 5-point Likert scale ranging from "Not at all" (1) to "To a very large extent" (5). Patient safety was measured with 12 items, while patient satisfaction, health benefit, and health level were measured with 1 item each. Background information, such as questions on whether or not the patient chose the hospital they were admitted to, was also included in the questionnaire.

2.3. Data Analysis

2.3.1. Preliminary Analyses

The study analysed the data with the aid of Microsoft Excel (Microsoft, Redmond, WA, USA), SPSS v.24 (IBM Corporation, Armonk, NY, USA), and AMOS v.25 (IBM Corporation, Armonk, NY, USA). Preliminary analysis (such as checking for normality, outliers, and missing value analysis) was conducted in SPSS. The missing values were found to be not at random, and therefore being mindful of how they were replaced was necessary. The study chose to use multiple imputations to replace them as recommended for non-randomness [28,29]. However, the 5 different imputations generated could not be pooled in AMOS as a single imputation for the estimation of the model. Thus, the missing values were eventually replaced with the series mean method. Analysis was performed mainly on the data with missing values due to their non-randomness and also due to the subject matter under investigation being patient experiences; as the study wanted to capture accurate measurements by the respondents. In order to ensure maximum privacy of respondents and still maintain relevant variables for analysis, departments for the analysis were aggregated into medical departments (Med) and surgical departments (Kir) across the hospitals based on the more specific and varied information on units in the hospitals provided by participants. This aggregation was performed according to the departmental codes for health institutions provided by the Norwegian Health Authority.

2.3.2. Measurement Model Development

The initial measurement model (Model 1) was developed in AMOS without modification indices (due to the exclusion of missing values). Missing values were replaced with the series mean method after the estimation of the initial model to obtain modification indices for correlating error terms among the items and improving the fitness of the model (Model 2). It is noteworthy that the missing values were only replaced in order to generate a full estimation with modification indices for correlating the error terms. Although all subsequent models after the initial model were estimated with the correlated error terms, estimations were done on the data with missing values, with the aim of obtaining a more accurate fit of the data to the models.

The initial model with modifications (correlated error terms), Model 2, was compared with 6 other models (Models 3–8), obtained by combining some dimensions into a single factor to further justify the fitness of the modified initial model. These combinations were based on the correlation coefficients between the dimensions. In addition, a proposed model containing a second-order factor for "nurse services", "doctor services", "information", and "organization" was also developed and compared with the initial modified model based on the validity tests, correlation analyses, and theoretical justifications (wording of questions). Fitness of all the models was ascertained using the following indices: Comparative Fit Index (CFI), Tucker Lewis Index (TLI), Root Mean Square Error of Approximation (RMSEA), and the PCLOSE. The thresholds recommended by Hu and Bentler [30] are presented in Table 1.

Table 1. Fitness indices and acceptable thresholds.

Fit Indices	Acceptable Thresholds
CFI	>0.95, excellent; >0.90, acceptable
TLI	>0.95, excellent; >0.90, acceptable
RMSEA	<0.06, excellent; 0.06–0.10, moderate
PCLOSE	>0.05, excellent

Adapted from Hu and Bentler (1999).

2.3.3. Validity and Reliability

Validity in this study was ascertained using convergent, discriminant, and predictive validity tests. Convergent validity deals with the relationship between a latent construct (patient experience dimensions) and its items [31]. The average variance extracted (AVE) was used to check convergent validity, where values must be at least 0.50, indicating that at least half of the variance in the construct (dimension) is explained by its items. Discriminant validity focuses on a construct and its items in relation to other constructs—that is, how different one construct (or dimension) and its items are from other constructs in the model [31]. Discriminant validity was examined using the Fornell–Larcker procedure, where discriminant validity is supported when the square root of the AVEs is greater than the correlation coefficients between the constructs [32]. Predictive validity focuses on the ability of the measure and dimensions to relate to and predict previously ascertained outcomes in literature. This was determined through correlation and regression analyses between patient experiences (and dimensions) and outcome variables (patient satisfaction, health benefits, and health level) with the aid of SPSS. Reliability of the measurement model was also determined using composite reliability values for every dimension of the patient experience measure, with a recommended value of at least 0.70 to ascertain its repeatability in different contexts.

2.4. Ethical Considerations

This study, with regard to data collection, analysis, and compilation, was conducted within the ethical and legal provisions and guidelines of the Norwegian Institute for Public Health (NIPH) and the University of Stavanger. The Norwegian Data Protection Authority and the Norwegian Directorate of Health approved the procedures in the survey. The hospital data protection official assessed the data processing in the hospitals where survey extension took place. Informed consent was obtained from participants in the survey. Respondents were informed that participation was voluntary and they were assured of confidentiality of the information they will provide. Respondents were also informed that they could opt out of the survey at any point as well as the procedure for opting out if they wished. Data was stored in a safe repository with a password, only accessed by the researchers. This study did not present results that revealed patients' identities, thus maintaining anonymity of respondents and confidentiality of responses. All relevant ethical requirements were duly upheld.

3. Results

3.1. Preliminary Analysis and Sample Characteristics

The study made use of responses from 4603 participants. Outliers were recorded for some of the questions, but this was to be expected considering the varied background characteristics, such as age and number of days spent in the hospital, which could influence participants' experiences. Nonetheless, most of these outliers were not deemed extreme based on the 1.5 and 3.0 interquartile ranges. Normality was also ascertained, using the −2 and +2 range [33], for all items of patient experience, except the kurtosis value for one item on "nurse services" and one item on "doctor services". Overall, the data could be said to be normally distributed to a large extent. The sample for the study was taken from five hospitals and characterized by a somewhat fair age distribution of patients across three groups: 60 years and below, between 61 and 73 years, and 74 years and above. Most of the respondents were admitted for three or fewer days, and more of them were also admitted to the medical department aggregate (Med). Table 2 presents the sample characteristics for this study.

Table 2. Sample characteristics.

Variables	Frequency	Valid Percent
Age		
Less than 61 years	1502	32.6
61–73 years	1528	33.2
73 years and above	1573	34.2
Days spent in hospital		
Less than 4 days	2630	57.1
4 or more days	1973	42.9
Department aggregates		
Medical (Med)	2468	53.6
Surgical (Kir)	2135	46.4
Hospitals		
Hospital 1	2067	44.9
Hospital 2	1084	23.5
Hospital 3	193	4.2
Hospital 4	794	17.2
Hospital 5	465	10.1

3.2. Initial Measurement Model Development, Modifications, and Comparisons

The initial CFA model (Model 1, Table 3), with the eight dimensions of patient experience, was then developed to be tested. The model showed acceptable fitness to the data based on fitness indices (CFI = 0.91; TLI = 0.89; RMSEA = 0.06; PCLOSE = 0.00). Nonetheless, there was a need to improve the fitness through modifications in order to reduce measurement errors and to obtain more accurate loadings of the observed items on their dimensions. Some modifications were made by drawing covariance between some error terms on the same dimensions with the rationale that, by virtue of sharing commonalities on the dimension, they are more justified to share similar error terms, thus reducing duplications of random measurement error of items. In total, 19 modifications were made based on the covariance coefficients, with the highest coefficient as 895.667 between S2 and S4 ("standard") and the lowest as 40.390 between D4 and D7 ("doctor services"). Aside from the coefficients, these modifications were theoretically justified. For example, the item D2 was worded, "Did you find that the doctors took care of you?", and D4 was worded as "Did the doctors have time for you when you needed it?" Participants may have given closely related responses due to the phrases "taking care" and "having time when you needed"; therefore, it was no surprise that they shared similar error terms, leading to considerable covariance coefficient. These statistical and theoretical justifications were made for each covariance drawn. The most modifications were made to "doctor services" (seven), followed by "standard" (five), "nurse services" (four), "information" (two), and "organization" (one). No modifications were made to "next of kin", "discharge", or "interaction", owing to very low covariance coefficients (below 20). The initial model with these modifications (Model 2 in Table 3) thus produced excellent fitness values for all indices. Furthermore, the model was compared with six other models (see Section 2), where the initial model with modifications showed the best fitness to the data. The fitness indices of the initial model before and after modifications, as well as those of the six alternative models for comparisons, are presented in Table 3.

Table 3. Fitness results for all models.

Fit Indices	Model 1—Initial Model without Modifications	Model 2 *—Model after Modifications	Models 3–8 *—Alternative Models	Model 9 *—Configural Invariance	Model 10 *—Model after Item Deletion	Model 11 *—Proposed Model
			1st 2nd 3rd 4th 5th 6th			
CFI	0.91	0.95	0.91 0.91 0.92 0.88 0.86 0.85	0.95	0.95	0.96
TLI	0.89	0.94	0.89 0.89 0.90 0.85 0.84 0.82	0.94	0.94	0.95
RMSEA	0.06	0.04	0.06 0.06 0.05 0.07 0.07 0.07	0.03	0.04	0.04
PCLOSE	0.00	1.00	0.00 0.00 0.00 0.00 0.00 0.00	1.00	0.99	0.98

Note: * These models were assessed with the modification estimates. 1st—nurse and doctor into one factor; 2nd—nurse, doctor and organization into one factor; 3rd—nurse and organization into one factor; doctor and information into one factor; 4th—nurse, doctor, organization, and information into one factor; next of kin and standard into one factor; discharge and interaction into one factor; 5th—nurse, doctor, organization, information, next of kin, and standard into one factor; discharge and interaction into one factor; 6th—all dimensions into one factor.

3.3. Measurement Invariance across Hospital Departments Aggregated into Two Groups

Model 2 was further examined for invariance across three categories: configural, metric, and scalar. Measurement invariance tests seek to ascertain whether the measurement model differs across variant groups in a data. The goal is to achieve little or insignificant variance across these groups in order to inspire confidence in the ability of the measure to generate accurate responses and assessments across groups [34]. Configural invariance results (see Model 9, Table 3) showed that the model had acceptable-to-excellent fitness to the data, thus ascertaining configural invariance for the eight-factor patient experience measure across the two hospital department aggregates. With regard to metric invariance, the chi-squared test showed that the fully constrained model and the unconstrained mode were different across the department groups and, thus, not metrically invariant. However, MacKenzie et al. [35] maintained that "full metric invariance is not necessary for further tests of invariance and substantive analyses to be meaningful, provided that at least one item (other than the one fixed at unity to define the scale of each latent construct) is metrically invariant" (p. 325). Thus, the critical ratios test was performed to examine whether the dimensions and the items were metrically invariant enough for further meaningful analyses. The analysis revealed that for all dimensions, with the exception of "next of kin", there was at least one item that was not statistically significant (metrically invariant) besides the item that was constrained for that dimension in the model. This means that the two items on the "next of kin" dimension had significantly different loadings (parameters) across the aggregated departments. Nonetheless, this test showed the model was metrically invariant across the departments to a large extent. The results of this test are presented as a supplementary table (Table S1). Scalar invariance was then examined for the model based on the differences in the measurement intercepts. The analyses showed that the model did not have scalar invariance. Differences in intercept estimates of items between the departments were computed, showing that almost all the items did not have scalar invariance across the two departments. The results are presented as a supplementary table (Table S2).

3.4. Reliability

Reliability for the measure was ascertained using composite reliability (CR) values. Generally, CR values above 0.70 are deemed acceptable to justify reliability. From Table 4, it is seen that all the dimensions recorded CR values above 0.70, with the highest being "doctor services" (0.92) and the lowest being "interaction" (0.72).

Table 4. Correlations, reliability, convergent, and discriminant validity before item deletion (Model 2).

	CR	AVE	1	2	3	4	5	6	7	8
1. Nurse services	0.90	0.57	**0.76**							
2. Doctor services	0.92	0.64	0.80	**0.80**						
3. Information	0.87	0.70	0.77	0.82	**0.83**					
4. Organization	0.81	0.53	0.85	0.80	0.79	**0.73**				
5. Next of kin	0.83	0.70	0.69	0.59	0.63	0.71	**0.84**			
6. Standard	0.82	0.44	0.65	0.57	0.56	0.73	0.60	**0.67**		
7. Discharge	0.87	0.77	0.57	0.56	0.63	0.58	0.49	0.44	**0.88**	
8. Interaction	0.72	0.57	0.57	0.58	0.56	0.63	0.53	0.50	0.56	**0.75**

Note: CR—composite reliability; AVE—average variance explained; figures in bold are the square roots of the AVEs for discriminant validity (using the Fornell–Larcker procedure; discriminant validity is supported when the square root of the AVEs are greater than the correlation coefficients between the constructs).

3.5. Convergent and Discriminant Validity

Convergent validity was examined using the AVE values, where an AVE value of at least 0.50 is considered acceptable [31]. Table 4 shows that all dimensions, with the exception of "standard", recorded values above 0.50, thus ascertaining convergent validity. Discriminant validity was ascertained using the Fornell–Larcker procedure. There, discriminant validity is supported when the square root of the AVEs is greater than the correlation coefficients between the constructs [32]. From Table 4, it is seen that discriminant validity issues were observed for "doctor services" (in relation to "information"); "organization" (in relation to "doctor services", "nurse services", and "information"); and "standard" (in relation to "organization"). This means that these three dimensions were not distinct from the others enough for each to measure the different sub-concepts under patient experience.

3.6. Construct Validity, Item Loadings, and Deletion

Construct validity for the items was examined by checking item loadings (parameter estimates) on their dimensions. Generally, good loadings were recorded as a majority of the items had loadings above 0.60. The item loadings ranged from 0.88 (on "discharge") to 0.55 (on "standard"). Two items had loadings below 0.60: 0.58 (ORG 2) and 0.55 (ST 5). Based on the suggestion of the master validity tool [36], these items together with a third (ST4) were deleted in a bid to boost the validity of the measure. Item loadings before and after deletion are presented in Table 5. After deletion, the dimension "standard" recorded an increase in AVE value, indicating that the remaining four items explained more variance in the dimension than the original six items, seen in Table 6. Figure 1 presents the model after item deletion as well as validity and reliability checks. See Model 10 in Table 3 for the fit indices of this model.

Table 5. Standardized factor loadings (before and after item deletion) and missing values.

Dimensions and Items	Factor Loadings			Missing Values N (%)
	Model 2	Model 10	Model 11	
Nurse services				
N1. Did the nursing staff talk to you so you understood them?	0.67	0.66	0.67	287 (6.2)
N2. Did you find that the nursing staff cared for you?	0.80	0.80	0.79	293 (6.4)
N3. Do you have confidence in the professional skills of the nursing staff?	0.78	0.78	0.78	282 (6.2)
N4. Did you tell the nursing staff everything you thought was important about your condition?	0.72	0.72	0.72	340 (7.4)
N5. Did you find that the nursing staff were interested in your description of your own situation?	0.83	0.83	0.83	328 (7.1)
N6. Were you included in the advice on questions regarding your care?	0.70	0.70	0.68	427 (9.3)
N7. Did the nursing staff have time for you when you needed it?	0.77	0.77	0.78	297 (6.5)
Doctor services				
D1. Did the doctors talk to you so you understood them?	0.73	0.73	0.73	300 (6.5)
D2. Did you find that the doctors took care of you?	0.84	0.84	0.83	302 (6.6)
D3. Do you trust the doctors' professional skills?	0.77	0.77	0.77	299 (6.5)
D4. Did the doctors have time for you when you needed it?	0.82	0.82	0.82	415 (9.0)
D5. Did you tell the doctors everything you thought was important about your condition?	0.77	0.77	0.77	384 (8.3)
D6. Did you find that the doctors were interested in your description of your own situation?	0.84	0.84	0.85	378 (8.2)
D7. Did you find that the treatment was adapted to your situation?	0.79	0.79	0.76	321 (7.0)
Information				
IF1. Did you know what you thought was necessary about how tests and examinations should take place?	0.79	0.79	0.85	320 (7.0)
IF2. Did you know what you thought was necessary about the results of tests and examinations?	0.85	0.85	0.86	334 (7.3)
IF3. Did you receive sufficient information about your diagnosis or your complaints?	0.86	0.86	0.87	326 (7.1)
Organization				
OR1. Did you find that there was a permanent group of nursing staff that took care of you?	0.67	0.67	0.68	121 (2.6)
* OR2. Did you find that one doctor had the main responsibility for you?	0.58	-	-	130 (2.8)
OR3. Did you find that the hospital's work was well organized?	0.81	0.82	0.82	107 (2.3)
OR4. Did you find that important information about you had come to the right person?	0.82	0.81	0.81	204 (4.4)

Table 5. Cont.

Dimensions and Items	Factor Loadings			Missing Values N (%)
	Model 2	Model 10	Model 11	
Next of kin				
NK1. Were your relatives well received by the hospital staff?	0.84	0.84	0.84	1362 (29.6)
NK2. Was it easy for your relatives to get information about you while you were in the hospital?	0.83	0.83	0.83	1732 (37.6)
Standard				
S1. Did you get the impression that the hospital equipment was in good condition?	0.71	0.72	0.78	108 (2.3)
S2. Did you get the impression that the hospital was in good condition?	0.77	0.78	0.86	122 (2.7)
S3. Was the room you were in satisfactory?	0.67	0.65	0.74	80 (1.7)
* S4. Was the opportunity for rest and rest satisfactory?	0.62	-	0.66	90 (2.0)
* S5. Was the food satisfactory?	0.55	-	-	122 (2.7)
S6. Was the cleaning satisfactory?	0.65	0.66	0.60	89 (1.9)
Discharge				
DC.1 Were you informed of what you could do at home in case of relapse?	0.87	0.87	-	1327 (28.8)
DC2. Were you informed of what complaints you could expect to receive in time after your hospital stay?	0.88	0.88	-	1195 (26.0)
Interaction				
IT1. Do you find that the hospital has worked well with your GP about what you were admitted to?	0.82	0.81	-	2523 (33.9)
IT2. Do you feel that the hospital has cooperated well with the home or other municipal services about what you were admitted for?	0.69	0.69	-	3401 (54.8)
Treatment services				
Nurse services			0.92	
Doctor services			0.86	
Information			0.84	
Organization			0.93	

Note: Items marked with * had the lowest loadings.

Table 6. Correlations, reliability, convergent, and discriminant validity after item deletion (Model 10).

	CR	AVE	1	2	3	4	5	6	7	8
1. Nurse services	0.90	0.57	**0.76**							
2. Doctor services	0.92	0.64	0.80	**0.80**						
3. Information	0.87	0.70	0.77	0.82	**0.83**					
4. Organization	0.81	0.59	0.87	0.78	0.79	**0.77**				
5. Next of kin	0.82	0.70	0.69	0.59	0.63	0.72	**0.84**			
6. Standard	0.80	0.50	0.64	0.56	0.55	0.74	0.59	**0.70**		
7. Discharge	0.87	0.77	0.57	0.56	0.63	0.56	0.49	0.44	**0.88**	
8. Interaction	0.72	0.57	0.57	0.58	0.56	0.62	0.53	0.47	0.56	**0.75**

Note: CR—composite reliability; AVE—average variance explained; figures in bold are the square roots of the AVEs for discriminant validity (using the Fornell–Larcker procedure; discriminant validity is supported when the square root of the AVEs are greater than the correlation coefficients between the constructs).

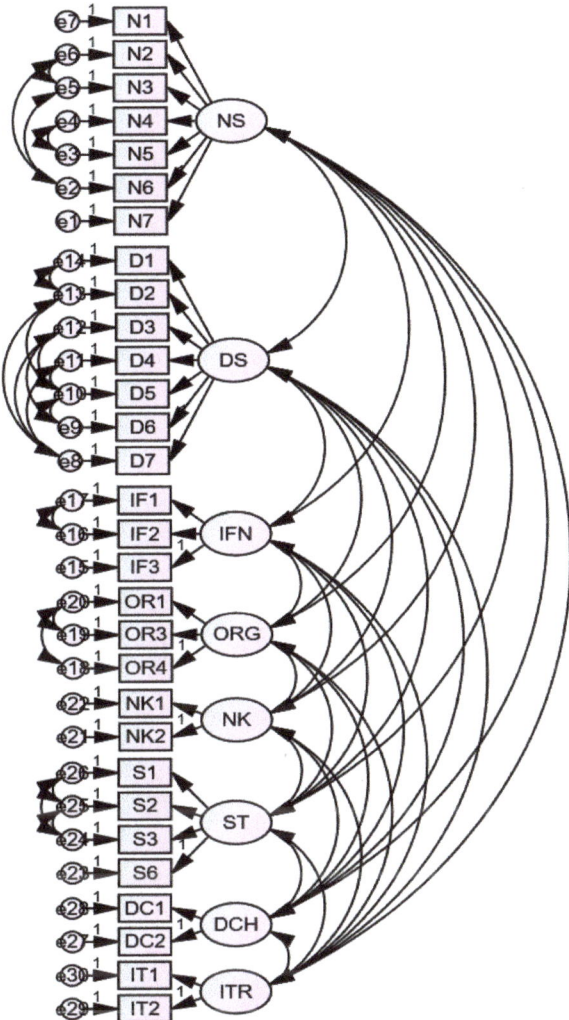

Figure 1. Model after validity checks and item deletion. Note: NS—nurse services; DS—doctor services; INF—information; ORG—organization; ST—standard; NK—next of kin; DCH—discharge; ITR—interaction.

3.7. Criterion-Related Validity

The study then assessed the predictive validity of the model based on its ability to relate to and predict outcome variables ascertained in existing literature. Overall satisfaction, health benefits, and health level were used as outcome variables while the patient experience measure and its dimensions were used as predicting variables. Patient experience measure and dimensions were computed with retained items after item deletion, and multiple linear regression was performed with age and number of days spent in hospital as control variables. The results showed that overall patient experience and each individual dimension related to and predicted at least one outcome variable positively and significantly. These results are presented in Table 7.

Table 7. Regression results for criterion-related validity.

	Model 10			Proposed Model (Model 11)			
	Satisfaction	Health Benefits	Health Level		Satisfaction	Health Benefits	Health Level
	Predictors				Predictors		
Overall patient experience	0.52 ***	0.47 ***	0.19 ***	Treatment services	0.57 ***	0.50 ***	0.28 ***
Nurse services	0.35 ***	0.18 ***	0.10 ***	Standard	0.20 ***	0.10 ***	0.00
Doctor services	0.07 ***	0.12 ***	0.10 ***	Next of kin	0.02	0.01	−0.07 ***
Information		0.09 ***					
Organization	0.19 ***	0.10 ***					
Next of kin			0.07 ***				
Standard	0.17 ***	0.08 ***					
Discharge		0.09 ***	0.13 **				

*** $p < 0.001$; ** $p < 0.01$; empty fields are not significant at 0.05 level; Treatment services—second order factor comprising nurse services, doctor services, information, and organization.

3.8. Proposed Measurement Model

A proposed model (Model 11) was developed, taking into consideration the frequencies of missing values for the items and the discriminant validity concerns. Items with missing values of more than 20% were excluded; therefore, the dimensions of "discharge" and "interaction" were removed from the model. The items on "next of kin" had more than 20% but the dimension was maintained. The questions were the following: "NK1: Were your relatives well received by the hospital staff?" and "NK2: Was it easy for your relatives to get information about you while you were in the hospital?" These questions were maintained because, unlike the other dimensions, relating and answering them depended on factors that are largely beyond the control of the patient, such as whether or not the patient had any relatives alive who visited the hospital and whether the patient stayed in the hospital long enough for relatives to visit the hospital. A second-order factor was added in the proposed model for "nurse services", "doctor services", "information", and "organization", collectively labelled "treatment services". This was based on the discriminant validity results, correlations among them, and the nature of the questions asked under these dimensions. The two lowest loading items (ORG 2 and ST 5) that were previously deleted were still excluded from this model. The proposed model showed excellent fitness to the data (similar to Model 10) and also met convergent, discriminant, and criterion-related validity requirements. See Figure 2 for the proposed model. Table 8 presents comparisons of tools and findings between the validation study by Pettersen et al. [8] and the current study.

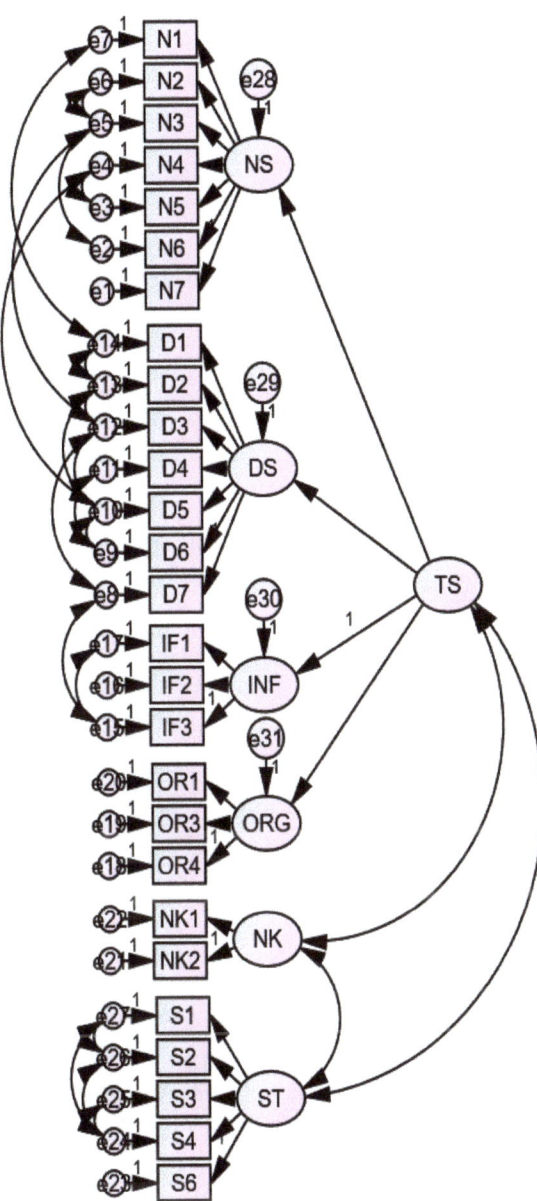

Figure 2. Proposed measurement model. Note: NS—nurse services; DS—doctor services; INF—information; ORG—organization; ST—standard; NK—next of kin; TS—treatment services (second-order factor).

Table 8. Tools and findings in the earlier validation study and the current study.

Study	Psychometric Tools Used	Findings
Pettersen et al. (2004)	Exploratory factor analysis Cronbach's alpha test Test-retest reliability Construct validity	10 factors (including general satisfaction) Confirmed Confirmed Achieved
Current study	Confirmatory factor analysis Model comparisons Measurement invariance Composite reliability test Convergent validity Discriminant validity Construct validity Criterion-related validity Second-order factor analysis	8 factors (excluding general satisfaction) Initial model was found to be best Configural and Metric achieved, Scalar not achieved Confirmed Confirmed for all except one factor Confirmed for all except three factors Achieved Achieved Achieved composite reliability, convergent validity, discriminant validity, construct validity and criterion related validity

4. Discussion

This study presents some major findings. First, the study confirmed that the eight-factor model showed good fitness to the data. The model achieved configural and metric invariance but not scalar invariance. The study also found that reliability values were all acceptable and all the dimensions, except "standard", attained the recommended 0.50 AVE value for convergent validity. With regard to discriminant validity, "doctor services" (in relation to "information"), "organization" (in relation to "doctor services", "nurse services", and "information") and "standard" (in relation to "organization") had issues. Construct validity and criterion-related validity were supported for majority of the results. One item each under "standard" and "organization" had the lowest loadings. Finally, a model including a second-order factor was proposed. The second-order factor, named "treatment services", consisted of four first-order factors: "nurse services", "doctor services", "information", and "organization". Moreover, the dimensions of "standard" and "next of kin" were included in this final model, but "discharge" and "interaction" were excluded. Hence, the final model included one second-order factor comprising four sub-factors as well as "standard" and "next of kin".

The dimensions with associated items found in this study were similar to those found by Pettersen et al. [8] while some dimensions, such as "doctor services", "nurse services", "organization", "information", and "hospital standards", overlapped with dimensions found by other studies [5,18,23]. Invariance tests conducted in the present study were absent in the study by Pettersen et al. [8], which marks a good contribution of this study. The tests showed that the model achieved invariance across the aggregated departments with regard to structure and pattern (configural) as well as the loadings of the items on their respective dimensions (metric). However, scalar invariance was not achieved for this model. Considering the diverse nature of the sample, as well as the aggregation of the departments into broad categories, this finding was expected. Putnick and Bornstein [37] asserted that scalar invariance is the most stringent compared with configural and metric, and instances of rigid scalar non-invariance could mean that the construct is generally variant across different groups. The findings also showed that reliability was good, based on composite reliability values, similar to the Cronbach's alpha values obtained by Pettersen et al. [8].

With regard to validity tests, the study found that all the dimensions, except "standard", attained the recommended 0.50 AVE value for convergent validity, similar to other related studies that examined similar dimensions using other instruments [4]. However, discriminant validity issues were found for "doctor services" (in relation to "information"), "organization" (in relation to "doctor services", "nurse services", and "information") and "standard" (in relation to "organization"). Discriminant validity was also missing in the study by Pettersen et al. [8], thus indicating another good contribution of this study. Examining the wordings of their items gives some possible explanation for this finding. For instance, D1 under "doctor services" was worded as "Did the doctors talk to you so you understood them?", while questions under "information" included "IF2. Did you know what you thought was necessary about the results of tests and examinations?" and "IF3. Did you receive sufficient information about your diagnosis or your complaints?" It is highly likely that patients will receive information on results and diagnosis mainly from their doctors and, as such, answering questions under "information" may be significantly influenced by the perception of how well the doctors spoke to these patients. Similarly, questions under "organization" were "OR1. Did you find that there was a permanent group of nursing staff that took care of you?", "OR2. Did you find that one doctor had the main responsibility for you?", "OR3. Did you find that the hospital's work was well organized?", and "OR4. Did you find that important information about you had come to the right person?" These questions feature clear wording relating to "nurse services", "doctor services", "information", and "standard", and it is therefore not surprising that no clear distinctions were found among them as constructs. Construct validity was also achieved with a majority of the items recording loadings of above 0.60. This was also achieved in the validation study by Pettersen et al. [8] using a different method and in related studies using other instruments with similar dimensions [5,18]. One item on "standard" and one on "organization" were, however, deleted due to loadings below 0.60, while another on "standard" was deleted in a bid to improve the discriminant validity. Perhaps the wording of these questions made them difficult for patients to understand clearly and respond accordingly. For instance, item S5 was framed as "Was the food satisfactory?" Patients may be left to decide what is meant by "satisfactory", thus making the question too vague, or perhaps the different dietary requirements and preferences made this question more loosely defined. Again, item OR2 was framed as "Did you find that one doctor had the main responsibility for you?", a question probably dependent on the ailments of the patient and likely to be out of the control of hospital organization. Thus, if a patient's ailments require more than a single main doctor, then this question may suggest to the patient that having two or more main doctors reduces the ability of the hospitals to organize their work well. Criterion-related validity was ascertained for the overall measure as well as the dimensions in predicting at least one of the three outcome variables: satisfaction, health benefits, and health level, which is consistent with previous studies [2,38–40].

Lastly, a model with a second-order factor, "treatment services", for four of the dimensions was proposed based on the results of the validity and reliability analyses: "nurse services", "doctor services", "information", and "organization". This constitutes the most important contribution of this study since this possibility was not explored in the study by Pettersen et al. [8], perhaps owing to the absence of discriminant validity examinations in their study, and since this indicates a change in the factor structure of the PEQ. Rindskopf and Rose [41] observed that second-order factors reflect relationships among first-order factors. It is worth noting that related studies that developed other PREMs for generic and specific health issues also found these four dimensions in common [5,17,23]. Although these studies did not develop a second-order factor for these dimensions, this is indicative of the prominence of these four variables in measuring and understanding patient experiences. The current finding, therefore, builds on this prominence to illustrate the high interrelationships and inextricable links among these factors, which brings some theoretical and practical implications to the fore.

4.1. Theoretical Implications

This study brings a very important, yet mostly ignored, contribution to the patient experience and quality healthcare literature: a need for more validation studies and surveys on patient experiences. The study responds to the recommendation by Pettersen et al. [8] that existing PREMs require scrutiny and also tackles the research gap identified in the matrix by Beattie et al. [19], indicating that the PEQ by Pettersen et al. [8] lacked some validity analyses. This buttresses the claim that, indeed, changing statistical methods and tools can reveal weaknesses of measures; moreover, this should be countered by regular psychometric appraisals of these measures. The results also contribute to the views of some researchers [20,21], regarding the need to repeat patient experience surveys to generate more reliable data for policy-making. The assessment of patients' perspectives of hospital care would have to be reliable and valid enough in order to elicit accurate information about their experiences, constructs, and outcomes. Thus, it is imperative to ensure that these instruments always perform optimally and generate reliable information on how to improve quality of care and hospital experiences. These results, therefore, provide a background for further studies to be conducted on PREMs.

Another major contribution of this study is the finding of a second-order factor labelled "treatment services", which consists of four factors: "nurse services", "doctor services", "information", and "organization". This means that there exist strong and significant relationships among these dimensions [41]. This finding also means that a single dimension or factor could adequately account for all four dimensions and could be identified as a major sub-dimension that captures these four dimensions. The "treatment services" factor has implications for the conceptualization of patient-oriented hospital service climates. Patients in these hospitals may have highly overlapping experiences across "nurse services", "doctor services", "organization", and "information". In more specific terms, it can be said that these patients experience a main dimension that accounts for significant portions of the four dimensions, perhaps because of the way these factors play out in the hospitals. For instance, doctors provide information regarding patients' health, ailments, and treatments while nurses organize and assist patients with the treatment process. This is significant in advancing knowledge of patient experiences. The experience of these four dimensions may not be that distinct, and patients, in experiencing service climate in the hospitals, may not adequately distinguish their shared perceptions of "doctor services" from "information" or of "nurse services" from "organization", for instance. The climate in the hospitals during healthcare delivery may thus be experienced and perceived by patients as having two levels of factors. This contribution is also a major highlight when compared with the study by Pettersen et al. [8], in which discriminant validity was not examined and a resulting second-order factor analysis was not explored. This challenges the theoretical structure of the PEQ and theoretical distinctness among these factors. Therefore, this study suggests a change in the factor structure of the PEQ and the development of a second-order factor for these four dimensions in the general patient experience literature. These possibilities are worth exploring in further surveys and studies on hospital factors as patient experiences during the caregiving process.

4.2. Practical Implications

Quality healthcare delivery is not exclusive to a region or country but a general goal of all healthcare systems worldwide. This can be contributed to by generating accurate information on how healthcare users experience healthcare systems. The results from this study suggest that it is not enough to develop a good measure of patient experiences, but it is imperative to review and reassess the ability of the measure to keep generating accurate information on patients' experiences and health. The questions in the PEQ may have to be revised in order to elicit more concise and accurate information from patients. Furthermore, some dimensions, such as "next of kin", seemed not to be relatable to most of the patients, judging from the many missing values and invariance tests. In addition, the PEQ should be administered with the second-order factor taken into consideration. It is imperative to analyse "nurse services", "doctor services", "information", and "organization" as a second-order factor, as shown in the proposed model, due to the validity issues that were realized in the analysis. This can provide researchers and management with adequate knowledge on what patients experience during the caregiving process. Moreover, management must take the interrelationships in the second-order factor into account to make meaningful, informed, and sustainable changes in the hospitals for patients. The second-order factor must be considered as a single factor encompassing these four dimensions, where patients' perceptions and interactions with a dimension have a ripple effect on the others. Such considerations in policies and practice can help management and workers to reduce errors that may have dire consequences.

4.3. Limitations and Directions for Future Research

This study employs data that is not at the national level but from a health region in Norway. That notwithstanding, the study has good generalizability power owing to the similarity in hospital and healthcare systems across the regions in Norway. Generalizing to other countries, however, is difficult due to the differences in culture and healthcare systems. The findings require additional research in different countries for further justification. Therefore, future studies on reassessing psychometric properties of PREMs may want to employ larger data sets, for instance at the national level or across regions, to further investigate and develop the measurement quality of such surveys. Furthermore, future research should adopt the proposed model (with the second-order factor) from this study and examine it empirically to confirm it or otherwise, within health sectors across different countries. It is also worth noting that only nurses' and doctors' services were assessed but not the services of other healthcare professionals in hospitals. Future research on developing and improving PREMs should therefore incorporate questions that assess the experience of services of other professionals.

5. Conclusions

Hospital management should know and consider the views and experiences of the people they care for if their services are to be influential in improving patients' health. The results of this study show that changes in psychometric analytical tools and methods can indeed highlight possible weaknesses and inadequacies in measures, as seen with the PEQ. This is evident in analyses such as invariance, discriminant validity, and second-order factors conducted in the current study but absent in the earlier study. Therefore, repeated surveys with refined and further developed questionnaires are needed to hopefully improve the performance of the measures. The results also indicate possible changes with regard to dimensionality of PREMs, owing to the second-order factor finding. This calls for adequate attention, from researchers and hospital management alike, to the interrelationships among some of the dimensions, as this has important implications for theory and practice in healthcare. Management should consider these relationships in making decisions concerning the quality of care for patients, while researchers should delve more into studies that ascertain the psychometrics and dimensionality of PREMs.

Supplementary Materials: The following are available online at https://www.mdpi.com/1660-4601/18/13/7141/s1, Table S1. Metric invariance across department aggregates; Table S2. Scalar invariance across department aggregates.

Author Contributions: Conceptualization, S.A.A., E.O., and R.J.M.; methodology, S.A.A. and E.O.; formal analysis, S.A.A.; investigation, S.A.A.; data curation, E.O. and S.A.A.; writing—original draft preparation, S.A.A.; writing—review and editing, E.O. and R.J.M.; supervision, E.O. and R.J.M. All authors have read and agreed to the published version of the manuscript.

Funding: This research received no external funding.

Institutional Review Board Statement: This study, with regard to data collection, analysis, and compilation, was conducted within the ethical and legal provisions and guidelines of the Norwegian Institute for Public Health (NIPH) and the University of Stavanger. The Norwegian Data Protection Authority and the Norwegian Directorate of Health approved the procedures in the survey. The hospital data protection official assessed the data processing in the hospitals where survey extension took place.

Informed Consent Statement: Informed consent was obtained from all subjects involved in the study.

Data Availability Statement: The data presented in this study are available on request from the corresponding author. The data are not publicly available due to an ongoing research project.

Acknowledgments: This study used anonymous data from the Norwegian Institute of Public Health. The interpretation and reporting of the data are the responsibility of the authors. We thank Ingeborg Strømseng Sjetne for preparing the data for this study and for her useful comments and suggestions.

Conflicts of Interest: The authors declare no conflict of interest.

References

1. Joober, H.; Chouinard, M.-C.; King, J.; Lambert, M.; Hudon, É.; Hudon, C. The patient experience of integrated care scale: A validation study among patients with chronic conditions seen in primary care. *Int. J. Integr. Care.* **2018**, *18*, 1–8. [CrossRef] [PubMed]
2. Bjertnaes, O.A.; Sjetne, I.S.; Iversen, H.H. Overall patient satisfaction with hospitals: Effects of patient-reported experiences and fulfilment of expectations. *BMJ Qual. Saf.* **2012**, *21*, 39–46. [CrossRef] [PubMed]
3. Pitter, J.G.; Csanádi, M.; Szigeti, A.; Lukács, G.; Kovács, Á.; Moizs, M.; Repa, I.; Zemplényi, A.; Thomas Czypionka, T.; Kraus, M.; et al. Planning, implementation and operation of a personalized patient management system for subjects with first suspect of cancer (OnkoNetwork): System description based on a qualitative study. *BMC Health Serv. Res.* **2019**, *19*, 131. [CrossRef]
4. Garratt, A.M.; Bjærtnes Ø, A.; Krogstad, U.; Gulbrandsen, P. The OutPatient Experiences Questionnaire (OPEQ): Data quality, reliability, and validity in patients attending 52 Norwegian hospitals. *BMJ Qual. Saf.* **2005**, *14*, 433–437. [CrossRef]
5. Iversen, H.H.; Holmboe, O.; Bjertnæs, Ø.A. The Cancer Patient Experiences Questionnaire (CPEQ): Reliability and construct validity following a national survey to assess hospital cancer care from the patient perspective. *BMJ Open* **2012**, *2*, e001437. [CrossRef]
6. Jenkinson, C.; Coulter, A.; Bruster, S. The Picker Patient Experience Questionnaire: Development and validation using data from in-patient surveys in five countries. *Int. J. Qual. Health Care* **2002**, *14*, 353–358. [CrossRef] [PubMed]
7. Oltedal, S.; Garratt, A.; Bjertnæs, Ø.; Bjørnsdottir, M.; Freil, M.; Sachs, M. The NORPEQ patient experiences questionnaire: Data quality, internal consistency and validity following a Norwegian inpatient survey. *Scand. J. Public Health* **2007**, *35*, 540–547. [CrossRef]
8. Pettersen, K.I.; Veenstra, M.; Guldvog, B.; Kolstad, A. The Patient Experiences Questionnaire: Development, validity and reliability. *Int. J. Qual. Health Care.* **2004**, *16*, 453–463. [CrossRef]
9. Wolf, C.; Jason, A. Defining patient experience. *Patient Exp. J.* **2014**, *1*, 7–19.
10. Wagland, R.; Recio-Saucedo, A.; Simon, M.; Bracher, M.; Hunt, K.; Foster, C.; Downing, A.; Glaser, A.; Corner, J. Development and testing of a text-mining approach to analyse patients' comments on their experiences of colorectal cancer care. *BMJ Qual. Saf.* **2016**, *25*, 604–614. [CrossRef] [PubMed]
11. Donabedian, A. The quality of care: How can it be assessed? *Jama* **1988**, *260*, 1743–1748. [CrossRef]
12. Glickman, S.W.; Baggett, K.A.; Krubert, C.G.; Peterson, E.D.; Schulman, K.A. Promoting quality: The health-care organization from a management perspective. *Int. J. Qual. Health Care* **2007**, *19*, 341–348. [CrossRef]
13. Lawson, E.F.; Yazdany, J. Healthcare quality in systemic lupus erythematosus: Using Donabedian's conceptual framework to understand what we know. *Int. J. Clin. Rheumatol.* **2012**, *7*, 95. [CrossRef]
14. Netemeyer, R.G.; Bearden, W.O.; Sharma, S. *Scaling Procedures: Issues and Applications*; Sage Publications: Thousand Oaks, CA, USA, 2003.
15. DeVellis, R.F. *Scale Development: Theory and Applications*; Sage Publications: Thousand Oaks, CA, USA, 2016.
16. Bruyneel, L.; Tambuyzer, E.; Coeckelberghs, E.; De Wachter, D.; Sermeus, W.; De Ridder, D.; Ramaekers, D.; Weeghmans, I.; Vanhaecht, K. New Instrument to Measure Hospital Patient Experiences in Flanders. *Int. J. Environ. Res. Public Health* **2017**, *14*, 1319. [CrossRef] [PubMed]
17. Garratt, A.M.; Bjertnæs, Ø.A.; Barlinn, J. Parent experiences of paediatric care (PEPC) questionnaire: Reliability and validity following a national survey. *Acta Paediatrica* **2007**, *96*, 246–252. [CrossRef] [PubMed]
18. Garratt, A.M.; Danielsen, K.; Forland, O.; Hunskaar, S. The Patient Experiences Questionnaire for Out-of-Hours Care (PEQ-OHC): Data quality, reliability, and validity. *Scand. J. Prim. Health Care* **2010**, *28*, 95–101. [CrossRef] [PubMed]
19. Beattie, M.; Murphy, D.J.; Atherton, I.; Lauder, W. Instruments to measure patient experience of healthcare quality in hospitals: A systematic review. *Syst. Rev.* **2015**, *4*, 97. [CrossRef] [PubMed]
20. Haugum, M.; Danielsen, K.; Iversen, H.H.; Bjertnaes, O. The use of data from national and other large-scale user experience surveys in local quality work: A systematic review. *Int. J. Qual. Health Care* **2014**, *26*, 592–605. [CrossRef] [PubMed]
21. Manary, M.P.; Boulding, W.; Staelin, R.; Glickman, S.W. The patient experience and health outcomes. *N. Engl. J. Med.* **2013**, *368*, 201–203. [CrossRef]
22. Garratt, A.; Danielsen, K.; Bjertnaes, Ø.; Ruud, T. PIPEQ—A method for measurement of user satisfaction in mental health services. *Tidsskr. Den Nor. Laegeforening Tidsskr. Prakt. Med. Ny Raekke* **2006**, *126*, 1478–1480.
23. Sjetne, I.S.; Bjertnaes, O.A.; Olsen, R.V.; Iversen, H.H.; Bukholm, G. The Generic Short Patient Experiences Questionnaire (GS-PEQ): Identification of core items from a survey in Norway. *BMC Health Serv. Res.* **2011**, *11*, 88. [CrossRef]

24. Ahern, M.; Dean, C.M.; Dear, B.F.; Willcock, S.M.; Hush, J.M. The experiences and needs of people seeking primary care for low-back pain in Australia. *Pain Rep.* **2019**, *4*, e756. [CrossRef]
25. Bjertnaes, O.; Deilkås, E.T.; Skudal, K.E.; Iversen, H.H.; Bjerkan, A.M. The association between patient-reported incidents in hospitals and estimated rates of patient harm. *Int. J. Qual. Health Care* **2014**, *27*, 26–30. [CrossRef]
26. Bjorngaard, J.H.; Garratt, A.; Grawe, R.W.; Bjertnaes, Ø.A.; Ruud, T. Patient experiences with treatment in private practice compared with public mental health services. *Scand. J. Psychol.* **2008**, *49*, 385–392. [CrossRef] [PubMed]
27. Hinsley, K.; Kelly, P.J.; Davis, E. Experiences of patient-centred care in alcohol and other drug treatment settings: A qualitative study to inform design of a patient-reported experience measure. *Drug Alcohol Rev.* **2019**, *38*, 664–673. [CrossRef] [PubMed]
28. Hair, J.; Black, W.; Babin, B.; Anderson, R.; Tatham, R. *Multivariate Data Analysis*, 6th ed.; Pearson Prentice Hall: Hoboken, NJ, USA, 2006.
29. Schreiber, J.B.; Nora, A.; Stage, F.K.; Barlow, E.A.; King, J. Reporting structural equation modeling and confirmatory factor analysis results: A review. *J. Educ. Res.* **2006**, *99*, 323–338. [CrossRef]
30. Hu Lt Bentler, P.M. Cutoff criteria for fit indexes in covariance structure analysis: Conventional criteria versus new alternatives. *Struct. Equ. Modeling A Multidiscip. J.* **1999**, *6*, 1–55.
31. Hair, J.F., Jr.; Sarstedt, M.; Hopkins, L.; Kuppelwieser, V.G. Partial least squares structural equation modeling (PLS-SEM). *Eur. Bus. Rev.* **2014**, *26*, 106–121. [CrossRef]
32. Fornell, C.; Larcker, D.F. Evaluating structural equation models with unobservable variables and measurement error. *J. Mark. Res.* **1981**, *18*, 39–50. [CrossRef]
33. Tabachnick, B.G.; Fidell, L.S. *Using Multivariate Statistics*; Cal Harper Collins: Northridge, CA, USA, 1996.
34. Vandenberg, R.J.; Lance, C.E. A review and synthesis of the measurement invariance literature: Suggestions, practices, and recommendations for organizational research. *Organ. Res. Methods* **2000**, *3*, 4–70. [CrossRef]
35. MacKenzie, S.B.; Podsakoff, P.M.; Podsakoff, N.P. Construct measurement and validation procedures in MIS and behavioral research: Integrating new and existing techniques. *MIS Q.* **2011**, *35*, 293–334. [CrossRef]
36. Gaskin, J.; Lim, J. Master Validity Tool. *AMOS Plugin Gaskination's StatWiki*. 2016. Available online: http://statwiki.kolobkreations.com (accessed on 20 May 2017).
37. Putnick, D.L.; Bornstein, M.H. Measurement invariance conventions and reporting: The state of the art and future directions for psychological research. *Dev. Rev.* **2016**, *41*, 71–90. [CrossRef] [PubMed]
38. Blazquez, R.A.; Ferrandiz, E.F.; Caballero, V.G.; Corchon, S.; Juarez-Vela, R. Women's satisfaction with maternity care during preterm birth. *Birth* **2019**, *46*, 670–677. [CrossRef] [PubMed]
39. Taylor, F.; Halter, M.; Drennan, V.M. Understanding patients' satisfaction with physician assistant/associate encounters through communication experiences: A qualitative study in acute hospitals in England. *BMC Health Serv. Res.* **2019**, *19*, 603. [CrossRef]
40. Lapin, B.R.; Honomichl, R.; Thompson, N.; Rose, S.; Abelson, A.; Deal, C.; Katzan, I.L. Patient-reported experience with patient-reported outcome measures in adult patients seen in rheumatology clinics. *Qual. Life Res.* **2021**, *30*, 1073–1082. [CrossRef] [PubMed]
41. Rindskopf, D.; Rose, T. Some theory and applications of confirmatory second-order factor analysis. *Multivar. Behav. Res.* **1988**, *23*, 51–67. [CrossRef]

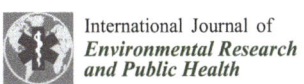

Article

Assessing Patient Experience and Attitude: BSC-PATIENT Development, Translation, and Psychometric Evaluation—A Cross-Sectional Study

Faten Amer [1,2,*], Sahar Hammoud [1], David Onchonga [1], Abdulsalam Alkaiyat [3], Abdulnaser Nour [4], Dóra Endrei [2] and Imre Boncz [2,5]

1 Doctoral School of Health Sciences, Faculty of Health Sciences, University of Pécs, H-7621 Pécs, Hungary; hammoud.sahar@etk.pte.hu (S.H.); onchonga.david@etk.pte.hu (D.O.)
2 Institute for Health Insurance, Faculty of Health Sciences, University of Pécs, H-7621 Pécs, Hungary; endrei.dora@pte.hu (D.E.); imre.boncz@etk.pte.hu (I.B.)
3 Division of Public Health, Faculty of Medicine and Health Sciences, An Najah National University, Nablus P.O. Box 7, Palestine; abdulsalam.alkaiyat@unibas.ch
4 Faculty of Economics and Social Sciences, An Najah National University, Nablus P.O. Box 7, Palestine; a.nour@najah.edu
5 National Laboratory for Human Reproduction, University of Pécs, H-7621 Pécs, Hungary
* Correspondence: amer.faten@etk.pte.hu

Abstract: Health care organizations (HCO) did not consider engaging patients in balanced scorecard (BSC) implementations to evaluate their performance. This paper aims to develop an instrument to engage patients in assessing BSC perspectives (BSC-PATIENT) and customize it for Palestinian hospitals. Two panels of experts participated in the item generation of BSC-PATIENT. Translation was performed based on guidelines. Pretesting was performed for 30 patients at one hospital. Then, 1000 patients were recruited at 14 hospitals between January and October 2021. Construct validity was tested through exploratory factor analysis (EFA) and confirmatory factor analysis (CFA). Additionally, the composite reliability (CR), interitem correlation (IIC), and corrected item total correlation (CITC) were assessed to find redundant and low correlated items. As a result, the scales had a highly adequate model fit in the EFA and CFA. The final best fit model in CFA comprised ten constructs with 36 items. In conclusion, BSC-PATIENT is the first self-administered questionnaire specifically developed to engage patients in BSC and will allow future researchers to evaluate the impact of patient experience on attitudes toward BSC perspectives, as well as to compare the differences based on patient and hospital characteristics.

Keywords: balanced scorecard; patient engagement; satisfaction; hospital; performance evaluation; quality

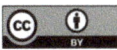

1. Introduction

1.1. Health Care System in Palestine

The performance of health care services is adversely affected by long waiting times, inefficiency, low productivity, burnt-out medical staff, and dissatisfied patients [1]. In addition to these universal challenges, the health care system in Palestinian territories has also been slapped by political and economic conflicts. Therefore, it is described to be incoherent and inadequate [2,3]. The 87 hospitals in Palestinian territories have five major types based on administrative type: 28 public, 39 nongovernmental organizations (NGOs), 17 private, two military, and one United Nations Relief and Works Agency for Palestine Refugees in the Near East (UNRWA) [4]. Military hospitals are not yet operating in West Bank. The bed percentage per administrative type is approximately 59% public, 26% NGO, 14% private, and 1% UNRWA [5]. These hospitals are distributed as seven in eastern Jerusalem, 53 in West Bank, and 30 in Gaza [6]. The geographic separation with the disrupted mobility between these territories, added to the blockade of the Gaza strip, the checkpoints in West Bank and Jerusalem, the separate de facto government health systems in Gaza and West Bank, the heavy reliance on external health financing, and the dependence on direct household expenditures imposed further challenges on improving the Palestinian health care system [2,7–9]. The spread of Corona virus-19 (COVID-19) has added an additional challenge. A recent study [10] referred to the COVID-19 era in conjunction with political conflict to have a double epidemic effect on Palestinian territories, which eventually impacted the Palestinian health system and health care organizations (HCO) performance during the pandemic.

1.2. History of Balanced Scorecard (BSC)

In 1992, Norton and Kaplan proposed the initial design of the balanced scorecard (BSC), which incorporated four perspectives: financial, customer, internal process, and knowledge and growth [11]. In some previous implementations of the BSC, the last perspective was also termed the learning, innovation, technology and development perspective [12].

The first generation of BSCs contained only the four perspectives steered by the organizational strategy. Figure 1 depicts the first generation of BSCs. In the second generation, researchers demonstrated the existence of causal links between the key performance indicators (KPIs) of these four perspectives [13]. These connections were referred to as BSC's strategic map. See Figure 2. The third generation, which incorporated objectives and action plans for each KPI, was then introduced.

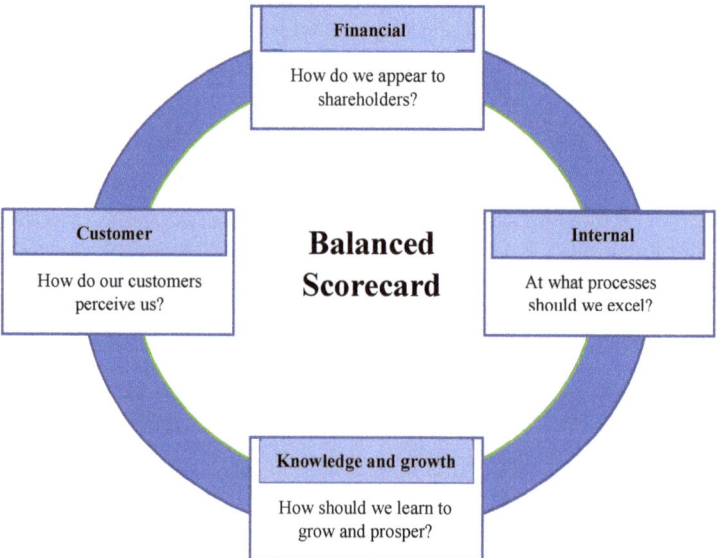

Figure 1. Balanced Scorecard perspectives [11].

The environmental and social perspective of sustainability was later added as the fifth pillar of BSC [14]. However, our recent systematic review of BSC implementations in the health care sector revealed that the management perspective should also be incorporated in BSC design. In this review, the 797 KPIs were reduced into 45 subdimensions after classification and regrouping. The reassembly of these subdimensions yielded 13 major dimensions:

Financial, efficiency and effectiveness, availability and quality of supplies and services, managerial tasks, health care workers' (HCWs) scientific development being error-free and safe, time, HCW-centeredness, patient-centeredness, technology, and information systems, community care and reputation, HCO building, and communication. See Figure 3.

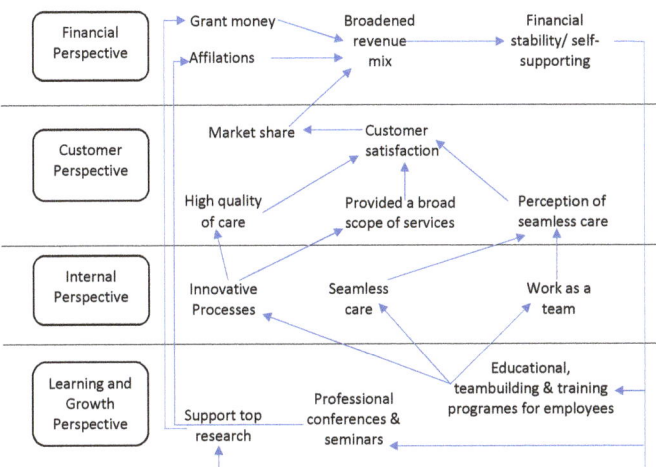

Figure 2. Duke University Health System Strategic Map [15].

We summarize the perspectives, major dimensions, and subdimensions that were more frequently used and deemed essential by health care managers worldwide.

1.3. The Impact of BSC

Two reviews focused on studying the effect of BSC, one of which analyzed the impact qualitatively [16] and the other presented a few instances of the positive influence [17]. This showed that no complete or rigorous scientific methodology has been reported until 2022 to evaluate the effect of BSC adoption in HCO. Given the lack of research on this topic, we performed a systematic review in which we assessed the impact of implementing the BSC on three attributes that represent the latest affected perspectives in the strategic maps [17,18]: HCWs' satisfaction, patient satisfaction, and financial performance. As a result, BSC implementation proved to positively improve the financial performance of HCOs [19]. Furthermore, we found that BSC was beneficial in enhancing the patient satisfaction rate. Additionally, BSC influenced the health care workers' (HCW) satisfaction rate, but to a lesser extent [19]. Despite the fact that BSC has a beneficial influence on patient satisfaction, prior implementations of BSC have solely focused on measuring patient satisfaction. One implementation at HCO in Afghanistan [20] created the community scorecard (CSC) to include the community in the assessment of the BSC. However, none of the studies included patients in the process of evaluating BSC [12,19,21]. Involvement of patients in this process could result in even higher levels of patient satisfaction. In addition, it will assist HCO managers and researchers in better understanding the BSC strategic maps as well as the causal links between KPIs based on the perceptions of patients.

In contrast to other performance evaluation (PE) tools, which primarily focus on analyzing the internal perspective, the BSC is regarded as a comprehensive approach for PE, as it involves the analysis of six perspectives [12]. For that, BSC implementations utilized different sources to conduct the PE of HCOs [12,19], including hospital records, patient satisfaction questionnaires, patient and HCW interviews, and observations. Additionally, BSC reviews [12,19] showed that only a few BSC implementations utilized validated scales to evaluate patient satisfaction, such as the Press Ganey questionnaires [22,23]. The patient satisfaction perspective is important since patients represent the hospitals' end receivers of health care services. However, researchers have pointed to the importance of the engagement of patients (EoP) in the process of health policy planning, evaluation, and delivery improvement [24,25]. Additionally, patient feedback was proven to positively impact performance in HCO [14]. Strategies to support EoPs include patient needs assessment, communication skills improvement, managing patient conflicts and complaints, maintaining patient confidentiality, patient training, and asking patients to review outputs by assessing their perceptions and experiences [25,26]. It is not sufficient to perform the PE of HCO based on manager and hospital records only; a focus on EoP among the selection of the KPIs at HCO was recommended [24]. However, BSC reviews referred to the lack of patient and family member involvement in the evaluation process of BSC [12,19,21,27].

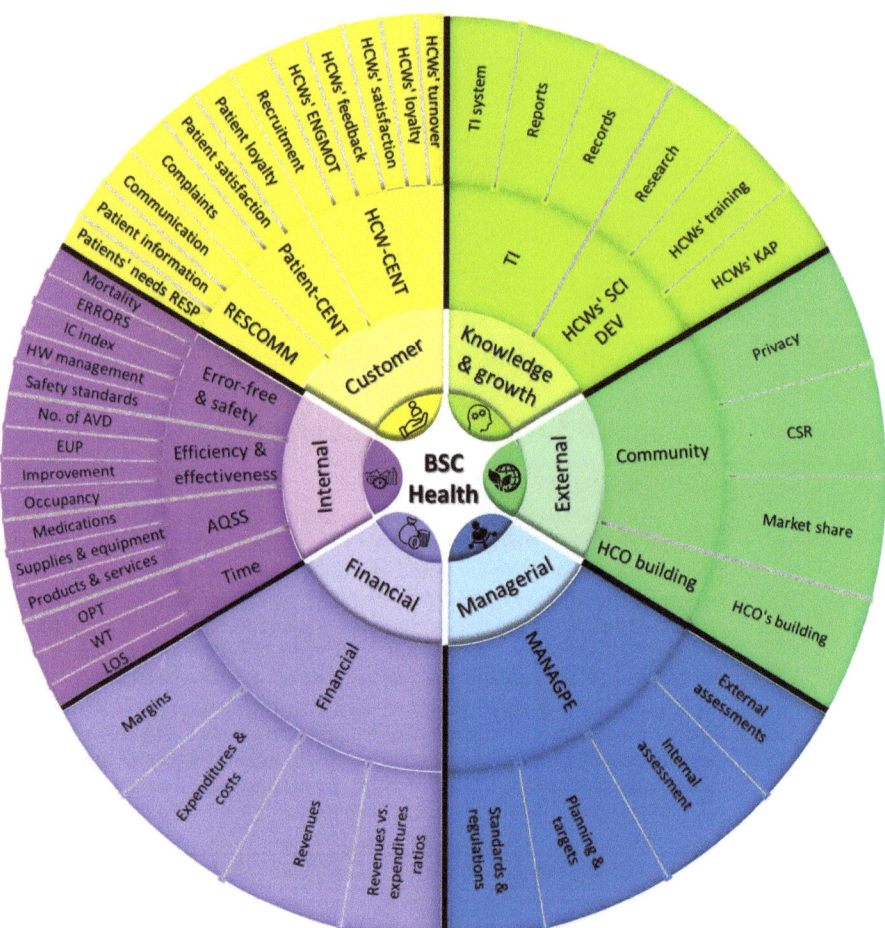

Figure 3. A summary of BSC perspectives in health care and their contents [12]. Figure legend: Summary of BSC perspectives and the underlying major and minor subdimensions for the PE of HCOs. Note: BSC, balanced scorecard; HCWs, health care workers; HCO, health care organization; IC, infection control; HW, health waste; WT, waiting time; LOS, length of stay; KAP knowledge, attitude, and practices; TI, technology and information; CSR, corporate social responsibility; ERRORS, errors, accidents, and complications; No. of AVD, number of admissions, visits, and diseases; EUP, efficiency, utilization, and productivity; AQSS, availability and quality of supplies and services; OPT, operation processing time; RESCOMM, response to patients' needs; Patient-CENT, patient-centeredness; ENGMOT, HCWs' engagement and motivation; HCW-CENT, HCW-centeredness; MANAGPE, managerial tasks and performance evaluation; SCIDEV, scientific development.

The first aim of this research was to develop a comprehensive instrument (BSC-PATIENT) that is able to assess: 1. patient experiences in light of BSC perspectives, 2. patient PI regarding BSC perspectives, and 3. patient satisfaction and loyalty attitude.

The second aim of this research was to customize the developed instrument at Palestinian hospitals, translate it into Arabic, and validate it.

2. The Conceptual Framework

In our conceptual model we considered the impact of BSC six perspectives which resulted at our previous systematic review and their underlying dimensions [12]. We also built it based on the psychological definitions of experiences and attitudes [28,29] and the previous literature regarding patient attitudes [28,30–33]. Experiences and perceptions enable people to act in a particular behavior and develop an image, satisfaction, or loyalty attitude [29]. Figure 4 represents our conceptual model.

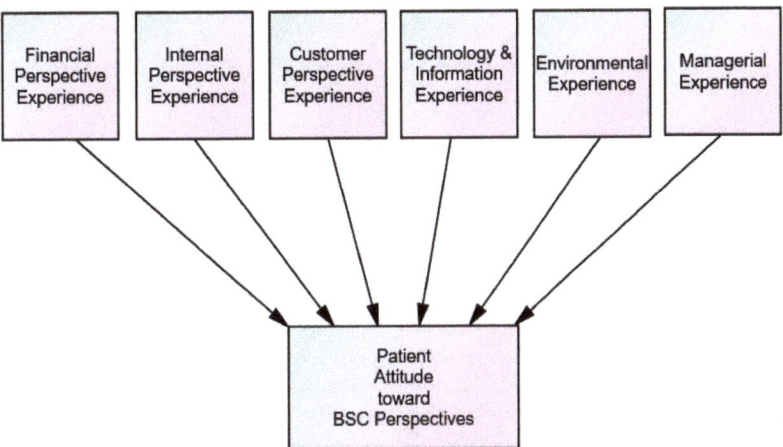

Figure 4. BSC-PATIENT conceptual model.

2.1. The Experience

Experience is defined as an event that was lived through [29]. Patient experiences at HCO are formed upon receiving the health care service or treatment. Becoming aware of the events, objects, or relationships utilizing senses or observation results in experience perceptions [29].

2.2. Attitudes

Attitudes form directly as a result of experiences. There are three types of attitudes, which are sometimes referred to as ABCs of attitude. First, the affective component is how the object, person, issue, or event makes someone feel. The behavioral component is how attitude influences someone's behavior. The cognitive component is someone's thoughts and beliefs about the subject. An example of attitude is image perception, satisfaction, and loyalty. Such evaluations are often positive or negative, but they can sometimes also be uncertain [28].

2.2.1. Patient Satisfaction Attitude

Satisfaction is the most commonly used metric by managers to assess customer perceptions [30]. Satisfaction does not always lead to loyalty. However, loyalty often begins with a sense of satisfaction [31]. Studies have found that patient satisfaction either plays a direct impact on loyalty attitudes or acts as a moderating variable between service quality and loyalty attitudes [32].

2.2.2. Brand Preference Attitude

Brand preference is the degree to which consumers prefer a specific brand relative to competing alternatives. It is considered an essential component of customer loyalty [30].

2.2.3. Perceived Quality (PQ) Attitude

Studies have proven that PQ exerts an indirect influence on patient loyalty. A rival hypothesis referred to satisfaction as a mediator between PQ and loyalty [32].

2.2.4. Perceived Image (PI) Attitude

A hospital PI was defined as the sum of beliefs, ideas, and impressions that a patient holds toward a particular hospital [34]. Patients usually form a PI of a hospital from their own past treatment experiences relative to the PIs of competing hospitals [33]. A positive PI of a bank was found to significantly improve the PQ. Therefore, in health care, a positive hospital PI may positively influence PQ. However, a recent review showed that this has not yet been studied [33].

2.2.5. Loyalty Attitude

A loyalty attitude is a behavioral intention that reflects faithfulness and allegiance to something [29]. In the marketing management field, Kotler and Keller (2015) defined loyalty as a deeply held commitment to rebuy or repatronize a preferred product or service in the future, despite influences to cause switching behavior [35]. A study revealed a need to use multiple indicators to predict customer loyalty behavior, such as customer satisfaction, brand preference against competitors, intention to return or repurchase, and willingness to recommend [30]. Moreover, customer behavior trends in the past were a good predictor of future customer behavior. It is important to emphasize that loyalty refers to customers' actual conduct, regardless of their attitudes or preferences. However, assessing customer loyalty attitudes can help predict their loyalty behavior in the future [36].

Repurchase Intention Attitude

Researchers have used repurchase intentions to help predict future purchasing behavioral intentions and loyalty [30]. On the other hand, customer retention behavior is defined as customers stating the actual continuation of a relationship with the organization. It is well known in marketing that past customer behavior tends to be a relatively good predictor of future customer behavior. However, most researchers focus on assessing repurchase intention attitudes and neglect assessing actual customer retention behavior [30].

Willingness to Recommend an Attitude

Word-of-mouth intention has been of importance to researchers in the past 30 years. Thus far, there is very little scientific research relating the intention of the recommendation to the actual recommendations [30].

3. Methods

3.1. Research Design

This is part of a broad project that aims to strategically develop Palestinian hospitals using BSC. This research is a cross-sectional study. The questionnaire was created and validated based on the key authors Kaplan and Norton's theortical framework [11] and the best practices for developing and validating health and behavioral scales [37].

3.2. Item Generation

The first panel consists of five authors in this research. Two researchers in health management (first and fourth), two hospital managers who are also expert researchers in health management (sixth and seventh), and one expert in the BSC tool (fifth) provided expert input on all stages of instrument development. First, we performed a systematic review [12], in which 797 KPIs were extracted from 36 BSC implementations at HCO worldwide. Then, categorization and regrouping of these KPIs resulted in 45 subdimensions and 13 major dimensions that are frequently used by health care managers and are important for PE and the strategic development of HCO [12]. Next, this panel performed a four-round Delphi method [38]. In the first round, the panel prepared a survey for hospitals' top managers to rate the resulting 45 subdimensions on a 10-point semantic scale, based on their importance for the strategic development of their hospitals. A description for each subdimension using the shortlisted KPIs was included in the manager survey. In the second round, the panelists reviewed the item face validity per subdimension [39]. Next, the first author asked a second panel consisting of 13 top hospital managers from 4 Palestinian hospitals to answer this survey individually. Additionally, hospital managers were asked to mention whether they considered any other subdimension or KPI that was not listed as essential. The subdimensions with an average score above 0.7 were chosen for the next step based on their ratings. In the third round, the first panel reviewed the resulting important subdimensions at the previous step and decided which subdimensions the patients could be engaged in their evaluation. As a result, 24 subdimensions resulted. In the fourth round, the panelists revised each item wording and clarity to patients. As a result, 52 items remained. In the fourth round, the panelists rated the relevance and importance for each remaining item based on four- and three-point ordinal scales, respectively [40]. Next, the first author calculated the content validity ratio (CVR), the item content validity index (I-CVI), the scale content validity index (S-CVI), and universal agreement among experts for the content validity index (CVI-UA) to assess the content validity per item and scale [40]. Only the items rated 0.99 or above in CVR were included as per Lawshe guidelines [41]. However, dimensions that scored 0.80–0.99 indicated the need to be revised. For the CVI, items that scored less than 0.60 were eliminated. Items that scored 0.6–0.79 were revised [40]. See Figure 5.

The panelists suggested using a three-point Likert scale: yes, neutral (I do not know), and no. This choice was due to the high number of the remaining items, the evidence of a high nonresponse rate of patients to the five-point Likert scale-validated tools [42–45], and the possibility for assessing item availability using yes/no questions. Additionally, this was found to lead to a faster and better item response, specifically considering the pandemic load on hospitals. All authors were asked to revise the instrument, and the final modifications were made accordingly.

3.3. Linguistic Validation and Translation

BSC KPI, balanced scorecard key performance indicators; CVI, content validity index; CVR, content validity ratio; CR, composite reliability; IIC, interitem correlation; CITC, corrected item-total correlation.

Since the dimensions resulting from the systematic review were in English, the questionnaire items were initially developed in English. Then, they were translated to Arabic. All translations were prepared as per the translation and validation guidelines [46]. The first author performed a final review to produce the final corrected translation. An expert checked the final form in the BSC, and minor modifications were recommended.

3.4. Pretest and Internal Consistency

The first version of the questionnaire was piloted in one NGO hospital in the south of West Bank. For that, 30 patients were asked to answer the first version of the questionnaire. They were asked to write their comments regarding language simplicity. The time needed to complete the questionnaire was also recorded. Items were coded before performing the analysis by IBM SPSS statistics 21 software. Then, Cronbach's alpha was calculated for each perspective to evaluate the internal consistency [47], and values above 0.6 were considered acceptable. Based on the results, some items were modified or deleted.

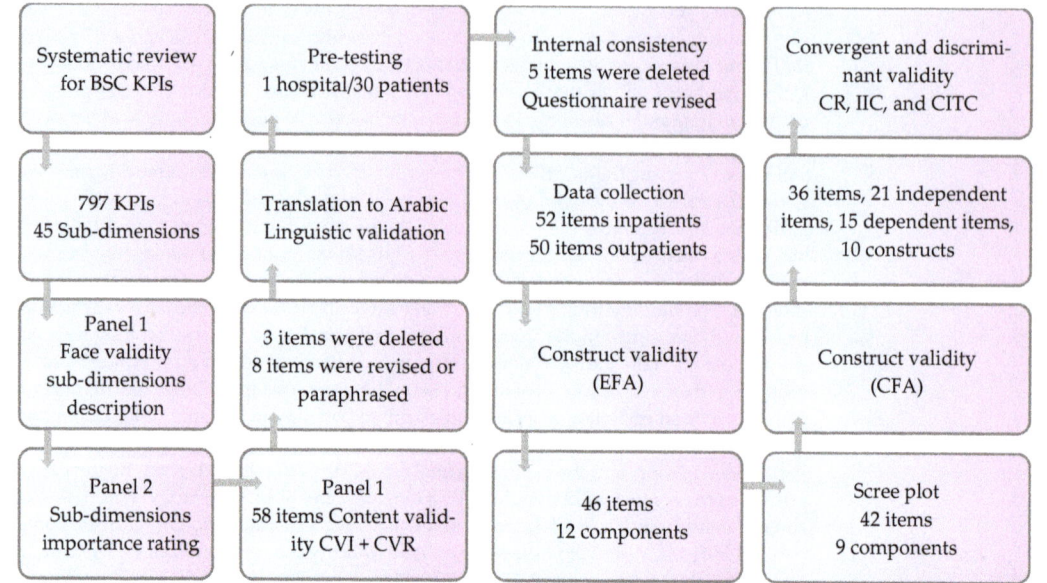

Figure 5. Flow chart for BSC-PATIENT development and psychometric validation.

3.5. Sampling Procedure and Power Calculation

Institutional Review Board (IRB) approval for this research was received on 31 May 2020. All methods described in this study were approved by the Research and Ethics Committee at the Faculty of Medicine and Health Sciences at An Najah National University with the reference code number (Mas, May/20/16). Afterward, requests at 15 hospitals in West Bank and three hospitals in Jerusalem were applied between June and December 2020. The hospitals were selected using a convenience sample. However, the total number of beds per administrative type and governorate was considered for choosing the participants (HCO and patients). Public hospital approval was first applied to the Palestinian Ministry of Health. Then, the request was applied to each hospital individually for all hospital types. The final form of the questionnaire was distributed between January and October 2021. The sample size was calculated according to the Steven K. Thompson sample size equation [48]:

$$n = \frac{N \times p(1-p)}{[N - 1 \times (d^2 \div z^2)] + p(1-p)}$$

where n is the sample size, N is the population size, p is the estimated variability in the population (0.5), d is the margin of error (0.05), and the z score is at the 95% confidence interval (1.96). In our study, N was the population volume in the Palestinian territories [4]. Therefore, the needed sample size was found to be $n = 385$ patients. Additionally, studies considered 300 participants as a good sample size to successfully run each exploratory factor analysis (EFA) and confirmatory factor analysis (CFA) or 5 respondents per parameter [49–51]. Splitting the sample to perform EFA and CFA is recommended to perform construct validity [52]. Therefore, a total of 1000 questionnaires were distributed, anticipating a lower response rate during the pandemic.

3.6. Data Collection and Participants

The first author and four medical students at An-Najah University collected the data. Each medical student received three hours of training on BSC and the data collection steps and ethics by the first author. Tasks and hospitals were delegated to them according to their living area: eastern Jerusalem and north, middle, and south of West Bank. The Gaza Strip was excluded due to the political situation and accessibility obstacles during the study. Moreover, five hospitals were excluded: two military hospitals that were not operating yet, one psychiatric hospital, and two rehabilitation hospitals. We sought variation in our sample regarding hospital size, area, and administrative type. For that, the maximum variation sampling strategy was used. The number of hospitals and the number of beds per administrative type were considered upon recruiting the sample [4]. The patients were conveniently chosen based on their willingness to participate in this research.

Printed questionnaires were distributed to respondents instead of sending the questionnaires via email to reduce nonresponse bias [53]. Additionally, all participants were asked to agree on participation in a consent form that is coherent with the Declaration of Helsinki ethical principles [54]. Patients were informed that participation was confidential. Additionally, all patients were informed that participation was voluntary, so they could refuse participation in the study or withdraw at any time. To reduce the response bias [53], the "I don't know (neutral)" answer was added as an option, since experiences and attitudes can sometimes be uncertain [28]. Second, the data collectors ensured that the number of missing answers was minimized by checking the questionnaires upon retrieval. In case of missing parts, they drew the participant's attention to answer them. When entering data, if any questions were found to be still missing, they were entered as I don't know.

The inclusion and exclusion criteria were set to be a Palestinian patient above 15 years old of any gender. Outpatients should have finished receiving medical care at the assessed hospital or had received medical care at least once previously and returned to the same hospital. Inpatients should have been admitted for at least one day. The following departments were included: emergency room, internal medicine, surgery, gynecology, and pediatrics. In the emergency department, the questionnaires were completed by the patient companions. Additionally, in the pediatric department, the questionnaires were completed by one parent of the child. For the rest, questionnaires were completed by patients themselves; unless they were unable to complete the questionnaire, the questionnaires were read to them by the data collector or a family member and completed according to patient answers. To distinguish, a question was added to ask the respondent if his responses were based on his own, family, or friends' experiences.

3.7. Statistical Analysis

Normality was tested using the Shapiro–Wilk test. The frequencies were used to analyze patient sociodemographics and the participating HCO characteristics. Our sample was split based on admission status to assess construct validity using EFA and CFA. EFA was performed for the inpatient sample using principal axis factoring with the Promax rotation method [55] in IBM SPSS statistics 21 software. The Kaiser–Meyer–Olkin (KMO) and Bartlett's sphericity tests were tested to determine the adequacy of the EFA [56]. The inclusion or exclusion of a component was determined by an eigenvalue ≥ 1 [57] and the visual assessment of Cattell's scree plot [58]. Item inclusion or exclusion was determined by a factor loading ≥ 0.50 and factor loadings on the assigned construct higher than all cross-loading of other constructs [50].

Second, CFA was performed for the components that resulted in EFA using the outpatient sample. The maximum likelihood estimation method in IBM Amos 23 Graphics software (IBM, Wexford, PA, USA) was applied. The goodness of fit for the competing models was evaluated through the most commonly used fit indices. Minimum discrepancies were divided by degrees of freedom less than five and closer to zero, p value higher than 0.05, goodness-of-fit index (GFI), comparative fit index (CFI), Tucker–Lewis's index (TLI), and cutoff values close to 0.95. Additionally, a root mean square error of approximation (RMSEA) <0.06 and standardized root mean square residual (SRMR) value <0.08 are needed before we can conclude that there is a relatively good fit between the hypothesized model and the observed data [59,60]. Item inclusion or exclusion in CFA was determined by a factor loading ≥ 0.50.

Third, the interitem correlation (IIC) and the corrected item-total correlation (CITC) were calculated [61]. In this study, items with a correlation higher than 0.9 were considered redundant and deleted [62]. A correlation of 0.3 was considered the lower limit. Additionally, the composite reliability (CR) per construct was evaluated after performing CFA. CR is preferred over Cronbach's alpha, specifically in structural equation modeling [63]. In the current study, a CR $\geq$ 0.6 was considered sufficient [64,65].

Finally, the Fornell-Lacker criterion was used to evaluate convergent and discriminant/divergent validities [66]. The average variance extracted (AVE) was considered adequate for convergent validity if it was higher than 0.5. However, if a value <0.5 with CR > 0.6, the convergent validity of the construct was still considered adequate [66]. To establish discriminant validity, the square root of the AVE (SQRT) should have a greater value than the correlations with other latent constructs [64]. Additionally, construct uniqueness was evaluated depending on the value of Spearman correlation (r) with other constructs at the same scale. Researchers recommended the separation of dependent and independent variables since the correlation between them can be misleading in assessing discriminant validity [67]. Therefore, we assessed r for the independent and dependent constructs separately. Then, r was described as negligible when r < 0.2, low (r = 0.2–0.49), moderate (r = 0.5–0.69), high (r = 0.7–0.85), or very high (r = 0.86–1.00). In this study, the absence of high or very high r between the subscale constructs indicated discriminant validity [68].

4. Results

4.1. Item Generation and Scoring

The demographics and characteristics of the second-panel hospital managers are shown in Table 1. The content validity resulted in removing one item and indicated that a revision is needed for eight items. The revised items required either further clarification and rewording or modification for specific participants. For example, the CVR results indicated that financial and price items should not be included for nonprofit hospitals. Additionally, the CVI results showed that particular items were relevant only to inpatients. This step raised the S-CVI, CVI-UA, and CVR from 0.90, 0.63, and 0.95 to 0.95, 0.78, and 0.97, respectively.

Table 1. Sociodemographic and characteristics of the second panel (executive managers).

Sociodemographic Characteristic		Panelists N	%	Sociodemographic Characteristic		Panelists N	%
Age				Position			
	30–39 years	4	30.7		CMO	3	23.1
	40–49 years	7	53.8		CFO	3	23.1
	60–69 years	2	15.4		CEO	3	23.1
Gender					Managing director	3	23.1
	Male	7	53.8		Operation manager	1	7.7
	Female	6	46.2	Highest degree			
Academic background					Bachelor degree	8	61.5
	Medicine	4	30.8		Master's degree	5	38.5
	Management	4	30.8	Administrative type			
	Accounting	3	23.1		Private	4	30.8
	Accounting and management	2	15.4		NGO	4	30.8
Years of experience					Public	5	38.5
	5–10 years	1	7.6				
	More than 10 years	12	92.3				

CMO, chief medical officer; CFO, chief financial officer; CEO, chief executive officer, NGO, nongovernmental organization.

4.2. The Instrument's Structure and Items

The patient sociodemographics and hospital characteristics section included age, gender, scientific degree, working sector, insurance availability, and type. Moreover, the number of visits to the evaluated hospital compares the attitudes of the new and previous customers. The number of earlier visits is considered necessary in the analysis since past customer behavior tends to be a good predictor of future behavior [19]. Moreover, the information source on which the respondent evaluation was built was recorded since perceptions and attitudes may emerge from direct personal experience or from observing other people's experiences, such as family and friends' experiences [20]. The second section of the questionnaire was designed to measure patient experiences in light of BSC perspectives and their attitudes toward them, including patient satisfaction, PQ, PI, and loyalty.

4.2.1. The Financial Perspective

It evaluated the health services and medication's price affordability. This section was answered only by patients who did not have insurance.

4.2.2. The Internal Perspective

This perspective assessed safety, time, and service availability. On the other hand, the PI of the cure rate, accuracy, complications, and PQ of services and medication were measured in the attitude section.

4.2.3. The Knowledge and growth Perspective

Information and training provided to patients were assessed in the experience section. Additionally, we assessed the PI of hospital technology and employee competencies in the attitude section.

4.2.4. The Customer Perspective

It assessed patient-centeredness and the HCW–patient communication experience. The attitude section assessed actual patient satisfaction and loyalty attitudes. In previous studies, validated items for loyalty measurement included satisfaction measurement and loyalty attitude measurement, specifically the recommendation and return intentions [30,33]. Using a single item to directly assess actual patient satisfaction was suggested to be better than its assessment through multidimensional items [69].

4.2.5. The Environmental Perspective

It evaluated the hospital building environment and hospital capacity, ease of access, and female concern experiences. On the other hand, a comparison with the other hospitals' medical and social PIs was included in the attitude section.

Finally, four items were reversed in the instrument, PIN9, which assessed the long waiting time. Additionally, PIN4, PIN5, and PIN6 assessed readmission, referral to other hospitals, and postoperative infection probability expectations, respectively.

4.2.6. The Managerial Perspective

As there is no direct contact experience between patients and hospitals' managers, we evaluated the hospital administrative type and the accreditation status in this perspective. So, we can study the impact of these factors on patient attitudes.

4.3. The Pretest and the Internal Consistency

The pretest was performed at one NGO hospital in the south of West Bank. Patients found the length of the questionnaire appropriate. Additionally, the layout was well accepted and clear. They gave specific minor comments that were incorporated. These corresponded to the rewording of a few items. The time for completing the questionnaire was less than 10 min.

Consequently, few modifications were made after piloting. Cronbach's alpha was calculated per BSC perspective. All perspectives had a Cronbach's alpha above 0.7 at the pretest, except for the environmental perspective, which was 0.59. Hence, some of its items were moved to other perspectives, and five items were deleted. As a result, 52 and 50 items remained for inpatients and outpatients, respectively.

4.4. Linguistic Validation and Translation

The final English and Arabic questionnaire forms were ready for use.

4.5. Sample Size and Characteristics

Since the research coincided during the COVID-19 pandemic, hospital approvals took six to nine months until they were received. Only 15 hospitals out of 18 agreed to participate. The UNRWA, The United Nations Relief and Works Agency for Palestine Refugees in the Near East; NGO, Non-Governmental Organization.

Data collection was performed between January and September 2021. The data from the pretest at one hospital were excluded. Next, we distributed 1000 questionnaires at the remaining 14 hospitals. As a result, 740 were returned (response rate was 74%). The characteristics and sociodemographics of the respondents are shown in Tables 2 and 3.

Table 2. Characteristics and sociodemographics of respondents (patients).

		Number of Patients (N = 740)	%			Number of Patients (N = 740)	%
Age (years)	Less than 20	63	8.5	Income (NIS)	Less than 1000	195	26.4
	20–29	209	28.2		1000–2000	98	13.2
	30–39	208	28.1		2001–3000	152	20.5
	40–49	159	21.5		3001–4000	140	18.9
	50–59	71	9.6		More than 4000	155	20.9
	60–69	24	3.2	Insurance type [#]	Public	492	66.5
	More than 70	6	0.8		Private	143	19.3
Gender	Females	325	43.9		UNRWA	63	8.5
	Males	415	56.1		No insurance	109	14.7
Highest degree	Elementary	85	11.5	Number of the current visit	First	227	30.7
	Secondary	217	29.3		Second	187	25.3
	Bachelor	366	49.5		Third	91	12.3
	Masters	63	8.5		Fourth	54	7.3
	PhD	9	1.2		Fifth	181	24.5
Working sector	Public	175	23.6	Admission status	Inpatients	350	47.3
	Private	183	24.7		Outpatients	390	52.7
	Free lancer	156	21.1	Respondent opinion is based on [#]	Personal experience	570	77
	Retired	17	2.3		Family experience	306	41.4
	Unemployed	209	28.2		Friends experience	96	13

NIS, New Israeli Shekel; UNRWA, The United Nations Relief and Works Agency for Palestine Refugees in the Near East; NGO, Non-Governmental Organization; [#], multiple response question.

Table 3. Number of patients and hospitals based on hospital characteristics.

		Number of Patients (N = 740)	%	Number of Hospitals (N = 14)	%
Administrative Type	Public	252	34.1	5	36
	NGO	277	37.4	5	36
	private	159	21.5	3	21
	UNRWA	52	7	1	7
City	Hebron	150	20.3	3	21
	Jerusalem	86	11.6	1	7
	Nablus	249	33.6	5	36
	Qalqilya	52	7	1	7
	Ramallah	151	20.4	3	21
	Tulkarm	52	7	1	7
Area	North	353	47.7	7	50
	Middle	237	32	4	29
	South	150	20.3	3	21

Table 3. Cont.

		Number of Patients (N = 740)	%	Number of Hospitals (N = 14)	%
Accredited hospital	Yes	185	25	3	21
	No	555	75	11	79
Size	Small (No. of beds <80)	241	32.6	5	36
	Medium (No. of beds 80–160)	261	35.3	5	36
	Large (No. of beds >160)	238	32.2	4	29

4.6. Statistical Analysis

The statistical analysis using the Shapiro–Wilk test showed that the data were not normally distributed, so nonparametric tests were used. Then, construct validation was assessed for the instrument.

4.6.1. Construct Validity in EFA

EFA resulted in 46 items with loadings higher than 0.50 for 16 components. Eigenvalues for all components were higher than one. The KMO was 0.813, reflecting a very high sampling adequacy [56,64], and Bartlett's test was also significant. The cumulative variance was 67.414%. See Table 4. The 12 components were patient attitude toward BSC perspectives (BSCP ATT), patient experience (PT EXR), service experience (SERV EXR), price experience (PR EXR), building experience (BUIL EXR), access experience (ACC EXR), complication perceived image (COMP IMAGE), technology experience (TECH EXR), information experience (INFO EXR), hospital social responsibility perceived image (HSRP IMAGE), and waiting time experience (WT EXR). One item (SAT2) loaded on the 12th component.

Table 4. Exploratory factor analysis (EFA).

Component	Item	Item Code	Component/Item Loadings											
			1	2	3	4	5	6	7	8	9	10	11	12
BSCP ATT	I will recommend this hospital to my family and friends.	SAT3	0.894											
	I believe I receive an accurate medical examination at this hospital.	PIN1	0.783											
	I will choose this hospital again when I need a medical consultation.	PEN2	0.754											
	I believe this hospital offers me better treatment than the other Palestinian hospitals.	PEN3	0.686											
	My overall satisfaction with this hospital's performance is high.	SAT1	0.683											
	I believe this hospital has a high cure rate.	PEN1	0.651											
	I will choose this hospital again when I need a medical consultation.	SAT2	0.579											
	I believe the staff at this hospital are competent, knowledgeable, updated, and skilled.	PLE1	0.537											
PT EXR	This hospital distributes surveys to assess my satisfaction before discharge.	PCU4		0.968										
	This hospital distributes surveys to assess my needs upon arrival to the hospital, admission, or during the stay.	PCU3		0.755										
	Separate male/female waiting area are available at this hospital.	PEN9		0.655										
	This hospital follows up with me after the discharge.	PLE11		0.645										
	My complaints are taken seriously into consideration and solved immediately at this hospital.	PCU5		0.601										
	I can book an online or a phone appointment at this hospital easily.	PLE7		0.586										
	Staff trained me on infection precaution measures such as hand hygiene, cough etiquette, isolation rational, personal protective equipment, etc.	PLE6		0.560									0.556	

Table 4. Cont.

Component	Item	Item Code	Component/Item Loadings											
			1	2	3	4	5	6	7	8	9	10	11	12
SERV EXR	Female doctors are available at this hospital.	PEN8			0.625									
	There are a variety of departments at this hospital.	PIN12			0.616									
	Services at night, vacations, and weekends are available at this hospital.	PIN18			0.556									
	There are a variety of specialties at this hospital.	PIN15			0.540									
PR EXR	I pay a reasonable price for the other medical services (laboratory, radiology, etc.) at this hospital.	PFI2				0.959								
	I pay a reasonable price for the medications at this hospital.	PFI3				0.888								
	I pay a reasonable price for the medical consultation at this hospital.	PFI1				0.848								
BUIL EXR	There is a sufficient number of chairs in the waiting area.	PEN13					0.639							
	The hospital has clean departments, corridors, rooms, bathrooms.	PEN12					0.585							
	The capacity of departments at this hospital including (ER, ICU, waiting room, etc.) is sufficient enough.	PEN14					0.562							
	This hospital has new building infrastructure (walls, ceiling, bathrooms, etc.).	PEN11					0.519							
ACC EXR	The accessibility to this hospital is easy by either public transportation or my car.	PEN4						0.910						
	The accessibility to this hospital in an emergency is easy.	PEN5						0.907						
COMP IMAGE	There is a probability for postoperative bacterial infection at this hospital	PIN6							0.765					
	There is a probability for case referral to another hospital	PIN5							0.752					
	There is a probability for case readmission at the same hospital	PIN4							0.602					
TECH IMAGE	This hospital use technology to link my prescriptions and tests with pharmacy and labs.	PLE9								0.842				
	This hospital use technology for saving my records.	PLE10								0.564				
INFO EXR	Information provided to me to be used after discharge is sufficient (medication and side effects, health condition, etc.).	PLE4									0.708			

Table 4. Cont.

Component	Item	Item Code	Component/Item Loadings											
			1	2	3	4	5	6	7	8	9	10	11	12
HSRP IMAGE	I believe this hospital offers social and volunteering activities to the community.	PEN7										0.601		
	I believe this hospital offers exemptions for poor patients.	PEN6										0.566		
WT EXR	I wait for a long time before receiving the medical service at this hospital.	PIN9											0.556	
	Percentage of Variance (%) Total variance = 63.29%		27.46	5.81	5.02	3.71	3.40	3.24	2.79	2.70	2.48	2.37	2.22	2.09
	Eigenvalues		14.28	3.02	2.61	1.93	1.78	1.69	1.45	1.40	1.29	1.23	1.16	1.10

Note: BSCP ATT, patient attitude toward balanced scorecard perspectives; PT EXR, patient experience; SERV EXR, services experience; PR EXR, price experience; BUIL EXR, building experience; ACC EXR, access experience; COMP IMAGE, complications perceived image; TECH IMAGE, technology perceived image; INFO EXR, information experience; HSRP IMAGE, hospital social responsibility perceived image; WT EXR, waiting time experience.

However, this item had a higher loading on the BSCP ATT. None of the specific inpatient items had loadings higher than 0.50. Moreover, the scree plot showed the necessity of deleting the last three components.

4.6.2. Construct Validity in CFA

The resulting nine components in EFA were tested in the Amos program. The model was edited based on the item loadings, model fit indices, and calculations in the convergent, discriminant, CR, IIC, and CITC at the next step until we arrived at the best model. First, adding two items that did not have loadings to the INFO EXR construct showed good loadings in CFA. The same was true for the BSCP ATT and TECH IMAGE constructs. Second, splitting the BUIL EXR component into two separate constructs, building environment experience (BUILENV EXR), and building capacity experience (BUILCAP EXR), improved the item loadings and the model fit. Third, PEN9 and PLE7 items were removed from the PT EXR construct because they have loadings lower than 0.50. On the other hand, PIN 14 and PIN 16 were added to BSCP ATT construct since both had loadings higher than 0.50 and improved the model fit. Moreover, merging the TECH IMAGE and COMP IMAGE items at the BSCP ATT construct resulted in loadings lower than 0.5 and IIC lower than 0.30. Hence, three separate constructs in the attitude section were decided. Finally, the modification indices in the Amos program were utilized to improve the model. The final model revealed that the CMIN/df, CFI, GFI, TLI, RMSEA, and SRMR indices in CFA were above or close to the cutoff points, reflecting a good fit model. Nevertheless, the p value was <0.001, which can be referred to as its sensitivity to normality. See Figure 6 and Table 5. To see the items which did not load in EFA, the items which were tested in CFA, and the final resulted items, refer to the Appendix A.

Table 5. Goodness-of-fit indices in EFA and CFA and results.

EFA [50,57]		CFA [70]	
Criteria for Good Fit [56,64]	Measurements	Criteria for Good Fit	Measurements
-KMO: 0.6: low adequacy 0.7: medium adequacy 0.8: high adequacy 0.9: very high adequacy -Bartlett's test p value < 0.05 -Inclusion/exclusion criteria for the components: 1. Eigenvalues ≥ 1 2. Visual assessment of Cattell's scree plot. -Inclusion/exclusion criteria for the items: 1- The factor loading ≥ 0.50. 2- Factor loadings on the assigned construct ≥ all cross-loading of other constructs.	-KMO = 0.901 (Chi square = 9052.693, degrees of freedom = 1326) -Bartlett's test p value < 0.001 -12 components which have Eigenvalues above 1 -Cumulative variance = 63.29%	- $\chi^2/df < 5$ and closer to zero - The p value > 0.05 - GFI - CFI - TLI - GFI, CFI, and TLI close to 0.95 - RMSEA < 0.06 - SRMR ≤ 0.08	$\chi^2/df = 1.58$ p value < 0.001 GFI = 0.901 CFI = 0.953 TLI = 0.944 RMSEA = 0.039 SRMR = 0.0439

Note: EFA, exploratory factor analysis; CFA, confirmatory factor analysis; KMO, Kaiser–Meyer–Olkin; χ^2/df, minimum discrepancy divided by its degrees of freedom; GFI, goodness-of-fit index; CFI, comparative fit index; TLI, Tucker–Lewis's Index; RMSEA, root mean square error of approximation; SRMR, standardized root mean square residual.

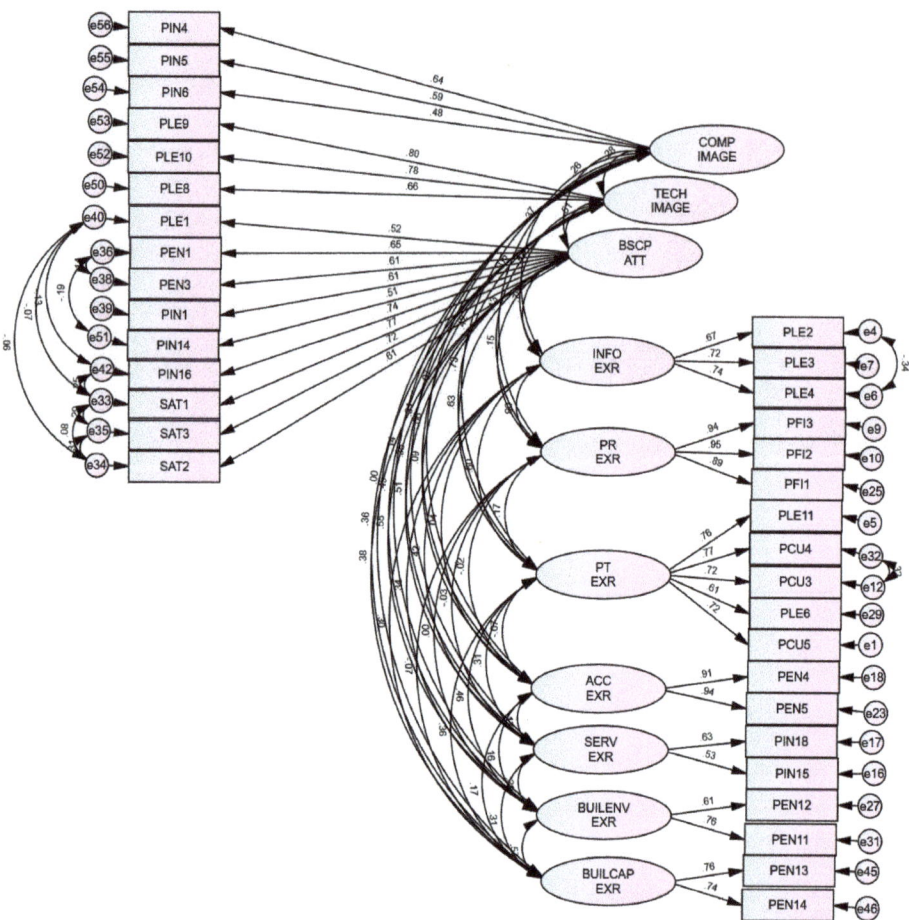

Figure 6. Confirmatory factor analysis (CFA). Independent items on the right side and dependent items on the left side. Note: COMP IMAGE, complications perceived image; TECH IMAGE, technology perceived image; BSCP ATT, patient attitude toward balanced scorecard perspectives; INFO EXR, information experience; PR EXR, price experience; PT EXR, patient experience; ACC EXR, access experience; SERV EXR, services experience; BUILENV EXR, building environment experience; BUILCAP EXR, building capacity experience.

4.6.3. Composite Reliability and Interitem Correlations

The composite reliabilities for all constructs were higher than 0.6 except the SERV EXR construct. However, this construct's IIC and CTIC were higher than 0.3. The other constructs also had IICs higher than 0.3, and their CITC ranged from 0.328–0.853, reflecting satisfactory IIC and CITC. See Table 6.

Table 6. Constructs IIC, CTIC, and CR.

Construct	IIC (Min.–Max.)	CTIC (Min.–Max.)	CR	N of Items (Total = 34)
COMP IMAGE	0.395–0.411	0.474–0.486	0.664	3
TECH IMAGE	0.390–0.594	0.486–0.642	0.794	3
BSCP ATT	0.328–0.641	0.505–0.735	0.861	9

Table 6. Cont.

Construct	IIC (Min.–Max.)	CTIC (Min.–Max.)	CR	N of Items (Total = 34)
INFO EXR	0.389–0.531	0.501–0.609	0.750	3
PR EXR	0.509–0.725 >>	0.596–0.760 >>	0.948	3
PT EXR	0.413–0.678	0.552–0.736	0.841	5
ACC EXR	0.853	0.853	0.906	2
SERV EXR	0.360	0.360	0.502	2
BUILENV EXR	0.412	0.412	0.643	2
BUILCAP EXR	0.527	0.527	0.721	2

COMP IMAGE, complications perceived image; TECH IMAGE, technology perceived image; BSCP ATT, patient attitude toward balanced scorecard perspectives; INFO EXR, information experience; PR EXR, price experience; PT EXR, patient experience; ACC EXR, access experience; SERV EXR, services experience; BUILENV EXR, building environment experience; BUILCAP EXR, building capacity experience; IIC, inter-item correlation; CITC, corrected item total correlation; CR, composite reliability; >>, was calculated only for patients who pay at the evaluated hospitals.

4.6.4. Convergent and Discriminant Validity

Convergent validity was less than 0.5 for BSCP ATT, BUILENV EXR, PTCOMINF EXR, SERV EXR, and COMP_IMAGE. However, the CR, IIC, and CITC showed satisfactory results [66], except for the SERV EXR, which had a CR equal to 0.50 but an IIC and CITC higher than 0.3. On the other hand, the square roots of the AVE were higher than the off-diagonal correlations between constructs. Additionally, a lower correlation between constructs indicates each construct's uniqueness. The correlations between the independent constructs were either negligible or low, except between two constructs, the PT EXR and INFO EXR, which were moderate. Merging the two constructs lowered the loadings and the model fit indices in CFA. The same was perceived regarding merging the BUILENV EXR and BUILCAP EXR constructs. Consequently, separate constructs were determined, as mentioned earlier. In regard to the independent constructs, negligible or low correlations existed among them. Neither high nor very high correlations existed between the independent constructs. Therefore, this establishes discriminant validity and the uniqueness of the independent constructs. The same holds true for the dependent constructs. In other words, convergent validity was met for all constructs except SERV EXR. In comparison, discriminant validity was met for all constructs, as shown in Tables 7 and 8.

Table 7. Convergent, discriminant, and divergent validity for the independent constructs.

Construct	AVE	INFO EXR	PR EXR	PT EXR	ACC EXR	SERV EXR	BUILENV EXR	BUILCAP EXR
INFO EXR	0.501	**0.708**						
PR EXR	0.858	*0.084* *	**0.926**					
PT EXR	0.515	*0.507* **	*0.095* *	**0.718**				
ACC EXR	0.828	*0.121* **	*-0.005*	*0.053*	**0.910**			
SERV EXR	0.337	*0.341* **	*0.002*	*0.242* **	*0.164* **	**0.581**		
BUILENV EXR	0.477	*0.302* **	*-0.006*	*0.336* **	*0.110* **	*0.209* **	**0.691**	
BUILCAP EXR	0.564	*0.288* **	*0.016*	*0.366* **	*0.164* **	*0.238* **	*0.394* **	**0.751**

Note: PT EXR, patient experience; INFO EXR, information experience; PR EXR, price experience; COMM EXR, communication experience; ACC EXR, access experience; BUILCAP EXR, building capacity experience; TECH EXR, technology experience; DEPV EXR, departments variety experience; SERV EXR, services; WT EXR, waiting time experience; BUILENV EXR, building environment experience; AVE, average variance extracted calculated by the average square of loadings at each construct and used to evaluate the convergent validity; **Bold**, square roots of the average variance extracted; *Italic*, Spearman correlations between independent constructs. Both are used to evaluate discriminant validity; *, $p < 0.05$; **, $p < 0.01$.

Table 8. Convergent, discriminant, and divergent validity for the dependent constructs.

Construct	AVE	BSCP ATT	TECH IMAGE	COMP IMAGE
BSCP ATT	0.413	**0.643**		
TECH IMAGE	0.564	*0.397* **	**0.751**	
COMP IMAGE	0.400	*0.216* **	*0.156* **	**0.633**

COMP IMAGE, complications perceived image; TECH IMAGE, technology perceived image; BSCP ATT, patient attitude toward balanced scorecard perspectives; AVE, average variance extracted calculated by the average square of loadings at each construct and used to evaluate the convergent validity; **Bold**, square roots of the average variance extracted; *Italic*, Spearman correlations between independent constructs, both are used to evaluate discriminant validity; **, $p < 0.01$.

5. Discussion

5.1. Discussion of the Main Results

In agreement with this paper's aim, it was possible to build a valid and reliable instrument. BSC-PATIENT is the first validated instrument to engage patients in the evaluation of hospitals by measuring their experiences and attitudes toward the hospital based on the BSC perspectives: the financial, internal, knowledge and growth, customer, and environmental perspectives. The deployment of this instrument at BSC implementations and PEs in general will improve patient satisfaction and allow a better understanding of BSC strategic maps based on patients' experiences and attitudes.

Our findings showed that patient attitude toward all BSC perspectives and dimensions loaded on one construct, except the images of technology and complications, loaded separately.

The instrument was customized to be compatible with Palestinian hospitals. Statistics revealed that out-of-pocket household payments constituted 39.8% of the Palestinian territories' total health care expenditures in 2018 [71]. This number is close to the results in our sample, which showed that 14.73% of patients did not have any insurance, and 19.32% had private insurance. Additionally, our analysis shows that another 35.41% or 1.49% of our sample had public or UNRWA insurance, respectively, but were receiving treatment at an NGO or private hospital at the time of the study. This situation indicates that the patients either made out-of-pocket payments or that the government paid a medical referral to private or NGO hospitals [4]. Therefore, incorporating the financial perspective consideration in this paper proved to be vital. Additionally, many BSC implementations in Afghanistan and Bangladesh revealed the need to consider the social and cultural perspective in evaluation, specifically female attentiveness concerns [20,72–75]. The authors believed that this was also the case in Palestine, so the BSC-PATIENT included such items. However, in different cultures, this may not be important. Hence, these items can be removed or replaced with other customized environment-related items. Finally, the technology perspective varies among Palestinian hospitals. Even though the Ministry of Health Hospitals and many other private hospitals have adopted the health medical information system for years, some hospitals still use the manual system for documentation. The authors also considered this perspective important in this evaluation.

The causal relationships between BSC dimensions that were described in BSC strategic maps may impose a challenge on producing a good fit model, specifically discriminant validity. Despite this challenge, our model proved satisfactory construct, convergent, and discriminant validity. The composite reliability was higher than 0.6 for all constructs except the SERV EXR construct. This may indicate that a separate evaluation for this construct item is needed. Moreover, the IIC and the CITC were satisfactory. In general, this questionnaire proved reliable and valid for engaging patients in hospital evaluations by measuring their experiences and attitudes toward Palestinian hospitals.

5.2. Comparison with BSC Implementations

The review of the dimensions utilized in BSC implementations [12] revealed that 77 percent of the implementations did not engage patients at any point in the assessment process. Instead, they relied only on hospital records and reports to evaluate the BSC perspectives. Patients were included in the remaining 22 percent of BSC implementations [72,74–80] to analyze only the patient satisfaction perspective. Although 11% of BSC implementations [20,74,80] included community members in the BSC perspective evaluation, none of the BSC implementations engaged patients in this process. In addition, patient interviews were utilized in each of the 22 percent of BSC deployments, but patient surveys were never used. This highlights both the significance of the BSC-PATIENT development and the originality of the study being conducted.

5.3. Comparison with Other Validated Instruments

5.3.1. Service Quality Scale (SERVQUAL)

One of the most popular models to measure service quality is the 44-question SERVQUAL instrument [81]. However, SERVQUAL has been criticized for encountering various shortcomings [82,83]. First, numerous studies have questioned whether SERVQUAL is applicable as a generic scale for measuring service quality in all settings [82], as it was not initially designed for hospitals. In contrast, BSC-PATIENT was explicitly designed for hospitals. Second, the concept of "subtraction" in the SERVQUAL model is not equivalent to psychological function [82]. However, BSC-PATIENT was designed to be coherent with psychological definitions by distinguishing between experience observations and attitudes. Third, researchers uncovered some shortcomings of the discriminant validity at SERVQUAL [82]. They explained that reliability, responsiveness, assurance, and empathy dimensions were not distinct from each other and loaded into one factor in many studies due to the high degree of intercorrelation [82]. All BSC-PATIENT constructs passed discriminant validity. Fourth, SERVQUAL has been criticized for focusing on functional quality, not reputational quality [83]. This challenge was overcome in BSC-PATIENT through the separation of observations and attitudes.

5.3.2. Press Ganey

Another commonly used instrument is Press Ganey [84], a 21-question instrument explicitly developed to measure hospital patient experience. However, Press Ganey also has a few shortcomings. Many studies using this instrument reported evidence of nonresponse bias [42,43]. The response rate for BSC-PATIENT was 75% despite the COVID-19 situation. Many patients commented that the questionnaire was interesting to complete. This can also be referred to as the simplicity of the three-point scale, unlike the five- and seven-point Likert scales, which can contribute to greater respondent burden and fatigue and may lead to higher refusal rates [69]. Finally, building, services, technology, price experiences assessing items, and patient attitudes were not considered necessary in Press Ganey.

5.3.3. Hospital Consumer Assessment of Health Care Providers and Systems (HCAHPS)

The 29-question Hospital Consumer Assessment of Health Care Providers and Systems (HCAHPS) [85] is widely used in the United States of America (USA) to evaluate patient experiences. It incorporates eight dimensions. However, the response rate for this instrument was found to be low [44,45]. Additionally, accessibility, price, and technology experiences were neglected. Moreover, HCAHPS allows researchers to evaluate the overall patient satisfaction rate based on their subratings for different experience constructs, such as communication with HCW perception [44,45,86]. Although experience perceptions can predict patient attitudes, including satisfaction, a separate evaluation of experiences and satisfaction and a direct satisfaction assessment were recommended [69]. This point was taken into account when designing the BSC-PATIENT.

5.4. Strengths and Limitations

In general, this paper has several strengths. First, BSC-PATIENT is the first instrument that engages patients in BSC perspective assessment. Second, this instrument can determine patient attitudes, including PI toward BSC perspectives, PQ, and satisfaction and loyalty. Third, to our knowledge, this is the first paper to distinguish between patient experiences and patient attitudes, which will allow us to study the relationship between patient experiences and attitudes in future studies. Fourth, this instrument was customized to be used for all insurance, leadership, and admission statuses. Fifth, this instrument was designed based on KPIs extracted from BSC implementations in primary, secondary, and tertiary health care settings in low-, middle-, and high-income countries worldwide. Hence, the implementation of BSC-PATIENT can be generalized to different health care settings and countries. However, the instrument may need some customization based on the health care setting strategy and the country's properties. For example, we customized the BSC-PATIENT at the environmental perspective based on Palestinian culture, the financial perspective based on administrative type, the knowledge and growth perspective based on the health information system in Palestine, and the few items specific for inpatients based on admission status. Finally, this paper offers a comprehensive hospital assessment from patient perspectives during COVID-19. To date, no study has assessed Palestinian hospital performance during this era. However, this instrument has some limitations. Despite this instrument assessing items such as patient education on infection control measures, it lacks COVID-19-specific items, as this instrument was designed before the COVID pandemic, so COVID-19-related items can be considered in future versions of the BSC-PATIENT instrument. Second, patient literacy was not assessed. However, the academic qualifications were evaluated at the demographics to be considered in the analysis. Third, measuring patient experiences in the past may involve a bias of recall. Additionally, participant bias may have occurred since the sample was convenient and the included hospitals agreed on participation. However, the high percentage of the included hospitals (30%) from the total number of hospitals at West Bank, and including all administrative type types from all regions, may have reduced the selection bias. Another limitation is that we could not validate this instrument in English due to our inaccessibility to English-speaking patients. Future research needs to consider testing the psychometric properties of BSC-PATIENT in an English-speaking country.

5.5. Practical Implications

Researchers and HCO managers are advised to utilize the BSC-PATIENT instrument in future BSC implementations. First, HCO managers will be able to highlight the strengths and weaknesses in BSC dimensions based on patients' perspectives. Second, analysis of the BSC strategic maps based on patients will allow managers to highlight the predictors of patient satisfaction and loyalty. Third, HCO managers will be able to distinguish between the patients' actual experiences and their attitudes. Analyzing the causal relationships between experiences and attitudes will provide insight for managers into which experiences should be improved to enhance patient attitudes. This will also guide managers in building their future action plans and how to allocate resources. Fourth, BSC-PATIENT can be utilized in the PE of HCO in general to evaluate a variety of dimensions instead of focusing only on patient satisfaction. The comprehensive analysis provided by this instrument will contribute to the health management field in general and will enhance patient satisfaction.

6. Conclusions

The BSC-PATIENT instrument was developed to engage patients in the PE of hospitals. This instrument was validated in Arabic and customized for Palestinian hospitals. This is the first instrument to engage patients in evaluating their experiences and attitudes toward the BSC perspective. It consists of 36 items; 21 items assessing patient experience observations and 15 items assessing patient attitudes. Both experiences and attitudes were designed based on BSC perspectives. The findings of this research showed adequacy in the psychometric properties of this instrument and suggest some recommendations for future research. First, we tested the psychometric properties of the BSC-PATIENT in English and other languages in different countries. Second, we consider developing instrumental BSC perspectives to engage other stakeholders in the PE of hospitals, such as doctors, nurses, and managers. Third, this instrument was used to assess the impact of patient experience on patient attitudes toward the hospital, specifically the PI, PQ, and satisfaction and loyalty. Fourth, managers must consider using a comprehensive approach for the PE of hospitals instead of limiting it to financial or internal indicators. Fifth, we compared the differences in patient experience and attitudes based on patient and hospital characteristics. Finally, enhancing patient engagement in the evaluation process instead of focusing on satisfaction alone must be considered in future BSC and PE implementations. Involving stakeholders in BSC's comprehensive evaluation will lead to a better and deeper understanding of hospital PE.

Author Contributions: This paper's conception and design were planned by F.A., A.A., A.N., D.E. and I.B. Additionally, F.A. and A.A. were responsible for hospital approvals. F.A. was responsible for the data acquisition, statistical analysis, interpretation of data, and writing the final draft. A.A., A.N., D.E. and I.B. supervised this research. F.A., S.H., D.O., A.A., A.N., D.E. and I.B. substantially revised the final manuscript draft. F.A., S.H., D.O., A.A., A.N., D.E. and I.B. approved the submitted version (and any substantially modified version that involves the author's contribution to the study) and agreed to be personally accountable for the author's contributions, to ensure that the accuracy and integrity of any part of the work were appropriately investigated and resolved. All authors have read and agreed to the published version of the manuscript.

Funding: The research was financed by the Thematic Excellence Program 2021 Health Sub-programme of the Ministry for Innovation and Technology in Hungary, within the framework of the EGA-10 project of the University of Pécs. The research was financed by the National Laboratory for Human Reproduction as part of the "Establishment of National Laboratories 2020" program. Data collection expenses were personally funded by F.A.

Institutional Review Board Statement: The Institutional Review Board (IRB) was received from the Research and Ethics Committee at the Faculty of Medicine and Health Sciences at An-Najah National University with reference code number (Mas, May/20/16) on 31 May 2020. Additionally, approval was obtained from the Palestinian Ministry of Health and 15 hospitals individually. Informed consent was attached to the questionnaire for each patient, and they were asked to agree on participation. All methods were carried out in accordance with relevant guidelines and regulations.

Informed Consent Statement: Informed consent was obtained from all subjects involved in the study.

Data Availability Statement: The datasets generated and/or analyzed during the current study are not publicly available because the data are still not fully analyzed and the research is still in process but available from the corresponding author (F.A.) upon reasonable request, with the permission of the UNRWA, Palestinian Ministry of Health, and Al Makassed Hospital.

Acknowledgments: We would like to thank Saad Abuzahra, Yazan Al-Habil, Haroun Nairoukh, and Mofeeda Afifi for their contribution to the data collection and entry at the north, middle, and south of West Bank, and eastern Jerusalem, respectively. Additionally, we thank Duha Shellah for her contributions in revising this paper. Finally, we thank Bashar Farran for his effort in the translation of the questionnaire.

Conflicts of Interest: The authors declare no conflict of interest.

Appendix A

Table A1. Items with no loadings.

Code	Question
PIN16	The services provided to me at this hospital have high quality.>>
PCU1	The medical staff at this hospital speaks a simple language with me.
PEN10	The staff at this hospital protects and respect my privacy.
PIN19	The food offered to you at this hospital has high quality.

Table A1. *Cont.*

Question	Code
PCU2	The staff at this hospital are kind, deal with courtesy and respect, and have a good relationship with me and my family.
PIN17	The hospital staff can respond to my inquiries rapidly.
PLE8	I believe this hospital uses the newest technology and devices for diagnosing and treating patients. <<
PLE5	Patient counseling services are available at this hospital.
PIN14	I believe the medications prescribed to me at this hospital have good quality and efficacy. >>
PIN8	The doctors and nurses at this hospital spend sufficient time with me.
PIN7	The hospital staff applies safety standards (gloves, masks, hygiene, etc.).
PEN15	My room is calm and peaceful.
PIN13	The medications prescribed to me are available at the hospital's pharmacy.
PLE3	Oral and written information provided to me or my family during my hospital experience is sufficient. #
PLE2	Information and guidance provided at admission or the first visit are sufficient. #

Note: #, items were added to INFO EXR construct in CFA; >>, items added to BSCP ATT construct in CFA; <<, items were added to TECH IMAGE construct in CFA.

Table A2. Items tested in CFA.

Construct	Code	No.	Question
BSCP ATT	SAT3	Q1	I will recommend this hospital to my family and friends.
	PIN1	Q2	I believe I receive an accurate medical examination at this hospital.
	PEN2	Q3	I will choose this hospital again when I need a medical consultation.
	PEN3	Q4	I believe this hospital offers me better treatment than the other Palestinian hospitals.
	SAT1	Q5	My overall satisfaction with this hospital's performance is high.
	PEN1	Q6	I believe this hospital has a high cure rate.
	SAT2	Q7	I will choose this hospital again when I need a medical consultation.
	PLE1	Q8	I believe the staff at this hospital are competent, knowledgeable, updated, and skilled.
	PIN16	Q9	The services provided to me at this hospital have high quality.
	PIN14	Q10	I believe the medications prescribed to me at this hospital have good quality and efficacy.
PT EXR	PCU4	Q11	This hospital distributes surveys to assess my satisfaction before discharge.
	PCU3	Q12	This hospital distributes surveys to assess my needs upon arrival to the hospital, admission, or during the stay.
	PEN9	Q13	Separate male/female waiting area are available at this hospital.
	PLE11	Q14	This hospital follows up with me after the discharge.
	PCU5	Q15	My complaints are taken seriously into consideration and solved immediately at this hospital.
	PLE7	Q16	I can book an online or a phone appointment at this hospital easily.
	PLE6	Q17	Staff trained me on infection precaution measures such as hand hygiene, cough etiquette, isolation rational, personal protective equipment, etc.
SERV EXR	PEN8	Q18	Female doctors are available at this hospital.
	PIN12	Q19	There are a variety of departments at this hospital.
	PIN18	Q20	Services at night, vacations, and weekends are available at this hospital.
	PIN15	Q21	There are a variety of specialties at this hospital.

Table A2. Cont.

Construct	Code	No.	Question
PR EXR	PFI2	Q22	I pay a reasonable price for the other medical services (laboratory, radiology, etc.) at this hospital.
	PFI3	Q23	I pay a reasonable price for the medications at this hospital.
	PFI1	Q24	I pay a reasonable price for the medical consultation at this hospital.
BUIL EXR	PEN13	Q25	There is a sufficient number of chairs in the waiting area.
	PEN12	Q26	The hospital has clean departments, corridors, rooms, bathrooms.
	PEN14	Q27	The capacity of departments at this hospital including (ER, ICU, waiting room, etc.) is sufficient enough.
	PEN11	Q28	This hospital has new building infrastructure (walls, ceiling, bathrooms, etc.).
ACC EXR	PEN4	Q29	The accessibility to this hospital is easy by either public transportation or my car.
	PEN5	Q30	The accessibility to this hospital in an emergency is easy.
COMP IMAGE	PIN6	Q31	There is a probability for postoperative bacterial infection at this hospital
	PIN5	Q32	There is a probability for case referral to another hospital
	PIN4	Q33	There is a probability for case readmission at the same hospital
TECH IMAGE	PLE9	Q34	This hospital use technology to link my prescriptions and tests with pharmacy and labs.
	PLE10	Q35	This hospital use technology for saving my records.
	PLE8	Q36	*I believe this hospital uses the newest technology and devices for diagnosing and treating patients.*
INFO EXR	PLE4	Q37	Information provided to me to be used after discharge is sufficient (medication and side effects, health condition, etc.).
	PLE3	Q38	*Oral and written information provided to me or my family during my hospital experience is sufficient.*
	PLE2	Q39	*Information and guidance provided at admission or the first visit are sufficient.*
HSRP IMAGE	PEN7	Q40	I believe this hospital offers social and volunteering activities to the community.
	PEN6	Q41	I believe this hospital offers exemptions for poor patients.
WT EXR	PIN9	Q42	I wait for a long time before receiving the medical service at this hospital.

Note: *italic* items did not load in EFA but were re-grouped to CFA constructs.

Table A3. Final resulted items.

Construct	Code	No.	Question
PT EXR	PCU4	Q1	This hospital distributes surveys to assess my satisfaction before discharge.
	PCU3	Q2	This hospital distributes surveys to assess my needs upon arrival to the hospital, admission, or during the stay.
	PLE11	Q3	This hospital follows up with me after the discharge.
	PCU5	Q4	My complaints are taken seriously into consideration and solved immediately at this hospital.
	PLE6	Q5	Staff trained me on infection precaution measures such as hand hygiene, cough etiquette, isolation rational, personal protective equipment, etc.
PR EXR	PFI2	Q6	I pay a reasonable price for the other medical services (laboratory, radiology, etc.) at this hospital.
	PFI3	Q7	I pay a reasonable price for the medications at this hospital.
	PFI1	Q8	I pay a reasonable price for the medical consultation at this hospital.
BUILENV EXR	PEN13	Q9	There is a sufficient number of chairs in the waiting area.
	PEN12	Q10	The hospital has clean departments, corridors, rooms, bathrooms.

Table A3. *Cont.*

Construct	Code	No.	Question
BUILCAP EXR	PEN14	Q11	The capacity of departments at this hospital including (ER, ICU, waiting room, etc.) is sufficient enough.
	PEN11	Q12	This hospital has new building infrastructure (walls, ceiling, bathrooms, etc.).
ACC EXR	PEN4	Q13	The accessibility to this hospital is easy by either public transportation or my car.
	PEN5	Q14	The accessibility to this hospital in an emergency is easy.
INFO EXR	PLE4	Q15	Information provided to me to be used after discharge is sufficient (medication and side effects, health condition, etc.).
	PLE3	Q16	Oral and written information provided to me or my family during my hospital experience is sufficient.
	PLE2	Q17	Information and guidance provided at admission or the first visit are sufficient.
SERV	PEN8	Q18	Female doctors are available at this hospital.
	PIN12	Q19	There are a variety of departments at this hospital.
	PIN18	Q20	Services at night, vacations, and weekends are available at this hospital.
	PIN15	Q21	There are a variety of specialties at this hospital.
BSCP ATT	SAT3	Q22	I will recommend this hospital to my family and friends.
	PIN1	Q23	I believe I receive an accurate medical examination at this hospital.
	PEN3	Q24	I believe this hospital offers me better treatment than the other Palestinian hospitals.
	SAT1	Q25	My overall satisfaction with this hospital's performance is high.
	PEN1	Q26	I believe this hospital has a high cure rate.
	SAT2	Q27	I will choose this hospital again when I need a medical consultation.
	PLE1	Q28	I believe the staff at this hospital are competent, knowledgeable, updated, and skilled.
	PIN16	Q29	The services provided to me at this hospital have high quality.
	PIN14	Q30	I believe the medications prescribed to me at this hospital have good quality and efficacy.
COMP IMAGE	PIN6	Q31	There is a probability for postoperative bacterial infection at this hospital
	PIN5	Q32	There is a probability for case referral to another hospital
	PIN4	Q33	There is a probability for case readmission at the same hospital
TECH IMAGE	PLE9	Q34	This hospital use technology to link my prescriptions and tests with pharmacy and labs.
	PLE10	Q35	This hospital use technology for saving my records.
	PLE8	Q36	I believe this hospital uses the newest technology and devices for diagnosing and treating patients.

References

1. Meena, K.; Thakkar, J. Development of Balanced Scorecard for Healthcare Using Interpretive Structural Modeling and Analytic Network Process. *J. Adv. Manag. Res.* **2014**, *11*, 232–256. [CrossRef]
2. Giacaman, R.; Abdul-Rahim, H.F.; Wick, L. Health Sector Reform in the Occupied Palestinian Territories (OPT): Targeting the Forest or the Trees? *Health Policy Plan.* **2003**, *18*, 59–67. [CrossRef] [PubMed]
3. Barghouthi, M.; Lennock, J. *Health in Palestine: Potential and Challenges*; Palestine Economic Policy Research Institute (MAS): Jerusalem, Israel, 1997.
4. PMOH. Health Annual Report, Palestine 2020. May 2021. Available online: https://Moh.Ps (accessed on 10 April 2022).
5. Sabella, A.R.; Kashou, R.; Omran, O. Assessing Quality of Management Practices in Palestinian Hospitals. *Int. J. Organ. Anal.* **2015**, *23*, 213–232. [CrossRef]
6. Palestinian News and Info Agency (WAFA) Hospitals in Palestine. Available online: https://info.wafa.ps/ar_page.aspx?id=14977 (accessed on 10 July 2021).
7. Regional Health Systems Observatory (EMRO). *Health Systems Profile: Palestine*; Regional Health Systems Observatory (EMRO): Cairo, Egypt, 2006.

8. World Health Organisation (WHO). *Vulnerability and the International Health Response in the West Bank and Gaza Strip*; An Analysis of Health and the Health Sector; World Health Organisation (WHO): Geneva, Switzerland, 2001.
9. World Health Organisation (WHO). *Health Conditions in the Occupied Palestinian Territory, Including East Jerusalem, and in the Occupied Syrian Golan Report*; World Health Organisation (WHO): Geneva, Switzerland, 2020.
10. Hammoudeh, W.; Kienzler, H.; Meagher, K.; Giacaman, R. Social and Political Determinants of Health in the Occupied Palestine Territory (OPT) during the COVID-19 Pandemic: Who Is Responsible? *BMJ Glob. Health* **2020**, *5*, e003683. [CrossRef] [PubMed]
11. Kaplan, R.; Norton, D. The Balanced Scorecard-Measures That Drive Performance. *Harv. Bus. Rev.* **1992**, *70*, 71–79. [PubMed]
12. Amer, F.; Hammoud, S.; Khatatbeh, H.; Lohner, S.; Boncz, I.; Endrei, D. A Systematic Review: The Dimensions to Evaluate Health Care Performance and an Implication during the Pandemic. *BMC Health Serv. Res.* **2022**, *22*, 621. [CrossRef]
13. Speckbacher, G.; Bischof, J.; Pfeiffer, T. A Descriptive Analysis on the Implementation of Balanced Scorecards in German-Speaking Countries. *Manag. Account. Res.* **2003**, *14*, 361–388. [CrossRef]
14. Kalender, Z.T.; Vayvay, Ö. The Fifth Pillar of the Balanced Scorecard: Sustainability. *Procedia Soc. Behav. Sci.* **2016**, *235*, 76–83. [CrossRef]
15. Duke-Children's-Hospital Duke Childrens' Hospital Case Abstract. Available online: https://thepalladiumgroup.com/download?file=AED_1551102784_116attachment_dubai_boot_camp_-_march_2019_opt.pdf%23Dubai_Boot_Camp_-_March_2019_opt.pdf (accessed on 15 May 2021).
16. Rabbani, F.; Jafri, S.M.W.; Abbas, F.; Pappas, G.; Brommels, M.; Tomson, G. Reviewing the Application of the Balanced Scorecard with Implications for Low-Income Health Settings. *J. Healthc. Qual.* **2007**, *29*, 21–34. [CrossRef]
17. Mcdonald, B. A Review of the Use of the Balanced Scorecard in Healthcare. *BMcD Consult.* **2012**, *2012*, 1–32.
18. Kaplan, R.S. Conceptual Foundations of the Balanced Scorecard. *Handbooks Manag. Account. Res.* **2009**, *3*, 1253–1269. [CrossRef]
19. Amer, F.; Hammoud, S.; Khatatbeh, H.; Lohner, S.; Boncz, I.; Endrei, D. The Deployment of Balanced Scorecard in Health Care Organizations: Is It Beneficial? A Systematic Review. *BMC Health Serv. Res.* **2022**, *22*, 65. [CrossRef]
20. Edward, A.; Osei-bonsu, K.; Branchini, C.; Yarghal, T.; Arwal, S.H.; Naeem, A.J. Enhancing Governance and Health System Accountability for People Centered Healthcare: An Exploratory Study of Community Scorecards in Afghanistan. *BMC Health Serv. Res.* **2015**, *15*, 299. [CrossRef] [PubMed]
21. Bohm, V.; Lacaille, D.; Spencer, N.; Barber, C.E. Scoping Review of Balanced Scorecards for Use in Healthcare Settings: Development and Implementation. *BMJ Open Qual.* **2021**, *10*, e001293. [CrossRef] [PubMed]
22. Fields, S.A.; Cohen, D. Performance Enhancement Using a Balanced Scorecard in a Patient-Centered Medical Home. *Fam. Med.* **2011**, *43*, 735–739. [PubMed]
23. Smith, H.; Kim, I. Balanced Scorecard at Summa Health System. *J. Corp. Account. Financ.* **2005**, *16*, 65–72. [CrossRef]
24. Gagliardi, A.R.; Lemieux-Charles, L.; Brown, A.D.; Sullivan, T.; Goel, V. Barriers to Patient Involvement in Health Service Planning and Evaluation: An Exploratory Study. *Patient Educ. Couns.* **2008**, *70*, 234–241. [CrossRef]
25. Anderson, N.N.; Baker, G.R.; Moody, L.; Scane, K.; Urquhart, R.; Wodchis, W.P.; Gagliardi, A.R. Approaches to Optimize Patient and Family Engagement in Hospital Planning and Improvement: Qualitative Interviews. *Health Expect.* **2021**, *24*, 967–977. [CrossRef]
26. Bellows, M.; Kovacs Burns, K.; Jackson, K.; Surgeoner, B.; Gallivan, J. Meaningful and Effective Patient Engagement: What Matters Most to Stakeholders. *Patient Exp. J.* **2015**, *2*, 18–28. [CrossRef]
27. Domecq, J.P.; Prutsky, G.; Elraiyah, T.; Wang, Z.; Nabhan, M.; Shippee, N.; Brito, J.P.; Boehmer, K.; Hasan, R.; Firwana, B.; et al. Patient Engagement in Research: A Systematic Review. *BMC Health Serv. Res.* **2014**, *14*, 89. [CrossRef]
28. David Susman Attitudes and Behavior in Psychology. Available online: https://www.verywellmind.com/ (accessed on 19 February 2022).
29. American Psychological Association APA Dictionary of Psychology. Available online: https://dictionary.apa.org/ (accessed on 19 February 2022).
30. Keiningham, T.L.; Cooil, B.; Aksoy, L.; Andreassen, T.W.; Weiner, J. The Value of Different Customer Satisfaction and Loyalty Metrics in Predicting Customer Retention, Recommendation, and Share-of-Wallet. *Manag. Serv. Qual. Int. J.* **2007**, *17*, 361–384. [CrossRef]
31. Genoveva, G. Analyzing of Customer Satisfaction and Customer Loyalty Based on Brand Image and Perceived Service Quality. *J. US-China Public Adm.* **2015**, *12*, 497–508. [CrossRef]
32. Zhou, W.-J.; Wan, Q.-Q.; Liu, C.-Y.; Feng, X.-L.; Shang, S.-M. Determinants of Patient Loyalty to Healthcare Providers: An Integrative Review. *Int. J. Qual. Health Care* **2017**, *29*, 442–449. [CrossRef] [PubMed]
33. Taneja, U. Brand Image to Loyalty through Perceived Service Quality and Patient Satisfaction: A Conceptual Framework. *Health Serv. Manag. Res.* **2021**, *34*, 250–257. [CrossRef] [PubMed]
34. Kotler, P.; Clarke, R.N. *Marketing for Healthcare Organizations*, 1st ed.; Prentice Hall: Englewood Cliffs, NJ, USA, 1987.
35. Kotler, P.; Keller, K. *Marketing Management*, 15th ed.; Prentice Hall: Saddle River, NJ, USA, 2014.
36. Peppers, D. Don Peppers Customer Loyalty: Is It an Attitude? Or a Behavior? *Retrieved Febr.* **2009**, *13*, 2012.
37. Boateng, G.O.; Neilands, T.B.; Frongillo, E.A.; Melgar-Quiñonez, H.R.; Young, S.L. Best Practices for Developing and Validating Scales for Health, Social, and Behavioral Research: A Primer. *Front. Public Health* **2018**, *6*, 149. [CrossRef]
38. Dalkey, N.; Helmer, O. An Experimental Apllication of Deplhi Method to Use of Experts. *Manage. Sci.* **1963**, *9*, 458–467. [CrossRef]

39. Simbar, M.; Rahmanian, F.; Nazarpour, S.; Ramezankhani, A.; Eskandari, N.; Zayeri, F. Design and Psychometric Properties of a Questionnaire to Assess Gender Sensitivity of Perinatal Care Services: A Sequential Exploratory Study. *BMC Public Health* **2020**, *20*, 1063. [CrossRef]
40. Zamanzadeh, V.; Ghahramanian, A.; Rassouli, M.; Abbaszadeh, A.; Alavi-Majd, H.; Nikanfar, A.-R. Design and Implementation Content Validity Study: Development of an Instrument for Measuring Patient-Centered Communication. *J. Caring Sci.* **2015**, *4*, 165–178. [CrossRef]
41. Lawshe, C.H. A Quantitative Approach to Content Validity. *Pers. Psychol.* **1975**, *28*, 563–575. [CrossRef]
42. Tyser, A.R.; Abtahi, A.M.; McFadden, M.; Presson, A.P. Evidence of Non-Response Bias in the Press-Ganey Patient Satisfaction Survey. *BMC Health Serv. Res.* **2016**, *16*, 350. [CrossRef]
43. Patel, A.B.; LaCouture, T.; Hunter, K.; Tartaglia, A.; Kubicek, G.J. Pitfalls and Predictors of Poor Press Ganey Patient Satisfaction Scores. *Int. J. Radiat. Oncol.* **2014**, *90*, S719–S720. [CrossRef]
44. Mann, R.K.; Siddiqui, Z.; Kurbanova, N.; Qayyum, R. Effect of HCAHPS Reporting on Patient Satisfaction with Physician Communication. *J. Hosp. Med.* **2016**, *11*, 105–110. [CrossRef] [PubMed]
45. Siddiqui, Z.K.; Wu, A.W.; Kurbanova, N.; Qayyum, R. Comparison of Hospital Consumer Assessment of Healthcare Providers and Systems Patient Satisfaction Scores for Specialty Hospitals and General Medical Hospitals: Confounding Effect of Survey Response Rate. *J. Hosp. Med.* **2014**, *9*, 590–593. [CrossRef] [PubMed]
46. Sousa, V.D.; Rojjanasrirat, W. Translation, Adaptation and Validation of Instruments or Scales for Use in Cross-Cultural Health Care Research: A Clear and User-Friendly Guideline. *J. Eval. Clin. Pract.* **2011**, *17*, 268–274. [CrossRef]
47. Cho, E.; Kim, S. Cronbach's Coefficient Alpha: Well Known but Poorly Understood. *Organ. Res. Methods* **2015**, *18*, 207–230. [CrossRef]
48. Thompson, S.K. *Sampling*, 3rd ed.; John Wiley & Sons, Inc.: Hoboken, NJ, USA, 2012.
49. Comrey, A.L.; Lee, H.B. *A First Course in Factor Analysis*; Psychology Press: London, UK, 2013; ISBN 9781315827506.
50. Williams, B.; Onsman, A.; Brown, T. Exploratory Factor Analysis: A Five-Step Guide for Novices. *Australas. J. Paramed.* **2010**, *8*. [CrossRef]
51. Bentler, P.M.; Chou, C.-P. Practical Issues in Structural Modeling. *Sociol. Methods Res.* **1987**, *16*, 78–117. [CrossRef]
52. Knafl, G.J.; Grey, M. Factor Analysis Model Evaluation through Likelihood Cross-Validation. *Stat. Methods Med. Res.* **2007**, *16*, 77–102. [CrossRef]
53. Sedgwick, P. Non-Response Bias versus Response Bias. *BMJ* **2014**, *348*, g2573. [CrossRef]
54. World Medical Association. World Medical Association Declaration of Helsinki: Ethical principles for medical research involving human subjects. *JAMA* **2013**, *310*, 2191. [CrossRef] [PubMed]
55. Mintzberg, H. Mintzberg on Management. Inside Our Strange World of Organizations 1989, New York and London: Free Press/Collier Macmillan. 418 pages. *Organ. Stud.* **1990**, *11*, 599. [CrossRef]
56. Kaiser, H.F.; Rice, J. Little Jiffy, Mark Iv. *Educ. Psychol. Meas.* **1974**, *34*, 111–117. [CrossRef]
57. Larsen, R.; Warne, R.T. Estimating Confidence Intervals for Eigenvalues in Exploratory Factor Analysis. *Behav. Res. Methods* **2010**, *42*, 871–876. [CrossRef] [PubMed]
58. Cattell, R.B. The Scree Test for the Number of Factors. *Multivar. Behav. Res.* **1966**, *1*, 245–276. [CrossRef]
59. Hooper, D.; Coughlan, J.; Mullen, M.R. Structural Equation Modelling: Guidelines for Determining Model Fit. *Electron. J. Bus. Res. Methods* **2008**, *6*, 53–60. [CrossRef]
60. Shi, D.; Lee, T.; Maydeu-Olivares, A. Understanding the Model Size Effect on SEM Fit Indices. *Educ. Psychol. Meas.* **2019**, *79*, 310–334. [CrossRef]
61. Cohen, J. Set Correlation and Contingency Tables. *Appl. Psychol. Meas.* **1988**, *12*, 425–434. [CrossRef]
62. Tavakol, M.; Dennick, R. Making Sense of Cronbach's Alpha. *Int. J. Med. Educ.* **2011**, *2*, 53–55. [CrossRef]
63. Peterson, R.A.; Kim, Y. On the Relationship between Coefficient Alpha and Composite Reliability. *J. Appl. Psychol.* **2013**, *98*, 194–198. [CrossRef]
64. Ab Hamid, M.R.; Sami, W.; Mohmad Sidek, M.H. Discriminant Validity Assessment: Use of Fornell & Larcker Criterion versus HTMT Criterion. *J. Phys. Conf. Ser.* **2017**, *890*, 012163. [CrossRef]
65. Hair, J.; Hult, G.T.M.; Ringle, C.S.M. *A Primer on Partial Least Squares Structural Equation Modeling (PLS-SEM)*; SAGE Publications, Incorporated: Los Angeles, CA, USA, 2014; ISBN 78-1-4522-1744-4.
66. Fornell, C.; Larcker, D.F. Evaluating Structural Equation Models with Unobservable Variables and Measurement Error. *J. Mark. Res.* **1981**, *18*, 39–50. [CrossRef]
67. Hair, J.; Wolfinbarger, M.; Money, A.H.; Samouel, P.; Page, M.J. *Essentials of Business Research Methods*; Routledge: England, UK, 2015; ISBN 9781317471233.
68. Bookter, A.I. *Convergent and Divergent Validity of the Learning Transfer Questionnaire*; Louisiana State University: Baton Rouge, LA, USA, 1999.
69. Willits, F.K.; Theodori, G.L.; Luloff, A.E. Another Look at Likert Scales. *J. Rural Soc. Sci.* **2016**, *31*, 126.
70. Hu, L.; Bentler, P.M. Cutoff Criteria for Fit Indexes in Covariance Structure Analysis: Conventional Criteria versus New Alternatives. *Struct. Equ. Model. A Multidiscip. J.* **1999**, *6*, 1–55. [CrossRef]
71. Palestinian Central Bureau of Statistics (PCBS) Percentage Distribution of Current Expenditure on Health in Palestine by Financing Schemes, 2017–2018. Available online: https://www.pcbs.gov.ps/ (accessed on 27 November 2021).

72. Rowe, J.S.; Natiq, K.; Alonge, O.; Gupta, S.; Agarwal, A.; Peters, D.H. Evaluating the Use of Locally-Based Health Facility Assessments in Afghanistan: A Pilot Study of a Novel Research Method. *Confl. Health* **2014**, *8*, 24. [CrossRef]
73. Khan, M.M.; Hotchkiss, R.D.; Dmytraczenko, T.; Zunaid Ahsan, K. Use of a Balanced Scorecard in Strengthening Health Systems in Developing Countries: An Analysis Based on Nationally Representative Bangladesh Health Facility Survey. *Int. J. Health Plan. Manag.* **2013**, *28*, 202–215. [CrossRef]
74. Peters, D.H.; Noor, A.A.; Singh, L.P.; Kakar, F.K.; Hansen, P.M.; Burnhama, G. A Balanced Scorecard for Health Services in Afghanistan. *Bull. World Health Organ.* **2007**, *85*, 146–151. [CrossRef]
75. Hansen, P.M.; Peters, D.H.; Niayesh, H.; Singh, L.P.; Dwivedi, V.; Burnham, G. Measuring and Managing Progress in the Establishment of Basic Health Services: The Afghanistan Health Sector Balanced Scorecard. *Int. J. Health Plan. Manag.* **2008**, *23*, 107–117. [CrossRef]
76. Josey, C.; Kim, I. Implementation of the Balanced Scorecard at Barberton Citizens Hospital. *J. Corp. Account. Financ.* **2008**, *19*, 57–63. [CrossRef]
77. Edward, A.; Kumar, B.; Kakar, F.; Salehi, A.S.; Burnham, G.; Peters, D.H. Configuring Balanced Scorecards for Measuring Health System Performance: Evidence from 5 Years' Evaluation in Afghanistan. *PLoS Med.* **2011**, *8*, e1001066. [CrossRef]
78. Mutale, W.; Stringer, J.; Chintu, N.; Chilengi, R.; Mwanamwenge, M.T.; Kasese, N.; Balabanova, D.; Spicer, N.; Lewis, J.; Ayles, H. Application of Balanced Scorecard in the Evaluation of a Complex Health System Intervention: 12 Months Post Intervention Findings from the BHOMA Intervention: A Cluster Randomised Trial in Zambia. *PLoS ONE* **2014**, *9*, e93877. [CrossRef] [PubMed]
79. Rabbani, F.; Pradhan, N.A.; Zaidi, S.; Azam, S.I.; Yousuf, F. Service Quality in Contracted Facilities. *Int. J. Health Care Qual. Assur.* **2015**, *28*, 520–531. [CrossRef] [PubMed]
80. Gao, H.; Chen, H.; Feng, J.; Qin, X.; Wang, X.; Liang, S.; Zhao, J.; Feng, Q. Balanced Scorecard-Based Performance Evaluation of Chinese County Hospitals in Underdeveloped Areas. *J. Int. Med. Res.* **2018**, *46*, 1947–1962. [CrossRef] [PubMed]
81. Parasuraman, A.; Zeithaml, V.A.; Berry, L.L. A Conceptual Model of Service Quality and Its Implications for Future Research. *J. Mark.* **1985**, *49*, 41. [CrossRef]
82. Ladhari, R. A Review of Twenty Years of SERVQUAL Research. *Int. J. Qual. Serv. Sci.* **2009**, *1*, 172–198. [CrossRef]
83. Buttle, F. SERVQUAL: Review, Critique, Research Agenda. *Eur. J. Mark.* **1996**, *30*, 8–32. [CrossRef]
84. Press Ganey Corporation Press Ganey Associates, Inc. Available online: https://www.pressganey.com/products/patient-experience (accessed on 20 November 2021).
85. Centers for Medicare & Medicaid Hospital Consumer Assessment of Healthcare Providers and Systems (HCAHPS). Available online: https://www.ahrq.gov/cahps/surveys-guidance/hospital/about/adult_hp_survey.html (accessed on 27 November 2021).
86. Bin Traiki, T.A.; AlShammari, S.A.; AlAli, M.N.; Aljomah, N.A.; Alhassan, N.S.; Alkhayal, K.A.; Al-Obeed, O.A.; Zubaidi, A.M. Impact of COVID-19 Pandemic on Patient Satisfaction and Surgical Outcomes: A Retrospective and Cross Sectional Study. *Ann. Med. Surg.* **2020**, *58*, 14–19. [CrossRef]

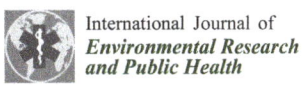

Article

Examining the Feasibility of an Application-Based Patient-Reported Outcome Monitoring for Breast Cancer Patients: A Pretest for the PRO B Study

Anna Maria Hage [1,†], Pimrapat Gebert [2,3,†], Friedrich Kühn [1], Therese Pross [1], Ulrike Grittner [2,3,†] and Maria Margarete Karsten [1,*,†]

1. Department of Gynecology and Breast Center, Charité—Universitätsmedizin Berlin, Charitéplatz 1, 10117 Berlin, Germany; anna-maria.hage@charite.de (A.M.H.); fiete.kuehn@gmx.de (F.K.); therese.pross@charite.de (T.P.)
2. Berlin Institute of Health at Charité—Universitätsmedizin Berlin, Charitéplatz 1, 10117 Berlin, Germany; pimrapat.gebert@charite.de (P.G.); ulrike.grittner@charite.de (U.G.)
3. Institute of Biometry and Clinical Epidemiology, Charité—Universitätsmedizin Berlin, Charitéplatz 1, 10117 Berlin, Germany
* Correspondence: maria-margarete.karsten@charite.de
† These authors contributed equally to this work.

Abstract: In preparation for the PRO B study which aims to examine the effects of an app-based intensified patient-reported outcome (PRO) monitoring for metastatic breast cancer patients, prior assessment of its feasibility was carried out. Sixteen breast cancer patients visiting the breast cancer unit at Charité were recruited and downloaded an app connected to an ePRO system. They received electronic questionnaires on two occasions (baseline and the following week) and were subsequently contacted for a semi-structured phone interview for evaluation. Eleven participants answered at least one questionnaire. Some participants did not receive any or only a part of the questionnaires due to technical problems with the app. Participants who completed the evaluation questionnaire ($n = 6$) were overall satisfied with the weekly PRO questionnaire. All interviewed ($n = 11$) participants thought it was feasible to answer the PRO questionnaires on a weekly basis for one year, as planned in the PRO B study. The pretest revealed a need for major technical adjustments to the app because push notifications about the receipt of new questionnaires were not displayed on some smartphone models. Due to the low number of participants, generalization of the findings is limited to our specific context and study. Nevertheless, we could conclude that if technical aspects of the app were improved, the PRO B study could be implemented as planned. The ePRO questionnaire was considered feasible and adequate from the patients' perspectives.

Keywords: patient reported outcomes; metastatic breast cancer; health apps; personalized medicine; ePROs; mobile health application; mHealth

Citation: Hage, A.M.; Gebert, P.; Kühn, F.; Pross, T.; Grittner, U.; Karsten, M.M. Examining the Feasibility of an Application-Based Patient-Reported Outcome Monitoring for Breast Cancer Patients: A Pretest for the PRO B Study. *Int. J. Environ. Res. Public Health* **2022**, *19*, 8284. https://doi.org/10.3390/ijerph19148284

Academic Editors: Andrea Glässel and Christine Holmberg

Received: 17 March 2022
Accepted: 4 July 2022
Published: 7 July 2022

Publisher's Note: MDPI stays neutral with regard to jurisdictional claims in published maps and institutional affiliations.

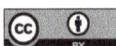

Copyright: © 2022 by the authors. Licensee MDPI, Basel, Switzerland. This article is an open access article distributed under the terms and conditions of the Creative Commons Attribution (CC BY) license (https://creativecommons.org/licenses/by/4.0/).

1. Introduction

The use of electronic patient-reported outcome (ePRO) measures in the care of oncologic patients is being increasingly studied. ePROs can collect real-time data about the patients' general condition using digital surveys and, therefore, enable a fast and personalized monitoring strategy for various domains, such as symptoms, side effects of therapies, functioning, and/or quality of life (QoL). As physicians often underestimate the severity of symptoms and side effects [1,2], collecting information directly from patients might improve the accuracy of this subjective data and potentially improve the efficiency of clinical care [3]. Digital tools such as apps facilitate this process [4,5].

Patients with metastatic cancer are often affected physically and mentally because of the diagnosis itself, its treatment, or coexisting conditions [6]. Basch et al., used an intensified digital PRO-monitoring on 766 cancer patients under chemotherapy, and detected clinical benefits such as improved QoL and a reduction in unplanned hospitalization and ER visits [7], as well as a statistically significant increase in overall survival [8]. Another study by Denis et al. also examined an electronic PRO-monitoring with alerts in advanced-staged lung cancer patients, and found improvements in overall survival, as well as better performance status at the first relapse compared to standard care [9,10].

While designing the PRO B study [11] which aims to evaluate the effects of an app-based PRO-monitoring with alerts on metastatic breast cancer patients' fatigue levels and QoL, we modified an existing digital symptom monitoring tool specifically for the project. The adapted system measures ePROs weekly using an app, then graphically displays the results for clinicians in a web tool and generates alerts in the case of deteriorating ePROs. The alert notifies the treating physician to get in contact with the patient to determine if further interventions are necessary.

In preparation for the PRO B study, prior testing of the ePRO system was conducted and evaluated by breast cancer patients. The study team wanted to include patients' perspectives on the planned PRO B study, since patient-centered care is a critical component of care quality.

Although prior testing of such systems is often recommended [12,13], usability evaluation of eHealth apps has been an under-represented topic in publications [14].

2. Materials and Methods

2.1. Aim of the Study

The pretest aimed to explore the feasibility of the planned PRO B study. Therefore, the main areas of interest were the patient's experience with the app used in the study, the patient's experience with the PRO B study questionnaires, and the feasibility of the PRO B study from the patient's perspective.

Insights and conclusions from the pretest will serve as suggestions for adjustments before starting the main phase of the PRO B study.

2.2. Study Design

This pretest was a single-arm pilot study and took place at the Breast Center of Charité—Universitaetsmedizin Berlin between February and March 2021. The study was approved by the Charité Ethics board (No. EA1/318/20). Breast cancer patients were invited to participate. They were instructed to download the PRO application "*Patient-Concept*" on their smartphone or tablet after giving written informed consent. The app then automatically generated an ID, which served as a pseudonym in the study and was communicated to the study team so that no identifying personal data was included in the ePRO system.

The ePRO system assigned questionnaires to the IDs in conjunction with push notifications on the patients' smartphones. Questionnaires were available for 48 h and disappeared after the 48 h period. The survey was performed at baseline and one week later. At baseline, anamnestic, socio-demographic, and PRO questionnaires were sent from the ePRO system to the app. A week later, patients were asked to complete a second PRO assessment and an evaluation questionnaire inquiring about the pretest.

Afterwards, we also conducted semi-structured telephone interviews with the participants to further assess their feedback on the pretest to explore additional information that might not have been represented in the evaluation questionnaire (Figure 1).

2.3. Participants

Female breast cancer patients of legal age were eligible for participation. Moreover, the participants were required to have access to the internet via a smartphone or tablet and be able to consent to participation. Patients visiting the breast cancer unit at Charité were invited to participate. However, unlike the PRO B study, inclusion in the pretest included, not only metastatic breast cancer patients, but also, patients with early breast cancer.

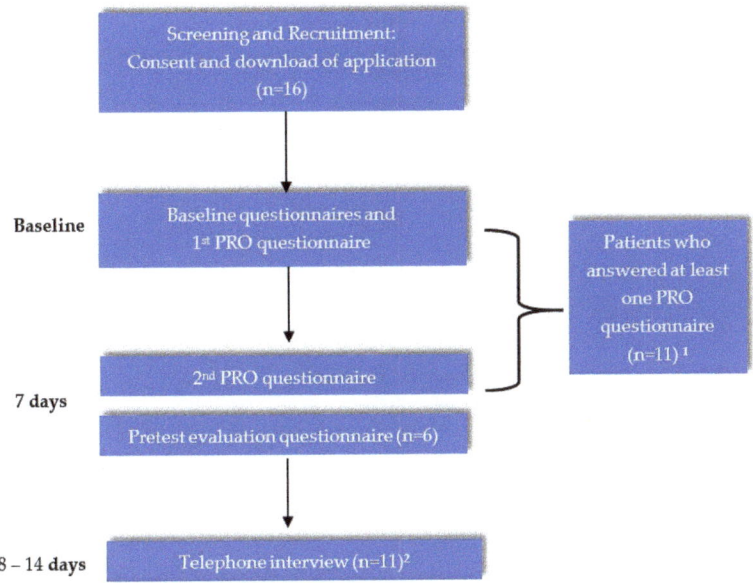

Figure 1. The pretest study flow. [1] Six out of eleven patients answered PRO questionnaires on both occasions; [2] The interview includes one patient who reviewed the questionnaires via e-mail and did not answer in the app.

2.4. Study Instruments

Baseline questionnaires collected data on medical history and socio-demographics [15].

PRO questionnaires for the PRO B study were compiled from items of the EORTC (European Organisation of Research and Treatment of Cancer) CAT (computerized adaptive testing) item bank [16]. Depending on the week, the number of questions asked ranged from 51 to 54 items concerning the domains QoL, physical, role, cognitive, emotional, and social functioning as well as the symptom scales of fatigue, pain, nausea/vomiting, dyspnea, insomnia, appetite loss, constipation, diarrhea, and financial difficulties. In the pretest, the questionnaires were assigned twice on a week interval.

The pretest evaluation questionnaire consisted of two parts: opinion about the weekly PRO questionnaire and opinion about the smartphone application. Both parts used closed questions with a Likert-scale and a few open questions (Supplementary File: Table S1). The first part was developed by the study team and consists of five questions with a 5-Likert scales. Internal consistency using Cronbach's alpha was 0.77 (acceptable). The second part was partly derived from the mHealth App Usability Questionnaire (MAUQ) [17] with a 7-point Likert-scale: 1 = strongly disagree to 7 = strongly agree) and the Cronbach's alpha was 0.87 (good internal consistency). Technical problems were assessed using open questions with a free text response option.

A semi-structured telephone interview guide was developed in a multi-stage consensus process by the study team, which included a senior breast surgeon/gynecologist, biostatisticians, a study nurse, and a psychologist pursuing a deductive and inductive strategy. Questions were developed attempting to verify hypotheses generated from the study teams' clinical expertise as well as being explorative in nature in order to freely capture the patients' perspective and gather information in addition to the quantitative assessment (Supplementary File: Table S2). The aim was to identify additional challenges that might not have been represented with the evaluation questionnaire.

2.5. Semi-Structured Interviews

The telephone interviews were conducted by two physicians (A.M. and F.K.) from the PRO B team using the developed guide. The physicians were not involved in the clinical care of the participants.

Participants were then interviewed individually by phone in German language. The interview questions are presented in the Supplementary data.

Since the interviews were not recorded and were only documented in the form of notes by the interviewing physicians, transcriptions were not available and, therefore, analysis was limited to a descriptive summary of the results.

2.6. Analysis

Exploratory statistics, such as median, minimum, maximum, and absolute and relative frequencies were used to describe quantitative data using Stata IC15 (StataCorp, 2017, College Station, TX, USA).

A biostatistician sorted the notes from the interviews into content domains (perception of workload and duration, perception of the PRO questionnaires, perception of using the application, general suggestions, and using the application in the future and recommendation) and summarized the results using frequency counts.

3. Results

Sixteen female patients were recruited. Four did not answer any questionnaires and were, therefore, excluded. Eleven patients answered questionnaires in the app at least once, and one patient received the questionnaires via e-mail due to technical problems. Mean age was 47 years (SD 11, range 31–70 years), two participants were diagnosed with metastatic disease, while 10 were diagnosed with early breast cancer.

Only six of the twelve participants answered the evaluation questionnaire at the end of the pretest.

Due to major technical problems, the app, in some cases, did not display notifications on the mobile phone, leaving the participants unaware that there were new questionnaires available, and the questionnaires expired unanswered after 48 h.

Nevertheless, we were able to include eleven patients in the semi-structured interviews to further assess the experience with the ePRO tool.

3.1. Results of the Evaluation Questionnaire

3.1.1. Patients' Experiences with the PRO B Study Questionnaires

Five out of six patients who answered the evaluation questionnaire were satisfied or very satisfied with the PRO questionnaires and the time spent on them. Four of the patients reported that the questions were very easy to understand and that they were able to concentrate the entire time. However, five patients reported that the questions were only moderately relevant to them (Table 1).

Table 1. General opinion about PRO B questionnaires in the application (n = 6).

General Opinion about PRO B Questionnaires	Very Much	Much	Moderate	A Little	Not at All
Overall satisfaction	3	2	1	0	0
The questions are understandable	4	1	1	0	0
The questions are relevant for breast cancer patients	0	1	5	0	0
I am able to concentrate while answering the questionnaires	4	1	1	0	0
Time needed to answer the questionnaires is appropriate	2	3	1	0	0

Two patients reported that some questions seemed very similar, e.g., regarding fatigue and physical functioning. Three patients answered that the survey lacked important aspects of chemotherapy-related side effects, e.g., polyneuropathy. One patient wished for more questions regarding psycho-oncology, e.g., on worry and anxiety.

3.1.2. Patients' Experiences with the Application

The results show that patients who were able to answer the questionnaires were overall very satisfied with using the app (median score of 7 points (7 = highest score)) (Table 2).

Table 2. Opinion on using the application (Likert scale ranges from 1 = totally disagree to 7 = totally agree) ($n = 6$).

Aspects	Questions	Median (Min, Max)
Ease of use and satisfaction	The app was easy to use	7 (5, 7)
	It was easy for me to learn to use the app	7 (7, 7)
	I like the interface of the app	6 (4, 7)
	The information in the app was well organized, so I could easily find the information I needed	6 (4, 7)
	I feel comfortable using this app in social settings	6 (4, 7)
	The amount of time involved in using this app has been fitting for me	7 (5, 7)
	I would use this app again	7 (4, 7)
	This app offers great opportunity to improve care for breast cancer patients	6 (4, 7)
	Overall, I am satisfied with this app	7 (5, 7)
System information arrangement	Whenever I made a mistake using the app, I could correct it easily and quickly	6.5 (1, 7)
	The navigation was simple and clearly structured	7 (5, 7)

3.2. Results of the Telephone Interview

The study team reached fourteen of the sixteen participants for the semi-structured telephone interview. Three of the participants did not participate in the telephone survey because they either did not receive any questionnaires ($n = 2$) or felt too ill to fill them out ($n = 1$). Overall, eleven patients were interviewed, of whom ten received and answered PROs at least once, and one participant reviewed the questionnaires after receiving them via e-mail instead of in the app (due to the technical problems).

- Perception of workload and duration

Out of eleven participants, all considered it feasible to answer all items once a week for a year as planned in the intervention group of the PRO B study. Most of the patients completed the questionnaires in around 5–20 min.

- Perception of the PRO questionnaires

After being asked if the PRO-questionnaires covered the most relevant aspects, patients responded positively, seven patients gave minor suggestions about what they would like to additionally see represented in the PRO-questionnaire. Side effects of treatment were mentioned most frequently ($n = 4$), and digestion, mental health, sexual and social aspects were also mentioned to better represent the patients' burdens. Four participants mentioned they felt that some questions seemed redundant and sounded too general. A participant remarked that the amount of housework varies for everyone and is, therefore, not a comparable term. One patient had a concern about emotional and financial problems related to the corona-virus pandemic, as it could have aggravated these problems. Another patient reported that it could be difficult to complete the quality-of-life questionnaire when a private event occurs that is not related to breast cancer. Moreover, one patient said that she was confused by the used ranking scale and remarked that she would feel more familiar with German school grades (1–6). However, all of the patients thought that the questions were helpful for the doctors to assess the patient's health status.

- Perception of using the application

Multiple patients reported having technical problems using the application, especially with getting push notifications. Therefore, they were left unaware of receiving questionnaires in the app. They had to check the app for the questionnaires frequently by themselves, otherwise the questionnaire would expire. No patient mentioned any problems in the app while answering the questionnaires.

- General suggestions from participants

All of the patients considered the system useful. One would have preferred a different color scheme, as the color blue seemed too sterile and reminded her of a hospital. A more personalized greeting would have been nice. Another patient would have liked to receive an additional notification on the second day to be reminded about the availability of questionnaires. It was also suggested to add a short explanation or instruction about the questions concerning health status. One patient would have liked to see the results of their health state assessment graphically displayed in the app and, if possible, receive a weekly report. She also suggested including a short explanation and information on each question in the app. Moreover, the patient would have liked to receive some information on the latest research in the app.

- Using the application in the future and recommending it to others

All but one of the patients interviewed (n = 10) would like to use the system and concept in the future and would recommend it to other patients. One patient reported that she already felt adequately treated and, therefore, would not need to use the application further in the future.

- Suggestions for motivating the control group

The control group in the PRO B study will answer questionnaires only quarterly, and alerts will not be generated in the case of deteriorating PROs [9]. The treating physicians will not have access to their answers during the study but will receive an overview at the end of the trial. As there is no primary benefit to answering the questionnaires for the control group, we wanted to examine if we should expect a high drop-out or non-compliance rate. Therefore, we asked the participants for suggestions on how to motivate the patients in the control group. Two participants mentioned that the control group could be questioned even more frequently. However, most of them suggested using a reminder notification and felt that the opportunity to contribute to research was incentive enough. For high compliance, the study team should explain the potential advantages of the project for future patients afflicted with metastatic breast cancer.

4. Discussion

In summary, the results show positive experiences in both the evaluation questionnaire and the telephone interview among participants who used the PRO B tool. Since interviews were not recorded and transcribed, the analysis is limited to descriptive summaries. Nevertheless, we could collect valuable insights from patients' perspectives and confirm the overall acceptability of the questionnaire and the PRO B study design. Participants were generally satisfied and found that the app could be useful for tracking their HRQoL and symptoms. The study team was previously concerned that the time spent on answering the questionnaires might be overwhelming. However, the pretest allayed those concerns. From the patients' points of view, answering the questionnaire on a weekly basis in the upcoming PRO B study is a tolerable burden that takes up a reasonable amount of time. Accordingly, after finding solutions to the severe technical problems, the app is feasible and possible to use for monitoring PROs in breast cancer patients. Moreover, downloading the *PatientConcept* application is free of charge and has been used to support communication between physicians and patients [18,19].

The pretest revealed a need for technical improvement to the ePRO system and app. Therefore, a function documenting the delivery of the questionnaires to the participants was established after the pretest. Most participants did not answer the full set of questionnaires during the pretest, mostly because they did not receive any or were not aware of them because of missing push-notifications. Receipt of push-notifications was improved in a subsequent app-update.

To ensure compliance in the upcoming PRO B study, non-responding participants will receive push notifications as a reminder after 24 h.

The limitations of this pretest are the small number of patients and short study period. Due to a longer than expected time for implementation of the ePRO system and the upcoming start of the PRO B study, the duration of the pretest was restricted. Also, most of the participants did not suffer from metastatic breast cancer—unlike the inclusion criteria of the PRO B study. Therefore, the patients' points of view and needs might differ.

Due to major technical problems with the app, we cannot draw conclusions about the response rate. Also, there was no testing of the alarm function in case of worsening scores because of the short study period. Moreover, qualitative assessment was not possible since the interviews were not recorded and transcribed. Nevertheless, we were still able to get an impression of the patients' views, and we consider their suggestions valuable.

5. Conclusions

As every medical procedure should primarily focus on the patient on whom it is performed, the inclusion of the patient's perspective in the development of new forms of care such as ePRO systems is crucial.

Unfortunately, in this pretest, findings from this study are limited to our specific study and context due to the low number of patients and the major unexpected technical problems with the app. Nevertheless, we note that none of the participants raised major concerns regarding the time spent answering the questionnaires via app or the content of the questionnaires. Therefore, we conclude that the PRO B study design and questionnaires are feasible and adequate to implement as planned. Major technical issues regarding push notifications in the app were identified and rectified after the pretest, but considerably delayed the start of enrollment for the PRO B study. When including new technologies in clinical studies, technical difficulties cannot be underestimated. Therefore, calculating a sufficient amount of time from pretest to enrollment is crucial.

Supplementary Materials: The following supporting information can be downloaded at: https://www.mdpi.com/article/10.3390/ijerph19148284/s1, Table S1: Pretest evaluation questionnaire; Table S2: A semi-structured telephone interview.

Author Contributions: Conceptualization, U.G. and M.M.K.; methodology, F.K., T.P., U.G., P.G. and M.M.K.; formal analysis, P.G.; writing—original draft preparation, A.M.H. and P.G.; writing—review and editing, F.K., T.P., U.G. and M.M.K. All authors have read and agreed to the published version of the manuscript.

Funding: This research was funded by a public grant from the Innovation Committee of the Federal Joint Committee ("Innovationsauschuss des Gemeinsamen Bundesausschusses", grant number 01NVF19013). The funder has no further role in the conduct of the study but must approve the changes of the protocol and financing.

Institutional Review Board Statement: The study was conducted according to the guidelines of the Declaration of Helsinki and was approved by the Institutional Review Board (or Ethics Committee) of Charité Universitätsmedizin Berlin (application number: EA1/318/20).

Informed Consent Statement: Informed consent was obtained from all subjects involved in the study. Written informed consent has been obtained from the patients to publish this paper.

Data Availability Statement: The data analyzed during this study are not permitted to be made publicly available.

Acknowledgments: We acknowledge the participants in the pretest, study nurses and the administrative and technical support from NeuroSys, the company working on the *PatientConcept* application. The authors would like to thank Felix Fischer and Alizé Rogge for their intensive reviews and suggestions.

Conflicts of Interest: The authors declare no conflict of interest. The funders had no role in the design of the study; in the collection, analyses, or interpretation of data; in the writing of the manuscript, or in the decision to publish the results.

References

1. Fromme, E.K.; Eilers, K.M.; Mori, M.; Hsieh, Y.C.; Beer, T.M. How accurate is clinician reporting of chemotherapy adverse effects? A comparison with patient-reported symptoms from the Quality-of-Life Questionnaire C30. *J. Clin. Oncol.* 2004, 22, 3485–3490. [CrossRef] [PubMed]
2. Laugsand, E.A.; Sprangers, M.A.; Bjordal, K.; Skorpen, F.; Kaasa, S.; Klepstad, P. Health care providers underestimate symptom intensities of cancer patients: A multicenter European study. *Health Qual. Life Outcomes* 2010, 8, 104. [CrossRef] [PubMed]
3. Basch, E.; Stover, A.M.; Schrag, D.; Chung, A.; Jansen, J.; Henson, S.; Carr, P.; Ginos, B.; Deal, A.; Spears, P.A.; et al. Clinical Utility and User Perceptions of a Digital System for Electronic Patient-Reported Symptom Monitoring During Routine Cancer Care: Findings From the PRO-TECT Trial. *JCO Clin. Cancer Inform.* 2020, 4, 947–957. [CrossRef] [PubMed]
4. Bae, W.K.; Kwon, J.; Lee, H.W.; Lee, S.C.; Song, E.K.; Shim, H.; Ryu, K.H.; Song, J.; Seo, S.; Yang, Y.; et al. Feasibility and accessibility of electronic patient-reported outcome measures using a smartphone during routine chemotherapy: A pilot study. *Support. Care Cancer* 2018, 26, 3721–3728. [CrossRef] [PubMed]
5. Benze, G.; Nauck, F.; Alt-Epping, B.; Gianni, G.; Bauknecht, T.; Ettl, J.; Munte, A.; Kretzschmar, L.; Gaertner, J. PROutine: A feasibility study assessing surveillance of electronic patient reported outcomes and adherence via smartphone app in advanced cancer. *Ann. Palliat. Med.* 2019, 8, 104–111. [CrossRef] [PubMed]
6. Reilly, C.M.; Bruner, D.W.; Mitchell, S.A.; Minasian, L.M.; Basch, E.; Dueck, A.C.; Cella, D.; Reeve, B.B. A literature synthesis of symptom prevalence and severity in persons receiving active cancer treatment. *Support. Care Cancer* 2013, 21, 1525–1550. [CrossRef] [PubMed]
7. Basch, E.; Deal, A.M.; Kris, M.G.; Scher, H.I.; Hudis, C.A.; Sabbatini, P.; Rogak, L.; Bennett, A.V.; Dueck, A.C.; Atkinson, T.M.; et al. Symptom Monitoring With Patient-Reported Outcomes During Routine Cancer Treatment: A Randomized Controlled Trial. *J. Clin. Oncol.* 2016, 34, 557–565. [CrossRef] [PubMed]
8. Basch, E.; Deal, A.M.; Dueck, A.C.; Scher, H.I.; Kris, M.G.; Hudis, C.; Schrag, D. Overall Survival Results of a Trial Assessing Patient-Reported Outcomes for Symptom Monitoring During Routine Cancer Treatment. *JAMA* 2017, 318, 197–198. [CrossRef] [PubMed]
9. Denis, F.; Lethrosne, C.; Pourel, N.; Molinier, O.; Pointreau, Y.; Domont, J.; Bourgeois, H.; Senellart, H.; Tremolieres, P.; Lizee, T.; et al. Randomized Trial Comparing a Web-Mediated Follow-up With Routine Surveillance in Lung Cancer Patients. *J. Natl. Cancer Inst.* 2017, 109, 1–8. [CrossRef] [PubMed]
10. Denis, F.; Yossi, S.; Septans, A.L.; Charron, A.; Voog, E.; Dupuis, O.; Ganem, G.; Pointreau, Y.; Letellier, C. Improving Survival in Patients Treated for a Lung Cancer Using Self-Evaluated Symptoms Reported Through a Web Application. *Am. J. Clin. Oncol.* 2017, 40, 464–469. [CrossRef] [PubMed]
11. Karsten, M.M.; Kuhn, F.; Pross, T.; Blohmer, J.U.; Hage, A.M.; Fischer, F.; Rose, M.; Grittner, U.; Gebert, P.; Ferencz, J.; et al. PRO B: Evaluating the effect of an alarm-based patient-reported outcome monitoring compared with usual care in metastatic breast cancer patients-study protocol for a randomised controlled trial. *Trials* 2021, 22, 666. [CrossRef] [PubMed]
12. Friis, R.B.; Hjollund, N.H.; Mejdahl, C.T.; Pappot, H.; Skuladottir, H. Electronic symptom monitoring in patients with metastatic lung cancer: A feasibility study. *BMJ Open* 2020, 10, e035673. [CrossRef] [PubMed]
13. Warrington, L.; Absolom, K.; Holch, P.; Gibson, A.; Clayton, B.; Velikova, G. Online tool for monitoring adverse events in patients with cancer during treatment (eRAPID): Field testing in a clinical setting. *BMJ Open* 2019, 9, e025185. [CrossRef] [PubMed]
14. Maramba, I.; Chatterjee, A.; Newman, C. Methods of usability testing in the development of eHealth applications: A scoping review. *Int. J. Med. Inform.* 2019, 126, 95–104. [CrossRef] [PubMed]
15. Bundesamt, S. *Demographische Standards, Ausgabe 2016*; Eine gemeinsame Empfehlung des ADM Arbeitskreis Deutscher Markt- und Sozialforschungsinstitute e.V., der Arbeitsgemeinschaft Sozialwissenschaftlicher Institute e.V. (ASI) und des Statistischen Bundesamtes. 6. überarbeitete und erweiterte Auflage. Statistik und Wissenschaft Band 17; Statistisches Bundesam: Wiesbaden, Germany, 2016. Available online: https://www.statistischebibliothek.de/mir/servlets/MCRFileNodeServlet/DEMonografie_derivate_00001549/Band17_DemographischeStandards1030817169004.pdf (accessed on 10 December 2020).
16. Petersen, M.A.; Aaronson, N.K.; Arraras, J.I.; Chie, W.C.; Conroy, T.; Costantini, A.; Dirven, L.; Fayers, P.; Gamper, E.M.; Giesinger, J.M.; et al. The EORTC CAT Core-The computer adaptive version of the EORTC QLQ-C30 questionnaire. *Eur. J. Cancer* 2018, 100, 8–16. [CrossRef] [PubMed]
17. Zhou, L.; Bao, J.; Setiawan, I.M.A.; Saptono, A.; Parmanto, B. The mHealth App Usability Questionnaire (MAUQ): Development and Validation Study. *JMIR mHealth uHealth* 2019, 7, e11500. [CrossRef] [PubMed]
18. Lang, M.; Mayr, M.; Ringbauer, S.; Cepek, L. PatientConcept App: Key Characteristics, Implementation, and its Potential Benefit. *Neurol. Ther.* 2019, 8, 147–154. [CrossRef] [PubMed]
19. Lang, M.; Ringbauer, S.; Mayr, M.; Cepek, L. How to improve disease management of chronically ill patients? Perception of telemetric ECG recording and a novel software application. *Clin. Res. Trials* 2019, 5, 1–6. [CrossRef]

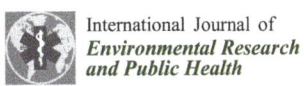

Article

National Profile of Caregivers' Perspectives on Autism Spectrum Disorder Screening and Care in Primary Health Care: The Need for Autism Medical Home

Sarah H. Al-Mazidi [1],* and Laila Y. Al-Ayadhi [2,3]

1 Department of Physiology, Faculty of Medicine, Imam Mohammed Ibn Saud Islamic University, P.O. Box 5701, Riyadh 11432, Saudi Arabia
2 Department of Physiology, Faculty of Medicine, King Saud University, P.O. Box 2925, Riyadh 11461, Saudi Arabia; lyayadhi@ksu.edu.sa
3 Autism Research and Treatment Centre, King Saud University, P.O. Box 2925, Riyadh 11461, Saudi Arabia
* Correspondence: s.almazeedi@gmail.com

Abstract: Although autism spectrum disorder (ASD) is a common developmental disorder, primary healthcare providers show a deficit in providing early diagnosis. To understand parents' experience and perspective in the diagnosis and intervention process of their children, a survey was deployed through social media to parents' with at least one child diagnosed with ASD. The survey included parents experience, satisfaction and perception in the diagnosis process and services provided for their children, stigma and type of support received. A total of 223 participants were enrolled. Although 62% of ASD patients were diagnosed by three years old, most diagnoses (66%) were non-physician initiated. Additionally, 40.8% of the parents reported that the services required for their child are available in their area of residence, but only 7.9% were satisfied with these services. Parents who received psychological support (9.9%) started early intervention, and their children have a better prognosis ($p \leq 0.005$). Stigmatized parents were more likely to delay intervention ($p \leq 0.005$). Parents' perception is to have qualified healthcare and educational professionals experienced in ASD. Our findings suggest that a specialized family-centred medical home for ASD patients would significantly benefit ASD patients, increase parents' satisfaction, reduce parents' stress, and ease their children's transition to adolescents.

Keywords: autism spectrum disorder; medical homes; autism; primary healthcare

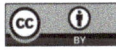

1. Introduction

Autism spectrum disorder (ASD) is a cluster of neurodevelopmental disorders which are characterized by restricted and repetitive behavioural patterns, and limitations in social interaction and communication [1]. Children with ASD have other comorbidities such as gastrointestinal problems, food and skin allergies, and epilepsy that needs direct medical attention [2]. According to the Centre for Disease Control and Prevention, the incidence of ASD has been estimated to be 1 in 54 children in the United States. The reason for this increase is not clear; it might be due to the changes in the diagnostic criteria or increased awareness of ASD among the community, medical professionals and educators [3,4]. Early diagnosis at three years old is crucial and significantly improves ASD patients' social behaviour and cognitive skills [5,6].

Since ASD has increased in the past decade, developing a special care system that provides optimal care for the children and their parents is essential. Although it is a common developmental disorder, primary health care providers show a deficit in providing early diagnosis. Physicians at the primary health care have a vital role in the early detection of ASD, which ensures optimal improvement for the children and reduces stress on caregivers [7].

Many diagnostic instruments are available for ASD, which includes validated scales, subscales, and checklists [8]. Ideally, diagnosis of ASD requires a multidisciplinary team of professionals specializing in the assessment of ASD [9]. This team includes a paediatrician, child psychiatrist, psychologist, speech-language pathologist, occupational and behavioural therapist [10]. Access to centres with a multidisciplinary team or experienced physicians in ASD is difficult and unavailable in all areas [11].

The American Academy of Pediatrics established special policies and standards for what is known as medical homes. A medical home is a specialized medical centre that is an accessible, coordinated and compassionate family-centred primary health care centre [12,13]. A medical home creates a partnership between caregivers and their paediatrician, clinicians, early childhood professionals, and educators, all of whom are specialized in ASD intervention [14]. Medical homes are cost effective, improve providers' and patients' satisfaction, reduce the psychological and financial burden on caregivers, and children are more likely to receive high-quality care [12,13,15]. Medical homes also provide healthcare providers trained to address medical and mental needs for ASD patients transitioning into adolescence and adulthood [16].

The aim of our study is to understand parents' experience in the diagnosis and intervention process of their children and their perspective of the best care for ASD children and their parents.

2. Methods

2.1. Study Design

We conducted a non-experimental, cross-sectional study of parents' satisfaction and perception of healthcare services for ASD patients. The study was approved by the Institutional Review Board.

2.2. Study Setting

This study sought to understand the parental experience of healthcare services provided for their ASD children in Saudi Arabia. Parents from different cities participated in this survey. The survey was distributed electronically to the families that have at least one child diagnosed with ASD through physicians, autism schools, autism centres, psychologists and educators using social media applications (Twitter, WhatsApp, and LinkedIn).

2.3. Participants and Procedures

Participant characteristics: Participants consisted of 224 parents of one or more children (males and females) with ASD diagnosed and treated in Saudi Arabia either by a physician or other healthcare provider (such as a psychologist).

The survey and consent: The survey had an introductory statement that describes the study's aims and that their participation was voluntary with complete anonymity ensured. It also stated that they were allowed to withdraw from the study at any time.

A 42 item self-administered online survey using Google Forms® (Google LLC, Mountain View, CA, USA) was prepared and administered via Google forms to the parents of ASD children. The survey was available from October 2020 to June 2021.

Six participants were invited to pilot-test the initial draft survey to validate it; minor modifications were made based on their feedback. Then, the survey was distributed using social media platforms, including Twitter, WhatsApp, and LinkedIn. The survey was sent three times to each potential participant to maximize our response rate.

2.4. Measures

The survey included both open-ended and closed-ended questions which evaluated the following:

2.4.1. Diagnosis Process and Referral Source

We asked the parents about the details that were experienced during the diagnosis and referral process of their children using closed-ended questions as follows: age of the child when diagnosed with ASD, the duration between the first visit to the healthcare professional and time they received the diagnosis, the healthcare professional that initiated the diagnosis, the main symptom that led to the diagnosis, the type of clinic that diagnosed their child, and the availability of the healthcare services in their area of residence to diagnose their child.

2.4.2. Parents' Satisfaction with the Service Provided for ASD Patients

Parents evaluated the health care services provided for their children according to the following: availability of the service in their area of residence, type of intervention received and treatment plan, emotional and psychological support received, subjective improvement after intervention as rated by the parents, type of follow-up clinic, early intervention (at the age of three years), yearly cost of their child intervention.

These questions were closed-ended, then an open-ended question was provided to explain the reasons for their dissatisfaction with the healthcare provided for their child. The open-ended question was qualitatively analysed using thematic framework analysis

2.4.3. Stigma and Stress Level of Parents

Parents rated their stress level during the diagnosis and intervention process of their children. All items were rated on a 5-point Likert scale, ranging from never (zero) to always (five), where higher scores indicated greater stress. We asked the parents if they are stigmatized with their child's diagnosis. Answers were provided as (Yes/No).

2.4.4. Parents' Perception of the Services That Should Be Provided for ASD Patients

To achieve patients' and parents' satisfaction with the available healthcare services, the parents were provided an open-ended question that explains their perspective on services that should be provided according to their point of view. This question was qualitatively analysed using thematic framework analysis.

2.5. Statistical Analysis

All the statistical tests were performed using the Statistical Package for Social Science (SPSS) software version 26. Descriptive statistical analysis was used to analyse the items included in the survey such as participants' demographics and other study outcomes. Responses were presented as frequencies and percentages. Chi-square and Fisher's exact tests were used to compare responses between variables in different categorical measures. p values that are equal to or less than 0.05 were considered significant. In the present study, saturation of data is the point at which no new themes were created [17]. The hybrid structure of our survey, with closed and open-ended questions, provided flexibility to apply both quantitative and qualitative analytic methods for analysis. After gathering the results, the quantitative data was tabulated, and the textual responses were collated for further qualitative analysis using a thematic analysis approach to identify themes and enable us to understand participants perspectives of health care services provided for their children.

3. Results

The survey was available for nine months (October 2020 to June 2021). Within the thematic analysis, we examined the recurrence of certain issues in the responses, that included (i) diagnosis, (ii) intervention, and (iii) quality of service. After reaching 200 participants, there were no new themes generated. Therefore, it was deemed that the data collection had reached a saturation point. We continued data collection for 24 more participants to ensure and confirm that no new themes are emerging.

3.1. Participant's Demographics

Survey Sample

A total of 224 participants (76.7% males) responded to the survey and completed a set of questions to screen for eligibility. Data saturation was reached and only one participant was excluded. Study demographic data are shown in Table 1. Male participants were significantly more than females. Participants' financial status was normally distributed. Table 2 shows family history. Most families have at least one working parent. The most reported disabilities of ASD siblings were learning disabilities (22.9%) and delayed speech (22.4%). The most reported diseases in the family were asthma (17%) and Rheumatoid Arthritis (10%).

Table 1. Demographics.

Characteristics	Variable	Percentage
Child Age (years)	1–3	1.3%
	4–6	13.9%
	7–9	20.7%
	10–12	35.4%
	13–15	18.8%
	More than 16	9.9%
Sex	Male	76.7%
	Female	23.3%
Area	Riyadh area	38.6%
	Dammam area	18.4%
	Abha and Jizan	2.3%
	Makkah area	16.2%
	Al-Khafji	1%
	Hail	1%
	Qassim	2.7%
	Madina	5.8%
	Al-Ehsaa	6.7%
Monthly Income	Low (less than 1500 $) SAR	27.8%
	Middle low (1500–2500 $)	24.3%
	Middle high (2600–4000 $)	25.1%
	High (more than 4000 $) SAR	22.2%
Property	Owned	53.4%
	Rented	46.6%

Table 2. Family History.

Characteristics	Variable	Percentage
Parents Related	Yes	38.6%
	No	61.4
Mothers Age	20–29	8.1%
	30–39	42.6%
	40–49	32.3%
	50–59	17%
Fathers Age	20–29	1.8%
	30–39	26%
	40–49	36.3%
	50–59	28.3%
	60+	7.6%
Mothers Education	Higher Education	3.9%
	University	47.1%
	Diploma	5.8%
	High school	43%
Fathers Education	Higher Education	8.4%
	University	32.7%
	Diploma	16.1%
	High school	41.7%
Work field Mother	Education	27.4%
	Health	6.7%
	Administrative	3.6%
	Self-Employed	5%
	Housewife	57.4%
Work field Father	Education	15.7%
	Health	1.8%
	Engineering	5%
	Administrative	17.5%
	Self-Employed	12.6%
	Unemployed	10.4%
	Other	35.4%
Siblings with other disorders	Developmental delay	4.9%
	Learning disabilities	22.9%
	Mental Disorder	8.5%
	Delayed Speech	22.4%
Parents with disorders	Delayed Speech	2.7%
	Learning Disabilities	2.7%
	Depression	2.3%
	Bipolar	1.3%
	Other psychological Disorders	4.9%
Family members disorders	Rheumatoid Arthritis	10.8%
	Multiple sclerosis	6.7%
	Alzheimer	4.9%
	Parkinson's Disease	2.7%
	Asthma	17.9%
	Psoriasis	3.1%
	Autoimmune Disease	4%

3.2. Survey Measures

3.2.1. Diagnosis Process and Referral Source

Descriptive information on the diagnosis process and referral source are shown in Table 3. The most common ASD symptoms reported within the children were delayed speech (70.9%), difficulties in communication with the child (61.9%), repetitive movements (50.7%) and abnormal playing behaviour (48%).

Table 3. Diagnosis and intervention.

Characteristics	Variable	Percentage
Childe age when diagnosed	1–3	64.1%
	4–6	32.3%
	7–9	3.5%
Child Education	Private School	13%
	Governmental School	17%
	Special needs school	46.6%
	Not at school Because:	
	Young Age	4.5%
	School not available	12.6%
	Other	6.3%
How long did it take to be diagnosed?	1 Month	23.5%
	1–3 Months	20.2%
	4–7 Months	11.7%
	8–12 Months	24.6%
	More than A year	20%
Type of clinic that made the diagnosis	Government	59.2%
	Private	40.8%
Service Available for diagnosis and treatment?	Yes	40.8%
	No	40.4%
	I don't know	18.8%
Once diagnosed, did he/she start treatment?	Yes	72.6%
	No	27.4%
Did the Childe improve after treatment?	Yes	74.9%
	No	25.1%
Did you receive the appropriate psychological support?	Yes	9.9%
	No	40.4%
	To some extent	49.7%
Satisfaction of services provided	Yes	7.2%
	No	49.8%
	To some extent	43%
Stigma	No	73.1%
	Yes	26.9%
Cost of Diagnosis	None	28.7%
	Up to 1000 SR	17%
	Up to 3000 SR	15.2%
	Up to 6000 SR	15.7%
	Up to 10,000 SR	23.3%
The primary symptom noticed	Speech delay	70.9%
	Communication issues	61.9%
	Repetitive movements	50.7%
	Different playing style	48%
	No danger senses	38.6%
	Socially isolated	35.4%
	Annoyed by sounds or colors	26%
	Learning problems	25.1%

According to the parents, only 32% were initially diagnosed by a paediatrician, while 46% were diagnosed by a psychologist and 22% by a speech therapist (Figure 1). About 64% of the ASD children received their diagnosis by the age of three-years-old, and 61% of them were diagnosed in a governmental medical facility. Only 40.8% of the parents reported that the services provided for their children were available in their area of residence. Additionally, many of the parents reported that the diagnosis process was long and costly (Table 3).

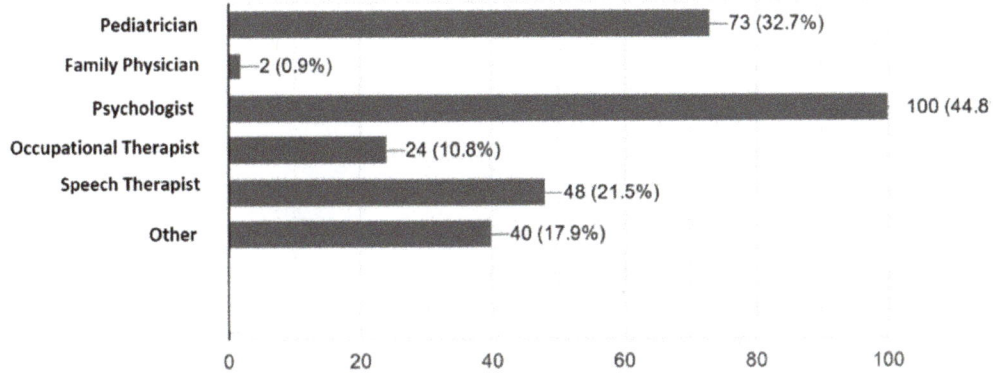

Figure 1. Healthcare professionals that initiated ASD diagnosis according to caregivers experience.

3.2.2. Parents' Satisfaction with the Service Provided for ASD Patients

Closed-ended questions were analysed to determine parents' satisfaction with the provided healthcare services. Then, an open-ended question was analysed using framework analysis, which led to the identification of categories within our themes as follows: (i) wrong initial diagnosis, (ii) availability of qualified healthcare professionals, and (iii) settings of healthcare centres for ASD.

The response to all themes was similar, but the frequency of participants with dissatisfaction with the settings of healthcare centres for ASD was found to be the greatest. For example, parents that reported the availability of services in their area of residence responded to the open question as follows:

- *There are many centres available for autism, but they are not as qualified as the centres in a neighbouring country.*
- *Unfortunately, there is no accurate diagnosis for our children, and the first diagnosis for my child was wrong.*
- *Unfortunately, there are no qualified healthcare professionals for the treatment and diagnosis of autism so far.*

Early intervention was significantly correlated with service availability ($p \leq 0.05$) and child improvement ($p \leq 0.03$). Table 3 shows that 72.6% of parents who reported that their child improved have started early intervention. Interestingly, most parents who started the intervention early work either in the health or education sectors (29.1%) compared to other parents ($p \leq 0.01$). There are 27% of parents who did not start intervention early. None of these parents work in the health sector (Table 2).

According to the parents point of view, which was subjectively based on their expectation of intervention, the most effective intervention was behavioural therapy (64.8%) followed by learning-directed therapy (52.4%). Other interventions include speech therapy (36.7%) and occupational therapy (41%) (Figure 2). Although 40.8% of the parents stated that the treatment and diagnostic services are available, only 7.9% were satisfied with the provided services.

We found that psychological support to the parents is crucial for their children's improvement. Only 9.9% of the parents received proper psychological support during their child's diagnosis and intervention process in the current study.

Parents who received psychological support were more likely to start early intervention (84%) than those who did not receive any psychological support ($p \leq 0.005$). Additionally, all parents who received psychological support reported that their children had improved, while 25.6% of parents who did not receive psychological support reported that their children had improved with the intervention ($p \leq 0.001$).

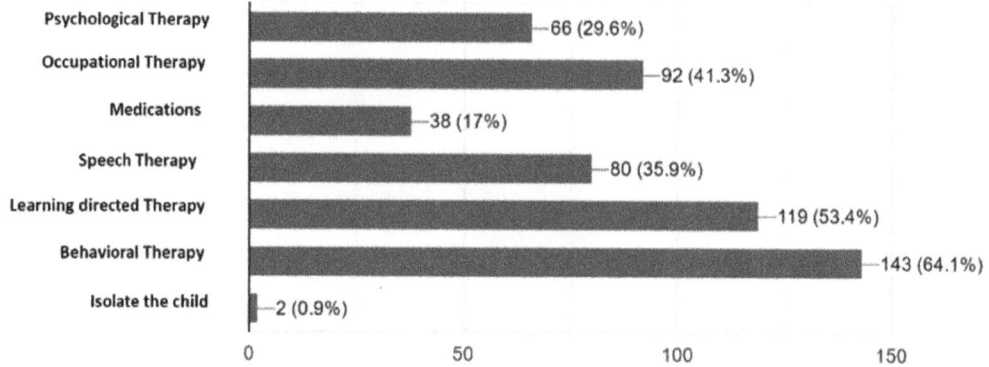

Figure 2. Caregivers subjective point of view on the most effective intervention for their children.

3.2.3. Stigma and Stress Level of Parents

The long duration until the official diagnosis was made had increased stress levels on the parents; for example, of all the 45.5% of total parents who reported extreme stress (Figure 3), 19.8% of them received the diagnosis within a month, while 40.6% of them received it after one year.

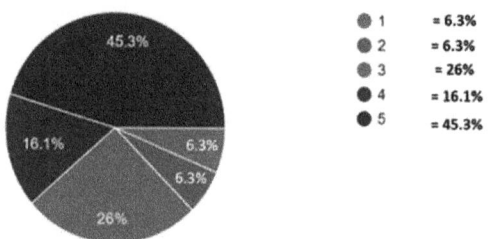

Figure 3. Stress level experienced by ASD caregivers. Level of stress indicated as 1 = Never and 5 = very often where higher score correlates to more stress.

Although most of our participants are not stigmatized by their child's diagnosis, we found that stigmatized parents did not start treating their children once they were diagnosed ($p \leq 0.005$).

3.2.4. Parents' Perspective on the Services That Should Be Provided for ASD Patients

The parents view and experiences and their perspectives on healthcare services for ASD children are similar in all cities in Saudi Arabia. There are three main categories within our themes analysed using framework analysis, and parents' responses were similar in each category.

We chose some of the parent's point of view as follows:

- View on diagnosis:

We hope to have excellent centers for children with mild autism and establish special schools to have curricula specialized in their way of thinking. I hope that autistic children get great attention in education, diagnosis, and training, because we, as parents, have been confused, and no guidance was provided to us, and access to services is still difficult for most of us.

We need the diagnosis to be immediate, accurate, with a precise treatment plan prepared by a specialized team, according to the needs of each child and immediately refer to an appropriate center, according to the specialists' point of view and not letting the parents struggle due to their lack of knowledge. Therefore, parents should be directed to the appropriate place that provides necessary services for their children.

We should emulate the experience of other countries and transfer knowledge and bring in the best experts in this field.

The difference of opinions during diagnosis has caused us great humiliation.

There should be an obligatory routine screening for autism in the preschool years.

- View on intervention

To have a complete center with all required medical, educational, social, and psychological consultants for parents and children. A center that would also prepare them for adulthood and merge smoothly into society and have jobs in the future.

To increase the governmental centers because the private centers cause a great financial burden on us.

Provide complete healthcare services that are accessible to all of the autism community.

- View on parents' support

In my opinion, the most important thing is the psychological stability of the parents.

We suffer from our preoccupation with our jobs for long periods, as we cannot take care of our autistic children as we should, and there is no safe place that accepts their presence for full working periods.

Increase awareness of autism and have special entertainment and sports centers for them.

4. Discussion

Whether there is an actual increase in the prevalence, or it is due to the awareness of ASD in the community, it is crucial to evaluate the current services offered to ASD patients and their parents to provide optimal care and increase their satisfaction with the offered services. This study aimed to evaluate the current healthcare services in the diagnosis and intervention of ASD and understand parents' perspectives on healthcare offered for them and their children. In our study, most parents reported that the services are unavailable in their area of residence or they are not aware of the available services. We also found that all parents working in the health field are treating their children, which indicates these healthcare services are not adequately promoted to the public. Moreover, most parents were not satisfied with the available services and reported that the diagnosis process was long and costly. The main reason for the high cost of ASD intervention is because it involves many specialized medical and educational services. One suggested solution to the high cost of intervention is to promote health care volunteering services at public clinics [18].

Parents of an ASD child experience chronic stress, especially during the diagnosis process [19,20]. Our results showed that psychological support is essential for ASD parents. Parents reported that the availability of high-quality services for their children might reduce the amount of stress they are experiencing. This finding is consistent with the results reported by Ault et al., who reported that ASD parents experience more stress and poor mental health when services are unavailable [21].

Prolonged duration until diagnosis and service availably are crucial to reduce parents' stress. In our study, some parents had multiple visits to the primary health care physician and paediatrician; it took as long as two years to have an official diagnosis and start intervention. This might be because most physicians in primary health care are not experienced in diagnosing ASD. This finding was supported by previous studies that reported that ASD is difficult to define, diagnose, and the physicians cannot translate their theoretical knowledge of ASD into their clinical practice, which shows a lack of experience in ASD diagnosis in primary health care physicians [22,23]. To overcome this, a previous study suggested a valid scale easily performed by any healthcare provider and does not require special training which might be distributed to primary health care and even to educators [5].

Early intervention has a significant impact on ASD patient's progress and improvement [24,25]. Although The American Academy of Pediatrics recommended routine screening of ASD for children aged from 18 months to 24 months, few centres or even countries follow this screening routine [26]. Early years educators can also be trained to use a simplified scale and report a possible ASD child. Teachers should also be trained to handle students with ASD and co-existing behaviours such as restrictive and repetitive behaviours and anxiety [27–29]. Although certification in special education is an advantage for ASD education, a study showed that special certification is not necessary for optimal academic outcomes in ASD students [30]. This is beneficial for some ASD children studying in regular schools or even merging some ASD children into the regular teaching system.

In our study, most parents were not stigmatized by their ASD child, and we found no correlation between stigma and service availability, income, or type of psychological support to the parents, and it did not affect their child's treatment or education. A multi-centre study reported that stigmatized parents need psychological support and that stigma increases with lower income and services availability [31]. Another study reported that parents who feel psychologically supported would positively impact their children's care, which was also a finding in our study [32]. This requires proactive action to develop a special psychological support service to help parents with their children's intervention.

Knowing the parents' experience is vital to evaluating our current diagnostic and intervention services and is the backbone of developing a satisfying healthcare system for parents, ASD patients and health care workers [33]. In our study, we asked for the parents' perspectives for ASD health care, which can be summarized as the following: there is a need for qualified paediatricians and primary care physicians to diagnose ASD and manage co-existing disorders such as gastrointestinal problems, seizures, allergies and to refer them to manage any behavioural or psychiatric disorders that co-occur in ASD such as attention-deficit hyperactivity disorder, anxiety, obsessive-compulsive disorder, and mood disorder. They also need a high-quality centre that meets the international standards in ASD intervention that includes psychologists, speech therapists, occupational therapists, and all medical tools and consults needed for their children that is accessible and affordable to all families. They also requested a centre that helps their children's transition into adolescence and adulthood and provides families with the necessary support.

All these suggestions fit into what is known as medical homes. A medical home is based on a partnership between physicians and parents. It is a society-based and coordinated primary healthcare centre that includes all care services that an ASD patient might need, such as qualified physicians, medical personnel, early educators and family support. All services and staff at a medical home are specifically trained to deal with ASD patients and co-existing medical and mental disorders and improve child and family diagnostic and intervention experience [34].

Recently, there is a global shift toward medical homes for ASD. It is cost-effective and relieves financial and psychological burdens on working parents. In our study, most parents reported that the services provided to their children were not satisfying, and many reported that they do not have access to healthcare services specific to ASD in their area. Our findings are consistent with a national survey in the United States, which found that ASD patients who do not have access to a medical home have higher burdens in all study indicators than those in a medical home [12]. Additionally, a study reported that parents of ASD children in medical homes are less stressed than the other ASD parents and reported improvement in their mental health [15]. Families are not aware of the concept of a medical home; thus, they lowered their expectation of healthcare services and did not expect to receive comprehensive care, and their treatment goals are limited to maintaining their children's current health [32,35].

In our study, most families reported that the diagnosis was non-physician initiated, which led to delayed diagnosis. The reason might be because the parents are more aware and educated, which makes them seek other health care professionals; as in our study, most parents reported that the primary source of information during the diagnostic process was gained from the internet. The difference in referral process in ASD was previously reported, which suggests that a medical home model may reduce the referral duration and reduce the chances that ASD patients are diagnosed as developmental delay cases [7]. In our study, parents were stressed during the diagnosis process, which would be significantly reduced in a family-based centre, as reported previously by Myers et al. [20].

5. Strengths and Limitations

Strengths of this study included a geographically diverse sample of parents and adequate sample size, a saturation of qualitative data, and the use of technology to recruit the participants, which decrease selection bias. Study limitations include the following: survey questions relied on parent self-report associated with recall bias. Future studies with larger samples size are needed to explore the relationship between types of health care services during the diagnostic and intervention process for ASD. Data collection was terminated because sample adequacy and saturation were reached, and no new insights were found during data analysis.

6. Conclusions

In this study, we used self-report measures to understand the parent experience during the diagnostic and treatment process and to seek their perspective in ASD healthcare services in their area of residence. Our findings suggest that a specialized family-centred medical home specific for ASD patients might have a significant impact in increasing parents' satisfaction with healthcare, reducing parents' stress, and easing the transition of their children to adulthood.

Author Contributions: S.H.A.-M.: Conceptualization, data collection, writing, review and editing, methodology, original draft preparation and software analysis. L.Y.A.-A.: Conceptualization, data collection, writing, review and editing. All authors have read and agreed to the published version of the manuscript.

Funding: This project was funded by the National Plan for science, Technology and Innovation (MAARIFAH), King Abdulaziz City for Science and Technology, Kingdom of Saudi Arabia, Award Number (08-MED 510-02).

Institutional Review Board Statement: The study was approved by the Institutional Review Board, Faculty of medicine, King Saud University (IRB number E-20-5158).

Informed Consent Statement: The survey has an introductory statement that describes the study's aims and that their participation was voluntary with complete anonymity ensured. It also stated that they were allowed to withdraw from the study at any time.

Data Availability Statement: Data in this research are available in tables section of this manuscript.

Conflicts of Interest: Authors declare that there is no conflict of interest.

References

1. Hodges, H.; Fealko, C.; Soares, N. Autism spectrum disorder: Definition, epidemiology, causes, and clinical evaluation. *Transl. Pediatr.* **2020**, *9*, S55–S65. [CrossRef]
2. Al-Beltagi, M. Autism medical comorbidities. *World J. Clin. Pediatr.* **2021**, *10*, 15–28. [CrossRef]
3. Saito, M.; Hirota, T.; Sakamoto, Y.; Adachi, M.; Takahashi, M.; Osato-Kaneda, A.; Kim, Y.S.; Leventhal, B.; Shui, A.; Kato, S.; et al. Prevalence and cumulative incidence of autism spectrum disorders and the patterns of co-occurring neurodevelopmental disorders in a total population sample of 5-year-old children. *Mol. Autism* **2020**, *11*, 35. [CrossRef]
4. Williams, J.G.; Higgins, J.P.; Brayne, C.E. Systematic review of prevalence studies of autism spectrum disorders. *Arch. Dis. Child.* **2006**, *91*, 8–15. [CrossRef] [PubMed]
5. Ramelli, V.; Perlini, R.; Zanda, N.; Mascetti, G.; Rizzi, E.; Ramelli, G.P. Early identification of autism spectrum disorders using the two-step Modified Checklist for Autism: Experience in Southern Switzerland. *Eur. J Pediatr.* **2018**, *177*, 477–478. [CrossRef] [PubMed]
6. Sutera, S.; Pandey, J.; Esser, E.L.; Rosenthal, M.A.; Wilson, L.B.; Barton, M.; Green, J.; Hodgson, S.; Robins, D.L.; Dumont-Mathieu, T.; et al. Predictors of optimal outcome in toddlers diagnosed with autism spectrum disorders. *J. Autism Dev. Disord.* **2007**, *37*, 98–107. [CrossRef]
7. Ming, X.; Hashim, A.; Fleishman, S.; West, T.; Kang, N.; Chen, X.; Zimmerman-Bier, B. Access to specialty care in autism spectrum disorders-a pilot study of referral source. *BMC Health Serv. Res.* **2011**, *11*, 99. [CrossRef]

8. Huerta, M.; Lord, C. Diagnostic evaluation of autism spectrum disorders. *Pediatr. Clin. N. Am.* **2012**, *59*, 103–111. [CrossRef] [PubMed]
9. Monteiro, S.A.; Dempsey, J.; Berry, L.N.; Voigt, R.G.; Goin-Kochel, R.P. Screening and Referral Practices for Autism Spectrum Disorder in Primary Pediatric Care. *Pediatrics* **2019**, *144*, e20183326. [CrossRef]
10. Alotaibi, A.M.; Craig, K.A.; Alshareef, T.M.; AlQathmi, E.S.; Aman, S.M.; Aldhalaan, H.M.; Oandasan, C.L. Sociodemographic, clinical characteristics, and service utilization of young children diagnosed with autism spectrum disorder at a research center in Saudi Arabia. *Saudi Med J.* **2021**, *42*, 878–885. [CrossRef]
11. Lappé, M.; Lau, L.; Dudovitz, R.N.; Nelson, B.B.; Karp, E.A.; Kuo, A.A. The Diagnostic Odyssey of Autism Spectrum Disorder. *Pediatrics* **2018**, *141*, S272–S279. [CrossRef]
12. Kogan, M.D.; Strickland, B.B.; Blumberg, S.J.; Singh, G.K.; Perrin, J.M.; van Dyck, P.C. A national profile of the health care experiences and family impact of autism spectrum disorder among children in the United States, 2005–2006. *Pediatrics* **2008**, *122*, e1149–e1158. [CrossRef] [PubMed]
13. Todorow, C.; Connell, J.; Turchi, R.M. The medical home for children with autism spectrum disorder: An essential element whose time has come. *Curr. Opin. Pediatr.* **2018**, *30*, 311–317. [CrossRef] [PubMed]
14. O'Dell, M.L. What is a Patient-Centered Medical Home? *Mo. Med.* **2016**, *113*, 301–304. [PubMed]
15. Limbers, C.A.; Gutierrez, A.; Cohen, L.A. The Patient-Centered Medical Home: Mental Health and Parenting Stress in Mothers of Children With Autism. *J. Prim. Care Community Health* **2020**, *11*, 2150132720936067. [CrossRef] [PubMed]
16. Harris, J.F.; Gorman, L.P.; Doshi, A.; Swope, S.; Page, S.D. Development and implementation of health care transition resources for youth with autism spectrum disorders within a primary care medical home. *Autism* **2021**, *25*, 753–766. [CrossRef]
17. Ando, H.; Cousins, R.; Young, C. Achieving Saturation in Thematic Analysis: Development and Refinement of a Codebook. *Compr. Psychol.* **2014**, *3*, CP.3.4. [CrossRef]
18. Bieleninik, Ł.; Gold, C. Estimating Components and Costs of Standard Care for Children with Autism Spectrum Disorder in Europe from a Large International Sample. *Brain Sci.* **2021**, *11*, 340. [CrossRef] [PubMed]
19. Whitmore, K.E. Respite Care and Stress Among Caregivers of Children With Autism Spectrum Disorder: An Integrative Review. *J. Pediatr. Nurs.* **2016**, *31*, 630–652. [CrossRef]
20. Myers, L.; Karp, S.M.; Dietrich, M.S.; Looman, W.S.; Lutenbacher, M. Family-Centered Care: How Close Do We Get When Talking to Parents of Children Undergoing Diagnosis for Autism Spectrum Disorders? *J. Autism Dev. Disord.* **2021**, *51*, 3073–3084. [CrossRef] [PubMed]
21. Ault, S.; Breitenstein, S.M.; Tucker, S.; Havercamp, S.M.; Ford, J.L. Caregivers of children with autism spectrum disorder in rural areas: A literature review of mental health and social support. *J. Pediatr. Nurs.* **2021**, *61*, 229–239. [CrossRef]
22. Jacobs, D.; Steyaert, J.; Dierickx, K.; Hens, K. Physician View and Experience of the Diagnosis of Autism Spectrum Disorder in Young Children. *Front. Psychiatry* **2019**, *10*, 372. [CrossRef] [PubMed]
23. Jacobs, D.; Steyaert, J.; Dierickx, K.; Hens, K. Implications of an Autism Spectrum Disorder Diagnosis: An Interview Study of How Physicians Experience the Diagnosis in a Young Child. *J. Clin. Med.* **2018**, *7*, 348. [CrossRef] [PubMed]
24. Kitzerow, J.; Hackbusch, M.; Jensen, K.; Kieser, M.; Noterdaeme, M.; Fröhlich, U.; Taurines, R.; Geißler, J.; Wolff, N.; Roessner, V.; et al. Study protocol of the multi-centre, randomised controlled trial of the Frankfurt Early Intervention Programme A-FFIP versus early intervention as usual for toddlers and preschool children with Autism Spectrum Disorder (A-FFIP study). *Trials* **2020**, *21*, 217. [CrossRef]
25. Constantino, J.N.; Abbacchi, A.M.; Saulnier, C.; Klaiman, C.; Mandell, D.S.; Zhang, Y.; Hawks, Z.; Bates, J.; Klin, A.; Shattuck, P.; et al. Timing of the Diagnosis of Autism in African American Children. *Pediatrics* **2020**, *146*, e20193629. [CrossRef]
26. McClure, L.A.; Lee, N.L.; Sand, K.; Vivanti, G.; Fein, D.; Stahmer, A.; Robins, D.L. Connecting the Dots: A cluster-randomized clinical trial integrating standardized autism spectrum disorders screening, high-quality treatment, and long-term outcomes. *Trials* **2021**, *22*, 319. [CrossRef] [PubMed]
27. Welsh, P.; Rodgers, J.; Honey, E. Teachers' perceptions of Restricted and Repetitive Behaviours (RRBs) in children with ASD: Attributions, confidence and emotional response. *Res. Dev. Disabil.* **2019**, *89*, 29–40. [CrossRef]
28. Adams, D.; MacDonald, L.; Keen, D. Teacher responses to anxiety-related behaviours in students on the autism spectrum. *Res. Dev. Disabil.* **2019**, *86*, 11–19. [CrossRef]
29. Love, A.M.A.; MToland, D.; Usher, E.L.; Campbell, J.M.; Spriggs, A.D. Can I teach students with Autism Spectrum Disorder?: Investigating teacher self-efficacy with an emerging population of students. *Res. Dev. Disabil.* **2019**, *89*, 41–50. [CrossRef]
30. Goldman, S.E.; Gilmour, A.F. Educating Students with Autism Spectrum Disorders: Is Teacher Certification Area Associated with Academic Outcomes? *J. Autism Dev. Disord.* **2021**, *51*, 550–563. [CrossRef]
31. Tilahun, D.; Hanlon, C.; Fekadu, A.; Tekola, B.; Baheretibeb, Y.; Hoekstra, R.A. Stigma, explanatory models and unmet needs of caregivers of children with developmental disorders in a low-income African country: A cross-sectional facility-based survey. *BMC Health Serv. Res.* **2016**, *16*, 152. [CrossRef] [PubMed]
32. Carbone, P.S.; Behl, D.D.; Azor, V.; Murphy, N.A. The medical home for children with autism spectrum disorders: Parent and pediatrician perspectives. *J. Autism Dev. Disord.* **2010**, *40*, 317–324. [CrossRef] [PubMed]
33. Jacobs, D.; Steyaert, J.; Dierickx, K.; Hens, K. Parents' views and experiences of the autism spectrum disorder diagnosis of their young child: A longitudinal interview study. *Eur. Child Adolesc. Psychiatry* **2020**, *29*, 1143–1154. [CrossRef] [PubMed]

34. Farmer, J.E.; Clark, M.J.; Mayfield, W.A.; Cheak-Zamora, N.; Marvin, A.R.; Law, J.K.; Law, P.A. The relationship between the medical home and unmet needs for children with autism spectrum disorders. *Matern Child Health J.* **2014**, *18*, 672–680. [CrossRef] [PubMed]
35. Russell, S.; McCloskey, C.R. Parent Perceptions of Care Received by Children With an Autism Spectrum Disorder. *J. Pediatric Nurs.* **2016**, *31*, 21–31. [CrossRef] [PubMed]

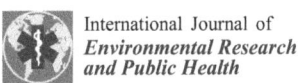

Article

Patient Navigation—Who Needs What? Awareness of Patient Navigators and Ranking of Their Tasks in the General Population in Germany

Susanne Schnitzer [1,*], Raphael Kohl [1], Hella Fügemann [2], Kathrin Gödde [3], Judith Stumm [4], Fabian Engelmann [5], Ulrike Grittner [6,7] and Nina Rieckmann [3]

[1] Charité—Universitätsmedizin Berlin, Corporate Member of Freie Universität Berlin and Humboldt Universität zu Berlin, Institute of Medical Sociology and Rehabilitation Science, Charitéplatz 1, 10117 Berlin, Germany; raphael.kohl@charite.de
[2] Brandenburg Medical School Theodor Fontane, Institute of Social Medicine and Epidemiology, 14770 Brandenburg an der Havel, Germany; hella.fuegemann@mhb-fontane.de
[3] Charité—Universitätsmedizin Berlin, Corporate Member of Freie Universität Berlin and Humboldt Universität zu Berlin, Institute of Public Health, Charitéplatz 1, 10117 Berlin, Germany; kathrin.goedde@charite.de (K.G.); nina.rieckmann@charite.de (N.R.)
[4] Charité—Universitätsmedizin Berlin, Corporate Member of Freie Universität Berlin and Humboldt Universität zu Berlin, Institute of General Practice and Family Medicine, Charitéplatz 1, 10117 Berlin, Germany; judith.stumm@charite.de
[5] Kassenärztliche Bundesvereinigung (KBV), Geschäftsbereich Sicherstellung und Versorgungsstruktur, Abteilung Versorgungsstruktur, 10592 Berlin, Germany; fengelmann@kbv.de
[6] Charité—Universitätsmedizin Berlin, Corporate Member of Freie Universität Berlin and Humboldt Universität zu Berlin, Institute for Biometry and Clinical Epidemiology, Charitéplatz 1, 10117 Berlin, Germany; ulrike.grittner@charite.de
[7] Berlin Institute of Health at Charité—Universitätsmedizin Berlin, Charitéplatz 1, 10117 Berlin, Germany
* Correspondence: susanne.schnitzer@charite.de

Abstract: The aim of the present study was to investigate the awareness of patient navigation (PN) in the general population in Germany and to assess which navigator tasks are considered most important. The analysis drew on a 2019 nationwide telephone survey of 6110 adults. We compared rankings of emotional support, administrative support and information among respondents with and without experience of patient navigation. One-fifth of the sample reported having heard of PNs; 13% of this group already had experience with PN. In both groups, the majority (>47%) considered assistance with applications to be most important. This was particularly the case among younger adults and those with a chronic disease. Within the inexperienced group, higher educated people had higher odds of ranking provision of information as most important for them, whereas women and those without a partner had higher odds of ranking emotional support as the most important task. This study shows that the majority of people predominantly expect PN services to offer administrative support, irrespective of their socioeconomic and health status. Whether these expectations are met by the diverse existing PN programs, which often have a strong focus on other tasks (e.g., increasing health literacy), has yet to be evaluated.

Keywords: patient navigation; health information; emotional support; social support; population survey; sociodemographic characteristics; chronic disease; subjective health

1. Introduction

A chronic disease raises a variety of questions for those affected. These may concern acute medical treatment, rehabilitation and other therapy. Furthermore, questions about social security, social benefits and assistance with everyday living/homecare may arise. In outpatient care, the degree of assistance that patients receive in managing and coordinating their own healthcare varies greatly between but also within healthcare systems. In many cases, patients are left unassisted in the coordination of all medical, psychological, social and legal aspects related to their disease management. The presence of multiple chronic conditions, absence of an informal support system and low health literacy may further complicate this. These barriers also exist in the German healthcare system. Above all, research has revealed that there is little coordination of patients' continued care in Germany [1], difficulties due to complex care in multimorbid patients [2], fragmentation of the German healthcare system and separate organization of the inpatient and outpatient sector [3,4]. In addition to these system barriers, on the patients' side, low health literacy [5]—especially of vulnerable groups, such as migrants or lower educated people [6,7]—or limited knowledge about further support offers [8–10] can restrict access to optimal healthcare.

In order to support patients over a longer period of time, patient navigation (PN) models have been deployed internationally and, more recently, in Germany [11–16]. Patient navigators (PNs) guide and support patients in gaining access to timely care and handling the increasingly complex healthcare system or treatment regimes [12,14,17]. They aim to support patients to organize their healthcare according to their individual needs and to optimize their care trajectory [11,14]. Patient navigators provide practical support (e.g., with applications, organization of appointments), give advice on social care issues and draw attention to existing support offers. In short, patient navigators (PNs) assist, inform, advise and guide patients through the healthcare system. They help patients to find their way through the healthcare and, if needed, adjacent care systems and support them in finding a competent institution or contact person for their concerns, needs and problems. Patient navigation ideally connects all healthcare sectors for patients, i.e., both in the hospital and at the doctor's office or in rehabilitation [18]. There is only a minimal consensus on the tasks and functions of PNs [19,20]. On the basis of qualitative interviews and focus group discussions with nurses, specialists and family doctors, Fillion and colleagues proposed a bi-dimensional framework that encompasses certain core tasks of navigators. The first dimension refers to the continuity of care, and the second dimension relates to patient and family empowerment [19]. Continuity of care was further divided into informational continuity (use of information, disease- or person-focused) and management continuity (e.g., matching unmet needs with services). The second dimension, empowerment, includes concepts such as supportive care, e.g., addressing patients' emotional and psychological needs [19].

In Germany, various—mainly indication-specific—patient navigation models have been developed in recent years and are currently being tested for their feasibility and efficiency [21,22]. These are model projects and patient navigation is currently not a widely implemented reimbursable service in statutory health insurance (in Germany, insurance is mandatory and about 90% of the population is covered by statutory health insurance). The majority of these patient navigation programs have been developed using an expert-driven approach and are based on the concept of 'ideal' patient pathways and evidence-based patient care for specific diseases. In this context, the roles and tasks of the navigators are defined a priori. However, to our knowledge, patients' perspectives on which tasks of patient navigation are most important have not been investigated systematically. In particular, this raises the question of the specific needs of different population groups or, in other words, who needs what most? The subjective needs of patients are an important requirement for the successful implementation of patient navigation models in healthcare practice. As there is little research on this topic, our study sheds some light on it.

Aim of the Study

The aim of the present study was to investigate the awareness of PN in the general population and to assess which navigator tasks are considered most important in several population subgroups according to sociodemographic and health status characteristics and previous experience with PN.

2. Materials and Methods

2.1. Study Design

Since 2008, an expert group of the German National Association of Statutory Health Insurance Physicians (Kassenärztliche Bundesvereinigung, KBV), in cooperation with the Institute of Medical Sociology and Rehabilitation Science of Charité University and the research institute Forschungsgruppe Wahlen (FGW), has conducted an annual representative population survey among all German-speaking adults living in households with a landline phone on various topics in outpatient healthcare. The analyses presented here are based upon the 2019 survey. A random sample was generated through regional stratification of the population, selection of landline phone numbers via randomized last digit dialing and selection of the respondent through the last birthday method. Computer-assisted telephone interviews (CATI) were conducted in the German language by the FGW between 11 March and 29 April 2019. The data were weighted for the number of landlines and persons per household, as well as for gender, age and education according to their nominal distribution across the adult population in Germany [23]. The weighted sample is representative for the German-speaking adult population and comprises 6110 persons (Table 1).

Table 1. Sociodemographic baseline data (weighted sample).

		n = 6110 *	% [95% CI]
Age	18–64	4294	70.3 [69.1; 71.4]
	65+	1815	29.7 [28.6; 30.9]
Sex	female	3196	52.3 [51.1; 53.6]
	male	2914	47.7 [46.4; 48.9]
Education	low	4122	68.3 [67.1; 69.4]
	high	1916	31.7 [30.6; 32.9]
Partnership	yes	4341	71.4 [70.2; 72.5]
	no	1741	28.6 [27.5; 29.8]
Region	East Germany	1063	17.4 [16.5; 18.4]
	West Germany	5047	82.6 [81.6; 83.5]
Urban/Rural	rural	1781	31.2 [30.0; 32.4]
	town	2603	45.6 [44.3; 46.9]
	big city	1326	23.2 [22.1; 24.3]
Chronic Illness	yes	2885	47.6 [46.3; 48.8]
	no	3177	52.4 [51.2; 53.7]
Subjective health	excellent/very good/good	4716	77.9 [76.8; 78.9]
	less well/bad	1342	22.1 [21.1; 23.2]

* Difference to 6110: missing data.

2.2. Assessment of PN Awareness and Importance of Navigator Tasks

Within an expert group of the NAVICARE research network (authors S.S., H.F., K.G., J.S.), the assessment of PN awareness and the most important tasks of PNs from the population's perspective were discussed. Finally, following the theoretical framework proposed by Fillion and colleagues [19], described above, and taking into account the results from a qualitative interview study with twenty lung cancer and twenty stroke patients [1], three main tasks of PNs were defined. Respondents were asked to select which one they consider the most important task. First, participants were asked whether they had heard of PNs before:

'In healthcare, there is a service provided by PNs who support and advise patients over a longer period of time after an acute illness/event such as stroke, or a longer-lasting disease such as cancer, e.g., in filling out applications. Have you heard of PNs?'

Subsequently, a filter was set: All those who answered 'yes' here were asked to indicate whether they had already had experience with a PN. This population constitutes the 'experienced' subsample in the present study. Respondents who had already heard of PNs but had not yet had any experience with PNs themselves constitute the 'inexperienced' subsample. Both subsamples were asked about their views on the most important task of PNs as follows: 'Which of the following three tasks of PNs would be/was most important to you?

- assistance with administrative matters, e.g., applications for rehabilitation care,
- provision of healthcare information,
- counseling and support for emotional problems resulting from the disease'.

Multiple answers were not possible, i.e., respondents had to choose one task.

2.3. Sociodemographic Characteristics and Health Status

PN awareness and the support needs/perception of the most important tasks may vary according to socioeconomic and health status. The following characteristics and subgroups were analyzed: Age (18–64/$\geq$65 years), gender (female/male), educational attainment (high school/no high school), current partnership (no/yes), region of current residence (East/West Germany), residential area (rural $\leq$ 5000; small town 5001–100,000; urban > 100,000), chronic illness (yes/no) and subjective health status (excellent, very good, good/less well, bad).

2.4. Statistical Analysis

For both subsamples (experienced/inexperienced), three dichotomous variables on the most important tasks (support with applications, provision of information, emotional support) were generated (0 = not most important/1 = most important). Associations with sociodemographic and health characteristics were analyzed using multiple binary logistic models. The analyses are considered exploratory. Altogether, we explored six models: M1a. application, M2a. information, M3a. emotional support (dependent variables of the inexperienced) and M1b. application, M2b. information, M3b. emotional support (dependent variables of the experienced). For each task, odds ratios (OR) and 95% confidence intervals (CI) were calculated. The two-sided level of significance was set at 5%. No adjustment for multiple testing was applied.

The number of refusers on the key variables were negligible, with 0.03% for knowledge of ('have you heard of PNs?') and 0.15% for experience with PNs ('have you already had experience with a PN?'). Respondents who refused to answer these questions were excluded from further analysis. In the experienced group, the rate of missing data on the question about the most important task of PNs was 9%; in the inexperienced group, it was 12%. Refusers on the questions on the most important tasks were included and coded as 0 (not most important) for each variable. Randomness of missing data was analyzed using the Chi^2 test with sociodemographic and health characteristics. Missing data occurred more often in older participants among the experienced ($p = 0.02$) and inexperienced group ($p < 0.001$) and in those with lower education among the inexperienced group ($p < 0.001$). All statistical analyses were performed using SPSS version 27.0 [24].

3. Results

About one-fifth of respondents (n = 1275/20.9%) had already heard of PNs. Of these, the majority had no prior experience with PN (inexperienced, n = 1105/86.8%), while a small group had prior experience (experienced, n = 168/13.2%).

3.1. The Most Important Tasks of PNs

In the inexperienced group, most people ranked support with applications (n = 525/47.5%) as the most important task of a navigator, followed by emotional support (n = 282/25.6%) and provision of information (n = 159/14.3%) (other support = 12.6%). In the experienced group, this ranking was slightly different. Support with applications was also ranked highest by about half of this subsample (n = 87/51.7%), followed by provision of information (n = 40/23.7%); few of the experienced ranked emotional support (n = 25/15.2%) as the most important task (other support = 9.4%).

3.2. Support with Applications

The descriptive results in Figure 1 show that within the inexperienced group, persons living in a partnership, younger respondents, men, chronically ill persons and respondents from rural regions assessed support with applications as the most important task of PNs (Figure 1). Younger respondents and chronically ill persons in the experienced group also answered more often than older respondents and persons without a chronic disease that support with applications is most important for them.

These results were confirmed by the results of the multiple regression models, with one exception: Within the inexperienced group, there was no substantial effect with city size after adjusting for the other characteristics. However, within the experienced group such an effect appeared: fewer people in rural areas (OR: 0.29; CI: 0.10, 0.89) and small towns (OR: 0.36; CI: 0.13, 0.98) than people in big cities assessed support with applications as most important (Table 2).

3.3. Provision of Healthcare Information

Within the inexperienced group, more highly educated than less educated persons and more persons with very good health than with poor health named the provision of health information as the most important task of PNs (Figure 1). In the experienced group, people from West Germany in particular assessed this task as the most important (Figure 1). The multiple regression analysis showed the same results. Within the inexperienced group, higher educated people had higher odds than lower educated people (OR: 1.55; CI: 1.06, 2.27) and people with bad health had lower odds than people with good health (OR: 0.54; CI: 0.32, 0.89) of ranking information as most important for them. Within the experienced group, more West than East Germans (OR: 3.59; CI: 1.06, 12.18) ranked information as the most important task (Table 2).

3.4. Emotional Support

For the inexperienced without a partner, emotional support from PN was identified as most important more often than for those with a partner. More women than men and more persons without a chronic disease compared with chronically ill persons rated emotional support as the most important task. The latter also applies to the experienced—more respondents without a chronic disease than with a chronic disease identified emotional support as the most important role of a PN. In the experienced group, the disproportionately high percentage of highly educated persons who stated that emotional support was most important is a striking result (Figure 1). Again, the results remained consistent in the multiple regression analyses. Within the inexperienced group, women, those without a partner and those without a chronic disease had higher odds of ranking emotional support as the most important task, whereas among the experienced, higher education was associated with emotional support as the most important task of a PN (Table 2).

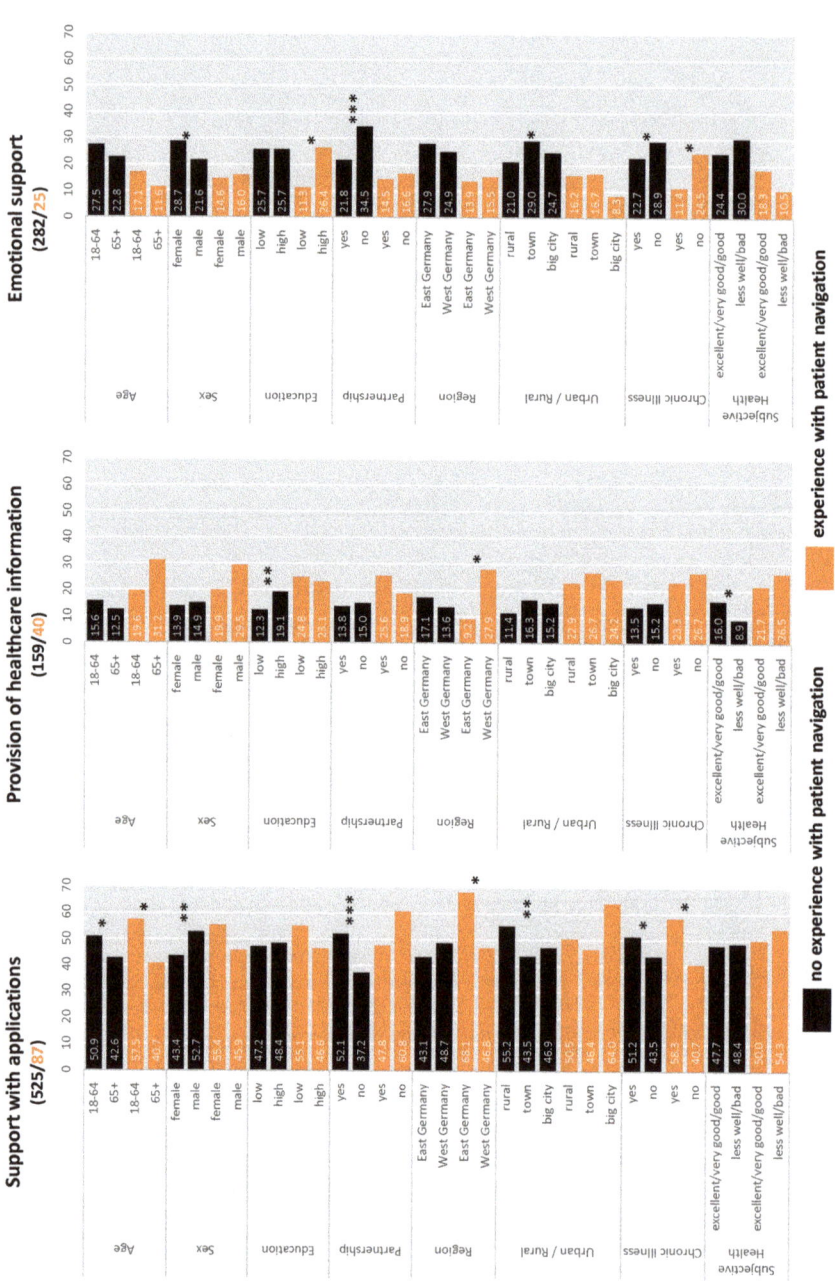

Figure 1. Differences (%, p) between the most important tasks and sociodemographic characteristics within both groups (persons with and without experience of patient navigation).

Table 2. Associations between the most important tasks within both groups and sociodemographic characteristics (multiple binary logistic regressions, OR 95% CI).

	No Experience with Patient Navigation			Experience with Patient Navigation		
	M1a. Application OR [95% CI]	M2a. Information OR [95% CI]	M3a. Emotional OR [95% CI]	M1b. Application OR [95% CI]	M2b. Information OR [95% CI]	M3b. Emotional OR [95% CI]
Age						
18–64	*1.33 [1.02, 1.74]*	1.15 [0.78, 1.69]	1.33 [0.97, 1.81]	*4.68 [1.86, 11.80]*	0.56 [0.22, 1.40]	0.64 [0.19, 2.17]
65+	1	1	1	1	1	1
Sex						
female	1	1	1	1	1	1
male	*1.55 [1.20, 2.00]*	0.98 [0.69, 1.40]	*0.66 [0.49, 0.89]*	0.48 [0.21, 1.07]	1.55 [0.68, 3.51]	1.27 [0.47, 3.45]
Education						
low	1	1	1	1	1	1
high	1.01 [0.76, 1.35]	*1.55 [1.06, 2.27]*	0.92 [0.66, 1.27]	0.56 [0.22, 1.45]	0.73 [0.27, 1.99]	*3.31 [1.05, 10.41]*
Partnership						
yes	*1.75 [1.32, 2.32]*	0.82 [0.56, 1.21]	*0.53 [0.39, 0.71]*	0.53 [0.23, 1.24]	1.66 [0.68, 4.07]	0.98 [0.33, 2.97]
no	1	1	1	1	1	1
Region						
West Germany	*1.40 [1.02, 1.92]*	0.70 [0.46, 1.06]	0.75 [0.53, 1.07]	0.38 [0.14, 1.01]	*3.59 [1.06, 12.18]*	0.90 [0.27, 2.97]
East Germany	1	1	1	1	1	1
Urban/rural						
rural ≤ 5000	1.33 [0.94, 1.88]	0.85 [0.52, 1.41]	0.84 [0.56, 1.26]	*0.29 [0.10, 0.89]*	1.03 [0.32, 3.24]	*3.15 [0.67, 14.67]*
town 5001–100,000	0.81 [0.59, 1.12]	1.14 [0.74, 1.76]	1.27 [0.89, 1.83]	*0.36 [0.13, 0.98]*	1.65 [0.59, 4.65]	1.82 [0.46, 7.25]
big city	1	1	1	1	1	1
Chronic illness						
yes	*1.68 [1.29, 2.20]*	0.91 [0.63, 1.32]	0.66 [0.49, 0.89]	*4.99 [2.01, 12.42]*	0.54 [0.21, 1.41]	0.37 [0.12, 1.17]
no	1	1	1	1	1	1
Subjective health						
less well/bad	1.00 [0.74, 1.37]	0.54 [0.32, 0.89]	1.30 [0.92, 1.84]	0.60 [0.26, 1.39]	1.46 [0.60, 3.53]	0.89 [0.28, 2.90]
excellent/very good/good	1	1	1	1	1	1
R^2 (Nagelkerke)	0.073	0.037	0.061	0.047	0.122	0.148

OR = odds ratios; 95% CI = and 95% confidence intervals, significant values at the 5% level are highlighted in italics.

4. Discussion

The present study provides evidence on the general population's views on PN tasks. Next to assessing the level of awareness of PNs in Germany, the objective of the study was to ascertain the most important tasks of PNs from the viewpoint of different population groups. 'Who needs what most?' was the guiding research question.

4.1. Comparison between Persons with and without Experience of PNs

Overall, about one-fifth of the population in Germany reported having heard of PNs, with 13% of this group already having had experience with this still fairly new care model. Assuming that prior experience with PNs has an influence on how the various tasks of navigators are prioritized by the patients, analyses were conducted separately for respondents with and without experience. The results show that there are both similarities and differences between the two groups. For both groups, it appears that the majority of respondents consider assistance with applications to be most important. For the inexperienced, however, emotional support is then cited second most often, while for the experienced, the second-ranked task was providing information.

There is wide evidence on the high relevance of health information as part of health literacy, which in turn influences people's health [7,25]. Broad activities have been carried out both nationally and internationally to disseminate health information to specific target groups or the general population—most recently during the COVID-19 pandemic [26–28]. However, the results of the present work indicate that in the case of a chronic illness or disease event, practical assistance in bureaucratic matters is even more important for patients than receiving information about their disease. Even though our results refer to Germany with its specific application system, e.g., in the field of rehabilitation care, studies from other countries also confirm the high relevance of bureaucratic support for patients in the healthcare system. A qualitative Canadian study explored caregivers' experiences caring for a child or youth with complex care needs, and their experiences and satisfaction as clients of a patient navigation center. As participants reported overwhelming organizational tasks, employed navigators supported the caregivers in bureaucratic matters and thus, among other things, improved the quality of life of the caring parents [29]. A study from the USA explored oncology navigators' perceptions of cancer-related financial burden and financial assistance resources via an online survey. Seventy-eight respondents participated in the survey, reporting that commonly identified barriers for patients obtaining assistance included lack of resources, lack of knowledge about resources and complex/duplicate paperwork [30]. This is in line with our study in which those with experience rated support with applications and the provision of information as most important for them more often than emotional support. Of course, this does not mean that emotional support is unimportant for this group of patients. One explanation for the relative lower ranking could be that this support need is currently better covered by existing support networks for chronically ill people and their psychological burdens. Psycho-oncology can be cited as a prominent example here [31]. In light of the current COVID-19 pandemic situation, the question which arises is whether respondents' prioritizing of PNs' tasks may change due to COVID's direct and indirect effects. In particular, it is conceivable that emotional support might be given a higher priority as people are more isolated and have more difficulties accessing support systems and healthcare. Simultaneously, it is possible that due to the increased barriers to gaining timely and adequate access to healthcare, people would rank practical/bureaucratic support as the most important tasks of PNs. Studies conducted during a future pandemic may use our binary coding system for a prompt assessment of the most important tasks of PNs; in such cases, the results should be analyzed depending on additionally integrated questions on the specific pandemic situation.

4.2. Support with Applications

In both groups there were associations with age and a chronic disease, i.e., regardless of experience with PN, support with applications was most important for younger respondents and respondents with a chronic disease. Thus, the priority here was not the need for health information, although a study showed that younger people in particular know little about health issues [32]. Due to their experiences, chronically ill patients, in turn, have a fairly good knowledge of health issues, so that their higher need for practical support seems plausible. This interpretation is in line with the results of a nationwide survey with chronically ill patients in the Netherlands [33]. In the experienced group, it is furthermore noteworthy that a high ranking for application support is particularly likely in big cities. Whether this is rooted in differences in individual support systems or an expanded understanding of healthcare providers' roles in rural versus urban areas in Germany has yet to be investigated.

4.3. Provision of Health Information

In the inexperienced group, the provision of health information by a PN is prioritized particularly often by well-educated respondents and respondents with good health. It is important to point out that a higher need for information does not necessarily mean a higher information deficit. On the contrary, with regard to educational attainment, various studies revealed a significant correlation between a high level of education and a high level of information, as well as a higher level of health literacy that goes along with it [32,33]. Health literacy includes the ability and desire to gather, obtain and understand health information [5,34,35]. In this respect, the results point to higher proactive behavior of higher educated people. This was confirmed by a study on informal caregivers based on a representative population survey in Germany. The results revealed that the odds of better educated people talking with their general practitioner about their burden of informal caregiving were significantly higher than for those with a lower education level [34]. These findings shed light on the needs of the population with low education levels, as they indicate lower proactive support seeking within this group. Studies in Germany showed that people with basic education are more likely to have difficulties in understanding health information than people with higher education [7,35]. This could be one reason for their lower proactive behavior compared to the higher educated. A study by Tille and colleagues in Germany revealed that health information seems to be insufficiently tailored to individuals aged 50 years and above as well as to those with intermediate and basic education [7]. Consequently, and in line with these results, it can be assumed that tailoring health information and materials to the competences of those with lower education may further facilitate these groups' understanding of health issues and foster patient empowerment.

The higher odds of people in West Germany than people in East Germany ranking the provision of information as a key task of PN is a noteworthy result in the experienced group. According to the results discussed above, this does not necessarily mean that there is a lower level of knowledge in West Germany. Also, it is possible that cultural differences due to previous exposure to differing healthcare systems in East and West Germany may account for this.

4.4. Emotional Support

The evaluation of emotional support was influenced by different characteristics—depending on already having had experience with PN or not. In the inexperienced group, women were more likely than men to prioritize emotional support. This result is confirmed by study results that show that women provide and receive more emotional support [36], which in turn can be explained by traditional role concepts and social norms [37–39]. However, it is notable that this association is no longer present in the experienced group. Here, the question that arises is whether the provision of a PN might have covered the emotional needs of women. The patient navigation studies currently being undertaken in Germany may well provide important insights here (for an overview of current patient navigation programs in Germany see [22]).

The protective effect of a partnership and social networks on health is confirmed by a number of studies [40–44]. Thus, the result is plausible that respondents without PN experience and without a partner were more likely than respondents with a partner to prioritize the emotional support of a PN. Analogous to the gender result discussed above, here too, the question is whether the support provided by a PN could have partly contributed to the result that respondents without a partner but with PN experience did not rank this form of support as a key task more often than respondents with a partner.

The result within the experienced group that better educated people rated emotional support as the most important task more often than less educated people points to a need for further research, as the background to this is unknown. A study by Oedekoven et al. on physical and mental burdens of informal caregivers showed that higher educated people were affected more often than lower educated people by mental burdens due to their caregiving situation [45]. According to these results, it seems that prevention measures and patient navigation programs should be tailored more precisely to the educational background of patients in order to meet their specific needs more effectively.

4.5. Strengths and Limitations

This study has substantial strengths, including a cohort of a large nationwide representative sample as well as the first ever assessment of patient navigation awareness and the population's view on PNs' most important tasks. Utilizing this sample, we provide evidence of the prioritized needs of different population groups regarding patient navigation. As a limitation of the study relating to the experienced group, the experience with navigation may be somewhat heterogeneous as patient navigation is not a care model that is regularly available to patients in Germany yet. On the one hand, the group may be comprised of participants from various model projects that are currently being evaluated in Germany. On the other hand, they may have experienced support from providers such as community care points or advice centers run by the Public Health Departments, which do not entirely fulfill the definition of patient navigation provided at the start of this paper but offer some forms of care management. Despite these differences, the study results indicate which support services patients seek most urgently.

Furthermore, the data were collected by telephone, and only people with a landline were contacted [7,23]. This might have resulted in a higher proportion of older persons being reached [46]. Older people refused to answer the question about the most important tasks of PNs more often than younger people (in both groups) and lower educated people more often than higher educated people (in the inexperienced group). Thus, differences in age and education may have been affected by differential refusal. However, as rates of missing data are low, we assume these effects are minor.

5. Conclusions

This study shows that the majority of people predominantly expect PN services to offer administrative support. However, there were variations in expectations by educational level, age, region and city size, health status, gender, marital status and prior experience with a patient navigation program. If no prior experience with PN programs exist, younger respondents and chronically ill people in particular prioritize support with applications as the most important task, while women and people without a partner rank emotional support and well-educated people the provision of health information as the most important task of a PN. If experience has already been gained with a PN, people in big cities rank support with applications most often as the most important task, while the provision of health information is prioritized more often by West than by East Germans and emotional support more often by better than by lower educated people.

In sum, results indicate that the social determinants of health, such as educational background, marital status or gender, should be recognized for tailored patient navigation models in order to provide better care and support to those in need. For successful broad-scale implementation of PN programs, it seems advisable to design the models flexibly so that the focus of the programs and navigators' tasks can vary depending on different population groups and their prioritized needs.

Author Contributions: Conceptualization, S.S. and N.R.; methodology, S.S. and U.G.; formal analysis, S.S. and R.K.; investigation, S.S. and F.E.; writing—original draft preparation, S.S.; writing—review and editing, S.S., R.K., H.F., K.G., J.S., F.E., U.G. and N.R.; funding acquisition, S.S. and N.R. All authors have read and agreed to the published version of the manuscript.

Funding: The present work is part of the research consortium 'NAVICARE—Patient-oriented health-services research'. NAVICARE is funded by the German Federal Ministry of Education and Research (01GY1911).

Institutional Review Board Statement: According to the local ethics committee of the Medical Faculty Charité—Universitätsmedizin Berlin, nonexperimental fully anonymized data do not require ethical approval according to national guidelines (2016/679 EU General Data Protection Regulation and Amtsblatt 230/2019, §2 Abs. 1. 2019). The KBV's Commissioner for Data Protection confirmed that all data protection standards have been met.

Informed Consent Statement: Informed consent was obtained from all subjects involved in the study.

Data Availability Statement: The datasets generated and analyzed during the current study will be stored in a non-publicly accessible repository. The access information is available from the corresponding author on reasonable request.

Acknowledgments: We thank Hillary Crowe for proofreading the final draft of the revised manuscript.

Conflicts of Interest: The authors declare no conflict of interest.

References

1. Fügemann, H.; Goerling, U.; Gödde, K.; Desch, A.K.; Müller-Nordhorn, J.; Mauckisch, V.; Siegerink, B.; Rieckmann, N.; Holmberg, C. What do people with lung cancer and stroke expect from patient navigation? A qualitative study in Germany. *BMJ Open* **2021**, *11*, e050601. [CrossRef] [PubMed]
2. Glaeske, G.; Hoffmann, F. Der Wettbewerb der Leitlinien bei älteren Menschen—Multimorbidität und Polypharmazie als Problem. *Neuro Geriatr.* **2009**, *6*, 115–119.
3. Ludt, S.; Heiss, F.; Glassen, K.; Noest, S.; Klingenberg, A.; Ose, D.; Szecsenyi, J. Patients' perspectives beyond sectoral borders between inpatient and outpatient care-patients' experiences and preferences along cross-sectoral episodes of care. *Gesundh. (Bundesverb. Arzte Offentlichen Gesundh. (Ger.))* **2013**, *76*, 359–365.
4. Nolte, E.; Knai, C.; Hofmarcher, M.; Conklin, A.; Erler, A.; Elissen, A.; Flamm, M.; Fullerton, B.; Sönnichsen, A.; Vrijhoef, H.J. Overcoming fragmentation in health care: Chronic care in Austria, Germany and The Netherlands. *Health Econ. Policy Law* **2012**, *7*, 125–146. [CrossRef] [PubMed]
5. Sørensen, K.; Van den Broucke, S.; Fullam, J.; Doyle, G.; Pelikan, J.; Slonska, Z.; Brand, H. Health literacy and public health: A systematic review and integration of definitions and models. *BMC Public Health* **2012**, *12*, 80. [CrossRef] [PubMed]
6. Schaeffer, D.; Berens, E.M.; Vogt, D. Health Literacy in the German Population. *Dtsch. Arztebl. Int.* **2017**, *114*, 53–60. [CrossRef]
7. Tille, F.; Weishaar, H.; Gibis, B.; Schnitzer, S. Patients' understanding of health information in Germany. *Patient Prefer. Adher.* **2019**, *13*, 805–817. [CrossRef]
8. Gödde, K.; Fügemann, H.; Müller-Nordhorn, J.; Grimberg, M.; Goerling, U.; Siegerink, B.; Rieckmann, N.; Holmberg, C. Structured Collection of Data on Support Offers for Lung Cancer and Stroke Patients in Berlin. *Gesundh. (Bundesverb. Arzte Offentlichen Gesundh. (Ger.))* **2020**, *84*, 35–42. [CrossRef] [PubMed]
9. Stumm, J.; Peter, L.; Sonntag, U.; Kümpel, L.; Heintze, C.; Döpfmer, S. Non-medical aspects in the care for multimorbid patients in general practice. What kind of support and cooperation is desired? Focus groups with general practitioners in Berlin. *Z. Evidenz Fortbild. Qual. Gesundh.* **2020**, *158*, 66–73. [CrossRef] [PubMed]
10. Stickel, A.; Gröpper, S.; Pallauf, A.; Goerling, U. Patients' knowledge and attitudes towards Cancer peer support programs. *Oncology* **2015**, *89*, 242–244. [CrossRef] [PubMed]
11. Carroll, J.K.; Humiston, S.G.; Meldrum, S.C.; Salamone, C.M.; Jean-Pierre, P.; Epstein, R.M.; Fiscella, K. Patients' experiences with navigation for cancer care. *Patient Educ. Couns.* **2010**, *80*, 241–247. [CrossRef] [PubMed]
12. Freeman, H.P. The origin, evolution, and principles of patient navigation. *Cancer Epidemiol. Prev. Biomark.* **2012**, *21*, 1614–1617. [CrossRef] [PubMed]
13. McBrien, K.A.; Ivers, N.; Barnieh, L.; Bailey, J.J.; Lorenzetti, D.L.; Nicholas, D.; Tonelli, M.; Hemmelgarn, B.; Lewanczuk, R.; Edwards, A.; et al. Patient navigators for people with chronic disease: A systematic review. *PLoS ONE* **2018**, *13*, e0191980. [CrossRef] [PubMed]

14. Peart, A.; Lewis, V.; Brown, T.; Russell, G. Patient navigators facilitating access to primary care: A scoping review. *BMJ Open* **2018**, *8*, e019252. [CrossRef] [PubMed]
15. Tan, C.H.; Wilson, S.; McConigley, R. Experiences of cancer patients in a patient navigation program: A qualitative systematic review. *JBI Database Syst. Rev. Implement. Rep.* **2015**, *13*, 136–168. [CrossRef]
16. van Ee, I.B.; Hagedoorn, M.; Slaets, J.P.; Smits, C.H. Patient navigation and activation interventions for elderly patients with cancer: A systematic review. *Eur. J. Cancer Care (Engl.)* **2017**, *26*, e12621. [CrossRef] [PubMed]
17. Freund, K.M.; Battaglia, T.A.; Calhoun, E.; Dudley, D.J.; Fiscella, K.; Paskett, E.; Raich, P.C.; Roetzheim, R.G.; Patient Navigation Research Program Group. National Cancer Institute Patient Navigation Research Program: Methods, protocol, and measures. *Cancer* **2008**, *113*, 3391–3399. [CrossRef] [PubMed]
18. Porzig, R.; Neugebauer, S.; Heckmann, T.; Adolf, D.; Kaskel, P.; Froster, U.G. Evaluation of a cancer patient navigation program ("Onkolotse") in terms of hospitalization rates, resource use and healthcare costs: Rationale and design of a randomized, controlled study. *BMC Health Serv. Res.* **2018**, *18*, 413. [CrossRef] [PubMed]
19. Fillion, L.; Cook, S.; Veillette, A.M.; Aubin, M.; de Serres, M.; Rainville, F.; Fitch, M.; Doll, R. Professional navigation framework: Elaboration and validation in a Canadian context. *Oncol. Nurs. Forum.* **2012**, *39*, E58–E69. [CrossRef]
20. Wilcox, B.; Bruce, S.D. Patient navigation: A "win-win" for all involved. *Oncol. Nurs. Forum.* **2010**, *37*, 21–25. [CrossRef] [PubMed]
21. Frick, J.; Schindel, D.; Gebert, P.; Grittner, U.; Schenk, L. Improving quality of life in cancer patients through higher participation and health literacy: Study protocol for evaluating the oncological social care project (OSCAR). *BMC Health Serv. Res.* **2019**, *19*, 754. [CrossRef] [PubMed]
22. Bundesverband Managed Care: BMC Lotsenprojekte in Deutschland. Available online: https://www.bmcev.de/wp-content/uploads/BMC-Lotsenlandkarte.pdf (accessed on 28 February 2022).
23. Kassenärztliche Bundesvereinigung. Versichertenbefragung der Kassenärztlichen Bundesvereinigung. 2019. Available online: https://www.kbv.de/media/sp/Berichtband_Ergebnisse_der_Versichertenbefragung_2019.pdf (accessed on 20 February 2022).
24. IBM Corp. *IBM SPSS Statistics for Windows. Version 27.0*; IBM Corp: Armonk, NY, USA, 2020.
25. Mackey, L.M.; Doody, C.; Werner, E.L.; Fullen, B. Self-Management Skills in Chronic Disease Management: What Role Does Health Literacy Have? *Med. Decis. Mak.* **2016**, *36*, 741–759. [CrossRef] [PubMed]
26. Nordanstig, A.; Asplund, K.; Norrving, B.; Wahlgren, N.; Wester, P.; Rosengren, L. Impact of the Swedish National Stroke Campaign on stroke awareness. *Acta Neurol. Scand.* **2017**, *136*, 345–351. [CrossRef]
27. Reilly, K.H.; Neaigus, A.; Shepard, C.W.; Cutler, B.H.; Sweeney, M.M.; Rucinski, K.B.; Jenness, S.M.; Wendel, T.; Marshall, D.M.; Hagan, H. It's Never Just HIV: Exposure to an HIV Prevention Media Campaign and Behavior Change among Men Who Have Sex with Men Participating in the National HIV Behavioral Surveillance System in New York City. *LGBT Health* **2016**, *3*, 314–318. [CrossRef]
28. Schaeffer, D.; Klinger, J.; Berens, E.M.; Gille, S.; Griese, L.; Vogt, D.; Hurrelmann, K. Health Literacy in Germany before and during the COVID-19 Pandemic. *Gesundheitswesen* **2021**, *83*, 781–788. [PubMed]
29. Luke, A.; Luck, K.E.; Doucet, S. Experiences of Caregivers as Clients of a Patient Navigation Program for Children and Youth with Complex Care Needs: A Qualitative Descriptive Study. *Int. J. Integr. Care* **2020**, *20*, 10. [CrossRef]
30. Spencer, J.C.; Samuel, C.A.; Rosenstein, D.L.; Reeder-Hayes, K.E.; Manning, M.L.; Sellers, J.B.; Wheeler, S.B. Oncology navigators' perceptions of cancer-related financial burden and financial assistance resources. *Support. Care Cancer* **2018**, *26*, 1315–1321. [CrossRef]
31. Lang-Rollin, I.; Berberich, G. Psycho-oncology. *Dialogues Clin. Neurosci.* **2018**, *20*, 13–22. [PubMed]
32. Schnitzer, S.; Kuhlmey, A.; Balke, K.; Litschel, A.; Walter, A.; Schenk, L. Kenntnisstand und Bewertung gesundheitspolitischer Reformen im Spiegel sozialer Determinanten. *Gesundheitswesen* **2011**, *73*, 153–161. [CrossRef] [PubMed]
33. Heijmans, M.; Waverijn, G.; Rademakers, J.; van der Vaart, R.; Rijken, M. Functional, communicative and critical health literacy of chronic disease patients and their importance for self-management. *Patient Educ. Couns.* **2015**, *98*, 41–48. [CrossRef]
34. Schnitzer, S.; Kuhlmey, A.; Engelmann, F.; Budnick, A. Informal caregivers and how primary care physicians can support them. *Dtsch. Arztebl. Int.* **2021**, *118*, 507–508. [CrossRef] [PubMed]
35. Schaeffer, D.; Vogt, D.; Berens, E.-M.; Hurrelmann, K. Gesundheitskompetenz der Bevölkerung in Deutschland: Ergebnisbericht. *Univ. Bielef. Fak. Für Gesundh.* **2016**, *28*, 2021. Available online: https://pub.uni-bielefeld.de/download/2908111/2908198/Ergebnisbericht_HLS-GER.pdf (accessed on 20 February 2022).
36. Dalgard, O.S.; Dowrick, C.; Lehtinen, V.; Vazquez-Barquero, J.L.; Casey, P.; Wilkinson, G.; Ayuso-Mateos, J.L.; Page, H.; Dunn, G.; Group, O. Negative life events, social support and gender difference in depression: A multinational community survey with data from the ODIN study. *Soc. Psych. Psych. Epid.* **2006**, *41*, 444–451. [CrossRef] [PubMed]
37. Addis, M.E.; Mahalik, J.R. Men, masculinity, and the contexts of help seeking. *Am. Psychol.* **2003**, *58*, 5–14. [CrossRef]
38. Mackenzie, C.S.; Gekoski, W.L.; Knox, V.J. Age, gender, and the underutilization of mental health services: The influence of help-seeking attitudes. *Aging Ment. Health* **2006**, *10*, 574–582. [CrossRef] [PubMed]
39. Seidler, Z.E.; Dawes, A.J.; Rice, S.M.; Oliffe, J.L.; Dhillon, H.M. The role of masculinity in men's help-seeking for depression: A systematic review. *Clin. Psychol. Rev.* **2016**, *49*, 106–118. [CrossRef] [PubMed]
40. Given, B.A.; Given, C.W.; Kozachik, S. Family support in advanced cancer. *CA Cancer J. Clin.* **2001**, *51*, 213–231. [CrossRef] [PubMed]

41. Schindel, D.; Schneider, A.; Grittner, U.; Jobges, M.; Schenk, L. Quality of life after stroke rehabilitation discharge: A 12-month longitudinal study. *Disabil. Rehabil.* **2021**, *43*, 2332–2341. [CrossRef] [PubMed]
42. Schneider, A.; Blüher, S.; Grittner, U.; Anton, V.; Schaeffner, E.; Ebert, N.; Jakob, O.; Martus, P.; Kuhlmey, A.; Wenning, V.; et al. Is there an association between social determinants and care dependency risk? A multi-state model analysis of a longitudinal study. *Res. Nurs. Health* **2020**, *43*, 230–240. [CrossRef] [PubMed]
43. Sparla, A.; Flach-Vorgang, S.; Villalobos, M.; Krug, K.; Kamradt, M.; Coulibaly, K.; Szecsenyi, J.; Thomas, M.; Gusset-Bahrer, S.; Ose, D. Individual difficulties and resources—A qualitative analysis in patients with advanced lung cancer and their relatives. *Patient Prefer. Adher.* **2016**, *10*, 2021–2029. [CrossRef]
44. Hajek, A.; König, H.-H. Longitudinal predictors of functional impairment in older adults in Europe–evidence from the survey of health, ageing and retirement in Europe. *PLoS ONE* **2016**, *11*, e0146967. [CrossRef]
45. Oedekoven, M.; Amin-Kotb, K.; Gellert, P.; Balke, K.; Kuhlmey, A.; Schnitzer, S. Associations between informal caregivers' burden and educational level. *GeroPsych* **2019**, *32*, 19. [CrossRef]
46. Jedro, C.; Holmberg, C.; Tille, F.; Widmann, J.; Schneider, A.; Stumm, J.; Dopfmer, S.; Kuhlmey, A.; Schnitzer, S. The Acceptability of Task-Shifting from Doctors to Allied Health Professionals. *Dtsch Arztebl. Int.* **2020**, *117*, 583–590. [CrossRef] [PubMed]

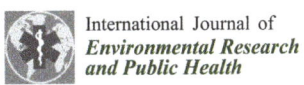

Article

How Is It to Live with Diabetes Mellitus? The Voices of the Diabetes Mellitus Clients

Charity Ngoatle [1,*] and Tebogo Maria Mothiba [2]

1. Department of Nursing Sciences, University of Limpopo, Polokwane 0727, South Africa
2. Faculty of Health Sciences, University of Limpopo, Polokwane 0727, South Africa
* Correspondence: charity.ngoatle@ul.ac.za; Tel.: +27-15-268-4652

Abstract: *Background*: Diabetes mellitus is described as a chronic disease resulting from failure of the pancreas to generate enough insulin or inability of the body to efficiently utilize the insulin it generates. Diabetes clients must adjust their lives to live healthy with the diseases for the rest of their lives. Optimizing diabetic knowledge and awareness among people living with diabetes will yield better health outcomes. This study seeks to investigate the knowledge, practices, and challenges of diabetes mellitus clients regarding management of the disease at selected clinics in the Capricorn District of Limpopo Province, South Africa. *Methods*: This study used a qualitative research approach and a phenomenological research design. A purposive sampling method was used to acquire the 18 participants for this study. Semi-structured interviews with a guide were used to collect data. Tesch's coding method was employed for data analysis. *Results*: The study findings revealed that there are comparable explanations of what it means to follow medication instructions by diabetes mellitus clients, and challenges living with DM. The findings also indicate that there are problems related to conceptualization of medication instructions among diabetes clients. *Conclusion*: This study indicated that diabetes mellitus clients have poor knowledge regarding management of the disease and its process, and problems related to medication instructions. Therefore, proper teaching of clients and guidance regarding diabetes and its management are required to improve compliance and delay of long-term complications.

Keywords: diabetes mellitus clients; diabetes mellitus; voices

1. Introduction

Diabetes is described as a chronic disease resulting from failure of the pancreas to generate enough insulin (type 1) or (type 1) inability of the body to efficiently utilize the insulin it generates [1]. The International Diabetes Federation (IDF) 2021 report recorded approximately 537 million individuals who are living with diabetes mellitus (DM) in worldwide [2]. The African continent claimed 24 million, with South Africa recording 4.5 million and the numbers continuing to rise [2]. The United Nations' (UN) Sustainable Development Goal (SDG) number 3.4 aims to reduce premature mortality from communicable diseases by one-third, by preventing, treating, and promoting mental health and well-being [3].

Since diabetes is a chronic disease, the clients must adjust their lives to live healthy with the diseases for the rest of their lives. Optimizing diabetic knowledge and awareness among people will yield better health outcomes for communities [4]. Increased diabetic knowledge is crucial for clients to enhance their lifestyle habits and improve medication adherence, resulting in better health benefits and delayed long-term complications [4]. Diabetes mellitus education is essential not only to the client but also to their families to adjust and manage the required lifestyle modification and offering psychological and dietary support [4].

Offering guidance to diabetes clients on where to source diabetes information is important to obtain credible knowledge. Most diabetes client obtain information from different

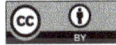

sources such as health professionals, educational sessions on DM, relatives, journals, television, websites and from other DM patients [5]. It has been found that good knowledge is linked to improved self-management practices and compliance to treatment in clients with diabetes mellitus [6].

Most diabetes clients in Iraq reported poor self-management practices due to a lack of proper knowledge because there are no educational programs on diabetes self-management strategies [7]. In Ethiopia, diabetes clients face challenges such as poor knowledge about diabetes, taking medication correctly, a lack of relationships with health professionals, poor support from friends and resulting loneliness with the disease [8]. Managing diabetes includes taking medication correctly and adopting a healthy lifestyle, which includes exercising and healthy eating [1]. The researchers wanted to understand what is the knowledge, practices and challenges of diabetes mellitus clients regarding management of the disease? This study sort to explore the knowledge, practices and challenges of diabetes mellitus clients regarding management of the disease at selected clinics in the Capricorn District of Limpopo Province, South Africa.

2. Methodology

2.1. Research Design

A qualitative, phenomenological, explorative, and descriptive research design was used to explore and describe the knowledge, practices, and challenges of clients regarding diabetes treatment at selected Clinics in the Capricorn District of Limpopo Province, South Africa. The design allowed the researcher to obtain an in-depth understanding of diabetic mellitus clients' knowledge, practices, and challenges of the disease and its treatment.

2.2. Study Setting

This study was conducted in four clinics (Dikgale clinic, Seobi-Dikgale clinic, Sebayeng clinic and Makotopong clinic) situated at the Ga-Dikgale village of the Capricorn District in Limpopo Province, South Africa. Dikgale is an established Health and Demographic Surveillance System (HDSS), which is run by the University of Limpopo with a high prevalence of NCDs, hence it was chosen as a study site.

2.3. Population and Sampling Strategy

The population of this study comprised all diabetes mellitus clients at Dikgale Village Clinics. The clinics cater for approximately 36,000 people and had 144 diabetes clients on treatment during the study period. Non-probability purposive sampling was used to acquire 18 participants who met the inclusion criteria and agreed to partake in this study. Participants who were free from hearing problems and psychologically sound were included in this study, whereas those who were physically unfit during the data collection period were excluded. The participants included sixteen (16) females and two (2) males. Data were collected in 2019 until saturation was reached.

Inclusion and Exclusion Criteria

Clients who were on treatment for more than a month and free from hearing problems were included. This study excluded diabetic clients who were physically unfit during the study period.

2.4. Data Collection Procedures

Semi-structured interviews using an interview schedule guide and audiotape were used to collect qualitative data. Field notes were taken to note down non-verbal cues which the voice recorder could not capture. A central question was posed in the same manner to each participant as follows: **"Could you please share with me how you take your medication"**? The central question was followed by probing questions after each participant's response. Data were collected until saturation, where no new information was coming up from the participants. The participants were also requested to hand in the packets of medications when they were explaining to compare what they were saying with what is written.

2.5. Data Analysis

The researchers applied Tesch's eight-step coding method to analyze the data as suggested by [9]. The researchers listened to the tape repeatedly and transcribed all information verbatim into a script. The transcripts and field notes were read to obtain a sense of the whole. The data were organized into themes and sub-themes. The researchers determined the most descriptive wording for the themes and sub-themes and the researchers re-coded existing material. The themes and sub-themes were summarized, and the data were sent to the independent coder.

2.6. Measures to Ensure Trustworthiness

Trustworthiness was ensured by applying the criteria of credibility, dependability, confirmability and transferability [9]. Credibility was ensured through engaging with the participants for approximately thirty minutes and conducting an audit trial. Dependability was ensured by use of the independent coder who is an expert in qualitative research to analyze data and a consensus meeting was held with the researchers to agree on the codes reached independently. Confirmability was ensured by providing a detailed methodology of this study. Transferability was ensured by providing enough details of the research methodology, which entails the research design, the population, the sampling method and the ethical considerations.

2.7. Ethical Clearance and Ethical Considerations

The researcher obtained ethical clearance from the University of Limpopo's Turfloop Research Ethics Committee (TREC), number: TREC/373/2017/PG. The researcher asked permission to conduct this study from the Department of Health Limpopo Province (approval number: LP_2017 11 016), Department of Health Capricorn District and the Nursing manager of the four Dikgale Village Clinics by writing requisition letters attached with research proposal.

The participants agreed to take part in this study voluntarily and were made aware that they could withdraw from participating at any time. Participants were also assured that their identity will not be revealed by assigning them codenames as their identification instead of their names.

3. Results

The results are presented below as reflected by diabetes mellitus clients. Table 1 presents the two themes and twelve sub-themes which emerged from this study.

Table 1. Themes and sub-themes.

	Themes		Sub-Themes
1.	Analogous explanations of what it means to follow medication instructions by diabetes mellitus clients	1.1	Adherence to medication instructions as directed by health professionals
		1.2	Questionable interpretation of adherence to medication instructions
		1.3	Description of the aspects to be considered when following medication instructions
		1.4	Lack of adherence to medication instructions viewed as "Digging a grave for self"
		1.5	Existence of daily health education sessions in clinics versus acceptance of medication instructions and related health advice as stipulated by nurses
		1.6	An explanation that there is a need versus no need for DMP to be assisted with adherence to medications
2.	Challenges experienced by DMP	2.1	Difficulties living with diabetes mellitus co-existing with other body ailments
		2.2	Socio-economic status versus adherence to medication
		2.3	Misunderstanding of medication instructions and the effect on treatment lifespan
		2.4	Lack of specific medication instructions provided by professional nurses
		2.5	Lack of specific medication instructions written on medication packages
		2.6	Illiterate DMP not catered for in medication instructions

3.1. Analogous Explanations of What It Means to Follow Medication Instructions by Diabetes Mellitus Clients

The study participants demonstrated an analogous explanation of what it means to follow medication instructions. This theme is supported by six sub-themes outlined in Table 2 below.

Table 2. Analogous explanations of what it means to follow medication instructions by diabetes mellitus.

	Theme 1		Sub-Themes
1.	Analogous explanations of what it means to follow medication instructions by diabetes mellitus clients	1.1	Adherence to medication instructions as directed by health professionals
		1.2	Questionable interpretation of adherence to medication instructions
		1.3	Description of the aspects to be considered when following medication instructions
		1.4	Lack of adherence to medication instructions viewed as "Digging a grave for self"
		1.5	Existence of daily health education sessions in clinics versus acceptance of medication instructions and related health advice as stipulated by nurses
		1.6	An explanation that there is a need versus no need for DMP to be assisted with adherence to medications

3.1.1. Adherence to Medication Instructions as Directed by Health Professionals

The findings show that participants adhere to medication instructions as directed by health professionals. This is evident in **Participant "D" saying** *"I take them the way they said should take them, i.e., two times, just that way. I would take them that way; in the morning and the evening. Is it that I would check them"*? **Participant "E" also gave their version, saying** *"It is just the fact that here at the clinic they said I should take the medication 3 times a day then I chose my times that I am going to take them when I wake up, during the day and in the evening before I sleep"*. **Yet Participant "H" said** *"We are guided by the nurses. The nurses teach us day by day that I should not at any time skip the time that I take the medication, and I should not at any time say I forgot them. Meaning lawfully our medication is taken daily and after meals"*.

3.1.2. Questionable Interpretation of Adherence to Medication Instructions

The study findings revealed that there is a questionable interpretation of adherence to the medications amongst diabetic clients. The interpretation includes the perception of how often the medication should be taken, the frequency explained is not clear and it differs from all the diabetes mellitus clients. This was manifested by **Participant "U" saying** *"I take my pills three times a day. I take them in the morning at 08:00, then at 13:00, and again at 18:00 in the evening"*. **Participant "U" further said** *"If they say I should take them four times, I should take them at around past 08:00, then at 11:00 I would take them. At 13:00 then I take the medications again and again at 17:00, then I would the medications again. It would be after taking food as it is time for food, then I would be done"*. **Participant "V" gave a diverse opinion but that did not differ much from the previous participant and said** *"My tablets, I take them at 07:00 am, again at 13:00, then lastly at 19:00"*. **Yet Participant "B" said** *"My diabetic medication, I am taking them in the morning around 08:00 or 09:00 is late and again at night when I go to sleep. I take them two times a day. "We were told the time when we were given the medications here at the clinic to take them in the morning and the evening"*. **Participant "H" also supports the previous participants and said** *"I eat in the morning at 07:00 and take the tablets, at 14:00 I would eat and take my tablets then in the late afternoon around 16:00 to 17:00 I would eat again and take my tablets"*.

3.1.3. Description of the Aspects to Be Considered When following Medication Instructions

The study findings also showed that there are certain aspects to considered when following medication instructions. This was seen in **Participant "C" highlighting that** *"When I take my first pill I eat first; we do not eat too much food because they said we must eat a fist-size pap and then wait for few minutes and take the medication. And they also said we should drink a lot of water so that the pills may be able to melt when they reach the stomach. Is it they say when the pills reach the stomach, they group themselves and sit"*? **Participant "H" also said** *"As I have already said that you give yourself time to say at such and such a time, I would take them* even when I visit places, I go with them in my bag. So, when that time arrives, I make sure that I ate something and take my pills so that I would not skip as it is not allowed". **Participant "M" gave their version, saying** "They said these medications should be taken after meals, so after eating we do take them". **Lastly, Participant "P" said** "I would take them in the morning and then again in the evening. Nonetheless, do not take them on an empty stomach; have something to eat then the pill will follow. That is how the doctor would have told, so you follow what the doctor would have told you".

3.1.4. Lack of Adherence to Medication Instructions Is Viewed by DMP as "Digging a Grave for Self"

The findings show that the participants view a lack of adherence to medication as digging a grave for self. This was seen in **Participant "P" saying** "The complications of not taking medication properly is that when the disease is going to come back to you, is it you would feel you are healed then feel like stopping the pills, most people stop. So, if they stop the pills; the next thing when the disease attacks again it becomes so hard where they would even fall. So, it does not want that when you use it then tomorrow say you no longer want the pill. Just continue until, it is your life, just accept yourself that this pill is your life". **Participant "T" said** "If you do not take them on time, they would not be able to control you well in the body because you would not be taking them on time. You might therefore come and say the pills are not working while the pills are working but the problem being you not taking them correctly. We might suffer dizziness and fall and then have problems. Sometimes your body might itch because you are not using your pills properly. So, it is needful that you use your pills correctly. Take them well in the morning, during the day and in the evening so that you might live well. So, for me to always be complicated it is because of not taking medication correctly, at correct times". **Yet Participant "U" alluded that** "I mean he would be affected badly because if you are not taking medication correctly you are making the disease to grow such that it would not be controlled. Because if you take them the day you like, you are not safe on the medications. It means you are just taking them because you collected them at the clinic while you are supposed to use them correctly and lawfully".

3.1.5. Existence of Daily Health Education Sessions in the Clinics Versus Acceptance of Medication Instructions and Related Health Advice as Stipulated by Nurses

The study findings revealed that there are health education sessions taking place daily at clinics. However, the findings also showed that some participants accept and follow medication instructions and related health advice given by nurses, whereas others do not. **Participant "C" said** "Yes, here at the clinic they are teaching us; after having a prayer, they then start teaching us about medication and say today is the day for Diabetes mellitus, tomorrow is for blood pressure, so on and so forth". **Participant "C" also indicated that they accept the health advice given by nurses and said** "Is it each time they teach us about sugar diabetes, I listen. Since I am suffering from it, I want to follow the instructions concerning it". **Participant "H" further said** "We are guided by the nurses. The nurses teach us day by day that I should not at any time skip the time that I take the medication, and I should not at any time say I forgot them". **Yet Participant "V" also said** "We come here at the clinic; here they tell us that the medications they give us, for diabetes mellitus we should take them three times a day. They teach us how we should take them". **On the contrary, participants do not follow medication instructions due to different reasons. Participant "D" alluded that** "We were told that we should take the medication continuously because if we stop, by the time we try them again they might not treat the disease well. But myself now I skipped a month to two because my husband was sick and I and to take care of him". **Participant "ZZ" mentioned that** "I cannot really say I am taking them properly. And yes, the sugar would not be at the required level because I am not taking them properly. Myself I have a machine for testing sugar. So, when I wake up in the morning, I check the sugar and if I find it to be around ke 10.5mmol or 11mmol or around 13mmol there, then, I get discouraged to eat. Because I will eat, and the sugar go a further higher. Then I tell myself not to eat until it goes a little bit down then eat later, because I will never take my medication without eating".

3.1.6. An Explanation That There Is a Need Versus no Need for DMP to Be Assisted with Adherence to the Medications

The findings illustrate that some participants need education on medication instructions, whereas others do not see the need. **Participant "N" indicated that they need assistance and said** *"Assistance like today we met a certain sister who is assisting us on how to take our medication. So, I feel we need assistance to be reminded of how we should take edications"*. **Participant "O" is aware that they are not taking medication correctly and hence need assistance,** *"Yes, I do need assistance because the way I am taking overdose is not correct"*. **Yet Participant "T" further said** *"I am not satisfied. I feel I need assistance on how I should eat and how to take medication correctly. I do not have such knowledge, I need it"*. On an obstinate, some participants indicated that they do not need assistance. **Participant "C" said** *"No, I do not think I need it because our nurses each time we come to collect medication, they give us a health talk about the different diseases and we get educated that people with this kind of disease take their medication like this, those with that disease they take their medication that way, so on and so forth"*. **Participant "V" also said** *"According to me, I do not need it because every day when we collect medications here at the clinic, they teach us how we should take the medication"*. **Yet Participant "U" said** *"No, I do not need it. I see myself taking the medications correctly, I am satisfied"*.

3.2. Challenges Experienced by Diabetes Mellitus Clients (DMPs)

The participants of this study exhibited that they are experiencing challenges related to medication instructions. This theme is supported by six sub-themes outlined in Table 3 below.

Table 3. Challenges experienced by diabetes mellitus clients (DMCs).

	Theme 2		Sub-Themes
2.	Challenges experienced by DMP	2.1	Difficulties living with diabetes mellitus co-existing with other body ailments
		2.2	Socio-economic status versus adherence to medication
		2.3	Misunderstanding of medication instructions and the effect on treatment lifespan
		2.4	Lack of specific medication instructions provided by professional nurses
		2.5	Lack of specific medication instructions written on medication packages
		2.6	Illiterate DMP not catered for in medication instructions

3.2.1. Difficulties in Living with Diabetes Mellitus Co-Existing with Other Body Ailments

The study results revealed that participants have difficulties living with diabetes mellitus while it co-exists with other body ailments. This is evident in **Participant "B"**, **who indicated that** *"Since I started with this medication, you see these fingers, they just get painful and swollen"*. **Participant "D" also had the same problem and said** *"Hmn . . . reality is that we want to be made whole even though when you try getting better other pains rise up"*. **Yet Participant "ZZ" indicated their frustration in this manner and said** *"The feet were swelling, and they even changed colour to black for many years until I decided to budget money for specialist. I wish they could stop swelling for good even though they are painful since the other one was once operated, and it is not completely healed, so the other one has to be operated as soon as the other is healed"*.

3.2.2. Socio-Economic Status versus Adherence to Medication

The study results revealed that the socio-economic status of the participants affects adherence to medication. **This is evident in Participant "A", who said** *"It may be that they say take your medication before you eat but when you have to take the medication you find that there is no food, you going to have to wait for the time there is food, and you eat and then take the medication, then do you see that the medication would not treat you well? Because one day it would reach 10:00 without you taking the medication while you will be waiting for the food then the medication is going to squeeze that one for 13:00"*. **Participant "I" supports this sub-theme and indicated that** *"Yes, we do take our diabetic pills, but my problem is that I would like to know that there were these diabetic pills that we were using on tea, but we are no longer being given them. I just want to know that since we are no longer given the tablets for tea, then could we go back to using sugar? So, "I do not know whether to go back to using sugar or not because those tea tablets* were fighting with sexual affairs and now that is a problem". **Yet Participant "J" said** *"Yes, I practice it. Do not you hear me when I say I do not want to lie to say I take them at 08:00 a.m., I could say I take them after each 08:00 a.m. So, I want to tell the truth that sometimes instead of taking the medication at 08:00, I take them after 08:00 a.m. whilst I will be busy with my child or I would be cooking. I would say I want to take the medication at 08:00 am but end up taking it at 09:00 a.m."*.

3.2.3. Misunderstanding of Medication Instructions and the Effect on Treatment Lifespan

Study findings revealed that participants misunderstood medication instructions and that results in a negative impact on client treatment lifespans. **Participant "M" said** *"The one that is called Metformin, I take it 3 times a day. I take it in the morning at 08:00, during the day at 13:00 and in the evening at 20:00. We just see us drinking them. We are not getting better, when you get heartburn, they say it is the sugar diabetes"*. **Participant "O" avows that** *"The one to be taken three times, I take it at 07:00 am, then at 13:00 and at 19:30. But I do not get better. I have lost a lot of weight; most of the time I lack appetite, I cannot eat but busy taking the pills"*. **Participant "I" also said** *"OH, I also take them after teatime in the morning between 09:00 and 10:00 am., then after lunch around 13:00 to 14:00 and in the evening around 18:00 to 19:00 before I sleep. I am troubled by one thing though, we do take the medications but Hai! They look like they are not working well because the disease just continues. Sometimes you just find yourself walking and you experience cramps or something like that"*.

3.2.4. Lack of Specific Medication Instructions Provided by Professional Nurses

The study results show that there is a lack of specific medication instructions provided by medication dispensers to the participants. **When Participant "G" was asked if it was explained to them how to use the medications, they said** *"No. They have never explained well to me, but they just said I should take the medication in the morning, during the day, and when I go to sleep"*. **Participant "C" also said** *"Myself, I was told to take my medication in the morning after eating and at night before I sleep"*. **Yet Participant "E" said** *"They said I should take the medication the way they are, but for the times and hours no. They just said in the morning, during the day, and at night"*. **Participant "Y" also added** *"No, they just say 'You know that you take you medication twice or thrice', so if you are taking them twice it means you will take them in the morning and evening and if it is three times, you will take them in the morning, afternoon and evening but the exact time they do not tell us"*. Participant "Y" went further to say that it was never explained to them how they should take the medication, and **Participant "B" said** *"They just write on the papers to say; once a day, three times a day or two times a day"*.

3.2.5. Lack of Specific Medication Instructions Written on Medication Packages

The study results show that there is a lack of specific medication instructions written on medication packages. **Participant "I" alluded that** *"I usually take them after tea in the morning and in the afternoon after eating, then would take another one, "No, I just see when they have written on the tablets packages; two times a day"*. **Participant "M" also said** *"The one that is called Metformin, I take it 3 times a day. I take it in the morning, during the day and in the evening. Is it, it is because it is written on the packaging"*! **Yet Participant "ZZ", with the same view, said** *"Is it they write on the packages that this one you take it twice a day, the other once daily after meals. They do not tell us the time to say that this one you should take it at 06:00, the other at 20:00. They just say take it twice daily meaning in the morning and evening. If it is three times it means is morning, afternoon, and at night when you sleep, but to say what time, no"*.

3.2.6. Illiterate DMP Not Catered for in Medication Instructions

The results show that illiterate diabetic clients are not catered for, in medication instructions written on the packaging and packet insert. This was specified by **Participant "T", who indicated that** *"I might not know because I cannot read. I only know the white big one. It is the one that I know I take it three times a day. All the others, they have even given me other pills, but I just do not know if they are related to diabetes mellitus because I am also suffering from high* blood pressure. I have two diseases". **Another participant, Participant "B", indicated that they cannot read English but can read the instructions and said** "Yes I can, even though I cannot read English. They write the instruction with a pen to say one tablet". **Participant "M" also said** "I do not know. These English things, where would we know them from"? **While Participant "T" elaborated** "Eish! Coming to the times I do not want to lie because I do not know the time, I have just timed that I take it around 09:00 am. Sometimes I forget and take it at 08:00 am or 09:00 am. The next dose I take at 14:00, I time the phone, if I see it written 1 and 4 (14), then I start to take it then in the evening when Muvhango starts then I take it. Those are the things I use to time my medication times because I cannot read".

4. Discussion

This study sought to investigate the knowledge, practices, and challenges of clients regarding diabetes treatment. The participants displayed adherence to treatment instructions as directed by medication dispensers. However, the information provided seemed inadequate, and this resulted in most participants not adhering to treatment through a lack of awareness. As a result, those participants did not think they need assistance with interpretation of medication instructions. In health care settings, medication adherence should be taken into account during the prescribing and dispensing process, and it should be given more attention [10]. Therefore, health professionals need to have higher levels of knowledge as they are the primary source of information for patients [4]. However, the authors of [4] found that health professionals in Saudi Arabia had low literacy levels related to diabetes mellitus. On the other hand, low patient knowledge such as stopping medication when feeling better and double dosing were found to be hindrances to treatment adherence [11].

The participants also highlighted some aspects which need to be considered when following treatments which enhance treatment compliance such as taking food before medication. These results concur with [12], where non-adherence to medication was linked to a lack of food as the food was supposed to be taken before medication. Socio-economic status has also been found to play a role in influencing treatment adherence in diabetes clients. Similar results have been recorded, where socio-economic circumstances were amongst the determinants of health in diabetes clients [13].

The participants exhibited a questionable understanding of how they view adherence. The way the participants were following their treatment showed that they do not understand the instructions even though they said they were adhering to them. Similar findings were observed by [14], where clients would leave their clinic visits not understanding health professional instructions related to treatment, even though they said they do. Adherence to treatment includes lifestyle modification, healthy eating and following recommendations related to medication on timing, dosage, frequency, and duration of medication use [15]. In another study, participants would stop medications when feeling better and some were not even aware of the implications thereof [11].

The participants had difficulty living with diabetes while having other body ailments. Similar results have been recorded, where participants had to take many medications for different ailments and ended up not taking diabetes medications as they did not know which one to take when [11].

The results also showed that participants misunderstood medication instructions and the effects on treatment lifespan. The same results were found where participants were following medication instructions but would stop when feeling better, and when they felt that the medication cost (price) was not equivalent to its effectiveness [11].

Some participants understand that non-adherence to treatment instructions is dangerous to their health and life, whereas some do not. Similar results were found where diabetes clients felt that adhering to treatment is difficult and overwhelming even though it was right to do so [16]. Another study found that diabetes clients had a misconception about treatment adherence, which led to non-adherence and poor health outcomes [17].

5. Summary

There were challenges faced by the participants in adhering to their treatment. A few aspects are worth mentioning as hindrances to adherence—low socio-economic status, misunderstanding of medication instructions, or non-existence of detailed medication instructions provided by professional nurses or on packages of medication, diabetes mellitus may also coexist with other body ailments, and illiteracy.

- The study site is overburdened with communicable diseases which are not controlled despite clients collecting their medications on monthly basis.
- There was no published data on how patients consume their medication and how professional nurses at primary care explain medication instructions to patients.
- What is the knowledge, practices, and challenges of diabetes mellitus clients regarding diabetes as a disease, its process and treatment?
- This study revealed that the medication dispensers at the primary health care level do not give in-depth education regarding diabetes and its treatment to the client.
- This study recommended that health care professionals should provide in-depth education about diabetes and its treatment, including explaining medication instructions to patients.

6. Limitations

This study was conducted in selected clinics in the Capricorn district of the Limpopo province of South Africa. Thus, the findings of this study cannot be generalized to other settings. The same methods, however, can yield similar results.

7. Implications of the Findings

The study findings confirm that continuous health education and guidance related to diabetes mellitus and its management should be underway.

7.1. The Health Care Professionals

Health professionals dispensing medications to diabetes clients should offer a thorough explanation and clarification of medication instructions to promote adherence. The explanation must include the lifestyle modifications and the disease process.

7.2. Limpopo Department of Health

The Limpopo department of health must conduct workshops for health care professionals on the interpretation of medication instructions and evaluate the effectiveness of the available self-management strategies for diabetes.

7.3. Department of Education

Health literacy related to interpretation of medication instructions must be incorporated in school curriculums for children to learn how medication is consumed properly and to teach other members at home.

8. Conclusions

This study indicated that diabetic clients have deficiencies in knowledge related to diabetes as a disease and treatment such as poor conceptualization of medication instructions and self-management strategies. Proper education regarding the disease and its management, including medication instructions, will improve adherence to treatment.

Author Contributions: Conceptualization, C.N. and T.M.M.; methodology, C.N. and T.M.M.; validation, T.M.M.; formal analysis, C.N.; investigation, C.N.; resources, C.N. and T.M.M.; data curation, C.N. writing—original draft preparation, C.N.; writing—review and editing, C.N. and T.M.M.; visualization, C.N.; supervision, T.M.M.; project administration, T.M.M.; funding acquisition, T.M.M. All authors have read and agreed to the published version of the manuscript.

Funding: This study was supported by the Flemish Interuniversity Council (VLIR UOS Limpopo project), grant number: ZIUS2018AP021, and an NIHSS Scholarship in association with SAWUDA (number: SDS17/1548).

Institutional Review Board Statement: Ethical clearance was obtained from the University of Limpopo's Turfloop Research Ethics Committee (TREC) (TREC/373/2017/PG). Permission to conduct this study was given by the Department of Health Limpopo Province (approval number: LP_2017 11 016), Department of Health Capricorn District and the Nursing manager of the concerned clinics.

Informed Consent Statement: Participants voluntarily participated in this study and signed informed consent. Information was provided to them to make informed decisions including the fact that their information will be published.

Conflicts of Interest: The authors declare no conflict of interest.

References

1. World Health Organisation. Diabetes. 2021. Available online: https://www.who.int/news-room/fact-sheets/detail/diabetes (accessed on 4 March 2022).
2. International Diabetes Federation. Diabetes Atlas. 2022. Available online: https://diabetesatlas.org/ (accessed on 4 March 2022).
3. United Nations. Department of Economic and Social Affairs Disability. 2022. Available online: https://www.un.org/development/desa/disabilities/about-us/sustainable-development-goals-sdgs-and-disability.html (accessed on 4 March 2022).
4. Alanazi, F.K.; Alotaibi, J.S.; Paliadelis, P.; Alqarawi, N.; Alsharari, A.; Albagawi, B. Knowledge and awareness of diabetes mellitus and its risk factors in Saudi Arabia. *Saudi Med. J.* **2018**, *39*, 981. [CrossRef] [PubMed]
5. Cantaro, K.; Jara, J.A.; Taboada, M.; Mayta-Tristán, P. Association between information sources and level of knowledge about diabetes in patients with type 2 diabetes. *Endocrinol. Y Nutr.* **2016**, *63*, 202–211. [CrossRef]
6. Chavan, G.M.; Waghachavare, V.B.; Gore, A.D.; Chavan, V.M.; Dhobale, R.V.; Dhumale, G.B. Knowledge about diabetes and relationship between compliance to the management among the diabetic patients from Rural Area of Sangli District, Maharashtra, India. *J. Fam. Med. Prim. Care* **2015**, *4*, 439.
7. Mikhael, E.M.; Hassali, M.A.; Hussain, S.A.; Shawky, N. Self-management knowledge and practice of type 2 diabetes mellitus patients in Baghdad, Iraq: A qualitative study. *Diabetes Metab. Syndr. Obes. Targets Ther.* **2019**, *12*, 1–17. [CrossRef] [PubMed]
8. Bhagavathula, A.S.; Gebreyohannes, E.A.; Abegaz, T.M.; Abebe, T.B. Perceived obstacles faced by diabetes patients attending university of Gondar Hospital, Northwest Ethiopia. *Front. Public Health* **2018**, *6*, 81. [CrossRef] [PubMed]
9. Creswell, J.W.; Creswell, J.D. *Research Design: Qualitative, Quantitative, and Mixed Methods Approaches*; Sage Publications: Thousand Oaks, CA, USA, 2017.
10. Celio, J.; Ninane, F.; Bugnon, O.; Schneider, M.P. Pharmacist-nurse collaborations in medication adherence-enhancing interventions: A review. *Patient Educ. Couns.* **2018**, *101*, 1175–1192. [CrossRef] [PubMed]
11. Naqvi, A.A.; Hassali, M.A.; Aftab, M.T.; Nadir, M.N. A qualitative study investigating perceived barriers to medication adherence in chronic illness patients of Karachi, Pakistan. *JPMA* **2019**, *69*, 216.
12. Imel, B.E.; McClintock, H.F. Food Security and Medication Adherence in Young and Middle-Aged Adults with Diabetes. *Behav. Med.* **2021**, 1–8. [CrossRef] [PubMed]
13. Walker, R.J.; Williams, J.S.; Egede, L.E. Influence of race, ethnicity and social determinants of health on diabetes outcomes. *Am. J. Med. Sci.* **2016**, *351*, 366–373. [CrossRef] [PubMed]
14. Bodenheimer, T. Teach-Back: A simple technique to enhance patients' understanding. *Fam. Pract. Manag.* **2018**, *25*, 20–22. [PubMed]
15. Jakovljević, M. Non-adherence to medication: A challenge for person-centred pharmacotherapy to resolve the problem. *Psychiatr. Danub.* **2014**, *26* (Suppl. S2), 2–7.
16. Mondesir, F.L.; Levitan, E.B.; Malla, G.; Mukerji, R.; Carson, A.P.; Safford, M.M.; Turan, J.M. Patient perspectives on factors influencing medication adherence among people with coronary heart disease (CHD) and CHD risk factors. *Patient Prefer. Adherence* **2019**, *13*, 2017. [CrossRef] [PubMed]
17. Islam, S.M.S.; Biswas, T.; Bhuiyan, F.A.; Mustafa, K.; Islam, A. Patients' perspective of disease and medication adherence for type 2 diabetes in an urban area in Bangladesh: A qualitative study. *BMC Res. Notes* **2017**, *10*, 131. [CrossRef] [PubMed]

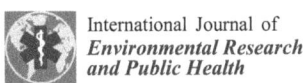

Article

"I Had to Rediscover Our Healthy Food": An Indigenous Perspective on Coping with Type 2 Diabetes Mellitus

Maya Maor [1,*], Moflah Ataika [2], Pesach Shvartzman [3] and Maya Lavie Ajayi [4]

1. Department of Sociology and Anthropology, Ariel University, Ariel 4070000, Israel
2. Clalit Health Services, Siaal Research Center for Family and Primary Care, Division of Community Health, Ben Gurion University of the Negev, Beer-Sheva 8410501, Israel; ataikam@bgu.ac.il
3. Pain and Palliative Care Unit, Siaal Research Center for Family Medicine and Primary Care, Division of Community Health, Ben Gurion University of the Negev, Beer-Sheva 8410501, Israel; pshvartzman@gmail.com
4. Gender Studies, Ben Gurion University of the Negev, Beer-Sheva 8410501, Israel; laviema@bgu.ac.il
* Correspondence: mayam@ariel.ac.il

Abstract: Type 2 Diabetes Mellitus (T2DM) is disproportionally prevalent among the Bedouin minority in Israel, with especially poor treatment outcomes compared to other indigenous groups. This study uses the perspective of the Bedouins themselves to explore the distinct challenges they face, as well as their coping strategies. The study is based on an interpretive interactionist analysis of 49 semi-structured interviews with Bedouin men and women. The findings of the analysis include three themes. First, physical inequality: the Bedouin community's way of coping is mediated by the transition to a semi-urban lifestyle under stressful conditions that include the experience of land dispossession and the rupture of caring relationships. Second, social inequality: they experience an inaccessibility to healthcare due to economic problems and a lack of suitable informational resources. Third, unique resources for coping with T2DM: interviewees use elements of local culture, such as religious practices or small enclaves of traditional lifestyles, to actively cope with T2DM. This study suggests that there is a need to expand the concept of active coping to include indigenous culture-based ways of coping (successfully) with chronic illness.

Keywords: diabetes; the Bedouin community; social inequality; active coping

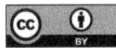

1. Introduction

Type 2 diabetes mellitus (T2DM) is disproportionally prevalent among indigenous groups, where its treatment outcomes are especially poor, and the complication rates are higher. This paper is based on the first qualitative study that is designed to explore the narratives of coping with T2DM by the Bedouin men and women from Israel. On the basis of a critical analysis of the literature in the field, we present a typology of the main theoretical approaches to the study of coping with T2DM among indigenous minorities: the biomedical approach, the minorities in transition approach, and the social justice approach. We explain the fundamentals of each approach and the reason behind our choice to employ the social justice approach in the analysis of our findings.

Following the presentation of the study's methodology, we demonstrate how listening to people's own narratives expands the previous understandings of indigenous culture in at least two ways. First, the influence of indigenous culture on coping is mediated through ethnic inequality, such as a lack of routine medical examinations or unsuitable living conditions. Thus, the negative influence of indigenous culture on coping is not predetermined. Second, indigenous narratives allow us to see how indigenous culture may be used in the service of optimal coping, e.g., using religious beliefs to counter T2DM-related stigmas or using traditional indigenous foods to control glucose blood levels. Together, these findings elucidate the critically important role of qualitative in-depth interviews in both explaining and targeting obstacles specific to indigenous groups that cope with T2DM, as well as utilizing indigenous groups' knowledge as resources for coping.

1.1. T2DM among Bedouins in Israel

Type 2 diabetes mellitus (T2DM) is the result of insulin resistance and is caused by the failure of the body's cells to use insulin properly, at times combined with an absolute insulin deficiency. It is the most common disease that has become a significant public health concern worldwide [1]. T2DM is associated with a series of significant health complications, as well as a significant economic burden [1,2]. Since some of the damage to health starts at a prediabetic stage, and since treating T2DM once it is diagnosed does not usually restore normal blood glucose levels, screening individuals at risk, and early diagnoses, are of crucial importance [1,2]. T2DM is closely associated with lifestyle choices, such as diet and exercise habits [3,4]. Social and cultural factors are dominant in the etiology, prevalence, and prognosis of T2DM, since the so-called lifestyle choices are often mediated by cultural and social contexts [2]. After a diagnosis, the modification of the individual's lifestyle, preferably through accessible and culturally relevant lifestyle modification programs, has been consistently found to be the best indicator of positive treatment outcomes [1,2]. Thus, understanding the complex interactions of culture and diabetes is of pivotal importance in the prevention, early detection, and treatment of T2DM.

Moreover, the interaction of culture and T2DM is even more significant, as T2DM is disproportionally prevalent among ethnic minorities and indigenous groups, e.g., African Americans [5] and Native Americans [6,7]. The high prevalence of diabetes among these groups is accompanied by especially poor treatment outcomes and higher complication rates in comparison to other social groups [5,7]. Poor treatment outcomes commonly lead to health complications such as kidney disease, blindness, limb amputation, nerve damage, heart disease, and cerebrovascular incidents [8].

The current study focuses on the Bedouin community of the Negev region of southern Israel. The Bedouin are a subset of the minority Arab community of Israel, and until relatively recently, they were a nomadic people. Since the establishment of the State of Israel in 1948, the Bedouin community has undergone a process of social and economic marginalization, influenced by a rapid—and at times, forced—transition to a semi-urban way of life [9]. Some moved to government-established townships, others to unrecognized villages that lack basic infrastructure and services, such as electricity, a water supply, educational institutions, and health care services, because the state disputes the legality of these settlements and, consequently, refuses to invest in basic infrastructure. Economically, the unrecognized villages are more disadvantaged than the legally recognized townships and are considered among the poorest settlements in Israel [8]. The transition to a semi-urban way of life has impacted changes in kinship structure, gender relations, economic structure, and political power [9].

T2DM is disproportionally prevalent in the Bedouin population of Israel, mirroring the experiences of indigenous and minority groups elsewhere in the Western world [10–12]. For example, a study from 2002 found that prevalence of T2DM among Bedouins in the Negev above the age of 35 years was as high as 7.3% for men and 9.9% for women [13]. A study from 2007 found the age-adjusted diabetes rate among Bedouins in Israel to be 12%, compared to only 8% among Jewish Israelis. The prevalence rate was especially notable among Bedouins between 40 and 49 years of age, where the prevalence rate was three times higher than in the Jewish population of the same age [14].

Treatment outcomes, as defined by the adherence to treatment, are poor, with 73% of Bedouin diabetes patients defined as not adhering to treatment [11]. Results remain poor when measured by diabetes controls, as one study found that only 29.3% of Bedouin patients had diabetes under control, compared to 46.7% among non-Bedouin patients [15].

1.2. Different Theoretical Approaches to T2DM among Bedouins in Israel

1.2.1. The Biomedical Approach

Most studies of coping with T2DM within the Bedouin communities in Israel employ the biomedical approach. According to this approach, which frames medical knowledge as objective and value-free, e.g., [8,14,16–18], coping and treatment outcomes are under the responsibility of the individual. According to this approach, negative treatment outcomes or complications are the result of the individual's lack of compliance with medical advice. For example, Tamir et al. assessed adherence to follow-up tests and drug treatments for a range of illnesses, including diabetes, in Bedouin communities in Israel and found that only 28% of diabetes patients complied with drug therapies [14]. They noted that the adherence to drug therapies and follow-up tests among Bedouin patients were alarmingly low in comparison to that of the Jewish Israeli population. At the same time, the authors' exclusive reliance on the analysis of data taken from medical records meant that they were not able to explore the underlying mechanisms that informed this low rate of compliance.

Studies that adopt the biomedical approach focus on individual factors as a potential explanation for poor coping, which is measured by the lack of adherence to treatment regimens and follow-up tests. These studies do not consider the wider social context as a possible explanation for distinctive coping strategies among the Bedouin. In fact, implementing this medicalized individual approach to understanding coping with diabetes among specific ethnic groups reflects a contradictory approach to ethnic identity. On the one hand, it recognizes that specific groups (e.g., Bedouins in Israel) have different experiences to those of Israel's ethnic majority in terms of diabetes rates and coping with diabetes. However, on the other hand, this approach does not recognize other forms of differences that may characterize these groups, including structural differences, such as different living conditions, that may make following biomedical advice very difficult. Instead, these approaches assign the responsibility for the possible difficulties in following medical advice to the individuals' lack of cooperation or their fatalistic approach.

1.2.2. The Minorities in Transition to Modernization Approach

We use the term "minorities in transition to modernization approach" to refer to the approach utilized in a cluster of studies that add an epidemiological focus to the individualized medical approach by specifically addressing the disproportionately high rates of diabetes and poor treatment outcomes among indigenous groups. An analysis of the theoretical underpinnings of this cluster of studies reveals a common narrative. According to the minorities in transition approach, the high prevalence of T2DM and the negative treatment outcomes among ethnic minorities in Western society are the result of a rapid transition from a nomadic agricultural lifestyle to a modern urban lifestyle, e.g., [13,19–21].

Like the biomedical approach, this approach is based on the understanding of a biomechanical model of disease, according to which, coping is an individual matter and optimal coping is manifested through an adherence to medical advice. Unlike the biomedical approach, studies that employ the "minorities in transition" approach address not only individual characteristics but also group or social/cultural characteristics, such as practices and beliefs shared by members of a specific community, as factors that may influence coping with T2DM.

Research by Yoel et al. included these two approaches [19]. Reflecting the biomedical rationale, they used questionnaires that accessed personal characteristics in an attempt to understand why some Bedouin patients fail to achieve optimal treatment outcomes. At the same time, the researchers moved beyond the biomedical model when they measured the extent to which Bedouin individuals held specific cultural beliefs that were attributed to the Bedouin community as a 'traditional community,' such as a suspicion towards Western medications or an inaccurate understanding of chronic illnesses. The researchers linked the extent to which patients held traditional beliefs and a noncompliance with treatment, and argued that traditional beliefs are the main obstacle to optimal treatment outcomes.

Another example of a study that used the minority in transition approach is the study by Dunton et al. who presented a case study of an influential patriarchal figure in a Bedouin community to demonstrate how traditional social and gender practices, within the wider setting of a rapid transition to modernization, can complicate coping with T2DM [21]. They focused on the social responsibility of the sheik (an honorific title in Arab culture commonly used to designate the ruler of a tribe/community) to host family, friends, and other influential figures in the community. The responsibility of hosting means frequent social gatherings in which the sheik and the guests feel a social obligation to eat foods rich in carbohydrates and sugars, as well as sugary drinks. They concluded their analysis with the claim that "These cultural norms present a challenge to diabetes care and management" [21] (p. 1). However, the researchers ignored the fact that before the disruption of the traditional nomadic lifestyle, sugary foods and drinks were not as central to social gatherings as they are today, and events were part of a lifestyle that included regular physical activity.

Other studies also explored the characteristics of Bedouin culture as a potential complicating factor. For example, in a paper that discussed the cultural modifications needed for an intervention program designed to facilitate coping with T2DM, traditional Bedouin nutrition is described as rich in carbohydrates and an obstacle to maintaining a suitable diet [22].

The minorities in transition approach expands the biomedical approach by exploring not only individual factors, but social practices and norms as well, taking a significant step in shedding light on coping among culturally different (i.e., not hegemonic Western) groups. Nonetheless, there are at least three major criticisms regarding the minorities in transition approach. First, this approach assumes that while Western communities have long been accustomed to a modern lifestyle and have therefore adopted practices and beliefs that balance the damaging effects of modern living conditions, such as the acceptance of biomedical knowledge, biomedical advice, the cooperation with the biomedical system, and self-monitoring, indigenous groups still live according to traditional norms and practices that were developed during the time when they lived nomadic lifestyles. In the future, when the transition to modernity is complete, indigenous groups will also incorporate so-called modern practices and beliefs; therefore, the prevalence of T2DM among them will decrease, and their treatment outcomes will improve.

Hence, this approach considers modern living conditions as the norm. Many studies acknowledge that a modern or urban lifestyle includes many risk factors for T2DM, such as a lack of physical activity or processed foods, but these elements are seen as necessary and inevitable, e.g., [19,21–23]. Since modern ways of life are seen as positive and the default in the Western world, traditional (i.e., non-Western) norms and practices are singled out as the problem.

Second, this approach views indigenous culture as having only negative influences on coping. Thus, it does not explore the possibility that elements of indigenous culture can yield effective coping strategies that may not have been taken into account by the biomedical model. For example, some studies acknowledge the need to change the healthcare system and suggest adapting biomedical intervention programs to the specific needs of the Bedouin community, e.g., [22,23]. However, none of these studies have examined coping options that go beyond those offered by the biomedical model, nor have they examined Bedouin culture as a potential source of such options.

Third, this approach does not pay sufficient attention to the economic, political, and social conditions that shape the context in which cultural norms are established. For example, in the case of hospitality and the serving of high carbohydrate foods, hospitality that involves the serving of foods and beverages that are detrimental to the health of diabetics may become more important as traditional social institutions associated with the nomadic lifestyle fade away [21]. In addition, poverty and the intermittent supply of electricity may increase a reliance on high-sugar and high-carbohydrate processed foods in the context of hospitality.

1.2.3. The Social Justice Approach

The fact that indigenous groups tend to be socially, economically, and culturally marginalized, and have a high incidence of poor treatment outcomes, has prompted researchers to explore how specific issues related to the social inequality of these groups may influence their ability to cope. Furthermore, some researchers argue that specific cultural norms and practices can, at least potentially, serve as a positive resource for the coping strategies that expand on those acknowledged by the biomedical approach. These works draw from a previous scholarly transition that shifted from the concept of the adherence to medical advice to the concept of active coping. Active coping is defined as the active and creative balance of medical advice and the fulfilment of personally, culturally, and socially valued activities, goals, and aspirations, while maintaining optimal health [24–26]. Since life goals and aspirations, as well as living conditions, are culturally mediated, the transition to active coping also allows researchers to make the connections between individual coping and the broader social, cultural, and ethnic factors.

We use the term "social justice approach" to refer to the approach used in a cluster of studies that explored how active coping is mediated and shaped by various social, economic, and cultural factors. These factors include the structural conditions of social inequality and oppression, which are especially prevalent in the lives of ethnic minorities and indigenous groups. The social justice approach criticizes the biomedical narratives of illness and coping by showing that the biomedical ideas regarding proper coping are often inapplicable to indigenous groups due to their everyday living conditions, and that the biomedical conceptualizations of coping are too narrow, as they rely solely on Western tradition, thus excluding coping strategies that draw on indigenous experience.

We argue that the social justice approach can be very useful in research regarding coping with T2DM in the Bedouin community in Israel, in light of existing structural, social, and health inequalities. The Bedouins are one of the most deprived population groups in Israel [27–29]. High poverty rates and poor nutrition can make it more difficult to balance blood glucose levels, purchase prescribed medication, or engage in regular physical activity [20,30]. Indeed, the typical Bedouin meal is low in protein, iron, and calcium content, but is rich in salt and calories [20,30].

In addition, beginning in the 1960s, the State of Israel initiated a process of urbanization and pressured the Bedouins to move into semi-planned towns. Many scholars claim this was done to move the Bedouin out of the Negev in order to allow Jewish Israelis to settle there [31,32]. The forced transition to the semi-planned towns exacerbated the existing social and economic deprivation and produced a social and cultural vacuum [9]. In addition, as of today, parts of the Bedouin community continue to live in unrecognized villages that lack standard government services and sufficient public infrastructure (e.g., water, electricity, public transportation, health services, and education services). Even recognized Bedouins towns and villages are offered significantly fewer healthcare services compared to other Arab and Jewish Israeli areas [33].

In this paper we argue, using the social justice approach, that what is often interpreted as personal or cultural noncompliance with treatment may, in fact, be related to a poor accessibility to medical services, high poverty rates, and other structural inequality factors.

Their similarities with indigenous groups in other parts of the world notwithstanding, the Bedouins in Israel are also characterized by distinct conditions that are not necessarily shared with other indigenous groups. These include increasingly high rates of polygamy [9], the unique structure of the Israeli health system, the specific historical modes of changes in living conditions [34], and a distinct cultural heritage. Thus, given the unique social, geographical, and cultural context of Bedouin groups in the Negev, insights gathered from an empirical study of this population, guided by a social justice framework, can contribute to the theoretical and empirical rigor of the social justice approach.

The goal of the present study is to utilize the social justice approach to understand coping with T2DM among Bedouins in Israel. Specifically, we aim to (1) explore the distinct challenges and barriers the Bedouin face in coping with T2DM and (2) to examine how successful coping can be conceptualized based on the perspectives of Bedouins in Israel. Thus, the section of the results will be divided into two main parts: the barriers to coping with T2DM in the Bedouin community, and the unique resources for coping with T2DM according to the two goals of the study.

2. Materials and Methods

The current study used the interpretative interactionism approach [35]. This approach, with its focus on the reciprocal relations between people and their social environments [35], was especially suitable for this study, because "it puts the patient at the center of the research process and makes visible the experiences of patients as they interact with the healthcare and social systems that surround them" [36] (p. 39). This approach includes a number of stages that are carried out as part of a circular process. The first of these is deconstruction, which consists of a critical review of the research literature to identify the preconceptions in the literature and existing tensions in interactions between patients, healthcare providers, and policies. The second is the epiphany, which consists of collecting stories that highlight the meanings attributed by participants to formative life experiences. The third is bracketing, which is analogous to data analyses. The fourth is contextualization, which involves taking into account the social, political, economic, and physical environments of participants, and contextualizing their stories within the wider context of inequality [35,36].

2.1. Participants and Recruitment

The interviewees were recruited through a clinic that is part of Clalit Health Services, the largest HMO in Israel, in the Bedouin city of Rahat, as well as through community projects run by the Arab-Jewish Center for Empowerment, Equality, and Cooperation (Negev Institute for Strategies of Peace and Economic Development). The inclusion criteria for participant selection were the self-identification as a Bedouin and having been diagnosed with T2DM for at least 6 months (to ensure a sufficient experience of coping with the illness).

The final study population consisted of 49 interviewees and was varied in terms of gender, age, geographical location, education, and socioeconomic status. After 49 interviews, the researchers determined through reflection on the data collection and analysis process that the saturation point (i.e., no new information was being received from participants) had been reached. Consequently, data collection ceased at this point.

The sample consisted of 34 women and 15 men. The mean age was 57 years, with a range between 18 and 78 years. Many of the interviewees had not completed high school, but several had an academic education. Thirty-six of the interviewees were married (mainly in polygamy marriages), seven were widowers, four were divorcees, and two were single.

2.2. Data Collection and Analysis

Ethical approval was obtained from our university's Human Subject Research Committee, and from the Helsinki Ethics Committee of the Clalit HMO, to allow for the recruitment of participants through different channels. We prepared information sheets in Arabic for distribution to the participants. All participants signed an informed consent form that was written in Arabic.

Qualitative semi-structured interviews were conducted in Arabic in the homes of the participants, or in the clinic, in accordance with the participants' preference. One female and one male research assistant who spoke both Arabic and Hebrew conducted the interviews. The interviews were based on the narrative approach [37]. Each interview began with a request to hear the illness narrative of the patient ("can you tell me your story of diabetes?"). When the interviewee completed the narration of their story, the interviewer asked supplementary questions (Interview guide) about signs and symptoms, tests, receiving the diagnosis, telling other people about it, any previous knowledge of diabetes, communication with health professionals, financial impacts, information and support needs, treatment decisions, and the use of complementary approaches.

All audiotaped interviews were transcribed and then translated into Hebrew. A thematic analysis was conducted [38]. The analysis was inductive, in that it relied on the use of emic codes that had emerged from the interviews, and deductive in that it was shaped by a critical literature review [34]. The data analysis was conducted in Hebrew and the quotes used in this manuscript were all translated into English by the authors.

3. Results

The analysis of the interviews produced many themes. In this paper, we focus on themes related to two questions: what are the unique barriers to coping with T2DM among Bedouins in Israel that result from physical and social inequalities? What are the unique resources of the Bedouin community for coping with T2DM?

3.1. Barriers to Coping with T2DM in the Bedouin Community

3.1.1. Physical Inequality: Land Dispossession

Beginning in the 1960s, the State of Israel initiated a process of urbanization and pressured the Bedouin to move into semi-planned towns. The forced transition to these towns prevented the Bedouin from sustaining a lifestyle based on traditional agriculture. This complicated the ability of patients to cope with T2DM on at least two levels. First, members of the Bedouin community could no longer engage in the daily physical activities involved in traditional agriculture. Second, they lost what is called "food sovereignty" [7]. Without the possibility of engaging in traditional agriculture, traditional foods (such as dried milk products or self-grown fruits and vegetables that are expensive to buy on the open market) were removed from their menu and replaced with processed cheap foods, as the following excerpt demonstrates:

> Before, we didn't have cancer or diabetes and now the Negev is full of diabetics, not because the Bedouin themselves have changed. What has changed is the lifestyle, the state has forced us to change [...]. The state took us and placed us in a town [...]. They changed us. We don't have lands to grow fruits and vegetables. In the past, we used to grow everything, also poultry and animals. The state fought us in every domain of life. We used to be a society that was based on production and now we're [a society] based on consumption. This [process] was initiated by the state. Even the fact that women are now inactive and idle is the result of the state changing our lifestyle (Jamila, a 67-year-old woman from a recognized settlement).

Jamila's words emphasize how state-imposed urbanization has reduced the ability of the community to cope with diabetes. These changes have hindered the ability of people to eat healthy fresh food. Furthermore, Jamila compares women's current status in the community to their status in the past, where they served a central role in the community thanks to their role in traditional agriculture [9]. In addition to the fact that traditional agriculture is no longer possible, gender norms, a lack of public transportation, and other factors complicate women's ability to work outside the home, and the result is that they have become physically inactive.

The transition from the production of foods to their consumption has complicated the ability to cope with T2DM in at least two additional ways. First, it has caused a decrease in the daily physical activity involved in traditional agriculture. Second, it has weakened the collective sense of meaning the community derived in the past from being productive. The following quote exemplifies the decrease in physical activity involved in everyday life:

> Today you have everything in the house and everything is [readily] available. When you go into the supermarket, you find a million things, take a few things and sit in front of the TV for three or four hours before bedtime. In the past, people went to sleep early, got up early, while today you sleep and get up and eat many diabetes-[inducing] foods (Tawfiiq, a 52-year-old woman from a recognized settlement).

The following quote demonstrates the decrease in the sense of collective meaning:

> Listen, there is a problem of house demolitions. We have children who won't have houses to live in in the future. There are unrecognized villages. The state confines us and leaves our needs as a society unfulfilled. They won't let us grow fruits and vegetables and derive self-satisfaction from production. In addition, we are dealing with an increase in the cost of living (Salim, a 46-year-old man from a recognized settlement).

Attending to the perspective of members of the Bedouin community makes it possible to identify barriers to coping that are currently not addressed or even perceived as such though the external prism of the biomedical approach. As seen above, some of the barriers are the experience of land dispossession, house demolitions, and a forced abrupt transition from a nomadic to semi-urban lifestyle.

3.1.2. Social Inequality: Inaccessibility to Health Care

Various researchers have linked the unfavorable treatment outcomes of T2DM to a lack of knowledge among members of the Bedouin community of "silent" diseases that may not cause symptoms at first (such as different types of cancer or diabetes), e.g., [13,19,21], thus attributing the unfavorable outcomes to a characteristic of the community itself. However, even if there is knowledge of the "silent" diseases, pre-symptomatic diagnoses (e.g., during routine screening tests) necessitates the accessibility to healthcare services. The inaccessibility of healthcare services was a subject that arose in many of the interviews. We noticed three reasons for inaccessibility: economic issues, a lack of health services in the region, and an inaccessibility due to communication problems.

Many interviewees recalled how the need to constantly work without taking leave prevented them from having a medical examination even years after the onset of significant symptoms. They sought medical assistance only after symptoms hindered their ability to work. For example, Khaled (a 67-year-old man from an unrecognized settlement) recounts how, despite having significant symptoms for years, he did not seek a medical examination. When asked why this was so, he responded:

> I don't know, I worked for many hours, day and night, never taking a day off, it was like that for several years. I worked as a security guard, [did] many shifts. I didn't sleep for more than two hours a day. I wanted to earn money.

In addition to the inaccessibility that stems from economic factors, various interviewees referred to a lack of availability of healthcare services in the areas where they resided. For example, they mentioned long waiting periods for appointments:

> We have difficulties in relation to healthcare services. We have only one physician, one administrator, one nurse, and one pharmacist [in the town], which causes a lot of difficulties [...] Getting an appointment requires a long waiting period (Abed, a 67-year-old man from a recognized settlement).

Interviewees from unrecognized settlements reported an even more severe lack of accessibility to healthcare services. They spoke of medication shortages, especially long waiting periods, and a lack of public transportation to medical facilities.

In order to cope optimally with T2DM, patients require knowledge about nutrition, physical activity, medical examinations and diagnoses, their eligibility for social rights, and more. Culturally relevant and accessible knowledge is key for both early detection and treatment as the participation in low-cost accessible lifestyle modification programs is one of the most effective indicators of successful treatment outcomes [1,2].

Many interviewees lacked such knowledge, as Sarab, a 53-year-old woman from a recognized settlement reported: "I have symptoms, but I didn't understand these symptoms." A lack of knowledge is related to a lack in resources that are suitable for the Bedouin community, such as Arabic language medical pamphlets, medical articles, and reports in the media, as well as culturally appropriate medical education workshops (e.g., on the topics of nutrition and physical activity), as the following excerpt demonstrates:

> Why is the Bedouin community neglected regarding this issue despite the fact that we are number one in relation to the ratio of those with diabetes? We have the highest percentages of diabetes [in relation to other communities/ethnic groups] [...]. We even lack publications in Arabic: all medical magazines are in Hebrew. Why don't we have pamphlets in Arabic to hand out to diabetics to save time for the dieticians? Why not publish a pamphlet of lifestyle recommendations for diabetic patients so that every physician could hand it out to his or her patients? (Aziza, a 48-year-old woman from a recognized settlement).

The Arabic language is still an official language in Israel, but government officials are not obliged to translate documents to Arabic and do so only in specific cases (Arraf-Baker, 2019). Moreover, patient illiteracy is also associated with a lack of knowledge regarding diabetes and how to cope with it:

> [How do you know about your rights?] I don't, I can't read, and I can't write [...] My physician told me that I was entitled to four hours a week assistance, but I asked for it twice and I was turned down. (Na'ama, a woman in her seventies [exact age unknown] from a recognized settlement).

> I'm very afraid of taking shots especially because I can't read or write I'm afraid that I will get confused and inject the wrong dosage. I'm afraid of the test I do with the glucometer as it is. . . . We need a solution for these patients, assistance in the form of someone who will inject them and support them. (Sarab, 53-year-old women from a recognized settlement).

The interview excerpts presented above demonstrate that the issues of poverty, social exclusion, and marginalization are critical to the understanding of late diagnoses and difficulties in coping. Even in the presence of stressful symptoms, some interviewees felt that they should not take leave from work to be tested, while others had no access to information in Arabic.

3.2. Unique Resources for Coping with T2DM

3.2.1. The Traditional Way of Life and Traditional Foods

In coping with diabetes day-to-day, one of the most dominant resources drawn from local indigenous culture was the traditional way of life. Various interviewees talked about how they used traditional methods of preparing food and ate traditional foods as a resource for coping with diabetes:

> There are many foods that I use to enhance my diabetes control. Cooked jerisha [wheat porridge], freekeh [roasted green wheat]. Foods that give energy, such as freekeh. Healthy foods. Food that strengthens my health, unlike fried food, salty pastries, and sweet foods that ruin my health ... I had to rediscover the [traditional Bedouin] healthy foods that we have always eaten (Fatma, a 50-year-old woman from a recognized settlement).

The words "I had to rediscover the healthy foods" demonstrates how any culture at a given date and time has a wide repertoire of cultural practices that include food practices. The interaction of the community with the physical, social, and political environments determines which practices take place and which do not.

In addition to eating traditional Bedouin foods, various interviewees told us how they still practiced some form of traditional agriculture (even partially) and, in this way, managed to incorporate the physical activity involved in traditional agriculture and household chores into their everyday lives:

> I see household chores as exercise for me. I raise chickens and goats. I get up for them sometimes. When a goat gives birth, every 24 h I go to see her and

return. Even household chores. I see them as exercise, even if they [healthcare professionals] say they are not exercise. (Fatma, a 50-year-old woman from a recognized settlement).

3.2.2. Traditional Practices of Healing

In addition to incorporating the physical activity involved in traditional agriculture and choosing healthy traditional foods, another resource related to indigenous culture is the cultivation of plants that serve as traditional herbal medicines. The following interviewee cultivates medicinal herbs and distributes them to friends free of charge. Cultivating traditional herbs allows her to combine a social activity with traditional healing practices:

I have herbal plants that I grow in my garden and boil, like hyssop. Everything is natural . . . I always liked having plants, but when I became ill I tried things and I learned what helps and what's good [with diabetes]. [How did you learn this?] Using my own personal experience, I tried things and I saw how it affected me, I also give people herbal infusions. [Do you also give people medicinal plants?] Yes, I give them infusions to try. I have a cousin with diabetes and I give her herbs, not instead of pills, but if you maintain a healthy diet and combine pills with herbs it goes well together. (Hanin, a 67-year-old woman from a recognized settlement).

Hanin suggests that her friends use herbs in addition to, and not instead of, Western medications. Similarly, other interviewees who said they used traditional herbs said they saw them not as a replacement for Western medications, but rather as a supplement.

3.2.3. Religion

Another dominant resource drawn from Bedouin culture is religion. The majority of the interviewees in our study explicitly stated that religious beliefs and practices significantly assisted them in coping with T2DM. The fact that participants employed religion in active coping, as we demonstrate below, is especially revealing in light of the fact that "minority in transition" studies tend to frame religion negatively as a factor that complicates coping and encourages passivity and fatalism, e.g., [13,19,21]. According to this view, religion encourages fatalism, which makes patients avoid taking steps to improve their health (ibid.). Our interviewees tell a different story about the role of religion in coping, adding to our understanding of how religion functions in this context. First, religious belief has a wider meaning than mere fatalism in relation to coping with T2DM. Many interviewees told us that religious beliefs improve their quality of life by instilling optimism in them and helping them to regularly incorporate physical activity in their everyday lives:

It's not good to lose hope. Belief in God strengthens hope and therefore believing is a positive force, a force that may help you cope, and religious belief really improves your morale. (Aadel, 59-year-old man from a recognized settlement).

In the context of the biomedical model, healthy diet instructions appear to lack any cultural connection. In contrast, our interviewees' stories demonstrate how individuals can employ various myths and cultural narratives to incorporate and practice useful techniques to cope with T2DM, such as "intuitive eating," which is the ability to remain attuned to one's body while eating, and to stop eating as soon as one feels satiated:

When the Prophet said "when eating one needs to make room for water, air and food," [he] didn't mean that one needs to eat until one is satiated. No, [one should] stop eating even if he is not satiated. In practice, I follow this advice because it makes me more comfortable; if I eat a lot, it keeps me from falling asleep at night. [Our] lifestyle has changed, but we have preserved some habits (Yasmine, a 52-year-old woman from a recognized settlement).

Yasmine draws on the local culture's resource of the Quran to instill meaning into changing her eating habits, specifically in the direction of intuitive eating, which is developing the ability to be attuned to one's bodily cues and sensations of hunger and satiation.

Local culture can be used as a resource to instill meaning into other health related practices, such as being physically active. According to the biomedical model, physical activity is practiced in order to keep the body healthy and not necessarily to achieve other goals (unlike spirituality in yoga, for example). In contrast, several interviewees described how they combined a routine of physical activity with their religious practice and, in doing so, managed to add personal and collective meaning to it. Ibrahim, a 62-year-old man from a recognized settlement reported: "Yes, every day I walk to morning prayer at the mosque one and a half kilometers and there and back. I try to walk regularly." In this context, Yamana noted the following:

> I pray, fast and observe religion. It helps me very much and calms me. I mean, if I didn't fast, I'd feel that everyone was fasting [except me] and that I was weak. That's why I fight my illness. The best proof [for that] is that now I fast, I fight my illness as vigorously as possible for my religion and for Allah. Because he who makes an effort for Allah, Allah will compensate him for everything. (Yamama, 50-year-old woman from a recognized settlement).

Beyond the possibility of taking part in different practices, such as fasting, religion provides different ways in which to contribute to the community. One participant learned to read as an adult and volunteers to heal people by reading verses from the Quran. Employing the Quran in a therapeutic manner enables her to creatively combine an emotional/supportive form of therapy with social activism in the community. Using religion as a healing resource, in this case by reading verses from the Quran, is a good example of a coping method that goes beyond the biomedical model:

> Every night I read verses from the Quran and it really helps me. I even heal other people with the Quran. I heal many people who approach me and I read instead of asking someone else to read and I don't charge for it. Thank God for everything (Ruan, a 48-year-old woman from a recognized settlement).

Beyond improving our interviewees' sense of well-being, increasing their optimism, contributing to their healing, and helping them to incorporate physical activity into their daily lives, religion assisted them in coping with the social stigma that surrounds T2DM. The social stigma of diabetes is a major force that complicates coping with T2DM in general, and in indigenous communities in particular. For example, many participants described how shame and fear of the social consequences of being identified as T2DM patients make them postpone or even relinquish important practices, such as glucometer testing, so as not to be seen engaging in them. Nevertheless, some interviewees describe how religious belief help them cope with the stigma attached to T2DM. For example, Na'ama, mentioned above, explained, "[I reveal the fact I have T2DM] to all of my friends and relatives ... Yeah, why should I be ashamed? It's from Allah."

To conclude, the interviewees' perspectives and experiences illustrate that local culture has the potential to facilitate coping with T2DM in at least two ways. The first of these is by inspiring them to use coping strategies not currently acknowledged by those who espouse the biomedical approach, such as engaging in traditional healing practices, traditional agriculture, and embracing a traditional lifestyle. The second is by enabling them to give culturally relevant meaning to coping practices, such as changing their eating habits and being physically active.

4. Discussion

4.1. Starting from the Indigenous Perspective: The Importance of the Coping Experience

The vast majority of studies that have examined coping with T2DM among the Bedouin in Israel have looked at the community from the outside. From this perspective, elements of local culture are seen mainly as obstacles or factors that interfere with optimal coping.

The transition from a nomadic to a semi-urban lifestyle is depicted as inevitable and tends to be generalized, as if such processes take place in different periods and geographical locations in an identical manner. The specific conditions under which the transition of the Bedouin community has taken place, and their own experience of it, are not addressed.

In contrast, the current study was conducted in close collaboration with the Bedouin community and a conscious decision was made to examine the issues at hand from the perspective of members of the Bedouin community (Etic). By attending to the insider perspective, we were able to hear different stories about the relationship between elements of local culture and coping with T2DM, as well as the experience of illness and coping with the illness itself.

4.2. Identifying "New" Barriers to Optimal Coping

Learning about the experience of members of the Bedouin community from their perspective allowed us to identify barriers to optimal coping that are currently not addressed or recognized though the external prism of the biomedical approach. Two such barriers to treatment are the experience of land dispossession and the rupture of caring relationships (Duwe, 2016).

Our interviewees described the way in which the forced transition to semi-planned towns undermined the community's ability to cope with T2DM by making it impossible to sustain a lifestyle based on traditional agriculture. In the context of a lack of employment opportunities and extreme poverty, cheap and processed foods replaced local agriculture. Poverty and the inability to engage in agriculture means that young women are forced to work long hours in low-wage jobs (if they are able to find employment at all), while the elderly (or other dependents) are left without support or social ties. This situation has resulted in various forms of spatial separation, such as house demolitions, which also have also disrupted the community's caring and supportive relationships.

The experience of transitioning from a nomadic to a sedentary lifestyle, as told by our interviewees, is not universal or inevitable. It occurred under specific conditions of external pressure, extreme poverty, a lack of suitable infrastructure, a lack of educational and employment opportunities, and experiences of discrimination and marginalization by other ethnic groups in Israel. It is therefore not surprising that, as other researchers have found, many interviewees experienced this transition as highly stressful, e.g., [39].

Examining issues from the perspective of the indigenous people themselves enhances our understanding of the barriers they face. For example, in interviewing Bedouin men and women about the perceived accessibility of healthcare, the researchers were able to break the concept of the inaccessibility of healthcare into three interconnected problems: the language barrier, cultural competency, and gender-based barriers [40]. Likewise, the stories of our interviewees suggest a more nuanced and complicated understanding of the "lack of awareness of the risk factors and complications of diabetes" often depicted as a significant barrier to treatment among indigenous groups, including the Bedouin community in Israel, e.g., [13,19]. By means of the interviewees' stories, it is possible to break this general barrier down into three interconnected problems. The first of these is the inaccessibility to healthcare due to economic problems. In such cases, even if individuals are aware of their symptoms and complications, their reluctance to take leave from work prevents them from seeking care. The second is a lack of informational resources tailored to the needs of the Bedouin community, such as medical pamphlets, medical articles, and media reports in Arabic. The third is the existence of significant rates of illiteracy.

As our findings show, illiterate patients experience great difficulties and high levels of anxiety over the daily management of T2DM. For example, they cannot properly read glucometers or medication package inserts. Literacy is not usually perceived as an urgent problem to solve in relation to coping with T2DM among indigenous patients. Likewise, a basic understanding of Hebrew is often taken as a given, but among elderly Bedouin women a lack of knowledge of Hebrew may lead to missed appointments or many hours wasted as they cannot understand they are being called through an automatic waiting room call system [40].

4.3. Transitioning from Compliance with Treatment to Active Coping and Identifying "New" Coping Strategies and Methods

There has been a transition from viewing optimal ways of coping with T2DM as (relatively passive) adherence to medical advice, to the active and creative balance of medical advice and the individual's valued activities and goals, often including what is called strategic non-compliance [24]. The concept of active coping has been central to this shift, as it has become widely understood that coping with a chronic disease cannot be reduced to adherence to medications or tests alone, but should be considered from the perspective of more holistic, alternative definitions of health and well-being [25,26]. The findings of the current study suggest that we should take the shift to active coping another step forward by changing the perception of what it means to (successfully) cope with chronic illness.

Making such a change invites us to recognize and learn from 'indigenous knowledge systems' [41]. By listening to how the interviewees use resources drawn from local culture, such as returning to certain elements of the traditional way of life of their community (e.g., by engaging in agriculture), or turning to traditional herbal medicine or religion, one can identify new ways in which to think about, and proactively cope with, T2DM.

Most studies that have examined the Bedouin community from the outside have related religion or religious faith to barriers to optimal ways of coping with T2DM, e.g., [13,19–21]. In stark contrast to this view, the majority of interviewees reported that religious faith was of great importance to them in coping with T2DM. Religious texts, practices, and beliefs gave new meaning to practices such as intuitive eating, changing eating habits, taking part in physical activity, and raising the collective awareness of the disease. Recognizing that disease management can have cultural and spiritual connotations is important in bridging the chasm between healthcare providers and indigenous people [41] and it is relevant to other ethnic communities. One can also think of organized walking to places of worship or organized physical activities inside places of worship as possibly culturally relevant resources for the promotion of physical activity in the ultra-Orthodox Jewish community, which also suffers extremely high rates of T2DM and poor outcomes [42].

In many cases, in their everyday coping with the disease, our interviewees combined life domains that are usually separated under the biomedical approach: religion, work, family, physical activity, and social activism. For example, the participant who learned to read as an adult and volunteers to heal people by reading verses from the Quran uses religion as a resource and a healing option while strengthening social ties in the community. Another example in combining religious practices with everyday coping, for example, controlling sugar levels in a way that allows religious fasting or the employment of religious beliefs to cope with social stigma. Creating small scale enclaves in which traditional agriculture can be practiced enables individuals to combine everyday physical activities with work.

4.4. A Multifaceted Approach to Promoting Health, Health Knowledge, and Health Equity: Bringing the Pieces Back Together

A multi-faceted approach to health requires bringing back together life domains that have been separated, at least in the context of health. For example, physical activity need not necessarily be a distinct activity, practiced in private spaces such as gyms (that are often expensive and inaccessible to different groups) in the evenings (often a time dedicated to social or familial actives) [40]. Initiatives that grant communities, families, and individual women small plots of land where they can engage in agriculture can increase opportunities for physical activity in a way that is attuned to the culture of the community. Similarly, encouraging religious leaders to speak about symptoms and coping with T2DM and other chronic diseases may also be useful in encouraging the integration of collective and individual religious practices with habits that support healthy lifestyles.

The movement towards cultural competence in healthcare is gaining attention and has been recognized both by researchers and policy makers [40,43,44]. A multi-faceted approach to health requires bringing back together life domains that have been separated, at least in the context of health. For example, this could include cookbooks that offer traditional dishes that are suitable for T2DM, or leaflets with recommendations for better food choices that take into account the availability of products and the local food culture.

A multi-faceted approach to health requires bringing back together life domains that have been separated, at least in the context of health and medicinal systems, rather than treating indigenous people only through the biomedical model [41].

5. Conclusions

Conducting the present study in close collaboration with the Bedouin community enabled us to hear different stories about the experience of T2DM and coping with it. The "insider'" perspective allowed us to identify barriers to coping that are currently not addressed by the literature, many of them directly related to the enforced transition to a semi-urban lifestyle, such as various forms of spatial separation as well as disruptions in the community's supportive relationships. By listening to how the interviewees use resources drawn from local culture, we have identified new ways in which to think about, and proactively cope with, T2DM. In addition, in their everyday coping with the disease, many of our interviewees combined life domains that are usually separated under the biomedical approach: religion, work, family, physical activity, and social activism. Accordingly, a multi-faceted approach to health requires bringing back together life domains that have been separated, at least in the context of health.

Supplementary Materials: The following supporting information can be downloaded at: https://www.mdpi.com/article/10.3390/ijerph19010159/s1, Interview guide.

Author Contributions: Conceptualization, M.M., M.L.A., P.S. and M.A.; methodology, M.M. and M.L.A.; investigation, M.M., M.L.A., P.S. and M.A.; resources, M.M., M.L.A., P.S. and M.A.; writing—original draft preparation, M.M. and M.L.A.; writing—review and editing, M.M., M.L.A., P.S. and M.A.; funding acquisition, M.M. and M.L.A. All authors have read and agreed to the published version of the manuscript.

Funding: This research was funded by Israel Science Foundation, grant number 713/16.

Institutional Review Board Statement: Helsinki committee of Clalit Health Services, approval code: 0015-17-COM-1, approval date: 30/5/2017; Human Subjects Research Committee at Ben Gurion Univerity of the Negev, approval code: 1422-2, approval date: 30/5/2017, 28/6/2016.

Informed Consent Statement: Informed consent was obtained from all subjects involved in the study.

Conflicts of Interest: The authors declare no conflict of interest. The funders had no role in the design of the study; in the collection, analyses, or interpretation of data; in the writing of the manuscript, or in the decision to publish the results.

References

1. Joshi, R.D.; Dhakal, C.K. Predicting Type 2 Diabetes Using Logistic Regression and Machine Learning Approaches. *Int. J. Environ. Res. Public Health* **2021**, *18*, 7346. [CrossRef]
2. Tuso, P. Prediabetes and lifestyle modification: Time to prevent a preventable disease. *Perm. J.* **2014**, *18*, 88–93. [CrossRef]
3. Mitchell, F.M. Reframing diabetes in American Indian communities: A social determinants of health perspective. *Health Soc. Work* **2012**, *37*, 71–79. [CrossRef]
4. Inouye, J.; Li, D.; Davis, J.; Arakaki, R. Ethnic and gender differences in psychosocial factors in native Hawaiian, other pacific islanders, and Asian American adults with type 2 diabetes. *J. Health Dispar. Res. Pract.* **2012**, *5*, 3. Available online: https://digitalscholarship.unlv.edu/jhdrp/vol5/iss3/3 (accessed on 12 January 2014).
5. Chard, S.; Harris-Wallace, B.; Roth, E.G.; Girling, L.M.; Rubinstein, R.; Reese, A.M.; Quinn, C.C.; Eckert, J.K. Successful aging Among African American Older Adults with Type 2 Diabetes. *J. Gerontol. Ser. B* **2017**, *72*, 319–327. [CrossRef]
6. Chino, M.; DeBruyn, L. Building True Capacity: Indigenous Models for Indigenous Communities. *Am. J. Public Health* **2006**, *96*, 596–599. [CrossRef]

7. Duwe, E.A.G. Toward a Story Powerful Enough to Reduce Health Inequities in Indian Country: The Case of Diabetes. *Qual. Inq.* **2016**, *22*, 624–635. [CrossRef]
8. Chlebowy, D.O.; Hood, S.; LaJoie, A.S. Facilitators and Barriers to Self-management of Type 2 Diabetes Among Urban African American Adults. *Diabetes Educ.* **2010**, *36*, 897–905. [CrossRef] [PubMed]
9. Abu-Rabia, R. Redefining polygamy among the Palestinian Bedouins in israel: Colonization, patriarchy, and resistance. *Am. Univ. J. Gend. Soc. Policy Law* **2011**, *19*, 459–480.
10. Yiftachel, O. Epilogue: Studying al-naqab/negev bedouins-toward a colonial paradigm. *Hagar* **2008**, *8*, 173–191.
11. Zucker, I.; Arditi-Babchuk, H.; Enav, T.; Shohat, T. Self-reported type 2 diabetes and diabetes-related eye disease in Jews and Arabs in Israel. *J. Immigr. Minor Health* **2016**, *18*, 1328–1333. [CrossRef] [PubMed]
12. Muhsen, K.; Green, M.S.; Soskolne, V.; Neumark, Y. Inequalities in non-communicable diseases between the major population groups in Israel: Achievements and challenges. *Lancet* **2017**, *389*, 2531–2541. [CrossRef]
13. Abou-Rbiah, Y.; Weitzman, S. Diabetes among Bedouins in the Negev: The transition from a rare to a highly prevalent condition. *IMAJ* **2002**, *4*, 687–689. [PubMed]
14. Tamir, O.; Peleg, R.; Dreiher, J.; Abu-Hammad, T.; Rabia, Y.A.; Rashid, M.A.; Shvartzman, P. Cardiovascular risk factors in the bedouin population: Management and compliance. *IMAJ* **2007**, *9*, 652–655. [PubMed]
15. Cohen, A.; Gefen, K.; Ozer, A.; Bagola, N.; Milrad, V.; Cohen, L.; Abu-Hammad, T.; Abou-Rabiah, Y.; Hazanov, I.; Vardy, D. Diabetes control in the Bedouin population in Southern Israel. *Med. Sci. Monit.* **2005**, *11*, CR376–CR380.
16. Murphy, E.; Kinmount, A.L. No symptoms, no problem? Patients' understandings of non-insulin dependent diabetes. *Fam. Pract.* **1995**, *12*, 184–192. [CrossRef] [PubMed]
17. Akbari, H.; Dehghani, F.; Salehzadeh, M. The impact of type D personality on self-care of patients with type 2 diabetes: The mediating role of coping strategies. *J. Diabetes Metab. Disord.* **2020**, *19*, 19,1191–1198. [CrossRef]
18. Knowles, S.R.; Apputhurai, P.; O'Brien, C.L.; Ski, C.F.; Thompson, D.R.; Castle, D.J. Exploring the relationships between illness perceptions, self-efficacy, coping strategies, psychological distress and quality of life in a cohort of adults with diabetes mellitus. *Psychol. Health Med.* **2020**, *25*, 214–228. [CrossRef]
19. Yoel, U.; Abu-Hammad, T.; Cohen, A.; Aizenberg, A.; Vardy, D.; Shvartzman, P. Behind the scenes of adherence in a minority population. *IMAJ* **2013**, *15*, 17–22.
20. Treister-Goltzman, Y.; Peleg, R. Health and morbidity among Bedouin women in southern Israel: A descriptive literature review of the past two decades. *J. Community Health* **2014**, *39*, 819–825. [CrossRef]
21. Dunton, S.; Higgins, A.; Amkraut, J.; Abu-Rabia, Y. Navigating care for Bedouin patients with diabetes. *BMJ Case Rep.* **2016**. [CrossRef]
22. Zilberman-Kravits, D.; Meyerstein, N.; Abu-Rabia, Y.; Wiznitzer, A.; Harman-Boehm, I. The impact of a cultural lifestyle intervention on metabolic parameters after gestational diabetes mellitus a randomized controlled trial. *Matern. Child Health J.* **2018**, *22*, 803–811. [CrossRef]
23. Fraser, D.; Bilenko, N.; Vardy, H.; Abu-Saad, K.; Shai, I.; Abu-Shareb, H.; Shahar, D.R. Differences in food intake and disparity in obesity rates between adult Jews and Bedouins in southern Israel. *Ethn. Dis.* **2008**, *18*, 13–18. [PubMed]
24. Campbell, R.; Pound, P.; Pope, C.; Britten, N.; Pill, R.; Morgan, M.; Donovan, J. Evaluating meta-ethnography: A synthesis of qualitative research on lay experiences of diabetes and diabetes care. *Soc. Sci. Med.* **2003**, *56*, 671–684. [CrossRef]
25. Maclean, H.M. Patterns of diet related self-care in diabetes. *Soc. Sci. Med.* **1991**, *32*, 689–696. [CrossRef]
26. Kelleher, D. Coming to terms with diabetes: Coping strategies and noncompliance. In *Living with Chronic Illness: The Experience of Patients and Their Families*; Unwin Hyman: London, UK, 1988; pp. 137–155.
27. Abu-Bader, S.; Gottlieb, D. Education, employment and poverty among Bedouin Arabs in southern Israel. *Hagar* **2008**, *8*, 121–135. (in Hebrew).
28. Muhammad, A.S.; Mansbach-Kleinfeld, I.; Khatib, M. A preliminary study of emotional and behavioral problems among Bedouin children living in 'unrecognized villages' in Southern Israel. *Ment. Health Prev.* **2017**, *6*, 12–18. [CrossRef]
29. Tubi, A.; Feitelson, E. Changing drought vulnerabilities of marginalized resource-dependent groups: A long-term perspective of Israel's Negev Bedouin. *Reg. Environ. Chang.* **2019**, *19*, 477–487. [CrossRef]
30. Cwikel, J.; Lev-Wiesel, R.; Al-Krenawi, A. The physical and psychosocial health of Bedouin Arab women of the Negev area of Israel: The impact of high fertility and pervasive domestic violence. *Violence Against Women* **2003**, *9*, 240–257. [CrossRef]
31. Kedar, A.; Amara, A.; Yiftachel, O. *Emptied Lands: A Legal Geography of Bedouin Rights in the Negev*; Stanford University Press: Redwood City, CA, USA, 2018.
32. Nasasra, M.; Richter-Devroe, S.; Abu-Rabia-Queder, S.; Ratcliffe, R. (Eds.) *The Naqab Bedouin and Colonialism: New Perspectives*; Routledge: London, UK, 2014.
33. Ministry of Health, Director of Strategic and Economic Planning. *Availability of Community Medical Services: Geographic Mapping*; Rev 01.2021. Available online: https://www.health.gov.il/publicationsfiles/availability_03122017.pdf (accessed on 12 December 2021).
34. Abu-Saad, I. Spatial transformation and indigenous resistance: The urbanization of the Palestinian Bedouin in southern Israel. *Am. Behav. Sci.* **2008**, *51*, 1713–1754. [CrossRef]
35. Denzin, N.K. *Interpretive Interactionism*; Sage: Thousand Oaks, CA, USA, 2001.

36. Tower, M.; Rowe, J.; Wallis, M. Investigating patients' experiences: Methodological usefulness of interpretive interactionism. *Nurse Res.* **2012**, *20*, 39–44. [CrossRef]
37. Rosenthal, G. Reconstruction of life stories: Principles of selection in generating stories for narrative biographical interviews. In *The Narrative Study of Lives*; Sage: Thousand Oaks, CA, USA, 1993; pp. 59–91.
38. Braun, V.; Clarke, V. Using Thematic Analysis in Psychology. *Qual. Res. Psychol.* **2006**, *3*, 77–101. [CrossRef]
39. Al-Said, H.; Braun-Lewensohn, O.; Sagy, S. Sense of coherence, hope, and home demolition are differentially associated with anger and anxiety among Bedouin Arab adolescents in recognized and unrecognized villages. *Anxiety Stress Coping* **2018**, *31*, 475–485. [CrossRef] [PubMed]
40. Shibli, H.; Aharonson-Daniel, L.; Feder-Bubis, P. Perceptions about the accessibility of healthcare services among ethnic minority women: A qualitative study among Arab Bedouins in Israel. *Int. J. Equity Health* **2021**, *20*, 1–9. [CrossRef]
41. Daschbach, A.B. All-Healing Weapon: The Value of Oplopanax Horridus Root Bark in the Treatment of Type 2 Diabetes. Master's Thesis, Western Washington University, Bellingham, WA, USA, 2019. Available online: https://cedar.wwu.edu/wwuet/886/ (accessed on 6 October 2021).
42. Leiter, E.; Finkelstein, A.; Greenberg, K.; Keidar, O.; Donchin, M.; Zwas, D.R. Barriers and facilitators of health behavior engagement in ultra-Orthodox Jewish women in Israel. *Eur. J. Public Health* **2019**, *29* (Suppl. 4), 186–455. [CrossRef]
43. Kalter-Leibovici, O.; Younis-Zeidan, N.; Atamna, A.; Lubin, F.; Alpert, G.; Chetrit, A.; Freedman, L.S. Lifestyle intervention in obese Arab women: A randomized controlled trial. *Arch. Inter. Med.* **2010**, *170*, 970–976. [CrossRef] [PubMed]
44. Daoud, N. Health equity in Israel. *Lancet* **2018**, *391*, 534. [CrossRef]

Article

Cultural Differences in Patients' Preferences for Paternalism: Comparing Mexican and American Patients' Preferences for and Experiences with Physician Paternalism and Patient Autonomy

Gregory A. Thompson *, Jonathan Segura, Dianne Cruz, Cassie Arnita and Leeann H. Whiffen

Department of Anthropology, Brigham Young University, 800 KMBL, Provo, UT 84602, USA
* Correspondence: greg.a.thompson@gmail.com

Abstract: Following up on previous research demonstrating the high level of care realized by a paternalistic Mexican physician, the present research further explored the hypothesis that there are cultural differences in preferences for and experiences with physician paternalism vs. patient autonomy in White American culture as compared with Mexican culture. In this research, we interviewed sixty (60) people including twenty (20) Mexican, twenty (20) Mexican American, and twenty (20) White American respondents. We asked these patients about their experiences with and attitudes towards paternalism and patient autonomy in healthcare interactions. With some caveats, our data showed strong support for both hypotheses while also suggesting a high level of care can be realized by paternalistic physicians when "paternalism" is understood in a cultural context. We close with a brief consideration of the implications of these findings.

Keywords: paternalism; patient autonomy; healthcare; culture; preference; practices; physician-patient interaction; White American; Mexican American; Mexican

1. Introduction

Is Autonomy a Cultural Universal?

Autonomy in healthcare has been widely accepted in Western medicine as one of the most important factors in bioethics [1–8]. Beauchamp and Childress included "Respect for autonomy" as one of their four key principles of biomedical ethics [9,10]. Beauchamp and Childress define the autonomous individual as someone who "acts freely in accordance with a self-chosen plan, analogous to the way an independent government manages its territories and sets its policies" [9] (p. 58). Although Beauchamp and Childress themselves argue that this definition of autonomy means that a patient choosing a paternalistic physician could be ethical even if it means a relative loss of that patient's autonomy in the physician-patient interaction, there has been some criticism of autonomy from within Western cultural contexts (e.g., most Western researchers and writers have considered paternalism in physician-patient interactions to be inimical to providing high quality care for patients [11–14]).

Respect for patient autonomy has also been central to principles and practices in healthcare in the West. For example, the Belmont Report (1979) names the "respect for persons" or autonomy, as its first basic ethical principle [15]. Article 5 in the UNESCO Universal Declaration on Bioethics and Human Rights (2009) states that: "The autonomy of persons to make decisions, while taking responsibility for those decisions and respecting the autonomy of others, is to be respected" [16] (p. 7).

Autonomy has been taken to be of such importance that it has often been thought to be ethically necessary to introduce it to other cultures where it is not highly valued. For example, while agreeing with Thompson and Whiffen's (2018) basic findings regarding a tendency towards paternalism in physician-patient interactions in Mexican culture [17], Lazcano-Ponce et al. (2020) argue that paternalism is equal to overprotection and they further argue that Mexican physicians need to more forcefully be "promoting autonomy in the doctor-patient relationship" [18] (p. 9). Yet, not everyone has been so sanguine about this kind of ethical imperialism. In arguing for a pluralistic view of ethical values, Shweder (2004) has suggested that it would be better to consider (at least) three ethics that can be taken as a preeminent value in a given culture and which can often contradict one another [19]. Autonomy is just one of these three ethics; community and divinity are the other two. As Jensen (2011) describes the pluralism of this approach: "The model, then, is not a simple one-size-fits-all, but rather accommodates the prevailing ethics of diverse peoples" [20] (p. 157). Many have noted that whereas Western culture values autonomy over both community and divinity, other cultures may place community or divinity as preeminent values in such a manner that those values can supersede autonomy. For our present purposes, this suggests that the preeminent ethical principle of autonomy in healthcare may not be a preeminent value in other cultures and that there may be other values that supersede patient autonomy [21–28].

In a similar vein, others have argued that because most research regarding physician-patient interactions has been conducted and interpreted from a Western perspective, paternalistic healthcare practices are regularly seen as negative even in cultures where paternalism is seen very positively [23,28,29]. A number of researchers have provided strong evidence that a paternalistic approach to healthcare is preferred in other countries. This research has included countries such as Ghana [29,30], Botswana [31], Ethiopia [32], Jamaica [33], Korea [34,35], China [36], India [27,37], Vietnam [28], Japan [38], Thailand [39,40], Pakistan [41], Turkey [42], Southern European Nations [43], and Mexico [17,24]. Others have pointed to the need to understand how physician-patient interactions are inflected by the values and ideals of the cultural contexts in which those interactions take place [21,28,30,31,34,44–46].

Taking just a few examples of how patient autonomy is often superseded by other values, Sousa (2011) shows how in India, physicians take the family's wishes into account, even when they may conflict with the patient's wishes [27]. Veatch (1985) documents a similar emphasis in China where it is common practice to inform the patients' families before speaking with the patient [46]. Ujewe (2018) and Payne-Jackson et al. (2004) have separately shown that there are similar ethical principles emphasizing community over autonomy in patient's interactions with healthcare providers in Africa and Jamaica [30,47]. Norman (2015) documented how Sub-Saharan African patients expect physicians to tell them what is wrong and that paternalism actually enhances the health seeking behavior of patients [29].

In direct contrast to those arguing for the imposition of autonomy in other cultures, others have even argued that applying an autonomous approach in healthcare in non-Western cultures leads to poor patient care [31,34,45]. In Botswana, Shaibu (2007) explains that autonomous decision-making in healthcare is not correlated to quality care and that the Western model contributes to "incongruence between the cultural values of Batswana (people of Botswana) and those of health workers as modeled on the western ethic" [31] (p. 503). Similarly, Betancourt (2000) relates the story of Mrs. Y, a sixty-year-old Japanese American woman, who visited an emergency room in the U.S. for a fever and bruises. When Mrs. Y's family were told her diagnosis of leukemia, they insisted that they had the right to withhold this diagnosis from Mrs. Y (in spite of the family's wishes, the American doctors told Mrs. Y her diagnosis, feeling that it was essential to let her make her own decisions about her care) [21]. Lai (1995) offers a similar example from Chinese culture where an autonomous approach disrupted emotional harmony by conflicting with the Confucian concept of *hsiao* [48]. McGrath et al. (2001) showed that participants from Indian, Filipino, Chinese, and Italian families described "The Western Way of informing people directly [about the terminal nature of an illness] was "too abrupt", "terrifying", and "blunt"" [44] (p. 307). Indeed, even some research from within Western contexts has suggested similar limits on the ethic of patient autonomy. Glaser and Strauss (1979) and Timmermans (1994) have separately demonstrated how the autonomy of dying patients can be limited by the awareness that is afforded them of their condition by others [49,50].

Taken together, this body of research offers strong evidence that patient autonomy is not necessarily the preeminent value in many healthcare settings around the world. Research on healthcare in Mexico suggests that Mexican healthcare is one of those cultural contexts in which physician paternalism may supersede patient autonomy.

Indeed, a number of researchers have shown that paternalistic practices are common in Mexican healthcare [51–55]. Garcia-Gonzalez (2009) found that the majority of patients who had chronic rheumatic diseases indicated they wanted to play a passive role and have the physicians make decisions for them [56]. Álvarez Bermudez (2018) analyzed interactions between nurses in Mexico and patients who had been hospitalized for more than three days and found that although less than half of those patients reported the nurses listening to their opinion, almost 70% of the patients characterized the attitude and communication of the nurses as "good" [57]. In a survey focusing on public perception and experiences of the Mexican healthcare system, Doubova et al. (2016) found almost 80% of their 1181 Mexican respondents reported receiving good quality care with 79.6% reported the primary care provider explains things in a way that is easy to understand; and 81% reported a primary care provider who solves most of the health problems [58] (p. 839).

Based on observations comparing over 40 physician-patient interactions of a Mexican physician with those of a White American physician, Thompson and Whiffen (2018) found that whereas the White American physician oriented to patient autonomy, the Mexican physician was paternalistic [17]. Importantly, they noted that far from appearing overbearing or domineering, the Mexican physician's paternalism was realized in a way that his Mexican patients appeared to appreciate as demonstrating a strong sense of care for his patients. These findings suggested that paternalistic physicians can demonstrate high quality care in Mexican culture. Thompson and Whiffen (2018) based this conclusion on observations of Mexican patients' reactions to their physicians [17]. Notably, due to IRB restriction and time challenges, their study lacked interview data with Mexican patients. The present research seeks to address this lack through interviews with sixty (60) participants from Mexican, White American, and Mexican American backgrounds regarding their preferences for as well as their experiences with patient autonomy and physician paternalism.

2. Methods

2.1. Participants

We completed a total of sixty (60) interviews with twenty (20) of the interviews coming from each of the following three groups: White American (note: We use the terms "White American", "Mexican", and "Mexican American" advisedly, recognizing the complex and potentially problematic nature of these terms. Both "White American" and "Mexican" are peculiar categories. Whereas the former is a racial category, the latter is a nation-state based category. Moreover, both categories have substantial intra-group diversity. Nonetheless, as we show in what follows, these problematic categorical boundaries correspond with substantial differences in preferences and thinking about autonomy and paternalism in relation to healthcare encounters. These differences are what we call "cultural differences". In doing so, we caution the reader to keep in mind intracultural variation so as not to overly reify or essentialize these "cultural" categories.), Mexican American, or Mexican. White American participants were U.S. citizens who self-identified as "White". Mexican American participants were born either in the U.S. and have parents or grandparents from Mexico or were born in Mexico. All Mexican American participants currently reside in the U.S. but citizenship status remained unidentified in case revealing that status might lead to harm (e.g., deportation). Mexican participants were born in Mexico and currently reside in Mexico. The participants came from several states in the U.S. and Mexico (see Table 1). Informed consent was obtained from all subjects involved in the study. The study was approved by the Institutional Review Board of Brigham Young University (approved 9 January 2021).

Table 1. Origin of Participants for the Three Groups.

White American		Mexican American		Mexican	
Location	Number	Location	Number	Location	Number
California	3	California	2	Hidalgo	16
Idaho	1	Kansas	2	Nuevo Leon	1
Texas	1	New Mexico	2	Tamaulipas	2
Utah	10	Texas	2	Veracruz	1
Washington	5	Utah	5		
		Washington	7		
Total	20		20		20

Participants were identified based on snowball sampling that began with researchers' acquaintances. 59 of the 60 interviews were conducted over Zoom. One interview was conducted in person due to their proximity to the interviewer. Interviews were conducted in the language of the participant's choice which was determined in the initial contact based on the participants' preference. All interviews with White American respondents were conducted in English; all interviews with Mexican respondents were conducted in Spanish, and 17 interviews with Mexican American respondents were conducted in English with only three conducted in Spanish. Due to IRB concerns with the immigration status of participants, we do not have precise data for Mexican American participants' length of time in the U.S. or of which generation they are. Nonetheless, the high proportion of Mexican American participants who chose English as their preferred language (17/20) suggests that these participants have been in the U.S. long enough to have substantially acculturated to mainstream American culture. This and other participant information including age, ratio of female-male, and interview duration is included in Table 2 below.

Table 2. Participant Information.

	Interview Language		Gender		Age		Interview Time
Group	Spanish	English	Female	Male	Range	Mean	Average (min:sec)
White American	0	20	12	8	30–58	47.5	36:39
Mexican American	3	17	15	5	31–60	48.6	39:27
Mexican	20	0	15	5	33–65	48.7	30:42
Total	23	37	42	18	30–65	48.2	35:36

2.2. Interview Questions

We had a basic interview protocol that we aimed to ask each participant (See Appendix A), but, due to time constraints, some less important questions needed to be skipped with some respondents. Most questions were open-ended questions seeking to assess participant's views, opinions, and experiences regarding patient autonomy and physician paternalism in their interactions with physicians, whether in the U.S. (for White American and Mexican American respondents), or Mexico (for Mexican and Mexican American respondents). Interviewers followed up these questions with unscripted probing questions to explore respondents' reasoning. These typically included questions such as:

'why do you prefer that?', 'can you give me an example?', or 'do you have good or bad experiences regarding that?'.

Regarding paternalism and autonomy specifically, we asked two main questions (see Questions 20 and 21 in Appendix A). Question 20 asks about their preferences for either paternalism or patient autonomy and 21 asks which one of these their physician most closely practices. Before asking any questions about paternalism and autonomy, we provided the following simple definitions of autonomy and paternalism:

Paternalism/*El Paternalismo*: A relationship in which the physician has substantial/most control and authority over the patient's healthcare decisions./*Una relación en la que el médico tiene un control sustancial/ mayor y más autoridad sobre las decisiones de atención médica del paciente.*

Autonomy/*La Autonomía*: A relationship in which the patient has substantial/most control and authority over their own healthcare decisions./*Una relación en la que el paciente tiene un control sustancial/ mayor y más autoridad sobre sus propias decisiones de atención médica.*

With these and other questions, we did not specify the context or the kind of physician. Rather, we left this up to the participants to define. Most talked about their primary care providers but some mentioned specialists of various kinds.

In addition to exploring these central questions, we also included an untested and exploratory method which involved a set of eight (8) "hypothetical" statements that were actual statements said in the physician-patient interactions described in Thompson and Whiffen (2018). For each of these hypothetical statements, patients indicated how unusual or weird they thought that statement would be if their doctor were to say it. Although the trend of those responses was in support of the cultural difference hypothesis, we did not have sufficient measures in place to ensure that participants understood the hypotheticals sufficiently well. As a result, in what follows, we have focused on participants' answers to and explanations of their answers to the central questions.

2.3. Methods of Analysis

The audio recordings of these interviews were transcribed using Otter.ai and Sonix.ai, and then corrections were made by a Research Assistant. These transcripts were then coded in MAXQDA (See Appendices B and C) based on basic principles of in vivo grounded theory.

We created two codebooks to organize the data. The first codebook (Appendix B) organized the data with basic codes such as: paternalism, autonomy, doctor authority, doctor professionalism, physical and emotional caring, moral advice, etc. Each of these codes was broken down into subcodes. For example, the code *Care1-Physical and emotional caring* was broken down into four subcodes: *Actions demonstrating lack of care, Interpretations of actions demonstrating lack of care, Actions demonstrating care 1*, and *Interpretation of actions demonstrating care 1*. The second codebook (Appendix C) aimed to separate and define patient autonomy and physician paternalism according to participants' descriptions. This included codes such as: *Autonomy—informed decision making* and *Paternalism—doctor's expertise*, as well as their preferences which were organized into *autonomy, paternalism,* or *mix*. Interviews were coded by each member of the research team, and each member of the research team checked the other member's codes to ensure that researchers' coding was consistent across researchers. Results relevant to the cultural difference hypothesis are described below.

3. Results

We begin with the quantitative data regarding respondents' preferences for patient autonomy vs. physician paternalism. We then explore these data further by describing our respondents' explanations of their answers to this question. In 3.2, we turn to respondents' answers to the question of actual experiences with physicians, again beginning with the quantitative data and then adding nuance and detail with the qualitative data describing their explanations for their answers. Because it is difficult to know how acculturated

Mexican Americans are to American culture, in order to best examine the cultural difference hypothesis, we will focus primarily on the comparison between the groups of White American and Mexican respondents when considering respondents' preferences for patient autonomy vs. physician paternalism. Yet, since Mexican Americans have experience with both White American *and* Mexican physicians, we include their responses in our analysis of respondents' experiences with their physicians.

One other caveat is in order. To be sure, our study is not intended as an hypothesis-testing study (which would require a more rigorous selection methodology and more rigorous statistical methods of analysis). Rather, our study is intended as an hypothesis-exploring study in as much as we explore the cultural difference hypothesis in light of our participants' responses. Our findings should be considered as preliminary findings and, we hope, serve as the basis for future hypothesis-testing research. However, we also feel that these data are quite compelling as they are.

3.1. Group Preferences Data

Figure 1 shows the number of respondents in each group expressing a preference for patient autonomy (please note that throughout the result section when we refer to "autonomy", we mean "patient autonomy"), paternalism (by which we mean "paternalism of the physician"), or a mix of both in their interactions with their physicians.

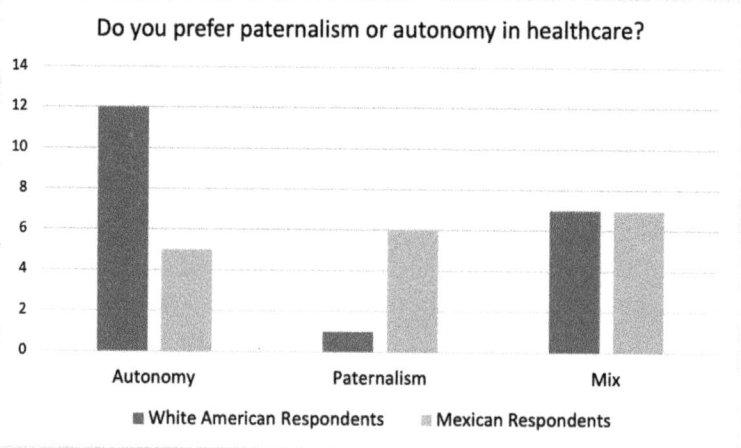

Figure 1. White American and Mexican Respondents' Preferences.

The cultural difference hypothesis that we explored in this study would suggest that White American respondents prefer "Autonomy" and the Mexican respondents prefer "Paternalism".

Our quantitative results provide modest support for this hypothesis (see Figure 1). Although only five of eighteen Mexican respondents said that they preferred "Autonomy", twelve of twenty of the White American respondents said that they preferred "Autonomy". Similarly, whereas only one of the twenty White American respondents said they preferred "Paternalism", six of the eighteen Mexican respondents said they preferred "Paternalism". Notably, seven White American respondents and seven Mexican respondents indicated that their preference was some kind of mix of both, something that we will explore further below.

A simple Chi-squared analysis of the responses of White American vs. Mexican responses produces a *p*-value of 0.012, suggesting that this difference is statistically significant (at the $p < 0.05$ level). Yet, as we will see next, when we dig into respondents' explanations of their answers to this question, the differences are even starker, especially for those who answered "Mix".

3.1.1. Group Preferences: White American Respondents

Beginning with White American respondents, 60% (12) said that they preferred "Autonomy". The most common aspects of autonomy mentioned by White American respondents were: *Informed decision making, doctor and patient as collaborators,* and *control over their body*. Ten White American respondents mentioned informed decision making, sixteen mentioned doctor and patient as collaborators, and ten mentioned the patient having control over their body. In addition to these common aspects of their descriptions of autonomy, a common logic emerged among White American respondents regarding their justifications for paternalism. This logic is roughly as follows: (1) they respect their physician's medical expertise, but (2) they are experts concerning their own bodies and (3) because bodily autonomy is paramount, they themselves should make the final treatment decision.

First, regarding their respect for their physician's expertise, many White American respondents who preferred "Autonomy", including Alyssa (30), Barbara (58), Megan (48), and Alexa (48), each noted the physician's medical expertise (note: all respondent names included in this article are pseudonyms). This is captured well by Barbara's comment: "The physician has the degrees, instruction, and knowledge on paper". While respecting and recognizing the value of their physician's medical training and expert knowledge, White American respondents also noted that this knowledge was not enough to justify locating the treatment decision with the physician.

Instead, White American respondents remarked that they are experts concerning their own bodies and that this knowledge is more important than the medical expertise of their physicians. As a result, these respondents felt that they themselves are the ones who should have the decision-making authority. Several White American respondents, including Irene (58), Julia (53), Alexa (48), and Jacob (32), each described the importance of their own knowledge regarding their bodies, summarized well by what Alexa said: "Because it's my life and my body, and I have the right to make those decisions ... They're just looking at it from a medical standpoint". Though the training and experience of the physician gives them some authority from a "medical standpoint", many White American respondents pointed that it is "their life", and "their body" and that this means that they should have the authority in the decision-making. Overall, White American respondents preferred being responsible for the final treatment decision.

Although "Autonomy" was the most common White American response, "Mix" was second with 35% (7) of White American respondents choosing "Mix". In their explanations of their responses, these respondents offered explanations that were very similar to the logic of the White American respondents who preferred "Autonomy". In their explanations of their decisions, Michelle (49), Emily (52), and Matthew (49) described a similar logic to those indicating a preference for "Autonomy". They "ultimately" preferred the locus of control and decision-making authority to be the patient. As Emily shared: "I really do like the doctor to give me their opinion, but I think that ultimately, it's the person's life and they need to choose what's best for them". Each shared that the "ultimate" decision-maker is the patient. In justifying this response, they gave similar reasonings such as bodily autonomy, it's the patient's life, or the patient is the expert regarding their body. Each of these definitions and reasonings are very similar to the definitions and reasonings given by the American respondents who preferred autonomy.

As one last example, Susan (51), a White American respondent who said she preferred "Mix" but leaned towards paternalism also sounds similar to these White American respondents who preferred "Autonomy". She shared: "I would want them [the physician] to be a little bit more in charge, but I would like to be a decision maker ... I think that we have ultimate say in our own treatment". Even though she said she leans toward paternalism, she explains that the patient still has the ultimate decision-making authority. Interestingly, she wants the physician to be "more in charge", but ultimately, she wants the final say.

The reasonings and definitions behind "Mix" for these White American respondents who chose "Mix" as their preference clearly point towards a more autonomy-oriented relationship with the physician. This further supports the idea that the White American respondents prefer an autonomy-focused physician-patient relationship.

Of course, as seen in Figure 1, one White American respondent, Abby (40), stated that she preferred "Paternalism" noting: "[I'm] going because [I] have a problem ... [I'm wasting my time] if I am not really going to do what they think is best for me, right?" Here Abby recognizes the medical experience and knowledge that the physicians have, yet she differs from the other White American respondents since she does not mention the importance of her knowledge of her body and life experience or of the importance of bodily autonomy. Instead, she leaves the final treatment decision with the physician. This offers an important reminder that the cultural difference hypothesis must not be *deterministic* in nature—as if culture necessarily determines behaviors. Rather, individual and intracultural variation must be acknowledged in any consideration of the role of culture in human behavior.

This deeper look into the White American respondents' descriptions and explanations of their preferences suggests a different organization of the quantitative data. Of the seven White American respondents who chose "Mix" as their preference, five actually described a preference for "Autonomy" in their explanations, and two describe something closer to "Paternalism". When considering their explanations for their answers, overall, seventeen White American respondents described a preference for "Autonomy" and three White American respondents described a preference that pointed more towards "Paternalism" (See Figure 2 below). This points towards a clear preference for patient autonomy among the White American respondents.

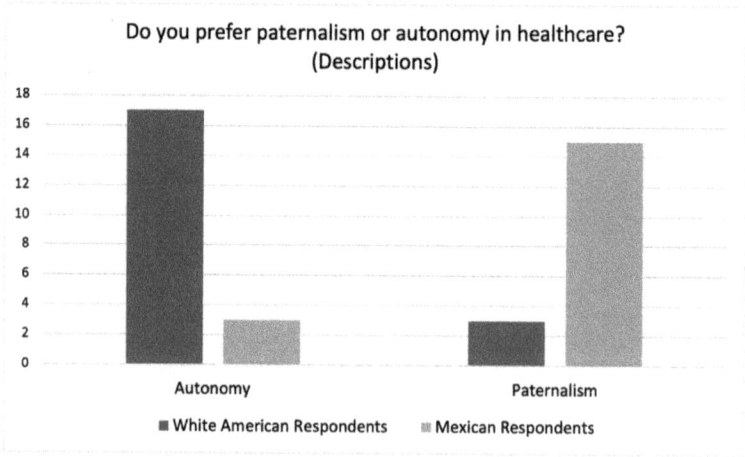

Figure 2. White American and Mexican Respondents' Preferences Based on Explanations.

3.1.2. Group Preferences: Mexican Respondents

As noted above, the most common preference described by Mexican respondents was "Mix" (39%, 7), with "Paternalism" being second (33%, 6), and "Autonomy" third (28%, 5). Although the distribution between these seems fairly even with only a slight preference for "Paternalism", as we will show below, the qualitative data illustrates an even stronger tendency towards a preference for "Paternalism" since in explaining their choices, several respondents who chose "Mix" actually described "Paternalism".

The overall logic of Mexican respondents' reasoning shared some similarities with the logic of White American respondents but differed in important ways. This logic could be roughly described as follows: (1) they respect their physician's medical expertise,

(2) although they have some knowledge of their own life experiences and bodies (3) their physician should have the final say in treatment decisions. An additional dimension of their logic was that qualities like trust, confidence, and obedience were crucial for their understanding of physician paternalism.

Similar to the White American respondents, several Mexican respondents who answered "Paternalism" for their preference noted a need to respect the physicians' expertise. Lucia (31), Diego (33), and Sara (43), each shared a sentiment that is well summarized by Josue's (52) simple statement: "They are the experts". These respondents described how the training, schooling, and experience of the physicians makes them the medical experts, something that the patient is decidedly not. When discussing their preferences for who makes the decision or if doctors should consult the patient, many Mexican respondents from those who preferred "Paternalism" or "Mix", including Isabela (47), Rosalia (52), Diego (33), and Samantha (55), reiterated the doctor's expertise such as what Samantha shared: "Pretending to take care of it without having the knowledge is impossible". Similarly, Diego shared: "I feel that they are the ones that know ... They have studied, they have the knowledge and experience necessary".

The Mexican respondents' descriptions point towards physicians' knowledgeability as qualifying the physicians to be the decision-maker. Anthony (50), Isabela, Rosalia, Josue, and Valeria (55), among others, ultimately shared that the locus of control should therefore be maintained by the physician and the physician should be the decision-maker. This is summarized well by what Rosalia shared: "The doctor is the one who decides ... because he is the one who knows". Furthermore, importantly, Lucia (48), and Camila (39), specifically pointed out that the doctor's training and experience gives each of them "confidence" in the physician as the decision-maker, as Lucia shared: "I trust that their study and their effort is really the best for me. I have confidence in my doctor regarding my health".

Regarding the seven Mexican respondents who stated "Mix" as their preference, six of them tended to lean towards paternalism or describe paternalistic characteristics that were similar to the Mexican respondents who preferred paternalism. In defining their "Mix", Camila, Yanira (40), Dexter (58), and Alvin (55), each shared how the physician is the one who knows and is the greater authority in making decisions. Yanira answered "Mix" as her preference, yet in her definition of what "Mix" means to her, she shared: "I like the part that the doctor gives you his indication and it is something that is not questionable. I understand that the doctor has to tell me what to do, but I also think that they could listen ... to what I have done or how I feel". Yanira clearly points to a paternalistic relationship as the doctor "has to tell [her] what to do"

Many of the Mexican respondents who said they preferred "Mix" actually described paternalism in their explanations. For example, Alvin, one of the Mexican respondents who preferred "Mix", stated: "I'd rather them give me the treatment because they're supposed to be the ones who know [best]", then later shared, "[Mix], because if I finish my medicine then I don't know what to get so I call the doctor and ask what does he suggest. They then tell me to buy this or that. So, that is when the decision is made between the both of us". Alvin indicates that his contribution as a patient is simply to let the doctor know that his medication has run out. The doctor will then "tell me to buy this or that". Here, Alvin clearly points to a paternalistic preference by his first statement even though he chose "Mix".

Although both Yanira and Alvin preferred "Mix", when specifically looking at the decision-making authority they clearly prefer paternalism. Other Mexican respondents who chose "Mix" as their preference later clarified that they leaned towards paternalism. These Mexican respondent's preferences, including Diana (38) and Angelica (37), are summarized well by what Diana shared. After having answered "Mix" as her preference Diana then shared that the doctor has more influence "because I think the doctor knows his job well and knows what he is doing".

In addition to these "Mix" responses that required some recoding, three of the five Mexican respondents who chose "Autonomy" as their preference actually described paternalism when explaining their preference. These respondents indicated that they have a choice whether or not to follow their physician's orders but that it is the physician's job to give orders and it is the patient's responsibility to follow those orders if they want to be healed. For example, Bella (44), who stated her preference as "Autonomy", shared: "I'm going to the doctor because I feel bad and I [want] him to help me. So, I have to do what he tells me if I want to feel good . . . In some way he'd have to explain it to me well so that I do it". Bella clearly points to paternalism as she admits that she has to do what the doctor says if she wants to feel good, yet the doctor still has to explain it well for her to fully comply. Her preference for "Autonomy" tended to relate more to compliance with the treatment, which she said depended on how well the physician explains his decision rather than who makes the decision. Similarly, Ana, a Mexican respondent who chose "Autonomy", said "there is always the security that [the] doctor has the ability and authority to recommend what is best for [the patient]". Here, as with a third Mexican respondent, we see the respondent who chose "Autonomy" is actually describing a relationship that is "Paternalistic".

In sum, six of the seven who answered "Mix" actually described paternalism and three of the five who answered "Autonomy" also emphasized paternalism. This means that when recounted according to their descriptions of their preferences, just three Mexican respondents preferred "Autonomy" while fifteen preferred "Paternalism" (See Figure 2).

When recounted to take into account what the respondents actually said (Figure 2), a strong trend emerges showing that whereas White American respondents strongly preferred autonomy, Mexican respondents strongly preferred paternalism. Although there were some important similarities in their explanations, such as the importance of the physician's expertise as well as the importance of the patient's knowledge of their own bodies, in the end these similar elements were interpreted quite differently. Whereas the White American respondents generally felt that the final treatment decision should be made by the patient due in large part to their rights, even responsibility, of bodily autonomy, the Mexican respondents felt that the physician should make the final treatment decision because their knowledge is far superior to that of the patient. The Mexican respondents also emphasized the importance of things such as the authority and trustworthiness of the physician, the obedience of the patient, and confidence in the physician.

3.2. Group Experiences Data

As will be shown below, the qualitative data on respondents' descriptions of group experiences was initially somewhat less clear regarding differences between White American and Mexican respondents' experiences. In particular, White American respondents' answers to the question of whether their physicians are oriented to autonomy or paternalism appeared to contradict the cultural difference hypothesis. We will thus begin our consideration of this data on respondents' experiences with physicians by presenting this apparently contradictory data.

3.2.1. White American Respondents Experiences of Paternalism with U.S. Physicians

As we can see in Figure 3, when comparing White American and Mexican respondents' answers to the question about whether the physicians that they have encountered are oriented to paternalism or autonomy, a very similar number of White American respondents viewed their doctors as paternalistic as did Mexican respondents (58% vs. 64%, or 79% vs. 82% if "Mix" is included).

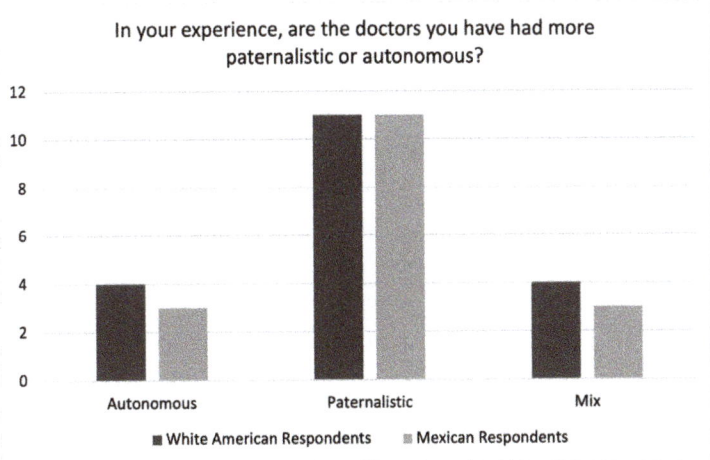

Figure 3. White American vs. Mexican Respondent Experiences.

This would appear to contradict the cultural difference hypothesis regarding respondents' actual experiences with physicians which would instead have suggested that White American respondents would describe their physicians as oriented to autonomy and Mexican respondents would describe their physicians as oriented to paternalism. Although it is of course possible that White American physicians are paternalistic, Mexican American respondents' answers suggest a different conclusion.

As noted above, we asked Mexican American respondents about their experiences with *both* American physicians and Mexican physicians. Considering that many of them had experience with physicians in both places, their responses provide the opportunity to directly compare experiences with Mexican and American physicians (see Figures 4 and 5).

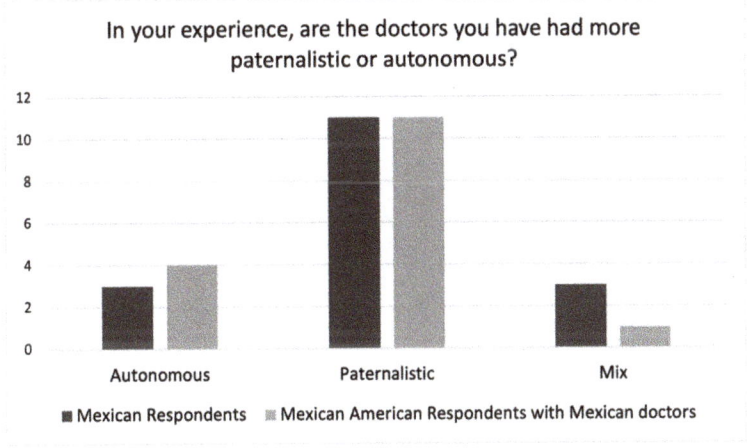

Figure 4. Mexican American vs. Mexican Respondent Experiences.

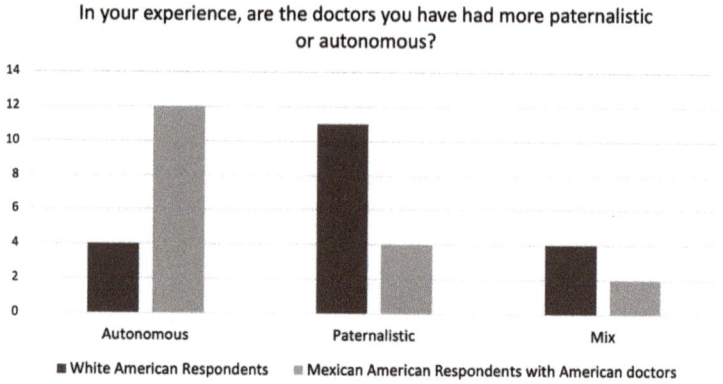

Figure 5. Mexican American vs. White American Respondents' Experiences.

Figure 4 shows Mexican American respondents' responses to this question regarding Mexican physicians as compared to Mexican respondents' responses with their Mexican physicians. The distribution between these two groups' responses is very similar with both groups describing Mexican physicians as paternalistic. Figure 5 shows Mexican American respondents' responses regarding American physicians as compared to White American respondents' responses with their American physicians. Here, the two groups differ rather significantly. Whereas the White American respondents tended to characterize American physicians as paternalistic, the Mexican American respondents tended to characterize their American physicians as autonomy-oriented. This of course raises an important question as to why these two groups characterize American physicians so differently?

3.2.2. Qualitative Data Explaining Respondents' Definitions of Paternalism

Respondents' explanations can help answer this question. As just noted, Mexican American respondents are particularly important in this regard since they had experience with both American and Mexican physicians and can provide a direct comparison. We will begin with their explanations.

Mexican American Respondents' Experiences with American and Mexican Physicians

In explaining their responses, several Mexican American respondents described the differences they saw between the physicians in the U.S. and Mexico. Mexican American respondents Victoria (37), and Andres (55), each said that in the U.S., doctors let patients decide what is best for them and give suggestions, but in Mexico it is "more obligatory" to follow the physician's treatment decision. Victoria pointed out that while a U.S. physician asks the patient if they agree with the given recommendation, a physician in Mexico gives more of a treatment directive leaving little room for the patient to contemplate whether or not to comply. Andres describes a very similar situation to Victoria, stating that Mexican physicians are much more insistent and authoritative by often making decisions before even asking the patient. Interestingly, Andres also notes that the authoritative physician who says "you have to do this" is "like a parent". Andres' and Victoria's descriptions highlight what many Mexican American respondents described as the differences between Mexican and American physician-patient relationships; whereas American doctors defer the final decision to the patient, Mexican doctors are the decision-making authority, often giving directives to the patient.

Moreover, this locating of the decision-making power with the physician was often viewed positively (e.g., "like a parent") while the reasons for American physicians' orientation to patient autonomy was viewed somewhat negatively. When explaining this difference, Gabriela (52) stated: "Here [in the U.S.], they are more afraid to try things . . .

in Mexico they are more open, more interactive ... " Gabriela goes on to point out that Mexicans are much more personal and open and thus can be rightfully more authoritative. In contrast to this, the "boundaries" in American culture, as she says, "limit" American physicians from being properly authoritative. Others offered similar descriptions that characterized Mexican physicians as able to be properly authoritative and American physicians as being held back or limited by the nature of American culture.

Regardless of how these qualities are valued, the Mexican American respondents make a strong case for the cultural difference hypothesis in as much as they describe American physicians operating very differently from Mexican physicians. Considering that these respondents are the only group who have experience with both American AND Mexican physicians, this offers strong support for the cultural difference hypothesis. However, it also raises another important question: what might the White American respondents mean by "paternalism" when they described their physicians as being paternalistic?

White American Respondents' Experiences with American Physicians

Interestingly, and in direct contrast to the Mexican American respondents' relatively positive descriptions of paternalism, when describing their American physicians as paternalistic, White American respondents overwhelmingly described this paternalism in very negative terms. Six White American respondents described paternalistic physicians as being arrogant and nine others described paternalism in terms of dismissiveness. Seven White American respondents described a physician who does not listen to or respect the patient or as only asking superficial questions as an example of a paternalistic and thus problematic physician. The lack of these "care" factors were a common reason why many White American respondents felt that their American physicians were paternalistic, and in a very negative sense.

Irene (58), Emily (52), Matthew (54), and Alexa (48), each mentioned arrogance as a characteristic of paternalism. Irene shared that she feels that doctors are paternalistic due to being "arrogant", because "they expect their patients to just do what they say and don't give their patients the opportunity to ask questions". Matthew offered a similar comment: "They [the doctors] kind of talk down to you ... they send the message that 'I'm the doctor, you're the patient. Just do what I say.'" These physicians acting paternalistically were seen as arrogant and therefore negative by these American respondents.

Another term that many White American respondents used to describe the paternalism of American physicians was "dismissive". This was used to describe situations where the doctor did not listen to the patient's concerns, opinions, or even their symptoms. Alyssa (30), Megan (48), Susan (51), Amanda (34), and Patricia (38), among others, gave experiences or descriptions of their physicians being dismissive. For example, Susan said: "The doctor would not listen to concerns. I didn't feel heard ... valued ... or trusted as somebody who knew symptoms ... His word was the final word, and nothing else". It should be clear here that dismissiveness is seen as one of the rather negative features of paternalism. Many of the other White American respondents mentioned that it is important that patients "feel heard" and "valued". In describing one of her experiences of paternalistic physicians, Amanda shared her story about being diagnosed with Polycystic Ovary Syndrome (PCOS). In giving her diagnosis, this physician did not provide her with the opportunity to ask questions about her diagnosis or treatment options. She felt overwhelmed and confused, stating: "I was crying on the way home because I thought I was deathly ill until, like, I researched it more". Here again, paternalism is being described in highly negative terms.

As we will see more clearly with the Mexican respondents, there are important differences in how the White American respondents describe paternalism as compared to how the Mexican and Mexican American respondents are describing it.

Mexican Respondents' Experiences with Mexican Physicians

Similar to the descriptions from the Mexican American respondents, many Mexican respondents described their Mexican physicians as often telling the patient what to do or deciding for the patient what the treatment will be. Instead of consulting and letting the patient decide, the physician takes the main or sole role in making treatment decisions. Samantha (55), Victoria (38), Rosalia (52), Diego (33), Yanira (40), and others, each said that their physicians tell them what to do. Samantha's description characterizes many of the Mexican respondent's experiences well when she said: "In most cases, they tell me what to do, how to do it and when to do it ... and in most cases they deliver". Here, Samantha points to a clear paternalistic relationship in which the physician is highly directive and has authority over the treatment decision. Yanira shared a similar sentiment: "Yes, they tell you what to do. They say: 'Do you want to be cured; you want to see a difference? Then you have to do this.'" Yanira points to the Mexican physicians as being highly directive. Yanira then further mentioned that she has confidence in and a preference for a paternalistic physician noting that if the patient doesn't get better, it's because they didn't follow the doctor's treatment decision. These experiences shared by the Mexican respondents clearly point to Mexican physicians as being paternalistic, while also indicating that these respondents appreciate their physicians' paternalism and view it positively.

There were a number of different aspects of this positive evaluation of paternalism. For example, Angelica (37) pointed out these characteristics as she describes her physician as: "very professional, so he always talks to me with a lot of respect and tries to explain everything. Obviously, there are terms that I don't understand because I'm not a doctor, but he tries to explain in simple terms my condition and what we'll do". As with the Mexican American descriptions of the paternalism of Mexican physicians, Mexican respondents often described their physicians' paternalism in very positive terms such as "very professional" and as treating their patients with "respect" while still being the decision-maker as the physician tells the patient "what we'll do".

Other positive evaluations of their paternalistic physicians by Mexican respondents included a strong sense that their physicians really care about them. For example, Maria (55) shared: "Yes, the doctor is sometimes like a spiritual father, like a priest or bishop in the church ... He also gives [personal] advice and sometimes you tell him personal things". Another Mexican respondent, Sara, who described her physicians as paternalistic shared: "Well, we talk about other things not related to my problem that I have at that moment and that makes me feel like he sees me as a person, not just as a disease". Samantha offered a similar sentiment about her physician who she described as paternalistic: "I have liked her [the physician] because ... she is interested in all aspects, emotional and physical ... She asks how you are, how's your daughter, how's work? She's a doctor that's very interested in her patients". Furthermore, Diana shared: "In my personal experience, they have always been kind and respectful ... [My doctor] always has a good attitude, he is looking me in the eye, he is attentive in the consultation".

As we can see, Mexican respondents evaluated their paternalistic physicians very positively. These descriptions demonstrate that they see these physicians as "like a spiritual father", caring, concerned, "attentive", "very interested" in their patients, and as someone who makes their patients feel seen as a person. What is most striking about these Mexican respondents' evaluations of their paternalistic physicians is that many of them are exactly opposite of the White American respondents' evaluations of their paternalistic physicians. Where the White American respondents described their physicians as not caring, inattentive, and uninterested, the Mexican respondents described their physicians as caring, attentive, and very interested in them as a person.

In sum, the Mexican respondents overwhelmingly described their physicians as being paternalistic, and in ways that were described positively and appreciated by these patients. Regarding the seemingly contradictory nature of the experience data, we will revisit this below in the discussion.

4. Discussion

Considering the relatively small (20) and non-random nature of our respondents in each group, our research should be understood to be exploratory and our findings preliminary. With this caveat in mind, our findings provide strong support for the cultural difference hypothesis, both in terms of White American vs. Mexican respondents' preferences for autonomy vs. paternalism (respectively) and in terms of differences of descriptions of experiences with Mexican vs. American physicians.

4.1. Differences in Preferences for Physician Paternalism vs. Patient Autonomy

Regarding the first, the White American respondents overwhelmingly said that they preferred a focus on patient autonomy with 60% choosing "Autonomy" and another 35% choosing "Mix" and just 5% choosing "Paternalism". When White American respondents described what they meant by "Mix", many of those who said "Mix" emphasized patient autonomy, making for a total of 17 out of 20 White American respondents who preferred "Autonomy". In their explanations of this preference, they described a situation where the physician shares their knowledge with the patient but the patient ultimately makes the final decision regarding treatment. These respondents felt that this was the preferred arrangement because the patients know best about their bodies and life experience and because they have a right, even an obligation, of bodily autonomy.

In contrast, the majority of Mexican respondents chose "Mix" with "Paternalism" coming in as a close second and "Autonomy" third. Yet, when they explained their choices, those who said "Mix" emphasized paternalism as did three of the five who said "Autonomy", making for a total of 15 out of 18 Mexican respondents who preferred "Paternalism". In their explanations, they described a situation where the patient shares their knowledge with the physician but the physician ultimately makes the final decision regarding treatment. These respondents felt that this was the preferred arrangement because the physicians are the experts and have the authority, even the obligation, to make treatment decisions for their patients.

Furthermore, the logic used by White American respondents to justify their preferences for patient autonomy was almost a mirror image of the logic used by Mexican respondents to justify their preferences for physician paternalism. Whereas White American respondents felt that the final treatment decision should be made by the patient who is informed by the physician of the necessary medical knowledge, the Mexican respondents felt that the final treatment decision should be made by the physician who is informed by the patient of the necessary bodily knowledge. This suggests a different organization of what is morally valued in these two cultural contexts. As such, it provides strong evidence for the cultural difference hypothesis regarding preferences for autonomy vs. Paternalism.

4.2. Cultural Differences in Experiences with Physician Paternalism vs. Patient Autonomy

Regarding respondents' experiences with autonomy and paternalism, responses to the question about whether their physicians were oriented towards autonomy or towards paternalism was, at first glance, less clear. Somewhat surprisingly given the findings in the literature on paternalism in American vs. Mexican healthcare, about the same number of White American and Mexican respondents described their physicians as paternalistic. At the same time, the Mexican American respondents contradicted the White American respondents' characterizations of American physicians as paternalistic, indicating that they are in fact oriented to patient autonomy. This raises an important question: what can explain these differences in respondents' characterizations of American physicians vis a vis paternalism?

A rather simple explanation might be to consider each group's experiences. Whereas the White American respondents only have experience with American physicians (this was clear in their responses), the Mexican American respondents have had experiences with both American and Mexican physicians and thus can compare each relative to the other (something that was evident in their responses when they asked whether we were talking about American or Mexican physicians). This would suggest that the Mexican American respondents have more context by which to judge American physicians and that American physicians are generally oriented to autonomy and that the White American respondents were simply using "paternalism" as a negative term to characterize their physicians. This is a plausible interpretation of the data but we would like to suggest a more nuanced interpretation that might provide a richer understanding of the ways in which culture is relevant to the question of autonomy vs. paternalism.

It may be that both the Mexican American and the White American respondents' characterizations of American physicians are accurate when considered relative to their own cultural frameworks. We can see two ways in which this cultural relativism works: first in how paternalism is defined and second in what it means when a physician acts paternalistically.

Regarding the first (i.e., what paternalism means), having seen the paternalism of Mexican physicians and with an understanding of the positive value of paternalism in that context, Mexican American respondents see American physicians as oriented to patient autonomy (in ways that are often seen negatively and thus in need of an excuse or explanation). On the other hand, White American respondents only have known American physicians and their own ideals of how a physician should act. Here, the ruling ideal is the autonomy of the patient and thus when White American respondents consider their physicians they find that their physicians do not compare well to their ideal of patient autonomy and conclude that their physicians are paternalistic. Thus, each group's characterization of American physicians vis a vis paternalism is relative to their experiences and cultural understandings of and ideals about what counts as paternalism, which appears to differ between these two groups.

Regarding the second (i.e., what it means for a physician to be paternalistic), we can see how the meaning of paternalism is evaluated differently in these two cultural contexts. Whereas the Mexican respondents consider their paternalistic physicians to be caring and concerned and very interested in them as a person, the White American respondents consider their paternalistic physicians who make decisions for them to be exactly the opposite—uncaring, unconcerned, and uninterested in them as a person and of their knowledge of their own bodies and of their bodily autonomy. This points to an important difference in the very moral evaluation of what it means for a physician to be paternalistic.

Both of these features point to more complex ways in which cultural differences function as fundamental organizing principles. This definitional question needs to be taken seriously by researchers. What is needed here is a rich understanding of what paternalism looks like in actual physicians' practices (e.g., Thompson and Whiffen 2018). The second concern of cultural relativism, what paternalism means, points to cultural differences in what it means to a patient to have an encounter with a paternalistic physician. Again, here it will be essential to observe patients' experiences with paternalistic physicians in order to explore and better understand those patients' reactions and characterizations of the encounter as well as the patients' consequent behaviors (esp. regarding things like treatment adherence and trust in their physician).

This also suggests that we consider paternalism in light of moral pluralism [19]. It should be clear that if we assume the White American respondents' characterizations of physician paternalism as uncaring, arrogant, disrespectful, dismissive, uninterested in the patient, and so on, then paternalism in a physician-patient relationship would in no way be a part of high-quality patient care. Yet, if we assume the Mexican respondents' characterizations of physician paternalism as caring, professional, respectful, "very interested" in their patients' lives, and so on, it would seem that physician paternalism is a necessary part of high-quality patient care. This again points to the importance of understanding the cultural contexts in which paternalism is defined and interpreted so that we can better understand the consequences that cultural differences will have for patients.

We would also like to note here that these findings raise important questions regarding why these Mexican respondents appear to have so much more positive relationships with their physicians as compared to the American respondents. These descriptions were particularly striking in light of the very negative, almost exactly opposite, descriptions that American respondents gave of American physicians. Although this quickly moves beyond the scope of the present study, our findings here do suggest that the paternalism of Mexican physicians demonstrates, for Mexican respondents, that Mexican physicians are highly caring, interested, and invested in their patients as individuals—a stark contrast with White American respondents' evaluations of their American physicians as uncaring, dismissive, and uninterested in them as patients.

We would further note that healthcare systems and institutions themselves contribute to the culture of healthcare in a given place. Thus there are likely other aspects of American healthcare systems and institutions, such as the proliferation of "defensive medicine" in response to a strong culture of litigation, that contribute to the emphasis on patient autonomy in the U.S. Importantly, this points to the fact that culture is not a simple matter of individual preferences or simply of good or bad physicians. Rather, cultural differences in physicians' practices are the result of a complex interaction between encultured individuals and encultured systems and institutions.

5. Conclusions

Based on our interviews with sixty (60) Mexican, Mexican American, and White American respondents, we found overall strong support for the cultural difference hypothesis with regard to preferences for and experiences of patient autonomy vs. physician paternalism. Whereas White American respondents preferred physicians oriented to patient autonomy, Mexican respondents preferred paternalistic physicians. With regard to their experiences, both White American and Mexican respondents tended to describe their physicians as paternalistic, only whereas the Mexican respondents described their physicians' paternalism in overwhelmingly positive terms, the White American respondents described their physicians' paternalism in overwhelmingly negative terms. Importantly, the Mexican American respondents, most of whom had experience with physicians in both places, indicated that whereas their American physicians were oriented towards autonomy, their Mexican physicians were oriented towards paternalism. This was in contrast to the White American respondents who tended to see their American physicians as paternalistic. As just outlined in our discussion, this provides further support for the cultural difference hypothesis by pointing to cultural differences in what paternalism means and what it means for a physician to be paternalistic.

The cultural difference hypothesis has some potentially important implications for healthcare practice. Two particularly important aspects that two of us previously proposed are demonstrations of physician care for patients and patients' treatment adherence (Thompson and Whiffen, 2018).

Regarding "care", our current study strongly suggests that physician paternalism is important for patients' perceptions of their physicians' care for them. Our data further suggest that these perceptions are determined relative to patients' cultural backgrounds. Whereas our White American respondents viewed paternalism as a deeply problematic physician behavior, our Mexican respondents viewed paternalism as a way that their physicians demonstrate their care for them as patients, as an indication of their interest in them as individuals. An understanding of how paternalism might be differently understood in different cultural contexts could have important implications for physicians interested in demonstrating care for and building trust with their patients.

Regarding treatment adherence, there was evidence pointing to the possibility that this cultural difference between Mexican patients and American physicians regarding how physicians interact with patients might result in lower levels of treatment adherence among these patients. In particular, the Mexican respondents repeatedly referred to paternalistic Mexican physicians in positive ways that indicated that the patients had confidence in the abilities of their Mexican doctors and that they saw them as trustworthy authorities that were supposed to be very directive when telling their patients what they needed to do. The Mexican American respondents also described what they saw as their American physicians' orientation to patient autonomy in negative terms that were in need of an explanation—as if they *should* be more directive but they cannot be more directive because it does not fit with the culture. This suggests that Mexican patients who are given treatment options by an autonomy-oriented physician might have less confidence in the authority of their physicians and thus be less likely to follow through with the treatment.

Minimally, both of these possibilities suggested by this and other research provide a strong argument for the importance of better understanding the role that cultural differences might play in healthcare practices. Our research here suggests that understanding these kinds of cultural differences is likely to be essential to improving treatment adherence while also creating trusting and caring physician-patient encounters.

Author Contributions: Conceptualization, G.A.T., L.H.W. and D.C.; methodology, G.A.T., L.H.W., D.C. and C.A.; formal analysis, G.A.T., J.S., C.A. and D.C.; investigation, J.S., D.C. and C.A.; writing—original draft preparation, J.S., D.C. and C.A.; writing—review and editing, G.A.T.; visualization, J.S. and G.A.T.; supervision, G.A.T.; project administration, D.C.; funding acquisition, G.A.T. and L.H.W. All authors have read and agreed to the published version of the manuscript.

Funding: This research was funded by Brigham Young University's Department of Anthropology Rust-Shallit Grant as well as a College Research Grant from the Family of Home and Social Sciences at Brigham Young University.

Institutional Review Board Statement: This study was approved by the Institutional Review Board of Brigham Young University (approved 9 January 2021).

Informed Consent Statement: Informed consent was obtained from all subjects involved in the study. All names included in this article are pseudonyms.

Data Availability Statement: The data presented in this study are available on request from the corresponding author pending IRB approval which must be submitted and completed by the requesting researcher. The data are not publicly available due to privacy and possible immigration information discussed in the IRB.

Acknowledgments: Early on, this research benefitted from the help of Breeze Parker. An earlier version of this paper was presented at the Society for Applied Anthropology and it has benefitted from feedback given by audience members. We are also grateful for the use of the John P. Hawkins Laboratory at Brigham Young University where the bulk of the data analysis was conducted.

Conflicts of Interest: The authors declare no conflict of interest. The funders had no role in the design of the study; in the collection, analyses, or interpretation of data; in the writing of the manuscript, or in the decision to publish the results.

Appendix A. Interview Questions

1. How many times would you say you've gone to see a doctor in the past year?
2. Do you usually go to the same doctor or do you see different doctors?
3. What is the ethnic background of the doctor that you usually see?
4. Describe the relationship that you have with the doctor you usually see. (Probes: Do they know much about you? Your family? Do you know much about them?)
5. How would you describe the personality of the doctor you usually see?
6. When your doctor gives you a diagnosis and a treatment plan:
    a. Does your doctor consult with you when deciding on a treatment plan? Which do you prefer (i.e., do you prefer that your doctor give you choices between treatments or would you prefer if they make the treatment decisions)?
    b. At the end of the day, who makes the final treatment decision, you or your doctor or both?
    c. Do you prefer to play a bigger part in the treatment decision making process, or do you prefer for your doctor to play a bigger part in the treatment decision making process?
    d. Do you prefer for your doctor to know a lot about you personally?

e. Is it weird if they ask about aspects of your personal life that are unrelated to the reason you are seeing the doctor? Do you prefer it when your doctor asks about your personal life?
f. Is it okay for your doctor to give you advice about aspects of your personal life that are unrelated to the reasons you are seeing the doctor? Do you prefer doctors that give such advice?
g. Have you ever questioned your doctor's treatment decision? For example, have you ever NOT taken a medicine that your doctor prescribed? If so, why did you choose not to? If not, can you imagine a situation in which you would not follow your doctor's orders for treatment?

7. Can you briefly describe the ethnic/cultural background of doctors that you have liked in the U.S. (or Mexico)? What was good about those experiences?
8. Can you briefly describe the ethnic/cultural background of doctors that you have not liked in the U.S. (or Mexico)? What was bad about those experiences?
9. For doctors with different/ethnic cultural backgrounds, of the doctors that you liked, are any of them from ethnic/cultural backgrounds different from your own?
10. (For American respondents) Do you have any Latinx friends?
    a. Have they ever shared anything with you about their experiences (good or bad) with doctors? If so, was the doctor American or another nationality/ethnicity? What did they say about it?

Hypotheticals

For each of the following situations, please tell me how normal or weird/awkward/unusual/strange (WAUS)
Scale:

1	2,3	4	5,6	7
perfectly normal	in between	a little WAUS	in between	highly WAUS

11. You are taking a medication that could cause depression and you tell your doctor that you don't want to take the depression medication and your doctor tells you "if you get depressed, you must take the medication". Why WAUS or why not?
12. You go to the doctor with your son and his hair is long and shaggy and your doctor tells you to get your son a haircut. Why WAUS or why not?
13. Your doctor tells you that you need to lose weight and then says "you have to exercise everyday". Why WAUS or why not?
14. During a regular check-up, your doctor tells you not to look at "very ugly things" (i.e., pornography) on the internet. Why WAUS or why not?
15. (Question only for women who have been pregnant) After an ultrasound, your doctor wipes off your abdomen and zips and buttons up your pants for you. Why WAUS or why not?
16. You go to the doctor with a particular concern (e.g., swelling in your feet) and your doctor asks you whether or not you *want* to take a medication (e.g., diuretic pills that help remove the liquid), would you think that is unusual? Why WAUS or why not?
    a. If you then agreed to the prescription and then you experienced side effects, would you be more or less likely to keep taking the medication if he asked if you wanted to take the medication rather than if he had told you "you must take the medication"?
17. Imagine you are a young single adult and go to your doctor and he tells you that you must get married. Why WAUS or why not?
18. Would you think it strange if you went to your annual check-up and your weight had been consistently increasing and your overweight doctor said to you "I'm not very good to talk about weight control to anybody" and then gave you basic advice about

a good diet? Why WAUS or why not? Would you be more or less likely to follow his instructions as compared to if the doctor had said "you are overweight and need to watch what you eat and make sure that you have a well-balanced diet"? Would it have seemed more strange if they were to have said that?

19. In your experience with American (or Mexican) doctors,
    a. RE: decision making, do they tell you what they want to do or do they give you information and let you decide what the best course of action is?
    b. RE: involvement/care, do they tend to know a lot about you personally? Do they ask a lot about you personally that may not be directly related to the reason you are seeing them?
    c. RE: advice-giving, do they tend to give you advice about your personal life and personal affairs even if it is not relevant to the reason you are seeing them?

- Define paternalism and autonomy

20. Do you prefer paternalism or autonomy in healthcare?
    a. Why?
21. In your experience, are mainstream American (or Mexican) doctors more paternalistic or autonomous?
22. (IF yes to 10) In your experience/understanding, are Mexican doctors more paternalistic or autonomous?

Appendix B. Codebook 1

1. Doctor Professionalism
    a. Lack of Professionalism: American
    b. Lack of Professionalism: Mexican
    c. American doctors
    d. Mexican doctors
2. Concerns about paternalism
    a. American doctors
    b. Mexican doctors
3. Concerns about autonomy
    a. Money concerns
    b. Lack of authority
        i. Actions showing lack of authority
        ii. Interpretation of actions
4. Support for paternalism
    a. American support
    b. Mexican support
    c. Authority of doctor
        i. Actions showing authority of doctor
        ii. Interpretation of actions showing authority
    d. Confident (vs. Uncertain or unsure)
    e. Decision-making
5. Support for autonomy
    a. American support
    b. Mexican support
    c. Shared decision-making
6. Mexican doctors are more paternalistic
    a. Actions supporting paternalism of Mexican doctors
    b. Interpretation of actions supporting paternalism of Mexican doctors

7. Care1-Physical and emotional caring
    a. Actions demonstrating lack of care1
    b. Actions demonstrating care1
    c. Interpretations of actions demonstrating care1
8. Care2-Personal business, moral advice
    a. Actions demonstrating care2
    b. Interpretation of actions demonstrating care2

Appendix C. Codebook 2
1. Characterizations of paternalism/autonomy
    a. Autonomy-informed decision-making
    b. Autonomy-doctor and patient as equals (collaboration)
    c. Autonomy-control over body
    d. Paternalism-authoritative doctor
        i. Arrogant
        ii. Dismissive
    e. Paternalism-familism
        i. Care for well-being
    f. Paternalism-doctor's expertise
        i. Patient decides if they agree with doctor
        ii. Patient admits they are unqualified
2. Autonomy
    a. People who say they prefer Autonomy, but describe something else
        i. Describe paternalism
        ii. Describe mix
    b. People who prefer autonomy (numbers and story)
        i. Mexican
        ii. Mexican-American
        iii. American
3. Paternalism
    a. People who say they prefer Paternalism but describe something else
        i. Describe autonomy
        ii. Describe mix
    b. People who prefer paternalism (numbers and story)
        i. Mexican
        ii. Mexican-American
        iii. American
4. Mix
    a. People who say P/A but give details as Mix
    b. Mix in middle
    c. Mix leaning toward autonomy
    d. Mix leaning toward paternalism
    e. Mix stories
    f. Mix preference
5. Narratives
    a. Very influential experiences
    b. Paternalism experiences
        i. Mix experiences

        ii.   Negative experiences
        iii.   Positive experiences
    c. Autonomy experiences
        i.   Mix experiences
        ii.   Negative experiences
        iii.   Positive experiences

References

1. Jennings, B. Autonomy. In *The Oxford Handbook of Bioethics*; Steinbock, B., Ed.; Oxford University Press: Oxford, UK, 2009.
2. Lewis, J. Getting Obligations Right: Autonomy and Shared Decision Making. *J. Appl. Philos.* **2020**, *37*, 118–140. [CrossRef]
3. Jennings, B. Reconceptualizing Autonomy: A Relational Turn in Bioethics. *Hastings Cent. Rep.* **2016**, *46*, 11–16. [CrossRef] [PubMed]
4. Macklin, R. Respect for cultural diversity and pluralism. In *Handbook of Global Bioethics*; ten Have, H.A.M.J., Gordijn, G., Eds.; Springer: New York, NY, USA, 2014; pp. 153–167. [CrossRef]
5. Sandman, L.; Munthe, C. Shared decision-making and patient autonomy. *Theor Med Bioeth* **2009**, *30*, 289–310. [CrossRef] [PubMed]
6. Schneider, C. *The Practice of Autonomy: Patients, Doctors, and Medical Decisions*; Oxford University Press: Oxford, UK, 1998.
7. Donnelly, M. *Healthcare Decision-Making and the Law*; Cambridge University Press: Cambridge, UK, 2010; Open WorldCat. Available online: http://www.myilibrary.com?id=296631 (accessed on 15 September 2021).
8. Entwistle, V.A.; Carter, S.M.; Cribb, A.; McCaffery, K. Supporting Patient Autonomy: The Importance of Clinician-Patient Relationships. *J. Gen. Intern. Med.* **2010**, *25*, 741–745. [CrossRef]
9. Beauchamp, T.L.; Childress, J.F. *Principles of Biomedical Ethics*, 7th ed.; Oxford University Press: Oxford, UK, 2013.
10. Coggon, J.; Miola, J. Autonomy, Liberty, and Medical Decision-Making. *Camb. Law J.* **2011**, *70*, 523–547. [CrossRef]
11. Beauchamp, T.; Childress, J. Principles of Biomedical Ethics: Marking Its Fortieth Anniversary. *Am. J. Bioeth.* **2019**, *19*, 9–12. [CrossRef]
12. Buchanan, D.R. Autonomy, Paternalism, and Justice: Ethical Priorities in Public Health. *Am. J. Public Health* **2008**, *98*, 15–21. [CrossRef]
13. Cooley, D.R. Elder Abuse and Vulnerability: Avoiding Illicit Paternalism in Healthcare, Medical Research, and Life. *Ethics Med. Public Health* **2015**, *1*, 102–112. [CrossRef]
14. Coulter, A. Paternalism or Partnership? *BMJ* **1999**, *319*, 719–720. [CrossRef]
15. National Commission for the Protection of Human Subjects of Biomedical and Behavioral Research. *The Belmont Report: Ethical Principles and Guidelines for the Protection of Human Subjects of Research*; U.S. Department of Health and Human Services: Elkredge, US, 1979. Available online: https://www.hhs.gov/ohrp/regulations-and-policy/belmont-report/read-the-belmont-report/index.html (accessed on 10 October 2021).
16. Ten, H.H.; Stanton-Jean, M. (Eds.) *The UNESCO Universal Declaration on Bioethics and Human Rights: Background, Principles and Application*; Unesco: Paris, France, 2009.
17. Thompson, G.A.; Whiffen, L.H. Can Physicians Demonstrate High Quality Care Using Paternalistic Practices? A Case Study of Paternalism in Latino Physician–Patient Interactions. *Qual. Health Res.* **2018**, *28*, 1910–1922. [CrossRef]
18. Lazcano-Ponce, E.; Angeles-Llerenas, A.; Rodríguez-Valentín, R.; Salvador-Carulla, L.; Domínguez-Esponda, R.; Astudillo-García, C.I.; Madrigal-de León, E.; Katz, G. Communication Patterns in the Doctor–Patient Relationship: Evaluating Determinants Associated with Low Paternalism in Mexico. *BMC Med. Ethics* **2020**, *21*, 125. [CrossRef] [PubMed]
19. Shweder, R.A. Moral realism without the ethnocentrism: Is it just a list of empty truisms? In *Human Rights with Modesty: The Problem of Universalism*; Springer: Dordrecht, The Netherlands, 2004; pp. 65–102.
20. Jensen, L.A. The cultural development of three fundamental moral ethics: Autonomy, community, and divinity. *Zygon®* **2011**, *46*, 150–167. [CrossRef]
21. Betancourt, J.; Green, A.; Carillo, J.E. The challenges of cross-cultural healthcare-diversity, ethics, and the medical encounter. In *Bioethics Forum*; Midwest Bioethics Center: Bethesda, MD, USA, 2000; Volume 16, pp. 27–32.
22. Buchholz, R.A.; Rosenthal, S.B. Toward a new understanding of moral pluralism. *Bus. Ethics Q.* **1996**, *6*, 263–275. [CrossRef]
23. Fernández-Ballesteros, R.; Sánchez-Izquierdo, M.; Olmos, R.; Huici, C.; Ribera Casado, J.M.; Cruz Jentoft, A. Paternalism vs. autonomy: Are they alternative types of formal care? *Front. Psychol.* **2019**, *10*, 1460. [CrossRef]
24. Finkler, K. *Physicians at Work, Patients in Pain: Biomedical Practice and Patient Response in Mexico*; Routledge: London, UK, 2019.
25. Ho, A. Relational autonomy or undue pressure? Family's role in medical decision-making. *Scand. J. Caring Sci.* **2008**, *22*, 128–135. [CrossRef]
26. Mitchell, P.; Cribb, A.; Entwistle, V.A. Defining What is Good: Pluralism and Healthcare Quality. *Kennedy Inst. Ethics J.* **2019**, *29*, 367. [CrossRef]
27. Sousa, A.J. *Pragmatic Ethics, Sensible Care: Psychiatry and Schizophrenia in North India*; The University of Chicago: Chicago, IL, USA, 2011.

28. Zivkovic, T. Lifelines and end-of-life decision-making: An anthropological analysis of advance care directives in cross-cultural contexts. *Ethnos* **2021**, *86*, 767–785. [CrossRef]
29. Norman, I. Blind trust in the care-giver: Is paternalism essential to the health-seeking behavior of patients in Sub-Saharan Africa? *Adv. Appl. Sociol.* **2015**, *5*, 94. [CrossRef]
30. Ujewe, S.J. Ought-onomy and Mental Health Ethics: From "Respect for Personal Autonomy" to "Preservation of Person-in-Community" in African Ethics. *Philos. Psychiatry Psychol.* **2018**, *25*, E-45. [CrossRef]
31. Shaibu, S. Ethical and cultural considerations in informed consent in Botswana. *Nurs. Ethics* **2007**, *14*, 503–509. [CrossRef]
32. Addissie, A.; Tesfaye, M. Ethiopia. In *Handbook of Global Bioethics*; ten Have, H.A.M.J., Gordijn, G., Eds.; Springer: New York, NY, USA, 2014; pp. 1121–1139. [CrossRef]
33. Aarons, D. Doctor-Patient Communication in Government Hospitals in JAMAICA. Ph.D. Thesis, McGill University, Montreal, QC, Canada, 2005.
34. Blackhall, L.J.; Murphy, S.T.; Frank, G.; Michel, V.; Azen, S. Ethnicity and attitudes toward patient autonomy. *Jama* **1995**, *274*, 820–825. [CrossRef] [PubMed]
35. Frank, G.; Blackhall, L.J.; Michel, V.; Murphy, S.T.; Azen, S.P.; Park, K. A discourse of relationships in bioethics: Patient autonomy and end-of-life decision making among elderly Korean Americans. *Med. Anthropol. Q.* **1998**, *12*, 403–423. [CrossRef] [PubMed]
36. Wang, Q. Doctor-Patient Communication and Patient Satisfaction: A Cross-Cultural Comparative Study between China and the U.S. Ph.D. Thesis, Purdue University ProQuest Dissertations Publishing, Bloomington, IN, USA, 2010. Available from ProQuest Dissertations and Theses Database. (Order No. 3444876).
37. Chattopadhyay, S.; Simon, A. East meets West: Cross-cultural perspective in end-of-life decision making from Indian and German viewpoints. *Med. Health Care Philos.* **2008**, *11*, 165–174. [CrossRef]
38. Ishiwata, R.; Sakai, A. The physician–patient relationship and medical ethics in Japan. *Camb. Q. Healthc. Ethics* **1994**, *3*, 60–66. [CrossRef] [PubMed]
39. Claramita, M.; Nugraheni, M.D.; van Dalen, J.; van der Vleuten, C. Doctor–patient communication in Southeast Asia: A different culture? *Adv. Health Sci. Educ.* **2013**, *18*, 15–31. [CrossRef] [PubMed]
40. Fadiman, A. *The Spirit Catches You and You Fall Down: A Hmong Child, Her American Doctors, and the Collision of Two Cultures*; Macmillan: New York, NY, USA, 2012.
41. Moazam, F. Families, patients, and physicians in medical decision-making: A Pakistani perspective. *Hastings Cent. Rep.* **2000**, *30*, 28–37. [CrossRef]
42. Kara, M.A. Applicability of the principle of respect for autonomy: The perspective of Turkey. *J. Med. Ethics* **2007**, *33*, 627–630. [CrossRef]
43. Gracia, D. The intellectual basis of bioethics in southern European countries. *Bioethics* **1993**, *7*, 97–107. [CrossRef]
44. McGrath, P.; Vun, M.; Mcleod, L. Needs and experiences of non-English-speaking hospice patients and families in an English-speaking country. *Am. J. Hosp. Palliat. Med.®* **2001**, *18*, 305–312. [CrossRef]
45. Nie, J.B. The plurality of Chinese and American medical moralities: Toward an interpretive cross-cultural bioethics. *Kennedy Inst. Ethics J.* **2000**, *10*, 239–260. [CrossRef]
46. Veatch, R.M. The ethics of critical care in cross-cultural perspective. In *Ethics and Critical Care Medicine*; Springer: Dordrecht, The Netherlands, 1985; pp. 191–206.
47. Payne-Jackson, A.; Alleyne, M.C. *Jamaican Folk medicine: A Source of Healing*; University of West Indies Press: Mona, Jamaica, 2004.
48. Lai, K.L. Confucian moral thinking. *Philos. East West* **1995**, *45*, 249–272. [CrossRef]
49. Glaser, B.G.; Strauss, A.L. *Awareness of Dying*; Transaction Publishers: Chicago, IL, USA, 1979.
50. Timmermans, S. Dying of awareness: The theory of awareness contexts revisited. *Sociol. Health Illn.* **1994**, *16*, 322–339. [CrossRef]
51. Lazcano-Ponce, E.; Angeles-Llerenas, A.; Alvarez-del Río, A.; Salazar-Martínez, E.; Allen, B.; Hernández-Avila, M.; Kraus, A. Ethics and Communication between Physicians and Their Patients with Cancer, HIV/AIDS, and Rheumatoid Arthritis in Mexico. *Arch. Med. Res.* **2004**, *35*, 66–75. [CrossRef] [PubMed]
52. Colmenares-Roa, T.; Huerta-Sil, G.; Infante-Castañeda, C.; Lino-Pérez, L.; Alvarez-Hernández, E.; Peláez-Ballestas, I. Doctor–Patient Relationship Between Individuals With Fibromyalgia and Rheumatologists in Public and Private Health Care in Mexico. *Qual. Health Res.* **2016**, *26*, 1674–1688. [CrossRef] [PubMed]
53. Armenta-Arellano, S.; Muños-Hernández, J.A.; Pavón-León, P.; Coronel-Brizio, P.G.; Gutiérrez-Alba, G. An Overview on the Promotion on Patient-Centered Care and Shared Decision-Making in Mexico. *Z. Für Evidenz Fortbild. Und Qual. Im Gesundh.* **2022**, *171*, 93–97. [CrossRef]
54. Brown, C.J.; Pagan, J.A.; Rodriguez-Oreggia, E. The Decision-Making Process of Health Care Utilization in Mexico. *Health Policy* **2005**, *72*, 81–91. [CrossRef]
55. Macklin, R. *Against Relativism: Cultural Diversity and the Search for Ethical Universals in Medicine*; Oxford University Press: Oxford, UK, 1999.
56. Garcia-Gonzalez, A.; Gonzalez-Lopez, L.; Gamez-Nava, J.I.; Rodríguez-Arreola, B.E.; Cox, V.; Suarez-Almazor, M.E. Doctor-Patient Interactions in Mexican Patients with Rheumatic Disease. *J. Clin. Rheumatol.* **2009**, *15*, 120–123. [CrossRef] [PubMed]

57. Bermudez, J.Á.; Carreño, J.P.S.; Rojas, J.A.V. Percepción de Los Pacientes Acerca de La Empatía de Las Enfermeras En Monterrey (México) = Perception of Patients about the Empathy of Nurses in Monterrey (Mexico). *Rev. Española De Comun. En Salud* **2018**, *9*, 46. [CrossRef]
58. Doubova, S.V.; Guanais, F.C.; Pérez-Cuevas, R.; Canning, D.; Macinko, J.; Reich, M.R. Attributes of Patient-Centered Primary Care Associated with the Public Perception of Good Healthcare Quality in Brazil, Colombia, Mexico and El Salvador. *Health Policy Plan.* **2016**, *31*, 834–843. [CrossRef]

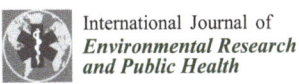

Article

What Patients Prioritize for Research to Improve Their Lives and How Their Priorities Get Dismissed again

Barbara Groot [1,2,*], Annyk Haveman [3], Mireille Buree [3], Ruud van Zuijlen [3], Juliette van Zuijlen [3] and Tineke Abma [1,2]

[1] Department Public Health and Primary Care, Leiden University Medical Centre, Leiden University, Albinusdreef 2, 2333 ZA Leiden, The Netherlands; abma@leydenacademy.nl
[2] Leyden Academy on Vitality and Ageing, Rijnsburgerweg 10, 2333 AA Leiden, The Netherlands
[3] Centrum voor Cliëntervaringen, Jacob Bontiusplaats 9 (INIT-gebouw), 1018 LL Amsterdam, The Netherlands; annyk.haveman@uiteigenbeweging.nu (A.H.); barbarazzi@hotmail.com (M.B.); info@vanzuijlen.dds.nl (R.v.Z.); barbarazzi@gmail.com (J.v.Z.)
* Correspondence: groot@leydenacademy.nl

Abstract: Health researchers increasingly work with patients in a participatory fashion. Active patient involvement throughout the research process can provide epistemic justice to patients who have often only had an informant role in traditional health research. This study aims to conduct participatory research on patient experiences to create a solid research agenda with patients and discuss it with relevant stakeholders. We followed a participatory research design in 18 sub-studies, including interviews and group sessions (n = 404 patients), and dialogue sessions (n = 367 professionals and directors in healthcare and social work, municipality civil servants, and funding agencies) on patient experiences with psychiatric care, community care, daycare, public health, and social work. Findings from the eight-year study show that four priorities stood out: attention for misuse of power and abuse; meaningful participation; non-human assistance, and peer support. Moreover, that: (1) patients, based on their experiences, prioritize different topics than experts; (2) most topics are trans-diagnostic and point to the value of a cross-disability approach; and (3) the priorities of patients are all too easily dismissed and require ethics work to prevent epistemic injustice. Long-term investment in a transdisciplinary community of practice offers a solid basis for addressing patient-centered topics and may impact the quality of life of people living with chronic illness, disability, or vulnerability.

Keywords: patient perspective; epistemic injustice; community of practice; participatory health research; co-researchers; assistance dogs; assistive technology; abuse; dependency; peer support

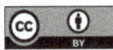

1. Introduction

There is increasing interest and support for the idea of patient and public involvement (PPI) in health services and, to a lesser extent, in health research. Examples are academics studying patient experiences and who identify as patients themselves [1–4] or who collaborate with people with lived experiences as their research partner or co-researcher [5–10]. More journals are also becoming patient-inclusive, such as the Patient Experience Journal with the Patients Included™ status. This status means that patients sit on the editorial board, routinely publish as authors, serve as peer reviewers, and provide open access. This all suggests a rising trend.

There are several arguments for including patients in research. Firstly, it is argued that patients possess unique experiential knowledge grounded in their lived experiences with the illness, vulnerability, or disability. This indicates that patients have singular perspectives on (coping with) their illness and treatment. This 'emic' or 'insider' perspective of patients is often as valuable and complementary to professionals' 'etic' or 'outsider' perspective [11]. When patients are involved in research, this will enhance the societal impact and relevance. Secondly, it is argued that patients as end-users should have a voice in research that ultimately affects their lives. This normative argument is closely related to the ideal of epistemic justice—a concept coined by philosopher and feminist Miranda Fricker [12,13]. Epistemic justice is a commitment to acknowledge the fundamental human right to be respected as a bearer of knowledge. In line with this ideal, patients should be given a say in knowledge production.

Although the arguments for PPI are compelling, day-to-day practice shows that involvement is not a straight-forward and smooth process. Studies demonstrate that PPI's implementation is highly uneven and that PPI is not yet firmly embedded or adequately formalized in European healthcare systems and research [14]. In practice, patients often do not have much influence or control over the research in which they are involved [15]. Patients, or clients who reflected on their experiences, are rarely engaged in a way in which their knowledge is valued equally and viewed as complementary in research, but are mostly involved at the levels of informing, consulting, and sometimes placation [16]. For example, patients are told about the study (informing), questioned in interviews or focus groups (consultation), and positioned on steering groups at specific moments in the research process (placation). In these settings, academics are still the initiators who determine the research agenda and control the research. Furthermore, patients living in vulnerable situations, that is, the 'seldom heard' [17], are rarely engaged [18].

The challenges of involving patients in research can be understood in the context of traditional power hierarchies in healthcare practices. Professional caregivers and health researchers have a privileged epistemic status based on expertise and thus risk (often unintentionally) downplaying patients' testimonies and interpretations. Some are not viewed as credible knowers because of a negative identity and prejudicial stereotypes in healthcare [19], especially in psychiatry [20], but also in child and youth care [21], chronic illnesses like chronic fatigue syndrome [22], and chronic pain [23]. Patients' testimonials can be disputed, for instance, because they do not follow the medical model [24]. Professionals may also (mis)judge patients' intelligence, credibility, and rationality based on their language skills and discourse [25]. Epistemic injustice thus impacts the quality and equity of care provided and limits research on patient experiences.

Recently, frameworks have been developed for PPI and, more for specifically, patient-led priority or research agenda-setting [26]. In these types of studies different groups, including patients, are involved in drawing up an agenda of topics that are important to investigate. These studies value patients' priorities as being of equal importance as the priorities of researchers and care professionals [27], and often focus on one diagnosis or patient group [28,29] or places and times defined by experts, like stays in a hospital [30]. Based on a systematic review of PPI frameworks, Greenhalgh and her team [26] suggest that researchers should develop and co-create a framework rather than choose one. How to co-create such a framework in a particular context, living up to the ideal of epistemic justice, and what kind of topics are prioritized when patients are genuinely involved in the agenda-setting from conception to conclusion, remains unclear.

The study presented in this article fills that void. It aims to create a solid patient-led research agenda amongst patients and discuss this agenda with relevant stakeholders (healthcare professionals, researchers, and funding agencies). We developed a framework together with stakeholders, including patients. Our findings show that (1) patients, based on their experiences, prioritize different topics than experts; (2) most topics are trans-diagnostic and point to the value of a cross-disability approach; (3) the priorities of patients are often too easily dismissed and require ethics work to prevent epistemic injustice.

When we use 'patients', we refer to people with chronic illnesses, psychiatric vulnerability, learning disabilities, or older adults currently receiving care. The term also refers those experiencing health problems due to poverty. 'Experts by experience' refers to patients who have reflected on their lived experiences, which are often life-changing. These experts often work as an advocate of the perspective of patients or use their skills and experiences to support peers and collaborate with professionals and researchers. We are aware that they may identify themselves as clients, users, end-users, service users, survivors, or people with an illness, vulnerability, disability, or living in poverty. In this article, we also use the term 'co-researcher' for anyone participating on equal footing with academics and who are often experts by experience.

2. Materials and Methods

2.1. Context: Learning Community on Patient-Led Care

In 2015, a small group of researchers and representatives of a patient advocacy organization with a shared mission to improve the quality of care for people living in vulnerable situations launched the Center of Client Experiences in the region of Amsterdam, The Netherlands (in Dutch: Centrum voor Cliëntervaringen, CvC for short; www.centrumvoorclientervaringen.com accessed on 5 February 2021). All members became 'partners' in the CvC learning community and strived for patient-led care, but felt alone in their mission. They often experienced resistance to their work that incorporated lived experiences or their collaboration with patients. The Center's researchers sought partners who shared their mission and wanted to build a community to learn with and from each other about patient-led care.

Between 2014 and 2021, the CvC network grew to include ten organizations as official community partners and 19 patient co-researchers. The community partners met in face-to-face work sessions. The workshops' agenda was decided by the group. We conducted sub-studies on patients' experiences in various contexts to improve care with and for patients, together with partners. In parallel, we hope this will create more room and acknowledgment for the client's perspective in care.

2.2. Methods and Analysis: Participatory Health Research

This article reports participatory health research (PHR) [31–33] in which 18 studies were conducted of lived experiences in psychiatric, community care, daycare, public health, and social work aimed to generate impact on the lives of patients (see Table 1). These 18 sub-studies drew on different groups of patients and co-researchers who all suffered from chronic illnesses or disabilities. In total, $n = 404$ patients shared their narratives in these sub-studies and $n = 367$ stakeholders (healthcare professionals, policymakers, funding agencies, municipal civil servants) were involved. The sub-studies' aim was not to compile a patient agenda, but to foster change in practice. This research presents an analysis and reflection on the significant topics on the group's agenda. In addition, the authors facilitated 12 three-hour work sessions at the CvC with 10–20 people each. The sub-studies and work sessions took place from 2014 to 2021.

The analysis was a collaborative and iterative process. In PHR, it is done with co-researchers and is an ongoing cyclical process of data generation and analysis over an extended period [31]. During this process, actions such as writing a research proposal also arise from the research, and are then reflected upon again. Important tenets of the analysis were: (1) that it was systematic; (2) that it occurred in collaborative dialogue and deliberation; (3) that findings were validated in the interim; and (4) that the process is replicable, as described below [56,57].

First, creative analysis methods were chosen in this study to analyze with co-researchers. This is common in participatory action research. Creative methods of analysis, such as the Critical Creative Hermeneutical Analysis (CCHA) [58], provided an opportunity to interpret experiences in an approachable way. We conducted this CCHA with co-researchers in each sub-study, in addition to thematic analysis [59] by the researcher(s). The CCHA and thematic analyses informed each other. As a result, extensive deliberation based on experiences (quotes from respondents) took place during all the sub-studies. Themes that emerged are described in the reports (see Table 1).

Secondly, a similar process occurred at a generic level, i.e., across all sub-studies. The first author was involved in all the studies discussed in this article. Over the past few years, she analyzed the reports thematically. The resulting themes were regularly discussed at work sessions at the Center for Client Experience. These were also the themes that were central to new research proposals written with co-researchers.

Finally, in November–December 2021, the first author thematically analyzed all reports, work session summaries, and draft research proposals and arrived at four themes, namely (1) attention to misuse of power and abuse; (2) meaningful participation; (3) alternative guidance or assistance; and (4) peer support. These themes were discussed with the co-authors (co-researchers) and validated in online meetings and telephone calls (due to the COVID-19 lockdown).

Table 1. The background of the 18 sub-studies.

Field of Experience	Participants and Co-Researchers	Methods	Patients Involved	Stakeholders Involved	Year	Dissemination	Funder
Community care	Patients with chronic diseases, physical impairments and older adults	Interviews and a dialogue session with stakeholders about the findings	$n = 32$	$n = 14$	2014–2015	Report [34]	A municipality
	Older patients with community care		$n = 29$	$n = 5$	2016	Report [35]	Care organization
	All patients with community care		$n = 85$,	$n = 79$	2017	Report [36]	A municipality
	Informal caregivers		$n = 49$	$n = 23$	2016	Report [37]	
	Informal caregivers of patients with dementia		$n = 19$	$n = 25$	2016	Report [38]	Social work organization
	Patients with a learning disability		$n = 20$	$n = 14$	2015–2016	Report [39]	A municipality
			$n = 20$	$n = 30$	2017	Report [40]	
			$n = 15$	$n = 8$	2019	Report [41]	
	Patients with a psychiatric vulnerability		$n = 5$	$n = 17$	2015	Report [42]	
	Patients who are dependent on assistive technology		$n = 6$	$n = 4$	2018–2020	Video [43]	Charitable foundation
General practitioners (GPs)	Frequent users of GPs		$n = 17$	$n = 5$	2019	Web text [44]	Health insurance company
Emergency psychiatric care	Patients who want to be admitted voluntarily		$n = 17$	$n = 32$	2019	Report [45]	Health insurance company
	Patients in psychiatric crisis		$n = 17$	$n = 28$	2017–2018	Report and articles [46,47]	Two psychiatric care institutions
Social work and public health	People ageing at home	(Online) Group sessions with session with stakeholders about the findings	$n = 40$	$n = 14$	2016–2020	Report [48]	A municipality & Applied University
	Patients in COVID-19 isolation		$n = 9$	$n = 21$	2020	Report [49]	Dutch Health Research Fund
	People living in poverty		$n = 6$	$n = 25$	2018	Report and articles [50–52]	Charitable foundation
	People without a job		$n = 10$	$n = 19$	2018–2019	Report and article [53,54]	A municipality
Hospital care	Youngsters with a respiratory disease		$n = 8$	$n = 4$	2018–2020	Article [55]	Dutch Foundation for Asthma Prevention

2.3. Author Team

The study's author team is a mix of academics and co-researchers. The first and final authors are academic participatory action researchers who facilitated building the CvC and were involved in all 18 sub-studies as a researcher. The second author is a change agent with a mix of patient identities. The third author is an expert by experience in having a learning disability, the fourth with a chronic disease and physical disability, and the fifth with informal caregiving of her husband. The second to fifth authors were all involved in one or more sub-studies. Additionally, they were engaged in the CvC from the start.

3. Results

The results firstly describe the topics on patients' research agenda for improving the healthcare system and policy (see Table 2). The shared topic of the agenda is 'dependency.' Patients are dependent on relatives, caregivers, organizations, procedures, and potential employers for (voluntary) jobs. Alternative support by peers, experts by experience, technology, and assistance dogs could support patients to become more independent. Patients' dependency is a vulnerability, and misuse of power could lead to abuse by others.

Table 2. The research agenda of patients based on 18 sub-studies.

Research Agenda of Patients	Explanation
Misuse of power and abuse	The misuse of power of (informal) caregivers and relatives on patients, with abuse (sexual, emotional, physical, financial) as a result
Meaningful participation	Support for patients to participate in a way that they are seen, heard, and belong to a bigger whole
Non-human assistance	Ways to implement alternatives support like assistance dogs and smart assistive technology
Peer support	Implementation on peer support and peer workers in settings like adolescent care, care for people with chronic illnesses or a learning disability, community care, and support for informal caregivers

The topics are not listed in a specific order; the first is not more important than the fourth. After the description of the research agenda, the findings from the dialogue with professionals on the agenda topics are shared.

3.1. Topics on the Patient Agenda

We describe four main topics of the patient agenda. These are the priorities of a broader list of issues. It is important to note that the topic of dealing with the restrictions, lockdowns, and other effects of the COVID-19 pandemic was critical at that moment. Still, we chose not to include pandemic topics in this patient agenda. More information on the priorities around COVID-19 from the patient perspectives of the CvC can be read in our report [49].

3.1.1. Awareness for Misuse of Power and Abuse

In many sub-studies, participants shared with us experiences about misuse of power and situations of abuse (sexual, emotional, physical, or financial) in their daily lives or in their past. Their dependency of caregivers, family, partner or friends was often the core of the experience.

> *"Our relationship? When it's good, it's very good. When it's terrible, it's very terrible. We can hurt each other a lot, but we also mean everything to each other. We will never forget that this is an abusive relationship, and like many abusive relationships, people fall away until at the end you are left with just the two of you."* A couple who receives community care.

> "Eventually, a group of 6–10 care professionals stood in the hallway to possibly jump on me. I found it threatening myself that they were all standing there. Then I ran away. Out of the door. The police went after me. I was taken away in handcuffs to the ambulance. Too bad. I found this very traumatic. I was crying. This is bad. I see that in the experiences of others too." A patient of emergency care.

> "Care professionals ask at the start of counseling if sexuality should be a topic in counseling. If the checkmark is 'off,' it is never brought up again. However, this can change in practice. Situations and wishes can change. But they do not. If the checkmark is 'off,' the topic is never brought up again. Although things happened . . . " A patient of community care.

In all cases, the topic was not on our prepared interview guide. Still, during interviews about experiences in life concerning their health status, participants mentioned one or more forms of abuse (sexual, physical, or emotional), usually when the audio recorder was stopped. For example, co-researchers often introduced themselves as persons with patient experiences and difficult moments in life. In the interview, many participants referred to their own hard lives. They did not share the experiences in detail, but named the topic of abuse in passing. Introducing the co-researchers seemed to encourage people to relate similar experiences. Some participants felt free to share details about abuse in the interview; some did not.

In all sub-studies involving people with a learning disability, many participants shared experiences of childhood abuse, misuse by their partner, or even abuse at the daycare facilities or by formal caregivers. Most of the time, the abuse was linked to the perpetrators' codependence. The perpetrators were often relatives, loved ones, or caregivers of people entirely dependent on them. However, most participants in this study did not expect to tell us about their experiences with abuse. We often heard that they had never told anybody in community care. They thus did not receive support for dealing with abuse and as a result, the incidents still impacted their health status significantly.

> "Nowadays, you can't just trust people. That's why I don't have any friends really. I used to go through a lot with friends, so you think..." A woman with a learning disability in an interview.

In another study in the context of GPs, we found they were most frequently used by women, and almost all of them had experiences of abuse in their daily lives or in their past. The abuse was a critical topic for them, but also taboo. It seemed challenging to share the issue with formal caregivers. Participants did not feel comfortable discussing it, although most had weekly contact with the GP.

3.1.2. Meaningful Participation

A second topic on the agenda is meaningful participation. In many sub-studies, patients share narratives about being a person who contributes to something or who cares for another. The topic of being seen, heard, and mattering emerged across almost all interviews. Many patients in the sub-studies cannot work in a paid or a voluntary job. Most organizations who provide a job are not as inclusive as patients wish and need. However, a job is an important way to build identity in Western society. A job ensures that you are seen (either positively or negatively), heard, and belong to a group or an organization, or enables you to break away from the patient role. A paid job can significantly improve quality of life and reduce dependence on a helping relationship. Besides, performing a task or helping someone, even if a small gesture, was a means to receive feedback and be part of a bigger whole.

> "When you are considered a vulnerable person, you have to work incredibly hard to be still able to do what you want to do. For example, if you're in a wheelchair, they talk about you with the person who pushes the wheelchair. Then you don't matter. So precisely when you're vulnerable, you have to work harder to matter still. Because of the vulnerability." A person with a physical disability in community care.

"I worked at the X [an organization that supports homeless people]. That was the only place I could go for a job. But those are all homeless people. I just wanted to get out of that circle. I slept with addicts and drug dealers. I wanted to get away from that. So I'd rather not go back into that again." A woman with a psychiatric vulnerability.

"I could start there, but on an on-call basis. (...) That doesn't really work for someone who needs a lot of structure." A man with a psychiatric vulnerability.

For example, in the sub-studies on people with psychiatric vulnerabilities, we heard several experiences of people who no longer socialized and have become isolated and afraid of meeting others. Some participants sought to have a meaningful life by providing daily care for various family members. Informal caregiving was a significant job for patients. In the studies on informal caregiving, we found that most informal caregivers were also patients themselves.

"I used to go to the snack bar a lot. But that all costs money. Sometimes I go to my mother's house for dinner a few times a week. My mother has an eye disease. I will take her to the hospital then. And sometimes she needs help reading because of her sight. Then I do that. Then I read to her." A patient with a psychiatric vulnerability.

In another study on experiences of community care for people with physical disabilities, patients shared stories about the role of caregivers in facilitating patients to participate in various activities. This included support for finding a (voluntary) job or hobby as well as with organizing the household and administration, so the patients had time to spend on social participation and volunteering. Many patients (would like to or did) managed their care to have energy left to spend on meaningful participation. A case illustrating this topic is a vivacious woman of 94, who spoke a lot about her activities and occupations. She has many social contacts, a good relationship with her son and daughter-in-law, and often goes out. For her, reciprocity is a significant value.

"I have many friends who keep coming. I am very proud of that. Sometimes I say, if it's too much trouble, you don't have to. But they even say, I look forward to it. It is always so nice. (...) They come here for fun. Thank goodness. They are busy enough." Woman with community care.

Her story shows that she can arrange her life, thanks to professional caregivers. A community caregiver supports her in her daily care, and (voluntary) organizations help her with transportation. Only in this way can she ease the burden on her family, monitor reciprocity, and participate in, what is for her, a meaningful way.

3.1.3. Non-Human Assistance

Patients, especially people with a chronic illness, disability, or vulnerability, note that medications and therapies do not always solve problems, help them in meaningful participation, reduce pain, or support recovery.

"Pills. Yes, I get those from the family doctor. But I don't take them. I don't want to. That's junk. but yes, I'm still in that pain." A woman who frequently comes to the GP.

In the sub-studies, we see that different people find support from animals like cats and assistance dogs, or smart assistive technology. This can be seen as non-human assistance. In the Netherlands, such support is not standard, as in the Dutch health system, assistance and support is mainly provided by humans, like physiotherapists, caregivers, physicians, social workers, etc. Non-human aid or support is often not evidence-based or accepted, and only a few healthcare organizations or foundations provide this type of care. It is thus difficult to arrange it without buying it yourself with private money.

To illustrate this topic, as an example, there is the fourth author, who has multiple sclerosis, cannot use his hands, and is dependent on a wheelchair. He found that devices with Bluetooth and WiFi connectivity can help him with many daily activities. In sub-studies, we also heard this from other patients:

"I can have a job due to voice-recognition software connected with my smartphone on my wheelchair. I write emails, and call people with the Siri assistant. I can organize my life from my smartphone. This makes me less independent of care." Man with assistive technology and community care.

However, in practice, the consumer devices that help patients with activities are not readily available at the municipality's care desk or through the health insurance provider. Most (female) caregivers are not interested in technology and are even afraid of pressing a button on the wheelchair or smartphone. Finally, nobody feels that they 'own' the topic of assistive technology. Therefore, change in this area is not occurring yet. All patients who could benefit from smart assistive technology need to reinvent the wheel.

Another example is the second author, who has a psychiatric vulnerability, received regular psychiatry treatments for years, had several crisis admissions, and eventually found support from an assistance dog. As an assistance dog for people with sight impairment or other physical disabilities, the dog also helps prevent psychosis. The author's dog is sensitive to her mood and trained to give signals that even she does not see. The dog becomes restless if she does not feel safe, so is a mirror for her well-being. In the sub-studies, we saw a valuable role for animals in support:

"I still have one cat, and luckily, she is very stable now, and I am very grateful for that. The other two, I had to finish their lives. Both had a cancerous tumor. Finally, the tumors killed them. They were so involved and intertwined with me because I cared so much about them, and they were my best therapists who helped me out of a deep valley and kept me on track." A woman with a psychiatric vulnerability.

However, this type of assistance is not a regular 'product' offered by the insurance provider or municipal support either. In different sub-studies with people with chronic psychiatric vulnerability, dogs are seen as a non-human form of assistance that is undervalued in the Dutch regular care system. These same experiences were shared in different studies, for example, where health professionals undervalue the impact of community garden projects, dancing projects, or yoga practices.

3.1.4. Peer-Support

In almost all studies, patients suggested that peers could be of value for them. Peers share a similar experience and situation. This identity of a peer is under-researched in healthcare. In psychiatric care, peer workers are increasingly part of healthcare teams. However, peer support is still new and undervalued in many other settings, such as healthcare for adolescents, chronic illnesses, people with a learning disability, and in community care or informal caregiving.

In a study of adolescents with respiratory disease, the participants shared experiences with peers in group sessions. They found this very useful, learned from each other, and received a different type of support from their peers. In healthcare, all treatments and therapies are solo, although these participants would love to share their experiences in a group. This could help them even more, they thought.

"You can tell your other friends, but they won't understand. You feel supported, since you are not the only one." Adolescent with a respiratory disease.

Patients in community care voiced similar feelings. The idea that people are eager to share their experiences in interviews with other co-researchers and love to join discussion groups is also a signal that peer support is valuable for them. According to patients, research on the value of peer support and the barriers of care professionals to be open to peer support is needed.

Peer support should not be confused with group therapy; it can also mean a group of people with a learning disability doing theater or a group of family caregivers engaging in a joint painting activity. It is not only about exchanging verbal experiences, but also about doing something together that allows the patient to meet people on a different level. Besides, peer support could inspire people or help them have hope for the future.

"Experiential experts are currently being used more and more in psychiatry. However, these have different statuses and power. The exchange is no longer 'really' reciprocal, like with peers." The second author in an analysis work session.

"I had an interview with an elderly lady that the kids did everything for. She felt like she couldn't do anything anymore. And then she saw me. A man in a wheelchair with many more limitations. And he comes independently by cab and does research. This inspired her enormously. She couldn't imagine a situation where she would ever have such a role, but I gave her hope for the future." Fourth author in a work session.

3.2. Reactions of Stakeholders on the Topics of the Agenda

Interestingly, some topics resonate more than others and were easier to follow up on.

3.2.1. Attention for Misuse of Power and Abuse

Many care professionals in support of people with a psychiatric vulnerability and learning disability know that misuse of power by others is a topic in the lives of their patients. However, for general practitioners, community care, researchers, and municipal civil servants, different kinds of abuse are less familiar, often taboo, which creates a gap between theory and practice. Most professionals mention that the topic of abuse is far from their lifeworld. It was not prominent in their education, and the majority think it is only a topic for psychiatrists. However, patients indicate that it is a theme, although complex, that should be given a place in healthcare because they perceive that many physical and mental problems are related to experiences of abuse. Engaging in a dialogue about these themes proved a challenge in this study. The question raised by professionals was: who is responsible for this topic and how do you start? Their practical expertise on this topic is limited, and they expressed hesitance. It was often coined as a wicked problem like systemic racism. Therefore, according to patients, besides better education and information on abuse, additional research is needed from patients' perspectives.

"Sexual abuse is still related to rapists—man in bushes. Or nowadays, people think of #MeToo. Men who rape in a working relationship. However, most abuse comes from men in relational sphere. At home. In families. Many professionals do not know this or understand that their patients are one of those people who are a victim. They often do now know what to do to empower these women." Change agent who summarizes the discussion in a dialogue session.

3.2.2. Meaningful Participation

Since 2014, healthcare policy in the Netherlands has focused on participation, thus there were funding opportunities for participation in the period of this study. For care professionals and policymakers, the focus was on 'more' participation, regardless of the activity. For patients, however, emphasis was on 'meaningful' participation, which was defined as generating a sense of belonging or activities that contribute to society as a whole. Stability of a (voluntary job) was also as important for patients. Professionals and policymakers welcomed the insights from the patients' perspective:

"The titles of your reports 'Not only participation works, but meaningful participation works' and 'Self-reliance, thanks to care' make it clear to us that the principles of our policy work out differently in practice. This is an eye-opener for us." An municipality civil servant.

3.2.3. Non-Human Assistance

On the topic of 'non-human assistance,' some alternatives resonate with stakeholders more than others. For example, assistive technology seems to fit policy priorities and funding opportunities. As a team, we succeeded in funding one small project to study the experiences of people who could not use their hands with assistive technology. During this process, it became clear that, in practice, there is often insufficient knowledge among healthcare professionals to implement technology successfully. We also found a gap between what municipalities and health insurers offer and what is required in practice.

As far as our attempts to find funding for a study on assistance dogs and the value of animals in support, we found none. Although there is a growing literature on the value of assistance dogs and animals for health, care professionals were not eager to join us in this topic, and funders were not keen to finance this study proposal.

> "There are two types of assistance dogs: more task-oriented and more sensitive dogs. The task-oriented dogs are used by people, for example, with vision impairments and police and ambulance personnel. The more sensitive dogs are more focused on interdependence and working with people with trauma, veterans and/or psychotic symptoms. In uniform professions, people who work with these dogs increasingly receive financial assistance to purchase dogs. Unfortunately, this is not the case for patients with psychosis susceptibility or PTTS. However, dogs can play a vital role in reducing re-experiences of the traumas, panic attacks, and expensive compulsory treatment, and can prevent traumatic admissions. In addition, assistance dogs can provide a solution since the new law in the mental health sector, where patients are forcibly treated at home. Patients today are often administered their mandatory medication at home, where their own home is no longer considered a safe place. The assistance dog can help to experience and support safety. Unfortunately, psychiatry is still secondary to the care of people with visible disabilities or physical impairments. That's also where the money for research is. That's where the priority lies. Moreover, many do not see animals as complete: people can do it better, they think." One of the co-researchers after the unsuccessful process of funding a proposal on assistance dogs for patients with psychosis susceptibility and or other mental health issues.

3.2.4. Peer Support

Finally, the topic of 'peer support' is associated with the topic of meaningful participation. This study found that being an expert by experience could be a meaningful and recovery-promoting activity for clients. While the recommendations of our studies in 2014–2017 were at the time 'new' to stakeholders, since 2018, experts by experience have become a hot topic in social work. However, peer workers or the contribution of experts by experiences and research opportunities on experiences are still rare in hospitals, community care, at the GP, and in healthcare for adolescents.

> "Initiating an advisory board with patients is already a big deal in the department. But now, we also have to do something with the advice of these people. That is often quite difficult to achieve. So working together with experts by experience or peer support groups is a bridge too far." Physician in an academic hospital.

> "The fact that we are researching patients' experiences in psychiatric crises is already very innovative. If we do participatory research, I am not taken seriously. In the department here, hierarchy is still important and also the gold standard of medical research. It is challenging to fit participatory research in this system. Maybe in a few years..." Emergency care professional in an academic hospital.

Moreover, organizing peer support groups requires facilitation. In healthcare, most professionals say they lack training for this—it is considered a social work activity. What is needed here is interdisciplinary collaboration to organize peer support. Therefore, patients see the urgency to study this topic.

4. Discussion

This study created a solid research agenda of patients. Findings show that patients prioritize four topics that related to dependency: research on (1) awareness of potential misuse of power by others and abuse (sexual, emotional, physical, or financial) as a result; (2) support for meaningful participation of patients; (3) ways to implement non-human support and assistance; and (4) the implementation of peer support groups and peer workers in healthcare. Surprisingly, these topics were easily dismissed again in dialogue with stakeholders like health professionals, policymakers, and funding agencies. Below, we present the expert knowledge available of the priorities placed on the agenda by patients and how their priorities relate to and are handled by the academic community.

Available knowledge on patients' priorities, and an action-orientation that is missing.

The priorities set by the patients in our studies are not (entirely) new for academics. For example, several review studies show the long-term health consequences of physical and emotional abuse, neglect, and sexual abuse [60–62], its prevalence [63], and disclosure [64]. However, research on economic abuse for adults in vulnerable situations is still a growing field [65]. Interestingly, most research on abuse had a low level of patient involvement. Furthermore, many of these studies recommend more randomized control trial studies (RCTs) and high-quality meta-studies to choose promising interventions for patients.

We see a similar pattern regarding 'alternative support and assistance'. Here, we also identify a gap between the priorities of patients and the recommendations for further studies in reviews. Many reviews and qualitative studies show the benefits for health of assistive technology [66–68], assistive dogs [69–72], or companion animals in general [73–77], but recommend gaining more knowledge from quantitative research designs. Only a few studies propose a national policy on a topic, for example, assistive technology or the development of a framework for changing its implementation, e.g., [77].

We have shown that patients' priorities are only partly covered in the literature, as scholars focus on more and better evidence assuming this will lead to a better quality of care by proven interventions. Patients are action-oriented and want academic research that stimulates tangible response to improve their quality of life. Patients also seek to learn what works in practice and co-produce new interventions that are relevant for their situation. Experts are therefore invited by patients to pay more attention to implementing knowledge to support patients in daily life.

How the priorities set by patients was dismissed again.

Many patient priorities, especially 'the hard-to-reach,' differ from the topics highlighted by professionals and researchers. This is often the case in agenda-setting studies [78–81]. Topics prioritized by patients represent their needs and wishes regarding scientific research. These issues reveal white spots that have been bypassed or superficially covered to new lenses on chronic illness and disability. While health science researchers tend to focus on highly specialized topics, patients focus on a broad array of interrelated issues of living with a chronic illness or disability. Moreover, researchers tend to focus on (para)medical treatments and psychological interventions, while patients also draw attention to the existential and social world of illness or disability [82]. In fact, patients constantly stress the importance of not being reduced to their patient role, but being seen as persons in their lifeworld context. As these issues are interrelated, researchers are invited to collaborate on the interface of humanistic and social scientific research with (bio)medical research. This requires transdisciplinary collaborations between academics, healthcare professionals and practitioners, and patients.

A systematic evaluation showed that one of the biggest challenges with patient-led research agenda-setting is that the topics generated may not be picked up by the funding agencies and researchers [83]. This was partly the case in our projects: some issues were well-received; others did not resonate with these stakeholders. In all instances, the facilitators teaming up with other partners in the community had to play a key role. They took responsibility for tying a certain topic to the scope of a funding agency. In the cases of assistive technology and meaningful participation, this was successful [54]. In the other instances, the facilitators looked for opportunities, but failed (thus far) to find resources to study the topics put on the agenda by patients. This leads to the conclusion that opening spaces for patient knowledge within academia is precarious and requires 'ethics' work to address power issues [5,84–87].

Finally, often patients are no longer involved in studies on the topics they prioritized [88]. In our case, the PPI and partnership had a more enduring status and resulted in a stable inclusion of patients in decision-making processes in a community of practice at the Center for Client Experiences (CvC) [84]. The partners were all willing to play a role as change agents toward a more inclusive healthcare and society. They were intensively involved and continued to act as advocates for the research agenda's implementation and patient participation in health research. The CvC became a strong community; patients are well-informed, articulate, ambitious, and willing to participate in a study. These patients are strong players in terms of self-organization, self-awareness, and assertiveness, which are sometimes lacking in other instances where patients are not well integrated. The CvC is thus an ideal community with members capable of becoming and remaining equal partners in research.

5. Conclusions

Initiating involvement and partnerships between patients and parties with different scopes, interests, and research agendas can be challenging. The research agenda-setting presented showed that patients as part of a larger community can be connected in a process to begin an exchange and broaden perspectives on health research agendas. This led to a new set of research topics that mattered to patients and covered several domains of life, extending beyond specific diagnoses. Yet, these priorities were easily dismissed again. We thus recommend a cross-disability, participatory, and deliberative-dialogical approach as a framework for agenda-setting in the future to generate research priorities resulting from a deliberative-dialogic process facilitated by, and embedded in, a stable transdisciplinary community.

Author Contributions: Conceptualization, B.G. and T.A.; formal analysis, B.G., A.H., M.B., R.v.Z., J.v.Z. and T.A.; funding acquisition, B.G. and T.A.; investigation, B.G., A.H., M.B., R.v.Z., J.v.Z. and T.A.; methodology, B.G. and T.A.; supervision, T.A.; validation, B.G.; writing—original draft, B.G.; writing—review and editing, B.G., A.H., R.v.Z., J.v.Z. and T.A. All authors have read and agreed to the published version of the manuscript.

Funding: This research received no external funding for writing this article. In Table 1, the funders of the different sub-studies are mentioned.

Institutional Review Board Statement: The study was conducted in accordance with the Declaration of Helsinki and approved by the Institutional Review Board (or Ethics Committee) of VU Medical Centre, protocol code: 2015485. They decided that the Medical Research Involving Human Subjects Act (WMO) does not apply to this research.

Informed Consent Statement: Informed consent was obtained from all subjects involved in the study.

Acknowledgments: We would like to acknowledge all community partners, co-researchers, and research colleagues who contribute(d) to the Centre of Client Experiences.

Conflicts of Interest: The authors declare no conflict of interest.

References

1. Fixsen, A. Communitas in Crisis: An Autoethnography of Psychosis Under Lockdown. *Qual. Health Res.* **2021**, *31*, 2340–2350. [CrossRef] [PubMed]
2. Richards, D.P.; Jordan, I.; Strain, K.; Press, Z. Patient partner compensation in research and health care: The patient perspective on why and how. *Patient Exp. J.* **2018**, *5*, 6–12. [CrossRef]
3. Schipper, K.; Abma, T.A.; van Zadelhoff, E.; van de Griendt, J.; Nierse, C.; Widdershoven, G.J. What Does It Mean to Be a Patient Research Partner? An Ethnodrama. *Qual. Inq.* **2010**, *16*, 501–510. [CrossRef]
4. Teunissen, G.J.; Lindhout, P.; Abma, T.A. Balancing loving and caring in times of chronic illness. *Qual. Res. J.* **2018**, *18*, 210–222. [CrossRef]
5. Groot, B.C.; Vink, M.; Haveman, A.; Huberts, M.; Schout, G.; Abma, T.A. Ethics of care in participatory health research: Mutual responsibility in collaboration with co-researchers. *Educ. Action Res.* **2019**, *27*, 286–302. [CrossRef]
6. Malterud, K.; Elvbakken, K.T. Patients participating as co-researchers in health research: A systematic review of outcomes and experiences. *Scand. J. Public Health* **2020**, *48*, 617–628. [CrossRef] [PubMed]

7. McCarron, T.L.; Clement, F.; Rasiah, J.; Moran, C.; Moffat, K.; Gonzalez, A.; Wasylak, T.; Santana, M. Patients as partners in health research: A scoping review. *Health Expect.* **2021**, *24*, 1378–1390. [CrossRef]
8. Nierse, C.J.; Schipper, K.; Van Zadelhoff, E.; Van De Griendt, J.; Abma, T.A. Collaboration and co-ownership in research: Dynamics and dialogues between patient research partners and professional researchers in a research team. *Health Expect.* **2012**, *15*, 242–254. [CrossRef]
9. Shen, S.; Doyle-Thomas, K.A.; Beesley, L.; Karmali, A.; Williams, L.; Tanel, N.; McPherson, A.C. How and why should we engage parents as co-researchers in health research? A scoping review of current practices. *Health Expect.* **2017**, *20*, 543–554. [CrossRef]
10. Smith, E.; Bélisle-Pipon, J.C.; Resnik, D. Patients as research partners; how to value their perceptions, contribution and labor? *Citiz. Sci. Theory Pract.* **2019**, *4*, cstp.184. [CrossRef]
11. Caron-Flinterman, J.F.; Broerse, J.E.; Bunders, J.F. The experiential knowledge of patients: A new resource for biomedical research? *Soc. Sci. Med.* **2005**, *60*, 2575–2584. [CrossRef] [PubMed]
12. Fricker, M. *Epistemic Injustice: Power and the Ethics of Knowing*; Oxford University Press: Oxford, UK, 2007.
13. Fricker, M. Epistemic justice as a condition of political freedom? *Synthese* **2013**, *190*, 1317–1332. [CrossRef]
14. Biddle, M.S.; Gibson, A.; Evans, D. Attitudes and approaches to patient and public involvement across Europe: A systematic review. *Health Soc. Care Community* **2013**, *29*, 18–27. [CrossRef] [PubMed]
15. Bombard, Y.; Baker, G.R.; Orlando, E.; Fancott, C.; Bhatia, P.; Casalino, S.; Onate, K.; Denis, J.-L.; Pomey, M.P. Engaging patients to improve quality of care: A systematic review. *Implement. Sci.* **2018**, *13*, 1–22. [CrossRef]
16. Arnstein, S.R. A ladder of citizen participation. *J. Am. Inst. Plan.* **1969**, *35*, 216–224. [CrossRef]
17. Groot, B.; Abma, T. Boundary Objects: Engaging and Bridging Needs of People in Participatory Research by Arts-Based Methods. *Int. J. Environ. Res. Public Health* **2021**, *18*, 7903. [CrossRef]
18. Goedhart, N.S.; Pittens, C.A.C.M.; Tončinić, S.; Zuiderent-Jerak, T.; Dedding, C.; Broerse, J.E.W. Engaging citizens living in vulnerable circumstances in research: A narrative review using a systematic search. *Res. Involv. Engagem.* **2021**, *7*, 1–19. [CrossRef]
19. Carel, H.; Kidd, I.J. Epistemic injustice in healthcare: A philosophial analysis. *Med. Health Care Philos.* **2014**, *17*, 529–540. [CrossRef]
20. Crichton, P.; Carel, H.; Kidd, I.J. Epistemic injustice in psychiatry. *BJ Psych. Bull.* **2017**, *41*, 65–70. [CrossRef]
21. Carel, H.; Györffy, G. Seen but not heard: Children and epistemic injustice. *Lancet* **2014**, *384*, 1256–1257. [CrossRef]
22. Blease, C.; Carel, H.; Geraghty, K. Epistemic injustice in healthcare encounters: Evidence from chronic fatigue syndrome. *J. Med. Ethics* **2017**, *43*, 549–557. [CrossRef] [PubMed]
23. Buchman, D.Z.; Ho, A.; Goldberg, D.S. Investigating trust, expertise, and epistemic injustice in chronic pain. *J. Bioethical Inq.* **2017**, *14*, 31–42. [CrossRef]
24. Heggen, K.M.; Berg, H. Epistemic injustice in the age of evidence-based practice: The case of fibromyalgia. *Humanit. Soc. Sci. Commun.* **2021**, *8*, 1–6. [CrossRef]
25. Peled, Y. Language barriers and epistemic injustice in healthcare settings. *Bioethics* **2018**, *32*, 360–367. [CrossRef] [PubMed]
26. Greenhalgh, T.; Hinton, L.; Finlay, T.; Macfarlane, A.; Fahy, N.; Clyde, B.; Chant, A. Frameworks for supporting patient and public involvement in research: Systematic review and co-design pilot. *Health Expect.* **2019**, *22*, 785–801. [CrossRef] [PubMed]
27. Manafò, E.; Petermann, L.; Vandall-Walker, V.; Mason-Lai, P. Patient and public engagement in priority setting: A systematic rapid review of the literature. *PLoS ONE* **2018**, *13*, e0193579. [CrossRef] [PubMed]
28. Abma, T.A.; Broerse, J.E. Patient participation as dialogue: Setting research agendas. *Health Expect.* **2010**, *13*, 160–173. [CrossRef]
29. Nierse, C.J.; Abma, T.A.; Horemans, A.M.; van Engelen, B.G. Research priorities of patients with neuromuscular disease. *Disabil. Rehabil.* **2013**, *35*, 405–412. [CrossRef]
30. Nepal, S.; Keniston, A.; Indovina, K.A.; Frank, M.G.; Stella, S.A.; Quinzanos-Alonso, I.; McBeth, L.; Moore, S.L.; Burden, M. What Do Patients Want? A Qualitative Analysis of Patient, Provider, and Administrative Perceptions and Expectations About Patients' Hospital Stays. *J. Patient Exp.* **2020**, *7*, 1760–1770. [CrossRef]
31. Abma, T.A.; Banks, S.; Cook, T.; Dias, S.; Madsen, W.; Springett, J.; Wright, M. *Participatory Research for Health and Social Well-Being*, 1st ed.; Springer Nature: Cham, Switzerland, 2019.
32. Abma, T.A.; Cook, T.; Rämgård, M.; Kleba, E.; Harris, J.; Wallerstein, N. Social impact of participatory health research: Collaborative non-linear processes of knowledge mobilization. *Educ. Action Res.* **2017**, *25*, 489–505. [CrossRef]
33. ICPHR (International Collaboration for Participatory Health Research). *Position Paper 1: What is Participatory Health Research?* Version: May 2013; International Collaboration for Participatory Health Research: Berlin, Germany, 2013.
34. Groot, B.; Vink, M.; Abma, T. *Goede Zorg in de Wijk. Eindrapportage van het Onderzoek 'Transitie Vanuit Cliëntenperspectief'*; Centrum voor Cliëntervaringen: Amsterdam, The Netherlands, 2015.
35. Duijs, S.E.; Groot, B.; Peterman, M.; van Zuijlen, R.; Werner, A.; Flipsen, I. *Zelfredzaam, Dankzij de Zorg! Een Responsief Onderzoek naar de Betekenis van en Mogelijkheden voor Zelfredzaamheid Vanuit het Perspectief van Cliënten*; Centrum voor Cliëntervaringen: Amsterdam, The Netherlands, 2016.
36. Duijs, S.E.; Groot-Sluijsmans, B.C.; Abma, T.A. *Veerkracht in Beeld: Veerkracht Gezien Vanuit de Ogen van Amsterdammers in Kwetsbare Situaties*; Eindrapportage; Metamedica, VU Medisch Centrum: Amsterdam, The Netherlands, 2017.
37. Groot, B.C.; Vink, M.; Abma, T.A. *Zorgen voor, Zorgen dat, Zorgen om: Goede Zorg in de Wijk Vanuit het Perspectief van Mantelzorgers*; Centrum voor Cliëntervaringen: Amsterdam, The Netherlands, 2016.
38. Groot, B.C.; Vink, M.; Abma, T.A. *Aandacht voor Stil Verdriet: Co-Creatie Mantelzorgondersteuning dementie Amsterdam Noord*; Centrum voor Cliëntervaringen: Amsterdam, The Netherlands, 2016.

39. Groot, B.C.; Vink, M.; Abma, T.A. *Goede zorg in de Wijk II: Monitoring Pilots Wijkzorg voor en met Verstandelijk Beperkte Cliënten*; Centrum voor Cliëntervaringen: Amsterdam, The Netherlands, 2016.
40. Groot, B.; Vink, M.; Abma, T. *Anders Kijken, Anders Doen vanuit Cliëntenperspectief. De Kunst van Wederkerige Relaties en Contact*; Centrum voor Cliëntervaringen: Amsterdam, The Netherlands, 2017.
41. Breed, M.; Groot, B.C.; Aussems, K.; Abma, T.A. *Droomscenario Door de Ogen van Cliënten en Ervaringen van Cliënten Anno 2019*; Centrum voor Cliëntervaringen: Amsterdam, The Netherlands, 2019.
42. Duijs, S.E.; Vink, M.; Groot, B.C.; Abma, T.A. *Goede Zorg in de Wijk II: Monitoring Wijkzorgnetwerk voor en met GGZ-Cliënten*; Centrum voor Cliëntervaringen: Amsterdam, The Netherlands, 2015.
43. Centrum voor Cliëntervaringen. Assistive Technology. 2020. Available online: https://www.youtube.com/watch?v=pHpj921dYmA (accessed on 5 February 2021).
44. Centrum voor Cliëntervaringen. 180 Keer per Jaar naar de Huisarts. 2019. Available online: https://centrumvoorclientervaringen.com/2019/09/10/180-keer-per-jaar-naar-de-huisarts (accessed on 5 February 2021).
45. Vink, M.; Groot, B.C.; Willems, P. *Motieven en Drijfveren voor Opname*; Centrum voor Cliëntervaringen: Amsterdam, The Netherlands, 2019.
46. Vink, M.; Groot, B.; Schout, G.; Abma, T.; Huberts, M. *Goede Zorg Bij Crisis: Het Belang van Contact*; Centrum voor Cliëntervaringen: Amsterdam, The Netherlands, 2017.
47. Groot, B.C.; Vink, M.; Huberts, M.; Schout, G.; Abma, T.A. Pathways for Improvement of Care in Psychiatric Crisis: A Plea for the Co-Creation with Service Users and Ethics of Care. *Arch. Psychol.* **2020**, *3*, 3.
48. Team Ouderenvriendelijk Buitenveldert. *Ouderenvriendelijk Op Maat: Onderzoeksrapport van het Project Ouderenvriendelijk Buitenveldert*; Centrum voor Cliëntervaringen: Amsterdam, The Netherlands, 2017.
49. Willems, P.; Vlasman, E.; Buree, M.; Derks, N.; Huberts, M.; Peterman, M.; Varkevisser, K.; van Zuijlen, R.; Groot, B. *Maatifest: Ertoe doen, ook in Coronatijd. Oplossingen Co-Creëren in Corona-Tijden: Een Participatief Actieonderzoek met Mensen in Kwetsbare Situaties*; Centrum voor Cliëntervaringen: Amsterdam, The Netherlands, 2020.
50. Groot, B.; Nijland, A.; Waagen, S.; Abma, T. Partnerschap met gezinnen in armoede op beleids- of programmaniveau. *Tijdschrift Voor Gezondh.* **2021**, *99*, 128–131. [CrossRef]
51. FNO Klankbordgroep Gezonde Toekomst Dichterbij. *Je Ziet Het Niet*; FNO: Amsterdam, The Netherlands, 2019.
52. Groot, B.C.; Abma, T.A. Participatory Health Research with Mothers Living in Poverty in the Netherlands: Pathways and Challenges to Strengthen Empowerment; 59 paragraphs. *Forum Qual. Soc. Res.* **2020**, *21*, 8.
53. Groot, B.C.; Overbeek, F.; Weerman, A. *Werkplaats Ervaringskennis: Leven in de Bijstand*; Centrum voor Cliëntervaringen: Amsterdam, The Netherlands, 2019.
54. Groot, B.C.; Weerman, A.; Overbeek, R.; Abma, T.A. Making a Difference. Participatory Health Research with Unemployed Citizens and Policymakers. *Int. Rev. Qual. Res.* **2020**, *13*, 200–218. [CrossRef]
55. Groot, B.C.; Dedding, C.; Slob, E.; Maitland, H.; Teunissen, T.; Rutjes, N.; Vijverberg, S. Adolescents' experiences with patient engagement in respiratory medicine: Lessons from establishing a youth council. *Pediatric Pulmonol.* **2021**, *56*, 211–216. [CrossRef]
56. Guba, E.G.; Lincoln, Y.S. *Fourth Generation Evaluation*; Sage: London, UK, 1989.
57. ICPHR (International Collaboration for Participatory Health Research). *Ensuring Quality: Indicative Characteristics of Participatory (Health) Research*; International Collaboration for Participatory Health Research: Berlin, Germany, 2016; Available online: https://tinyurl.com/2fccmf5u (accessed on 23 January 2022).
58. Van Lieshout, F.; Cardiff, S. Innovative ways of analysing data with practitioners as co-researchers: Dancing outside the ballroom. In *Creative Spaces for Qualitative Researching*; Brill Sense: Leiden, The Netherlands, 2011; pp. 223–234.
59. Clarke, V.; Braun, V. Thematic analysis. In *Encyclopedia of Critical Psychology*; Springer: New York, NY, USA, 2014; pp. 1947–1952.
60. Norman, R.E.; Byambaa, M.; De, R.; Butchart, A.; Scott, J.; Vos, T. The long-term health consequences of child physical abuse, emotional abuse, and neglect: A systematic review and meta-analysis. *PLoS Med.* **2012**, *9*, e1001349. [CrossRef]
61. Hailes, H.P.; Yu, R.; Danese, A.; Fazel, S. Long-term outcomes of childhood sexual abuse: An umbrella review. *Lancet Psychiatry* **2019**, *6*, 830–839. [CrossRef]
62. MacGinley, M.; Breckenridge, J.; Mowll, J. A scoping review of adult survivors' experiences of shame following sexual abuse in childhood. *Health Soc. Care Community* **2019**, *27*, 1135–1146. [CrossRef]
63. Hughes, R.B.; Lund, E.M.; Gabrielli, J.; Powers, L.E.; Curry, M.A. Prevalence of interpersonal violence against community-living adults with disabilities: A literature review. *Rehabil. Psychol.* **2011**, *56*, 302. [CrossRef]
64. Tener, D.; Murphy, S.B. Adult disclosure of child sexual abuse: A literature review. *Trauma Violence Abus.* **2015**, *16*, 391–400. [CrossRef]
65. Postmus, J.L.; Hoge, G.L.; Breckenridge, J.; Sharp-Jeffs, N.; Chung, D. Economic abuse as an invisible form of domestic violence: A multicountry review. *Trauma Violence Abus.* **2020**, *21*, 261–283. [CrossRef] [PubMed]
66. Lenker, J.A.; Harris, F.; Taugher, M.; Smith, R.O. Consumer perspectives on assistive technology outcomes. *Disabil. Rehabil. Assist. Technol.* **2013**, *8*, 373–380. [CrossRef] [PubMed]
67. Güldenpfennig, F.; Mayer, P.; Panek, P.; Fitzpatrick, G. An autonomy-perspective on the design of assistive technology experiences of people with multiple sclerosis. In Proceedings of the 2019 CHI Conference on Human Factors in Computing Systems, Glasgow, UK, 4–9 May 2019; Association for Computing Machinery: New York, NY, USA, 2019; pp. 1–14.

68. Carver, J.; Ganus, A.; Ivey, J.M.; Plummer, T.; Eubank, A. The impact of mobility assistive technology devices on participation for individuals with disabilities. *Disabil. Rehabil. Assist. Technol.* **2016**, *11*, 468–477. [CrossRef] [PubMed]
69. Rodriguez, K.E.; Greer, J.; Yatcilla, J.K.; Beck, A.M.; O'Haire, M.E. The effects of assistance dogs on psychosocial health and wellbeing: A systematic literature review. *PLoS ONE* **2020**, *15*, e0243302. [CrossRef] [PubMed]
70. Bremhorst, A.; Mongillo, P.; Howell, T.; Marinelli, L. Spotlight on assistance dogs—Legislation, welfare and research. *Animals* **2018**, *8*, 129. [CrossRef]
71. Perkins, J.; Bartlett, H.; Travers, C.; Rand, J. Dog-assisted therapy for older people with dementia: A review. *Australas. J. Ageing* **2008**, *27*, 177–182. [CrossRef] [PubMed]
72. Lindsay, S.; Thiyagarajah, K. The impact of service dogs on children, youth and their families: A systematic review. *Disabil. Health J.* **2021**, *14*, 101012. [CrossRef]
73. McNicholas, J.; Gilbey, A.; Rennie, A.; Ahmedzai, S.; Dono, J.A.; Ormerod, E. Pet ownership and human health: A brief review of evidence and issues. *BMJ* **2005**, *331*, 1252–1254. [CrossRef]
74. DeMello, M. *Animals and Society*; Columbia University Press: New York, NY, USA, 2021.
75. Westgarth, C.; Christley, R.M.; Christian, H.E. How might we increase physical activity through dog walking? A comprehensive review of dog walking correlates. *Int. J. Behav. Nutr. Phys. Act.* **2014**, *11*, 1–14. [CrossRef]
76. Gilbey, A.; Tani, K. Companion animals and loneliness: A systematic review of quantitative studies. *Anthrozoös* **2015**, *28*, 181–197. [CrossRef]
77. MacLachlan, M.; Banes, D.; Borg, J.D.; Donnelly, B.; Fembek, M.; Ghosh, R.; Gowran, R.J.; Hannay, E.; Hiscock, D.; Hoogerwerf, E.J.; et al. Assistive technology policy: A position paper from the first global research, innovation, and education on assistive technology (GREAT) summit. *Disabil. Rehabil. Assist. Technol.* **2018**, *13*, 454–466. [CrossRef] [PubMed]
78. Abma, T.A. Dialogue and deliberation: New approaches to including patients in setting health and healthcare research agendas. *Action Res.* **2019**, *17*, 429–450. [CrossRef]
79. Nierse, C. Collaborative User Involvement in Health Research Agenda Setting. Ph.D. Thesis, Vrije Universiteit, Amsterdam, The Netherlands, 2019.
80. Hilverda, F.; van der Wouden, P.; van der Heijden, G.J.M.G.; Pittens, C.A.C.M. A research agenda on oral health care as a boundary object that unites the perspectives of patients and practitioners. *Health Expect.* **2021**, *24*, 1701–1712. [CrossRef] [PubMed]
81. Schölvinck, A.F.M.; Pittens, C.A.; Broerse, J.E. Patient involvement in agenda-setting processes in health research policy: A boundary work perspective. *Sci. Public Policy* **2020**, *47*, 246–255. [CrossRef]
82. Carel, H. *Illness. The Cry of the Flesh*, 2nd ed.; Routledge: London, UK, 2008.
83. Teunissen, G.J. Values and Criteria of People with a Chronic Illness or Disability: Strengthening the Voice of Their Representatives in the Health Debate and the Decision Making Process. Ph.D. Thesis, Free University, Amsterdam, The Netherlands, 2014.
84. Groot-Sluijsmans, B.C. Ethics of Participatory Health Research: Insights from a Reflective Journey. Ph.D. Thesis, Vrije Universiteit, Amsterdam, The Netherlands, 2021.
85. Groot, B.C.; Abma, T.A. Ethics and Participatory Health Research. In *Handbook of Social Inclusion*, 1st ed.; Liamputtong, P., Ed.; Springer Nature: Cham, Switzerland, 2021; Volume 1, pp. 1–17.
86. Groot, B.C.; Haveman, A.; Abma, T.A. Relational, ethically sound co-production in mental health care research: Epistemic injustice and the need for an ethics of care. *Crit. Public Health* **2020**, 1–11. [CrossRef]
87. Abma, T.; Groot, B.; Widdershoven, G. The ethics of public and service user involvement in health research: The need for participatory reflection on everyday ethical issues. *Am. J. Bioeth.* **2019**, *19*, 23–25. [CrossRef]
88. Abma, T.A.; Pittens, C.A.C.M.; Visse, M.A.; Elberse, J.E.; Broerse, J.E.W. Patient involvement in research programming and implementation. *Health Expect.* **2015**, *18*, 2449–2464. [CrossRef]

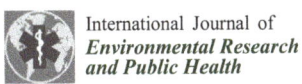

Article

Evaluating the Effect of Kaftrio on Perspectives of Health and Wellbeing in Individuals with Cystic Fibrosis

Sean A. Aspinall, Kelly A. Mackintosh, Denise M. Hill, Bethany Cope and Melitta A. McNarry *

Applied Sports, Technology, Exercise and Medicine (A-STEM) Research Centre, Faculty of Science and Engineering, Swansea University, Fabian Way, Swansea SA1 8EN, UK; 921125@swansea.ac.uk (S.A.A.); k.mackintosh@swansea.ac.uk (K.A.M.); denise.hill@swansea.ac.uk (D.M.H.); 982528@swansea.ac.uk (B.C.)
* Correspondence: m.mcnarry@swansea.ac.uk

Abstract: Background: Modulator therapy represents a significant step forward in CF care and is expected to have a significant impact on the health and mortality of many individuals with CF. Studies have predominantly explored the physiological effects of modulator therapy on clinical outcomes, with little consideration of the individual lived experience of modulator therapy among adults with Cystic Fibrosis. Methods: To explore this, semi-structured interviews were conducted with 12 individuals currently taking Kaftrio, which were subsequently thematically analysed. Results: Three overarching themes were identified: (i) positive perception of Kaftrio, (ii) negative perception of Kaftrio, and (iii) the relationships with the clinical team. The experience of modulator therapy should be recognised as being unique to the individual, with perceptions of illness, self-identity, and outcomes strongly dictating the lived experience. Conclusions: There is a consensus that, while for many, the quality of life is evidently increased through the use of Kaftrio, this is not without its own challenges. This highlights the need for both individuals with CF and their clinical teams to learn to navigate this new disease landscape.

Keywords: chronic illness; lived experience; qualitative analysis; modulators; trikafta; semi-structured; self-identity; quality of life

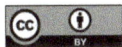

1. Introduction

Cystic Fibrosis (CF) is the most common and severe autosomal, recessive genetic disorder in the Caucasian population, currently affecting over 10,000 individuals in the UK [1]. Complications caused by a compromised function of the Cystic Fibrosis Transmembrane Regulator (*CFTR*) gene result in impaired chloride ion transport in the epithelial cells, affecting pancreatic, respiratory, gastrointestinal, reproductive, and skeletal function [2]. Despite the fact that CF is a multi-organ disease, respiratory failure represents the main cause of morbidity and mortality. Specifically, the absence or dysfunction of the CFTR protein results in abnormal mucus secretion, recurring infections, inflammation, airway obstruction and, ultimately, progressive decline in pulmonary function [3–7].

The majority of treatments available for CF treat the complications and symptoms associated with the disease, independent of the genetic defect. However, over the last decade, treatment has gradually been directed towards restoring CFTR protein function, thus targeting the underlying cause of the disease [8,9]. CFTR modulators are targeted therapies that increase the processing and delivery of CFTR to the cell surface (correctors) and increase the flow of ions through activated CFTR proteins at the cell surface (potentiators) [10]. The introduction of Ivacaftor for individuals with class III and residual function mutations (e.g., G551D), followed by Tezacaftor/Ivacaftor combinations in individuals homozygous for F508del, have evidenced significant improvements in sweat chloride, pulmonary function, body weight, and overall quality of life (QoL) [9,11,12]. As of June 2020, NHS England and the European Medicines Agency (EMA) approved the use of the highly effective triple modulator therapy Tezacaftor/Ivacaftor/Elaxacaftor in individuals over the age of 12-years who present with at least one F508del mutation [8].

It is widely purported that initiating triple modulator therapy (Kaftrio) will change the course of CF lung disease for many individuals. Indeed, triple modulator therapy has been shown to have beneficial effects not only in those with mild-to-moderate CF but also in those with more severe pulmonary status [13]. Whilst current research is unequivocal in its evidence for positive respiratory outcomes, we are yet to truly understand the effects that chronic triple therapy treatment has on patient outcomes related to mental health and quality of life. Di Mango et al. [14] reported that three months of treatment with Elexacaftor/Tezacaftor/Ivacaftor resulted in significant improvements across the majority of domains of the CFQ-R questionnaire, with the exception of emotional functioning, health perceptions, body image, and digestive symptoms. However, such objective data fails to explore the intricacies of the true patient experience, which remain unknown. Given the diverse nature of CF, it is imperative to understand patients' perspectives of the impact of Kaftrio in order to inform and shape future clinical practice.

Whilst the introduction of modulator therapy brings hope for many, there remain many unanswered questions. Given the magnitude that such a therapy is expected to have on an individual's day-to-day life, understanding the real-world experience is key. Prior to therapy, previous lived experience has described CF as unpredictable and challenging, with individuals striving for equality and desiring to experience the opportunities that their healthy peers take for granted [15]. As individuals begin to experience the physiological effects of the treatment, this study aims to explore the effect these changes have on an individual's perception of reality and to what extent the modulator has changed their life beyond just the physical aspects.

2. Methods

Twelve individuals (10 Females; 28.1 ± 6.4 years) with CF were recruited via social media and provided informed consent to participate in the study. Eight individuals had received treatment for 6-months prior to the interview, two individuals for 10-months prior on compassionate grounds, and two individuals had been prescribed Kaftrio for over one year as part of phase 3 clinical trials. The study was approved by the Research Ethics Committee at Swansea University (Ref: MN_22-10-22).

To explore the individuals' experiences and perceptions of Kaftrio (ELX/TEZ/IVA, Vertex Pharmaceutical), participants were asked to take part in a semi-structured interview with the first author via video conferencing software (Zoom, Zoom Video Communications Inc., San Jose, CA, USA) lasting up to 60 min. The flexible interview guide was devised in line with Evans et al. [16] to facilitate an in-depth discussion of the personal experiences of Kaftrio and was pilot tested to ensure that the questions were sensitive and appropriate. The interview involved the exploration of commonly reported benefits and side-effects of Kaftrio, with social challenges, disease management, anxiety, and identity explored in line with existing literature [17]. To maintain anonymity, individuals were given a pseudonym so as not to be identifiable within the manuscript. Whilst the interviews probed both positive and negative effects of Kaftrio, participants were prompted to expand on how these personal experiences shaped their perceptions of Kaftrio.

The interviews were recorded and subsequently transcribed verbatim. All of the data were analysed through qualitative content analysis by the first author [18]. The data were subject to line-by-line coding to identify appropriate and accurate themes. These codes identified features of the data that the first author considered pertinent to the research question. A member of the research team independently verified that these themes were reflective of the narrative, thus representing the data appropriately. The first author then identified quotes that were congruent with the overarching themes. These quotes were then grouped into subthemes which were aligned with the overarching themes and related to the overall story and research question. These extracts aimed to identify issues within the theme to provide a clear example of the individual's point.

3. Results

The main themes identified were: (i) a positive perceptions of Kaftrio, (ii) a negative perceptions of Kaftrio, and (iii) the relationship with the clinical team, as shown in Table 1.

Table 1. Identified themes regarding individual's perceptions of Kaftrio.

Perception of Kaftrio	
Dimension	Theme
Perceived Positive	Improved Quality of Life
	Pulmonary Function and the Purge
	Reduced Rate of Exacerbation
	A Sense of Normality
Perceived Negative	Side Effects
	Removal
	Loss of Identity
Relationships	Clinical Team
	Psychological Support

3.1. Positive Perceptions of Kaftrio

Of the study population, 10 individuals demonstrated positive perceptions towards Kaftrio, with many rereferring to an increase in quality of life as the main positive outcome. Health prior to Kaftrio therapy appeared to be a strong indicator of perception, with those of poorer health perceiving themselves to have more substantial increases in their quality of life.

3.1.1. Improved Quality of Life

All individuals who identified an increased quality of life stated that they noticed the positive effect of Kaftrio on multiple aspects of day-to-day living within a few days of treatment commencement. Specifically, participants cited: (i) reduced coughing, (ii) reduced breathlessness, (iii) more energy, (iv) increased appetite, (v) improved sleep duration and quality, and (vi) the ability to complete daily tasks easier. Angie described:

"... a week in I would say I didn't coughdotso I'd get up in the morning and cough for hours ... now I test my cough and be like, god can I actually still cough?"... Also, there's a block that we walk now and I never in a million years thought I would ever be able to walk around that ... now I walk around it and I'm like what? I've just walked that I can't believe it."

Craig also noted the profound effect Kaftrio had on sleep quality:

"... one of the major things is sleeping at night and not coughing. So, I would be tossing and turning and coughing ... even when I went on antibiotics. My second night on Kaftrio ... I just hadn't coughed yet. Even to this day [over six months] it's the same and it's something I can't get my head around."

One outcome that resonated with all participants, regardless of pulmonary function, was the obvious change in energy levels on a day-to-day basis. As an example, Ben, suggested:

"I am fitter and healthier now than I've ever felt in my entire life. Like on Saturday I rode 50 miles on a bike. Could never comprehend that in my entire life. Like ever doing that."

3.1.2. Pulmonary Function and the "Purge"

Prior to taking Kaftrio, many individuals expressed concern at watching their pulmonary function regularly decline. For those who had not yet experienced a significant decline in forced expiratory volume (FEV_1), they believed it was 'only a matter of time' until their condition deteriorated significantly. Self-reported increases in pulmonary function varied substantially between individuals, ranging from 1 to 20%. For many, an increase in pulmonary function brought comfort that Kaftrio was making a substantial difference at a cellular level. Marin spoke of her recent changes in pulmonary function:

> "Pre-Symkevi I was 55%, Symkevi gave me 10%. Kaftrio pushed me to numbers I had had when I was 13 [years old]—the best was 83% and now it's more around 78–80%... all those percentages mean a lot don't they?"

Prior to this increase, many individuals highlighted experiencing the infamous 'purge', whereby individuals expectorate large quantities of mucus from their lungs in the 24–72 h after they commenced Kaftrio treatment. Many individuals placed value on this as a sign that the medication was starting to work:

> "Had the purge, enjoyed it! It only lasted around 12–24 h, my lungs felt so much clearer than ever before, I thought wow this is fast acting but you don't believe it somehow. My lung function increased straight away. I stopped coughing within a week."

However, the percentage increase in FEV_1 was not the main positive health outcome expressed by participants. Many found value in the perception that Kaftrio would help preserve their lung function, thereby reducing anxiety associated with pulmonary function tests, as they now placed less significance on test outcomes given their increased quality of life. Individuals often professed that clinical perceptions of health and decisions on their care were determined based on pulmonary function alone, without taking the patient perceptions into consideration when evaluating health and quality of life. Indeed, an absence of acknowledgement concerning the effects that pulmonary function readings had on anxiety and an individual's mood had led some individuals in the past to actively avoid clinic visits. Participants noted that a low FEV_1 value during routine clinic visits when they felt otherwise well had been mentally challenging. Hence, critically, Kaftrio was suggested to provide some confidence that these decreases in FEV_1 may be less frequent, with Cynthia discussing how recent infections and declines were hopefully not going to have too much of an impact now:

> "Over the last year I was suffering more with haemoptysis and I got MRSA (methicillin-resistant Staphylococcus aureus) and NTM (Nontuberculous mycobacteria) all in one year. I could see edging toward 30 [years old] that this is going to be the decline basically and I was hoping that it [Kaftrio] would sort of, not let it [lung function] go down too much."

3.1.3. Reduced Rate of Exacerbations

A characteristic of CF is that many individuals experience frequent exacerbations that may require hospitalisation for intravenous (IV) antibiotic therapy. Depending on disease severity, individuals spoke of how they can experience IV therapy every four to 12 weeks. For Ben and Charlie, who had previously been under frequent antibiotic regimes, Kaftrio significantly reduced the need for hospital visits. Ben described:

> "They [the clinical care team] have tried to put me on IV's at least four times this year because they said to me, you 'normally' have them every three months. I have now accepted to go on it, but [since Kaftrio] that will be almost a full year without them, which is unheard of for me."

Similarly, Charlie spoke of the decreased frequency of her hospital visits:

> "I was in hospital like four or five times per year ... [on Kaftrio] about 14 months is the longest I have been without and that's the longest it's been for seven years."

Whilst individuals accept that their CF is not cured and that they may be prone to IV treatment in the future, the significant reduction in treatment burden brought the participants a sense of relief. Whilst the requirement for IV treatment echo's life pre-Kaftrio, it is something Rosie is willing to live with if it remains as infrequent:

"... the other part of me was like, if I only have IV's once a year for the rest of my life, then that's cool, I can totally accept that."

3.1.4. A Sense of Normality: Independence, Opportunity and Hope

The accumulative perceived effects of improved quality of life and management of pulmonary function had substantial effects on the mental state of many individuals. Angie spoke of how she feels ever closer to living a 'normal' lifestyle—or a lifestyle closer to that of her peers:

"It does gives us that chance, like I can be like everyone else ... .as a woman, I can start to think about having kids, the door is still open for me now ... I have more chances to take risks. Whereas before, I would just not even consider attempting things ... there is nothing there now to stop me, these things are in my hands."

Individuals commonly mentioned the increased *choice* they had. Cynthia believed that whilst choices were not specifically taken away from her, her CF played a substantial, subconscious role in the choices and decisions that she made:

"With time extending [due to Kaftrio] it just means you are like, 'oh well maybe I could get that retirement plan, maybe I should think about that'. I never got a lifetime ISA (Individual Savings Account) because I was never going to get to 50 [years] to use it. I thought I had another 15 years tops ... So I am sort of allowing myself to think about these things, whereas otherwise I would put them in a box."

Individuals felt the opportunities they had in life had increased considerably. Videl, for example, explained that she is starting to make plans to participate in activities that her CF had previously placed restrictions on:

"... so I have ridden dressage for years ... and that has slowly decreased because of my health ... I had lost sight of everything that was important to me because I was so poorly ... I dreamt about it (competing) but now I am like, come on, you can do it ... I feel like I am making up for lost time."

For most within the study, Kaftrio represented the catalyst for a new illness narrative that was characterised by a sense of hope. Hence, Kaftrio signified a 'new start', where CF did not play such a critical role in their life. Kaftrio also represented substantial advances in treatment in a short space of time, with the hope that this may just be the beginning of further successful treatment options until the point that diagnosis with CF is no longer a "life sentence".

3.2. Negative Perceptions of Kaftrio

The experiences associated with the negative perceptions of Kaftrio centred around: (i) side effects, (ii) the removal of therapy, and (iii) a loss of identity. Whilst most individuals spoke of side effects, a truly negative experience was found in six individuals. It was noted that two individuals had had to cease Kaftrio therapy due to both physiological and psychological side effects.

3.2.1. Side Effects: A Decrease in Quality of Life

Those who displayed predominately negative perceptions of Kaftrio had experienced serious side effects, wherein their quality of life had deteriorated below that of the pre-Kaftrio period. Katie noted that she had tried to persist with the treatment for 10-months despite side effects, which included debilitating migraines, 'brain fog', and sound sensitivity, but eventually chose to stop treatment as her quality of life had become so poor that getting out of bed was difficult:

"I was elated. It felt like I didn't have CF but the headaches started on day one—we know migraines now. I would have to go be in a dark quiet room. That helped me a little... I did not feel like I was on this planet. I forgot my date of birth and sound sensitivity was crazy, even talking became a struggle ... I went on for 10 months, I felt ungrateful. I thought this was how my new life was supposed to be (before I decided to come off it). I have no regrets—it is easier to live with CF than on Kaftrio."

Rachel documented the significant effect Kaftrio had on her body image, perception of self, and confidence, to the point where, despite her improved pulmonary function, she chose to cease treatment in the hope that she could better manage her weight and mental health:

"I felt every time I was going to clinic, it was a few more kilograms ... then it reached the point where I was the heaviest I have ever been and was really not comfortable. My lungs got better but I couldn't enjoy and reap the benefits because I was putting on all this weight. I was looking at myself and wanting to cry because I was so unhappy in how I looked."

3.2.2. Removal: Returning to a Life Pre-Kaftrio

Unpleasant side effects were something that many individuals within the study were willing to live with, given the trade-off for long-term health benefits. However, others worried that the potential side effects would mean that they had to discontinue Kaftrio. Similarly, all participants were wary of the effect that Kaftrio had on their liver, with the worry that potential increases in liver enzymes would result in their team removing access to modulator therapy. Laura, who had CF-related liver disease, noted that Kaftrio had elicited major positive changes to her pulmonary health, but she was concerned that this might only be short-lived should her liver status change:

"Back in 2020, around June, my liver disease became fatal and failed ... after being on it [Kaftrio] for a couple of weeks ... my liver function rose ... for me it was very stressful ... The liver thing is never going to get better, that's always going to be there. I have got the fear that ... because your liver function can just go up, I get scared in case they stop you ... would I revert back to how I was and everything that has improved be ripped away from me?"

Accordingly, as many participants had seen the positive changes that Kaftrio had on their day-to-day life, a number of participants lived in fear of Kaftrio subsequently being removed due to other health complications. For many, returning to a life pre-Kaftrio was now unimaginable, with Ben describing:

"I think my main anxiety comes from the fact that I've now been given this opportunity or like dangled carrot of, look what your life could be like, and in the back of my mind is when is it going to go away. All the time."

These feelings were echoed by Marin:

" ... It's all riding on it [Kaftrio] now ... there's no other alternatives ... and if it stops working, where do you go, even in your head with that?"

As a result, a sense of uncertainty around the future was something that the majority of individuals reported, regardless of their overall experience. These participants stated that the lack of available knowledge regarding the long-term efficacy of Kaftrio raised concerns that their health may start to deteriorate without warning. For older individuals, such as Katie and Marin, they referred to Kaftrio as their 'last chance', and Marin expressed a desire for additional understanding as to how their health may hypothetically look in the short-term future:

"What happens if I go back to where I was [pre-Kaftrio]? This was the be all and end all, this was supposed to solve all my problems and if this doesn't work then what? I have had to speak with a psychologist... It is [the worry] more the idea of what happens when this goes away—how long is that going to be there? Nobody knows."

Many described CF as a proverbial rollercoaster, with emotional highs and lows. The participants were accustomed to "looking over their shoulder" for negative health outcomes to present themselves, and Kaftrio was suggested to represent for some a scenario that was almost too good to be true and *"something that never happens to us [CF individuals]"*. As such, individuals consistently professed they were *"not allowing themselves to get carried away"*.

3.2.3. Loss of Identity

For some, modulator therapy resulted in an "identity crisis" and a feeling of being overwhelmed. Four individuals noted an understanding as to the path in which their life was following pre-therapy; however, the prospect of an extended life left a lot of unanswered questions and thoughts regarding both short- and long-term goals. Individuals spoke about how their CF has always been 'road mapped' out, whereas, since Kaftrio, the road was unclear. Ben spoke about his struggles of having to alter his perception of self:

" . . . this is how I summed it up. I completely lost my identity. Like, I didn't know who I was or what I am doing or what is going on . . . I felt like my identity was my health and my job and now they are not the same."

Indeed, the concept of a loss of identity highlights that, for some, Kaftrio may represent a period of trauma in which individuals find it hard to manage or conceptualise their new health status. For two participants, the issues lay in having to disassociate with the person they were and the life they were used to when the future remained so uncertain.

Overall, the perceived negative impacts of Kaftrio found within this sample were mainly focused on the side effects, having the taste of a 'normal' life cruelly removed, and fear and uncertainty regarding a drug in its infancy, which left the participants unable to let themselves become *"too carried away"*.

3.3. *Relationship with Clinical Teams and Psychological Support*

As life with CF begins to change following Kaftrio, some participants called for a change in their clinical care, with participants expressing a desire for their clinical care teams to listen more to their views. For those participants who were more confident, Kaftrio initiated a desire to take charge of their health and make decisions they felt were in their best interest, with Rachel expressing her hope that her input could be taken seriously:

"I want my input to mean something to my clinic team—at the moment they roll their eyes as if to say, oh here she goes again. I feel judged, I might not know the science, but they forget I am the one living with the condition daily. I am hoping that with Kaftrio I can have a firmer stance on things I do not agree with—I hope it gives me the chance to show them I actually am right."

However, Rachel spoke of how her previous experience with the clinical care team had prevented her from reaching out for the support she needed while taking Kaftrio:

"[In the past] I called my psychology team nearly in tears, I was really struggling. All they told me was that the waiting list was long and that I would likely not be seen for at least eight weeks . . . if that was someone's cry for help, there is no-one listening. With Kaftrio, I lost my identity straight away, I was overwhelmed and didn't know where to turn—I didn't even try to phone clinic as I knew no-one would answer."

Charlie also called for psychological support to be routinely available at clinic visits, alongside the dieticians, physiotherapists, and consultants:

"The teams need to do more. This is a life changing event that we have just been told to be grateful for and get on with it—I don't know how to get on with it."

For those struggling with weight and their perception of self, CF dietary care was quoted as being *'not the best'*, with individuals feeling as though the concept of nutrition/dieting and CF has a stigma attached to it, even in the face of Kaftrio. With the introduction of Kaftrio, some individuals within the current study were seeking methods to control their weight, though they were met with a lack of importance placed on weight and physique by their clinical team. Rachel spoke of her experience when she met her team to raise weight-related concerns:

> "I told them I was struggling with perception of self. I did not like how I looked, it was damaging my confidence. I have always struggled with weight and managed to lose some of it myself pre-Kaftrio. But when I gained weight on Kaftrio, the only thing they had to say to me was, 'no don't worry, . . . your lung function looks great'. That's not what I needed to hear—I felt lost."

Other individuals acknowledged the great work their clinical care teams undertook for them, but there was a consensus that there needed to be a deeper empathetic understanding of the new psychological and physical challenges that come with the use of Kaftrio. Hence, there was a call from the participants for care teams to gain a further understanding of the existential concerns regarding the dramatic change of health status for many (but not all) in an extremely short time period.

3.4. A Message to the 10%

Finally, all of the participants explained their hope that, as with themselves, one day there would be a treatment available for the 10% whose genetic mutation does not support therapy with Kaftrio. Many referenced a phenomenon they described as similar to 'survivor's guilt'. They alluded to how difficult they would find it, looking in from the outside, whilst somebody with the 'same' condition was starting to make plans about their new life. Individuals currently taking Kaftrio alluded to the fact that they wanted to make the most out of Kaftrio and adopt further health-seeking behaviours in honour and respect of those that were not able to take Kaftrio. For those who had ceased treatment with Kaftrio, they felt guilty that they were choosing to discontinue something that another individual would wish to have. Importantly, Kaftrio was not simply seen as just 'another treatment' but as a gift that they had to cherish.

> "I've got so much guilt that I can't think about it too much. I have this like, it's not survivors' guilt but something along those lines . . . They [the ineligible] are just watching it all unravel. They [Vertex] have to do something for them."

Accordingly, the participants receiving Kaftrio felt a sense of responsibility to those who were unable to receive the therapy. Given the positive changes that it had provided to many participants' quality of life, they felt they owed it to those not taking Kaftrio to try and live life to the fullest. At the same time, all individuals expressed sorrow that not everyone would tolerate or could take Kaftrio. The individual messages aimed at the 10% were that of belief, hope, and a will to keep fighting, as all individuals believed it was only a matter of time before they had alternative treatment. For most, their personal adherence to Kaftrio was in honour to them as a way to ensure they never take this 'gift' for granted.

4. Discussion

By employing a qualitative approach, this study has offered a unique, in-depth insight into the lived experience of modulator therapy for CF individuals, highlighting the multi-faceted implications associated with the changing landscape of the disease and its treatment. The participant narratives revealed the positive impact that Kaftrio had on the individual's disease state, with an improved overall quality of life and a significant reduction in 'classical' CF challenges. Moreover, the accumulative effect of these positive changes was reported as facilitating a sense of hope, normality, and independence, thereby allowing individuals to live a lifestyle which they considered to resemble that of their healthy peers. However, individuals also narrated negative experiences associated with the therapy, revealing significant inter-patient variability outside the physiological context [19]. The current narrative was ultimately dictated by an individual's ability to tolerate the therapy, with individuals expressing feelings of fear and resignation. Some individuals expressed increased anxiety and distress in relation to uncertainty around the removal of therapy and, for some, dealing with a redefining of one's identity. Regardless of perception, individuals mentioned their relationships with their clinical teams and called for additional counselling and psychological support to be offered to meet the new psychological needs of the individual, given the significant change in the landscape of the disease.

The implementation of Kaftrio represented a positive shift in the illness narrative of those who were able to tolerate the therapy. For example, for the first time, many individuals noted a sense of control and optimism for the future due to Kaftrio's substantial effect on their quality of life. Indeed, many participants viewed Kaftrio as a second chance at life in which individuals had the opportunity to use previously negative experiences to reconstruct a positive self-transformation for the future they did not previously have [20]. Although the data on modulator therapy and life expectancy is not yet available, Kaftrio gave individuals hope and a representation of trust in an imagined future. Given the life-limiting nature of CF, individuals spoke of how they did not trust in their future enough (pre-Kaftrio) to believe they would reach milestones such as retirement and parenthood. The implementation of Kaftrio elicited a reality-based belief that a positive future did exist in which an individual could now plan for life events they previously perceived as impossible.

Drawing on experience, individuals recounted the limiting effect CF had on their life prior to modulator therapy, with many professing that they had lost sight of things that were important to them due to poor health status. The implementation of Kaftrio was the catalyst for a reduction in traditional CF challenges, which decreased the burden that CF had on individuals' day-to-day lives. Gratitude was expressed for this sudden respite, with individuals speaking of how thankful they were to have their *lives back*. Longitudinal analysis has shown that gratitude is associated with a number of positive traits such as increases in self-esteem, satisfaction with life and fewer symptoms of depression [21,22], suggesting that as well as positive physical change, modulator therapy may also enhance an individual's mental well-being. As in Davidai and Gilovich [23], CF forced individuals to focus on the obstacles and difficulties in life, given that they demanded immediate action. Kaftrio represented a metaphorical tailwind, in which individuals were given a reprieve [24] and a chance to focus on the things in life that bring them positive emotions. For those who felt they had been simply existing, Kaftrio represented an opportunity in which they could now truly live.

Although, for many, the experience of modulator therapy was a predominately positive one, for some, the sudden change in perspective had negative psychological effects. Whilst individuals expressed hope and gratitude, the narrative highlighted the difficulty of dealing with this rapid change in health, with individuals experiencing anxiety and fear, as seen in cancer survivors, in response to uncertainty, unanswered questions, and fear of relapse [25]. The current study identifies that modulator therapy may elicit feelings of anxiety associated with the overwhelming and uncertain future individuals now face in regards to themselves, their identity, and their future. As reported in those who receive a non-diagnosis of Huntington's Disease, the prospect of a prolonged life can be one that is intimidating and stressful, as individuals perceive demands that they now must do something they were unprepared for, extraordinary and/or meaningful with their new, longer lives [26].

In the context of planning their new lives, some spoke of a loss of identity and a need to redefine their sense of self. As with other chronic conditions, one's illness identity is dictated by the degree to which the disease has affected the way they see themselves and that the illness is integrated into one's sense of self [27]. Whilst many professed a state of acceptance around their CF, for those who felt their illness dominated their identity, the shift in health, and thus identity, was described as "almost post-traumatic". For those who experienced a change in identity, albeit one of positive health, there was a need for meaning reconstruction, which elicited emotions commonly associated with the grieving process and the loss of self [28]. It is worth noting, however, that whilst the initial loss of identity can be a negative experience, as individuals construct new meaning to their new lives, Tedeschi and Calhoun [29] argue that this process can breed positivity through the phenomenon of post-traumatic growth (PTG). Through continuous reappraisal of themselves, individuals who do experience PTG report feelings of becoming more resilient, confident, and independent whilst also developing a greater awareness of life's fragilities [28]. Whilst many had developed coping strategies for their CF, they felt surprised and unprepared to deal with this emotion in response to a wholly positive event. Given that PTG can initiate feelings of stress and anxiety, the development of psychological programs promoting coping strategies should be considered in the management of life post-initiation of therapy, as it is likely that this initial transition is met with fear and uncertainty [30,31].

It is clear from this present study that the effect of modulator therapy had a strong impact on the relationship an individual had with their clinical team, with individuals stressing that their clinical teams failed to understand them as an individual or the effect their authoritarian decisions had on their physical and mental well-being. As such, many individuals felt that they did not have input in their own treatment decisions or did not feel confident in disagreeing for fear of judgement or guilt. This experience has been identified within the broader literature, with CF individuals often finding difficulty in communicating with their clinical teams due to how they discuss sensitive topics [32]. Whilst clinical teams understand CF as an *illness*; there is often a failure to understand how each individual conceptualises the disease [33]. Given that many individuals receiving Kaftrio will now have to contest with the phenomena of survivorship, it is key for clinical teams to consider the psychological effects that this can have. Common concerns within this narrative mirror that of cancer survivors, with issues around managing stress, fear of recurrence [or in this instance, treatment removal] and living with uncertainty [30]. As individuals begin to redefine their constructs of reality without the burden of CF, there is a need for clinical teams to understand the new existential concerns of living with CF to ensure the post-Kaftrio era is not defined by poor clinical relations. As such, this study has implications for service delivery, with a heavier focus needed on the team's understanding of the complexities and new challenges facing those with CF [33], enabling more meaningful relationships with clinical teams. Whilst clinical care teams perceive the life-changing nature of Kaftrio to be one of positivity for the CF individual, it must be understood that simply increasing one's quantity of life does not necessarily increase one's psychological wellbeing and quality of life in the long term [33].

The present study also identified feelings of survivor's guilt in both those who could and could not tolerate the therapy, a concept similarly reported in other life-limiting diseases [34,35]. The concept of survivor's guilt has been defined into four specific areas: *altered identity, altered relationships, mental health* and *physical symptoms*, and *resolution* [26,36]. The narrative identified each of these depictions aside from resolution (e.g., the feelings of guilt disappearing). Whether survivor's guilt underpins the psychological experience of modulators is yet to be established and cannot be concluded from this narrative. However, the study identified that individuals conceptualised survivor's guilt according to their treatment experience. For those able to tolerate therapy, feelings centred around a sense of substitute guilt or unfairness in relation to those who are ineligible or could not tolerate the therapy. Indeed, individuals manifested feelings of guilt due to the fact that they could now begin a life less compromised by CF, whereas others are not able to have that luxury. Similarly, as described in Hutson et al. [36], this shift in identity may have further repercussions when considering identification with others and feelings of belonging within the CF community. Alternatively, where the treatment failed, feelings of guilt centred around the idea that they were *ungrateful* or had *wasted* a treatment from which others could have benefited. The given individuals were aware of the substantial cost associated with the therapy, and the guilt was further exacerbated with perceptions of their personal burden on the healthcare system being heightened. As the occurrence of survival guilt in the context of modulator therapy is yet to be understood, there is a need for further research to ascertain when it occurs and develop potential preventative methods to aid patients.

5. Limitations

The perceptions of modulator therapy from this qualitative study were based on the lived experiences of 12 individuals, which led to data saturation, lending credibility to the findings. Whilst individuals were interviewed from across the United Kingdom and, therefore, from multiple different clinics, the study did not explore patient perspectives from other countries in which modulator therapy is available. Furthermore, the study population included significantly more females than males; as such, we are unable to ascertain whether these perspectives are also affected by sex or gender. Given both factors, the generalisability of this information is potentially limited.

Although genetic mutation was discussed, this was not a variable which was explored in detail. As suggested in Varilek and Isaacson [33], further research is needed to ascertain whether there are differences in the experience of modulator therapy between genotypes.

6. Conclusions

For many individuals, Kaftrio represents 'as close to a cure' as CF individuals will have access to in their lifetime, with substantial changes in their quality of life, opportunities, and optimism for the future. However, this does not come without negatives, with individuals experiencing anxiety with regards to side effects, the efficacy of long-term treatment, and a fear of a return to life pre-Kaftrio. For the few who feel left behind, those whom it did not work for, or for the 10% who are not eligible, the message remains one of hope. An important overarching theme is that more needs to be provided by clinical teams to help manage the magnitude of effect that Kaftrio has both physically and mentally. Whilst individuals express gratitude toward Kaftrio, for many, that does not come with an absence of negative emotions.

Author Contributions: S.A.A. was involved in the design, data collection, analysis, interpretation and writing of the manuscript; K.A.M. was involved in the conception, design, interpretation and writing of the manuscript; D.M.H. was involved in the design, analysis and reviewing of the manuscript; B.C. was involved in the analysis, interpretation and reviewing of the manuscript; M.A.M. was involved in the conception, design, analysis, interpretation, and reviewing of the manuscript. All authors have read and agreed to the published version of the manuscript.

Funding: This work was supported by the Knowledge Economy Skills Scholarships (KESS). KESS is a pan-Wales higher-level skills initiative led by Bangor University on behalf of the HE sector in Wales. It is part funded by the Welsh Government's European Social Fund (ESF) convergence programme for West Wales and the Valleys.

Institutional Review Board Statement: The study was conducted in accordance with the Declaration of Helsinki, and approved by the Institutional Ethics Committee of Swansea University (ref. number MN_22-10-22).

Informed Consent Statement: Informed consent was obtained from all participants involved in the study.

Data Availability Statement: The data presented in this study are available on request from the corresponding author. The data are not publicly available due to their sensitive nature.

Conflicts of Interest: None of the authors have any conflict of interest to declare.

References

1. Cystic Fibrosis Trust. *UK Cystic Fibrosis Registry Annual Report 2017*; Cystic Fibrosis Trust: London, UK, 2017.
2. Ridley, K.; Condren, M. Elexacaftor-Tezacaftor-Ivacaftor: The First Triple-Combination Cystic Fibrosis Transmembrane Conductance Regulator Modulating Therapy. *J. Pediatr. Pharm.* **2020**, *25*, 192–197. [CrossRef] [PubMed]
3. Cantin, A. Cystic Fibrosis Lung Inflammation: Early, Sustained, and Severe. *Am. J. Respir. Crit. Care Med.* **1995**, *151*, 939–941. [CrossRef] [PubMed]
4. Heijerman, H.G.; McKone, E.F.; Downey, D.G.; van Braeckel, E.; Rowe, S.M.; Tullis, E.; Mall, M.A.; Welter, J.J.; Ramsey, B.W.; McKee, C.M.; et al. Efficacy and safety of the elexacaftor plus tezacaftor plus ivacaftor combination regimen in people with cystic fibrosis homozygous for the F508del mutation: A double-blind, randomised, phase 3 trial. *Lancet* **2019**, *394*, 1940–1948. [CrossRef]
5. Kadoglou, N.P.; Iliadis, F.; Angelopoulou, N.; Perrea, D.; Ampatzidis, G.; Liapis, C.D.; Alevizos, M. The anti-inflammatory effects of exercise training in patients with type 2 diabetes mellitus. *Eur. J. Cardiovasc. Prev. Rehabil.* **2007**, *14*, 837–843. [CrossRef] [PubMed]

6. Lopes-Pacheco, M. CFTR Modulators: The Changing Face of Cystic Fibrosis in the Era of Precision Medicine. *Front. Pharmacol.* **2020**, *10*, 1662. [CrossRef]
7. Penketh, A.R.; Wise, A.; Mearns, M.B.; Hodson, M.E.; Batten, J.C. Cystic fibrosis in adolescents and adults. *Thorax* **1987**, *42*, 526–532. [CrossRef]
8. Elborn, J.S. Modulator treatment for people with cystic fibrosis: Moving in the right direction. *Eur. Resp. Rev.* **2020**, *29*, 200051. [CrossRef]
9. Paterson, S.L.; Barry, P.J.; Horsley, A.R. Tezacaftor and ivacaftor for the treatment of cystic fibrosis. *Expert Rev. Respir. Med.* **2019**, *14*, 15–30. [CrossRef]
10. Fredrick, G.; Hadida, S.; Grootenhuis, P. Pharmacological Rescue of Mutant CFTR Function for the Treatment of Cystic Fibrosis. In *Ion Channels*; Springer: Berlin/Heidelberg, Germany, 2008; pp. 91–120.
11. Ramsey, B.W.; Davies, J.; McElvaney, N.G.; Tullis, E.; Scott, C.; Bell, P.D.; Griese, M.; McKone, E.F.; Wainwright, C.E.; Konstan, M.W.; et al. A CFTR Potentiator in Patients with Cystic Fibrosis and theG551DMutation. *N. Engl. J. Med.* **2011**, *365*, 1663–1672. [CrossRef]
12. Connett, G.J. Lumacaftor-ivacaftor in the treatment of cystic fibrosis: Design, development and place in therapy. *Drug. Des. Dev. Ther.* **2019**, *13*, 2405–2412. [CrossRef]
13. Shteinberg, M.; Taylor-Cousar, J.L. Impact of CFTR modulator use on outcomes in people with severe cystic fibrosis lung disease. *Eur. Resp. Rev.* **2020**, *29*, 190112. [CrossRef] [PubMed]
14. DiMango, E.; Spielman, D.B.; Overdevest, J.; Keating, C.; Francis, S.F.; Dansky, D.; Gudis, D.A. Effect of highly effective modulator therapy on quality of life in adults with cystic fibrosis. *Int. Forum Allergy Rhinol* **2021**, *11*, 75–78. [CrossRef] [PubMed]
15. Knudsen, K.B.; Boisen, K.A.; Katzenstein, T.L.; Mortensen, L.H.; Pressler, T.; Skov, M.; Jarden, M. Living with cystic fibrosis-A qualitative study of a life coaching intervention. *Patient Prefer. Adherence* **2018**, *12*, 585–594. [CrossRef] [PubMed]
16. Evans, A.B.; Barker-Ruchti, N.; Blackwell, J.; Clay, G.; Dowling, F.; Frydendal, S.; Hybholt, M.G.; Lenneis, V.; Malcolm, D.; Phoenix, C.; et al. Qualitative research in sports studies: Challenges, possibilities and the current state of play. *Eur. J. Sport Soc.* **2021**, *18*, 1–17. [CrossRef]
17. Quittner, A.L.; Saez-Flores, E.; Barton, J.D. The psychological burden of cystic fibrosis. *Curr. Opin. Pulm. Med.* **2016**, *22*, 187–191. [CrossRef] [PubMed]
18. Hsieh, H.-F.; Shannon, S.E. Three Approaches to Qualitative Content Analysis. *Qual. Health Res.* **2005**, *15*, 1277–1288. [CrossRef]
19. Chevalier, B.; Hinzpeter, A. The influence of CFTR complex alleles on precision therapy of cystic fibrosis. *J. Cyst. Fibros.* **2020**, *19*, S15–S18. [CrossRef]
20. Pals, J.L. Narrative Identity Processing of Difficult Life Experiences: Pathways of Personality Development and Positive Self-Transformation in Adulthood. *J. Personal.* **2006**, *74*, 1079–1110. [CrossRef]
21. Lambert, N.M.; Fincham, F.D.; Stillman, T.F. Gratitude and depressive symptoms: The role of positive reframing and positive emotion. *Cogn. Emot.* **2012**, *26*, 615–633. [CrossRef]
22. McCullough, M.E.; Emmons, R.A.; Tsang, J.-A. The grateful disposition: A conceptual and empirical topography. *J. Personal. Soc. Psychol.* **2002**, *82*, 112–127. [CrossRef]
23. Davidai, S.; Gilovich, T. The headwinds/tailwinds asymmetry: An availability bias in assessments of barriers and blessings. *J. Personal. Soc. Psychol.* **2016**, *111*, 835–851. [CrossRef] [PubMed]
24. Bhalla, M.; Proffitt, D.R. Visual–motor recalibration in geographical slant perception. *J. Exp. Psychol. Hum. Percept. Perform.* **1999**, *25*, 1076–1096. [CrossRef] [PubMed]
25. Hewitt, M.E.; Bamundo, A.; Day, R.; Harvey, C. Perspectives on Post-Treatment Cancer Care: Qualitative Research with Survivors, Nurses, and Physicians. *J. Clin. Oncol.* **2007**, *25*, 2270–2273. [CrossRef] [PubMed]
26. Winnberg, E.; Winnberg, U.; Pohlkamp, L.; Hagberg, A. What to Do with a Second Chance in Life? Long-Term Experiences of Non-Carriers of Huntington's Disease. *J. Genet. Couns.* **2018**, *27*, 1438–1446. [CrossRef] [PubMed]
27. Charmaz, K. The Body, Identity, and Self: Adapting To Impairment. *Sociol. Q* **1995**, *36*, 657–680. [CrossRef]
28. James, G.; Neimeyer, R.A. Loss, Grief, and the Search for Significance: Toward a Model of Meaning Reconstruction in Bereavement. *J. Constr. Psychol.* **2006**, *19*, 31–65. [CrossRef]
29. Tedeschi, R.G.; Calhoun, L.G. The posttraumatic growth inventory: Measuring the positive legacy of trauma. *J. Trauma. Stress* **1996**, *9*, 455–471. [CrossRef]
30. Ness, S.; Kokal, J.; Fee-Schroeder, K.; Novotny, P.; Satele, D.; Barton, D. Concerns Across the Survivorship Trajectory: Results from a Survey of Cancer Survivors. *Oncol. Nurs. Forum* **2012**, *40*, 35–42. [CrossRef]
31. Rajandram, R.K.; Jenewein, J.; McGrath, C.; Zwahlen, R.A. Coping processes relevant to posttraumatic growth: An evidence-based review. *Support. Care Cancer* **2011**, *19*, 583–589. [CrossRef]
32. Eaton, C.K.; Beachy, S.; McLean, K.A.; Nicolais, C.J.; Bernstein, R.; Sáez-Clarke, E.; Quittner, A.L.; Riekert, K.A. Misunderstandings, misperceptions, and missed opportunities: Perspectives on adherence barriers from people with CF, caregivers, and CF team members. *Patient Educ. Couns.* **2020**, *103*, 1587–1594. [CrossRef]
33. Varilek, B.M.; Isaacson, M.J. The dance of cystic fibrosis: Experiences of living with cystic fibrosis as an adult. *J. Clin. Nurs.* **2020**, *29*, 3553–3564. [CrossRef] [PubMed]

34. Huggins, M.; Bloch, M.; Wiggins, S.; Adam, S.; Suchowersky, O.; Trew, M.; Klimek, M.; Greenberg, C.R.; Eleff, M.; Thompson, L.P.; et al. Predictive testing for Huntington disease in Canada: Adverse effects and unexpected results in those receiving a decreased risk. *Am. J. Med. Genet.* **1992**, *42*, 508–515. [CrossRef] [PubMed]
35. Valverde, K.D. Why Me? Why Not Me? *J. Genet. Couns.* **2006**, *15*, 461–463. [CrossRef]
36. Hutson, S.P.; Hall, J.M.; Pack, F.L. Survivor Guilt. *Adv. Nurs. Sci.* **2015**, *38*, 20–33. [CrossRef] [PubMed]

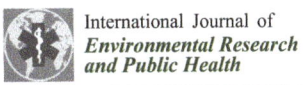

Article

Interprofessional Collaboration in Fall Prevention: Insights from a Qualitative Study

Isabel Baumann [1,2], Frank Wieber [1,3,*], Thomas Volken [1], Peter Rüesch [1] and Andrea Glässel [1,4]

1. Institute of Public Health, Zurich University of Applied Sciences (ZHAW), 8400 Winterthur, Switzerland
2. Center for the Interdisciplinary Study of Gerontology and Vulnerability, University of Geneva, 1205 Geneva, Switzerland
3. Department of Psychology, University of Konstanz, 78464 Konstanz, Germany
4. Institute of Biomedical Ethics and History of Medicine, University of Zurich, 8006 Zurich, Switzerland
* Correspondence: frank.wieber@zhaw.ch; Tel.: +41-58-934-43-47

Abstract: (1) Background and objective: to explore the experiences of Swiss health care providers involved in a community fall prevention pilot project on barriers and facilitations in interprofessional cooperation between 2016 and 2017 in three regions of Switzerland. (2) Methods: semi-structured interviews with health care providers assessed their perspective on the evaluation of jointly developed tools for reporting fall risk, continuous training of the health care providers, sensitizing media campaigns, and others. (3) Results: One of the project's strengths is the interprofessional continuous trainings. These trainings allowed the health care providers to extend their network of health care providers, which contributed to an improvement of fall prevention. Challenges of the project were that the standardization of the interprofessional collaboration required additional efforts. These efforts are time consuming and, for some categories of health care providers, not remunerated by the Swiss health care system. (4) Conclusions: On a micro and meso level, the results of the present study indicate that the involved health care providers strongly support interprofessional collaboration in fall prevention. However, time and financial constraints challenge the implementation. On a macro level, potential ways to strengthen interprofessional collaboration are a core element in fall prevention.

Keywords: fall prevention; interprofessional collaboration; qualitative research; focus groups; community health services; older adults; evaluation; physical therapy; occupational therapy; general practitioners

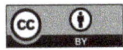

1. Introduction

1.1. The Risk of Falls among Older Adults

Falls are a major risk to the older adult's health. A Cochrane review indicates that among people over 65 years, the fall incidence is about 33% per year and among people over the age of 85, it is about 50% per year [1]. Data from Switzerland for 2013 indicates about 90,000 falls among people over 65 years registered at the Swiss Council for Accident Prevention (BFU) [2]. Falls often lead to fractures, in particular proximal femoral fractures. Besides the harm to the older adults who experience the falls, the subsequent treatment creates huge costs [3].

The risk of falls among older adults is multifactorial. Risk factors associated with falls include health-related factors such as poor nutrition [4], cognitive impairment [5–8], functional disabilities [6,9] and environmental factors such as home safety [10]. Due to this multifactorial nature of falls, different health care providers are involved in the prevention and the management of the fall risks [11,12]. Physical or occupational therapists carry out physical exercise programs or adjust home environments in a way to increase the older adults' safety [12–14]. Nurses provide regular health care for the older adults in hospitals and homes and are thus particularly aware of their needs in terms of reducing fall risks [5]. If medication or similar treatments are applied, general practitioners are usually involved [15].

Therefore, preventing and managing falls calls for an interprofessional approach not only in inpatient but also in outpatient or community settings [16]. Interprofessional collaboration, defined as an active relationship between health care providers to work together to solve problems or provide services and to focus on a common goal, has been found to have mixed but predominantly positive effects on health care provided to community-dwelling older adults [17,18].

1.2. Interprofessional Fall Prevention

In conventional community-based fall prevention, health care providers often work independently from each other. For instance, a review study that focused on general fall prevention found that non-medical health care providers are at times not equally included in decision-making processes [19]. Interprofessional fall prevention, in contrast, allows health care providers to not only exchange experiences but also patient-related information to develop a tailored health care program and shared decision-making processes. A small qualitative study from Canada found that health care providers feel more "on top of things" and can learn from each other if they work together with providers from other disciplines [20].

This exchange of experiences and information is smoother if health care providers know each other personally [21]. Personal contacts allow reducing misunderstandings and ineffective care. In addition, the literature suggests that interprofessional collaboration requires specific communication skills, for instance, a common language [22,23]. Technical terminology including abbreviations or jargon of some professionals may not be understood by others [24]. Introducing a common language is thus important and needs mutual communication and exchange. However, this may be perceived as a loss of professional identity [24].

Another important factor for a smooth functioning of the interprofessional collaboration is role clarity, i.e., the definition of the function of each team member and her/his contribution to the collaboration. Due to potential role conflicts between the members of an interprofessional team, a structured protocol with predefined division of roles and responsibilities is helpful [25,26]. Such protocols have to be negotiated among the team members, a participatory process which is usually carried out in interprofessional meetings that allow to plan and coordinate health care [27]. If roles and responsibilities are not explicitly defined, experience shows that the team members feel overlooked or overburdened [21]. In contrast, if team members have an equal status or a perception of balance within the team, they trust each other more, which leads to a better functioning of the interprofessional team [28].

As a challenge, a review study that focused on older people living in the community found that interprofessional collaboration is more time-consuming than multi- or non-interprofessional collaboration, which is often not adequately reimbursed [26]. In particular, the coordination between the team members consumes large amounts of time [28]. Consequently, time pressure renders interprofessional collaboration challenging [22].

In support of the interprofessional collaboration, many of the studied interprofessional teams describe that they use specific tools for exchange of information about patients [25,29]. Some use electronic health records, which facilitate coordination in times of the digitalization of health care [26]. These tools allow team members to know about the patient's health status and the other team members' care activities [27].

1.3. Primary Prevention Program in Switzerland

In Switzerland, the foundation of health promotion Switzerland ("Gesundheitsförderung Schweiz") launched the pilot project "Via Pilotprogramm Sturzprävention" between 2014 and 2016. The project aimed at improving fall prevention among community-dwelling older adults and particularly addressed older adults with a risk of falling or who have already fallen; it thus constitutes specific rather than general fall prevention. As part of this aim, it focused on improving the health care provision on fall prevention of older adults by building and strengthening the network between community health service providers based on standardizing interprofessional collaboration. The fall prevention pilot project was implemented in three regions in the German speaking part of Switzerland: two rural (regions 1 and 2) and one urban (region 3). The present study is the result of the qualitative research conducted in the context of a project evaluation.

The fall prevention pilot project followed a bottom-up approach. In each of the three different regions of Switzerland, it provided a tailored organizational structure to bring health care providers from different professions together to discuss and implement potential measures. Health care providers involved in this fall prevention pilot project were physicians (general practitioners (GP), geriatric specialists, and other specialists), physical therapists, occupational therapists, hospitals, home care providers, organizations of the civil society, and a senior citizens' organization. An overview over the health professions involved is provided in Figure 1. In each region, health care providers and institutions developed their own measures, although partly shared and adopted each other's measures. One measure consisted in organizing a continuous interprofessional training for health care providers in fall prevention. Another measure consisted in creating evidence-based tools (e.g., a registration form) to facilitate communication [30]. The interprofessional training included contents such as the recognition of stumbling blocks and the self-awareness of impaired vision in everyday life or exercises to train balance.

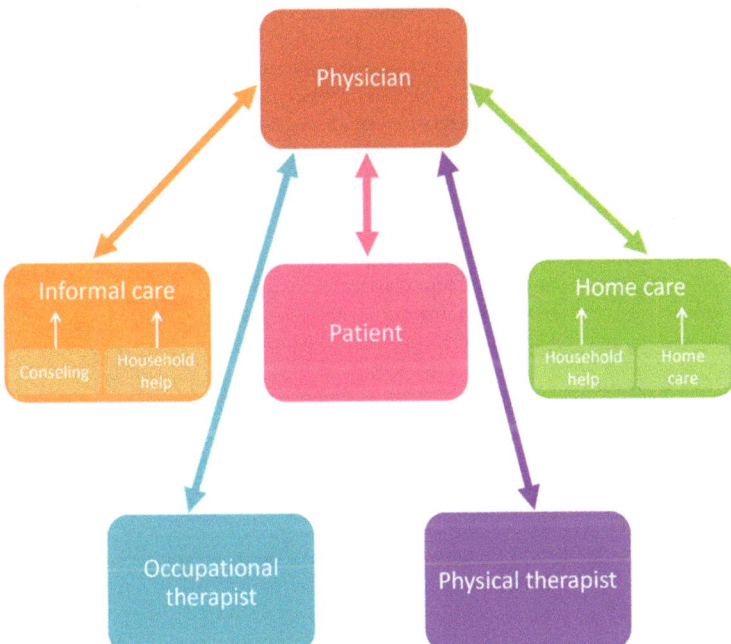

Figure 1. Overview of the health professions involved in the Swiss primary prevention program.

2. Materials and Methods

2.1. Study Design

In 2016, our research group was mandated by "Gesundheitsförderung Schweiz" to conduct a summative evaluation of the fall prevention pilot project. The design of our evaluation involved qualitative interviews and a focus group with several representatives of the five largest categories of health care providers, as well as a quantitative survey among all health care providers and representatives of the institutions involved in the fall prevention pilot project. The evaluation of the pilot project comprised six case studies: three in the pilot regions (regions 1 to 3) and three in comparison regions (regions 4 to 6). For each of the project regions, we included one comparison region with a similar socio-demographic structure and in a similar geographic setting (i.e., regions 4 and 5 are rural, region 6 is urban).

2.2. Methodology

In this paper, we focus on the results of the qualitative study. Therefore, the aim of our article is to explore the experiences of the health care providers involved in the fall prevention pilot project on barriers and facilitations in interprofessional cooperation in fall prevention in Switzerland. The results of the quantitative part of the evaluation have been presented in a report [31]. Qualitative methods offer the possibility to explore the research object from the perspective of those who experience an everyday relation to it, in the sense of the so-called user, consumer, or client perspective [32]. In contrast to the quantitative methodology, the qualitative approach promises greater openness to unexplored concepts or phenomena and focuses [33] on how people understand and interpret their social world [34].

2.3. Data Collection and Participants

Qualitative data were collected between September 2016 and March 2017 in individual telephone interviews and one focus group. In the pilot regions, participants were the members of the coordination group which was responsible for the implementation of the pilot project. The research team received a list of representatives of all occupations from the main representative responsible for the project. The researchers then contacted the representatives by email and telephone. In the control regions, the researchers browsed the internet to identify one representative of each occupation.

In each region, we aimed at interviewing one representative of the five largest categories of health care providers (physicians, physical and occupational therapists, home care nurses, and informal carers). In addition, a representative of a seniors' organization participated in the focus group in region 1. While in the pilot regions (regions 1–3) all of the contacted representatives of the health care providers participated in the focus group or the individual interview, in the control regions (4–6) it was more difficult to recruit participants. For this reason, we interviewed four rather than five representatives in the control region, because some of the contacted health care providers were not available for an interview (see Table 1). This difference may bias the results in the direction that more support for interprofessional fall prevention may be observed in the pilot region.

Two trained researchers conducted the focus group. The two researchers who conducted the individual interviews and focus groups had no prior personal relationships with the interviewees. Researcher 1 moderated the focus group discussion, which was based on a semi-structured guide of questions focusing on the following six main topics: (1) collaboration between health care providers in fall prevention, (2) use and evaluation of tools and processes, (3) communication with the public, (4) use and evaluation of further training, (5) cooperation in the coordination group, (6) the perceived direction and strength of changes through the fall prevention pilot project, as well as (7) the possibility to comment on the topic. Researcher 2 composed the written protocol of the focus group. For reasons of quality assurance, the focus group was completed with a joint debriefing of the two researchers, in which the main results were consolidated. The qualitative interviews followed the same interview guide. The focus group and the qualitative interviews were audio recorded and transcribed verbatim based on the defined rules [35].

Table 1. Overview of the participants in the focus group and interviews (note: NA—no answer).

Region	Organization/Occupation	Education	Year of Birth	Overall Occupational Experience (in Years)	Occupational Experience in Fall Prevention (in Years)
1 (pilot, rural)	Physician	GP	1970	-	6
1 (pilot, rural)	Occupational therapist	Occupational therapy HF	1978	-	10
1 (pilot, rural)	Occupational therapist	Occupational therapy HF	1967	-	15
1 (pilot, rural)	Physical therapist	Physical therapy	1964	-	3
1 (pilot, rural)	Informal care	Nursing sciences HF	1965	-	3
1 (pilot, rural)	Senior citizen	Apprenticeship	1939	-	3
2 (pilot, rural)	Physician	GP	1967	17	1
2 (pilot, rural)	Occupational therapist	BSc in Occupational therapy	1974	18	18
2 (pilot, rural)	Physical therapist	Physical therapy	1975	26	26
2 (pilot, rural)	Home care nurses	Nursing expert	1967	25	8
2 (pilot, rural)	Informal care	Adult sports trainer	1963	14	5
3 (pilot, urban)	Physician	GP	1965	23	20
3 (pilot, urban)	Physical therapist	Physical therapy	1988	NA	NA
3 (pilot, urban)	Occupational therapist	Occupational therapy HF	1961	25	13
3 (pilot, urban)	Home care nurses	Nursing sciences	1973	20	13
3 (pilot, urban)	Informal care	Adult sports trainer	1963	13	5
4 (control, rural)	Occupational therapist	Occupational therapy	1972	15	5
4 (control, rural)	Home care nurses	Nursing sciences	1992	3	2
4 (control, rural)	Physical therapist	Physical therapy	1958	36	27
4 (control, rural)	Physician	GP	1971	19	19
5 (control, rural)	Occupational therapist	Occupational therapy	1970	21	21
5 (control, rural)	Physician	GP	1954	38	38
5 (control, rural)	Informal care	NA	1962	32	11
5 (control, rural)	Physical therapist	Physical therapy	1961	30	30
6 (control, urban)	Physical therapist	Physical therapy	1953	39	2
6 (control, urban)	Physician	GP	1968	23	11
6 (control, urban)	Occupational therapist	Occupational therapy	1969	16	22
6 (control, urban)	Home care nurses	Nursing sciences	1984	8	3

2.4. Data Analysis

The data were analyzed using a qualitative content analysis based on Mayring [36]. The aim of this analysis is to reduce information from the participants' statements in such a way that the essential content remains and the structures and core characteristics become clearer. For this purpose, to develop a category system, an inductive procedure and a deductive procedure based on the six main topics of the semi-structured guide were used. The coding guide to create categories and the coding rules contained therein served as a basis for ensuring traceability and replicability of the procedure. The data analysis was managed by using the software MAXQDA version 12 (VERBI: Berlin, Germany).

2.5. Quality Assurance of the Data Analysis

For reasons of transparency and comprehensibility, the participants received the scripted interviews for reading aloud and for making comments called "member checking" of the transcripts. Data were analyzed by researcher 2 using a code book and building up a system of written memos. Data were grounded in the text by using original quotations of the anonymized participants of the interviews. A researcher handbook was used for notes during the process.

3. Results

Five main categories regarding interprofessional collaboration in fall prevention in Switzerland were identified in the study:

1. Information and communication;
2. Stakeholder and collaboration;
3. Cooperation between the health care providers;
4. Case-related cooperation;
5. Continuous training measures.

In the following, we report the results for each category. We first focus on hindering aspects that were perceived by the health professionals before we present the facilitating aspects that were mentioned.

3.1. Information and Communication

3.1.1. Barriers

The registration forms that were developed to facilitate the communication between the health care providers are not equally used in all regions and by all categories of health care providers. In fact, the registration forms are particularly often used by home care providers. The following statements about the registration forms show excerpts of the status of use in the pilot regions.

"I mean the registration sheets. So, they still have to prove themselves. It's not quite like that yet." (Region2_P1)

"From the registration forms I have received only two so far." (Region2_P5)

"At the moment I've actually had only a few of these messages. And the messages we sent to the doctors didn't come back. We didn't hear anything more." (Region2_P1)

3.1.2. Facilitators

Nevertheless, in general, the health care providers in the pilot regions rated the familiarity of the registration sheets for assessing the risk of falls as equally high and rated the preparation of the registration sheets as good.

"The registration sheet has proved its worth to the extent that it is now known to all participants, and it is clear what happens with it. There is still development potential in the fact that general practitioners distribute concrete tasks to [home care]. From October to December, we sent 36 registration forms, eight of them were provided with the concrete feedback by the family doctor and 21 came back without anything being written, [. . .] and for seven they did not receive patient's consent to be sent in." (Region3_P4)

In the three comparison regions, the health care providers were interviewed in the context of the qualitative interviews to assess their perceptions on the usefulness of the so-called registration form for their work. The structure and content of the registration form were briefly explained. In principle, the players in the comparison regions were open minded towards such a registration sheet and considered it to be useful.

3.2. Stakeholder and Collaboration

3.2.1. Barriers

In the interviews, it became clear that fall prevention as an isolated topic of cooperation is not the starting point, but it is considered in the context of more complex case-related questions of cooperation in care.

"One difficulty of the whole interview is that it focuses on the fall. We as family doctors and home care practices a comprehensive care and often fall is a topic among many. And this makes it a bit difficult to simply ask about falls. That is of course a topic. When I then talk to home care, it's a topic, how can you support. And in the palliative situation, of course, the patient is even worse 'weighed up' [. . .], do you need a round table with the relatives, for example? This is about bringing all professional groups together at one table. Why we don't do that is also the time. A round table is simply very time-consuming. It needs all the players, and you can only do that in individual cases." (Region6_P2)

The health care providers in the comparison regions also report existing networking and cooperation structures. They originate in other areas of health care, such as neurology or palliative care. These structures benefit the purpose of fall prevention. Cooperation usually refers to an exchange of information, which can take place orally at a round table, by telephone, in writing by e-mail, or in the form of reports. However, it is reported to not take place regularly or systematically and is still not paid or reimbursed by the Swiss health care system.

"There is little cooperation, and in most cases, this is an exchange of information but not effective cooperation. So, the information about medication, about diagnosis list, like for example with Parkinson's [disease], which also per se in the diagnosis contains a fall potential, or that one has prescribed physical therapy for this or that." (Region6_P2)

"No, and it's more for patients, too, in the palliative situation. So, it is not primarily about falls. But the round tables are rather for the overall situation: Is it still possible at home, what can you do with home care? And then the risk of falling is perhaps a sub-theme. […]. But there is practically no effective, coordinated cooperation only about falls." (Region6_P2)

3.2.2. Facilitators

In contrast, continuous training measures had a positive effect on networking and thus on cooperation between the actors in the pilot regions.

"You then get to know the people who work in the same city, in the same place. So, I felt that this was very positive […] and the exchange can take place." (Region3_P2)

"I think it's very important to bring everyone to one table so that the network can develop. And this is only possible through personal contacts, […] then it is easier to make contact. It is always positive to meet people from other professions not only for fall prevention. This also has positive effects on other things. If you know the people personally, then the threshold is lower to call or ask." (Region2_P1)

"It's always good to know the people [health care professionals] who are in contact with the general practitioner." (Region2_P4)

Personal contacts allowed removing interpersonal barriers, which facilitated queries and had a positive effect on the regional inter-professional cooperation. Specific details relevant to the health care provisioning can be exchanged more easily.

3.3. Cooperation between the Health Care Providers

3.3.1. Barriers

In one of the pilot regions, the project has led to little noticeable change from the point of view of doctors and occupational therapists. Nevertheless, contact was facilitated:

"We now know each other's face and thus the threshold for a telephone call is lowered." (Region3_P3)

In another pilot region, the project has hardly brought about any changes in the day-to-day practice of doctors, albeit in feedback. The cooperation with the core actors (physiotherapy, occupational therapy, hospital, and home care) has remained the same. However, the involvement of the optician has been positive and thus an increase in inter-professional collaboration is discernible.

"I have made positive experiences concerning the cooperation with the general practitioners, just by sending the registration form and the prescription actually came back, otherwise with the other instances [health care providers] the networking, at least in my environment, has not taken place." (Region3_P3)

In the comparison regions, the cooperation between the health care providers revealed a similar pattern as in the pilot regions. Certain professions are in closer contact with each other than others, such as physicians and physical therapists, or physicians and home care providers.

"Physical therapists who go home. We now also have occupational therapy in the region, which I have also referred patients to in rare cases. First and foremost, physical therapy and home care." (Region5_P5)

"We have very little contact with occupational therapy etc. We have now for the first time, the [nonprofit organization in health care] has now made such a campaign, where they offer inexpensive fall prevention measures. And there we came into contact for the first time." (Region6_P3)

3.3.2. Facilitators

In some of the pilot regions, the interprofessional fall prevention was assessed more positively.

"It has been interesting, watching different foci. And it certainly contributed positively to the cooperation." (Region2_P1)

Certain health care providers work more closely together, such as physicians and physical therapy, or physicians and home care. First networks are growing.

"That's why only [home care] and general practitioners work interprofessional now. So, we know from each other, and everyone has his share of what he perceives, but overall, the topic of fall prevention is still less important that other topics." (Region3_P4)

Case-related exchange and interprofessional cooperation are fostered by spatial proximity, for instance by being in the same village or in the same building. Here, group medical practices have an advantage over individual medical practices in using this potential for cooperation. An occupational therapist from a comparison region states:

"When patients come to us and they need physical and occupational therapists, they usually have both. This means that I am not at all in need of finding the telephone number of another physical therapist." (Occupational therapy_P4)

Coordinated communication between the health care providers is highly important. Tools such as the registration form, for instance, had a positive effect on collaboration between the general practitioners and the physical therapists, leading to prescriptions and follow-up prescriptions.

3.4. Case-Related Cooperation

3.4.1. Barriers

Skeptical assessments of case-related cooperation and networking have become apparent, which relate to existing framework conditions and the available time resources. The actors expressed the need for exchange:

"The physical therapist or even the general practitioner simply have no time, or rarely, to seek exchange. In their professional environment, where in both professions almost every tenth min has to be accounted for, I don't think that [cooperation] has much room." (Region3_P2)

"Not much has changed, we have always had a good cooperation between physical therapy, occupational therapy, hospital, home care and ourselves [. . .] If possible, we should prefer to do something electronically. The time resources of all participants are limited." (Region2_P5)

"Home care, we are dependent on working together with others. General practitioners prescribe home care, but general practitioners do not seek this form of interdisciplinary cooperation. It is a historical structure. This hierarchical thinking is certainly a hindrance. The only thing where this begins to dissolve is in palliative care, where general practitioners or doctors and nurses in psychiatry are dependent on each other. Is there an exchange [. . .], which significantly increases patient satisfaction and improves care when working together on an interdisciplinary basis? But there is little time for this." (Region3_P6)

3.4.2. Facilitators

However, there are also positive experiences with case-related cooperation. Case-related exchange between physical and occupational therapy is sometimes created without being explicitly triggered by fall prevention.

"The cooperation with physical therapists and occupational therapists is not structured at all. But we know that there are some [health care providers] who make similar efforts." (Region3_P6)

3.5. Continuous Training Measures

Most of the participants in the pilot regions responded positively to the continuous education training courses on fall prevention. The main reasons were that they enabled health care professionals to get to know each other and to establish networks. In addition, the courses employed an interdisciplinary approach to fall prevention.

3.5.1. Barriers

However, the continuous trainings offered only limited space to break down barriers for future collaboration or interprofessional exchange.

"I missed this opportunity to use it for an interdisciplinary meeting. They were physiotherapists and occupational therapists. But there was no moment when one could have exchanged ideas. I have already reported this." (Region3_P6)

In the comparison regions, continuing training about fall prevention was offered to individual professional groups in the past, for example in physiotherapy. Interprofessional continuing trainings were rarely attended.

"One could certainly do [interprofessional continuous training] on the field of fall prevention. But sometimes interprofessional continuous training is really difficult, because health care professionals bring along different conditions and have different needs." (Region6_P2)

3.5.2. Facilitators

Continuous training measures in the pilot regions had a positive effect on the cooperation between health care providers in these regions. Personal contact, getting to know each other, and the removal of barriers to making contact for queries facilitated interprofessional collaboration.

"You then get to know the people who work in the same city, in the same place. Well, I found that very positive […] and the exchange can take place." (Region3_P2)

"I think it's very important to bring everyone together at one table so that the network can develop. And this is only possible through personal contacts, if you know who is behind it, it is easier to make contact. It is always positive to meet people from other professions not only for fall prevention. This also has positive effects on other things. If you know the people personally, then the threshold to call or ask is lower." (Region2_P1)

"It's always good to know the people who have to do with the general practitioner and physical therapy is also a topic that runs parallel where [the home care organization] doesn't notice anything." (Region2_P4)

Content-related aspects that were perceived positively by the participants were:

"Positive impressions of the continuous training, which was simply clearly practice-oriented and caused aha-effects with the employees." (Region3_P6)

"Also, different workshops. One was with the optician, so this self-awareness, what it can mean with bad visibility, what effects it can have. That has already triggered something." (Region2_P4)

In conclusion, we can maintain that the qualitative interviews provide in-depth insights about the desirability of cooperation and obstacles in the feasibility of interprofessional collaboration in fall prevention. Our analysis highlights that cooperation between certain occupational groups—e.g., for all professions with home care has improved, whereas for others not much has changed through the project—e.g., between general practitioners and physical therapists.

4. Discussion

The present article aimed to explore how health care providers involved in a pilot project evaluate the impact of the project on the effectiveness of fall prevention in older adults in Switzerland regarding facilitators and barriers of interprofessional collaboration for building a professional network. Our study contributes to the literature by providing evidence on interprofessional collaboration in fall prevention, a field of study that has received little attention in Switzerland.

Three statements were evaluated as particularly relevant by most health professionals: First, interprofessional continuous trainings were highly appreciated. On the one hand, the trainings allowed health professionals to establish relevant networks. On the other hand, health professionals perceived improved quality of care due to an interdisciplinary approach to fall prevention. These findings are in line with previous research from the United States that emphasized how interprofessional education improved fall prevention by expanding health professional's disciplinary view and by improving communication between the disciplines [37,38].

Second, interprofessional collaboration was rated as resource intensive. To foster interprofessional collaboration in fall prevention, more time, financial resources, and/or more health care providers are needed. Previous research shows that a lack of human resources and financial compensation constitute serious barriers to interprofessional fall prevention programs [39–41]. A study from Switzerland highlighted that in the outpatient setting, remuneration for some tasks in interprofessional collaboration is provided only for some but not all health care professionals [39].

Third, defining the roles of health care professionals was evaluated as a major challenge for successful interprofessional fall prevention. These findings complement earlier research [38,39,42]. For instance, a study from Australia that was carried out in a similar setting as our study showed that overlapping roles led to a sense of competition and even rivalry between the professionals rather than to improved interprofessional collaboration, particularly if they competed for business [42].

Limitations

First, the present study employed a post hoc design, in which interviews in comparison regions served to provide insights into how the actual fall prevention practice in pilot regions might differ. However, this design does not allow drawing strong conclusions about the size and causality of the observed differences and similarities. Second, the small number of interviews and focus groups prevented the qualitative analyses form attaining a high level of saturation, in which the content and structure derived from earlier interviews and focus groups would have been confirmed and no new arguments were added by the later interviews and focus groups. The first and second limitations both may lead to results affected by information bias. Information bias arises if the data collected systematically deviate from the truth [43,44]. Such bias may be present in our data in particular for two reasons. First, respondents of the pilot study may have had an interest to report their work in a more positive light than they experienced because they may feel responsible for the implementation of the pilot project and interested in the continuation of the project. Second, participants in the focus group may have mutually influenced each other. The first source of bias was addressed in our study by using a control group. The second source of bias was partially addressed by using individual interviews.

A third limitation of the project was that the fall prevention pilot project was implemented in regions that had already pre-existing interprofessional networks. Thus, the transferability to other regions might be limited such that the implementation of the pilot project in regions without such interprofessional networks might turn out to be more difficult. In general, it should be noted that all interviews were conducted in the German-speaking regions of Switzerland and the results are not easily transferable to the French and Italian-speaking regions of Switzerland. A final limitation of the project is that the data stems from 2017 and is thus not very recent. Nevertheless, we consider our study as an important contribution to the field of fall prevention in Switzerland for two reasons. First, falls constitute the deadliest cause of all non-occupational injuries in Switzerland [45]. There is thus a need to better understand how fall prevention may be best addressed. Second, to our knowledge, besides one other project [46], the pilot project studied here is one of the only fall prevention programs that has been evaluated recently. In contrast to the other project mentioned, our study includes a control group (i.e., health professionals in the control regions) which allows to better capture a potential causal effect of the fall prevention program. Our study therefore fills a gap in the knowledge on fall prevention in the Swiss context.

5. Conclusions

With the increasing number of older adults in Switzerland as well as the continuously increasing life expectancy, the incident rates of falls are likely to increase. Given the often-severe consequences of falls in terms of individuals' health, fall prevention is a central topic from a health care as well as a health economic perspective. Although there is evidence on a micro and meso level demonstrating that fall prevention measures can improve older adults' health, quality of life, and independence, there is the need to complement these advances by improving the interprofessional collaboration in fall prevention on the macro level in the sense of public health policy.

Author Contributions: F.W. was the principal investigator of the study including funding acquisition, project administration, and supervision. I.B., T.V. and P.R. were substantially involved in the conceptualization and study design. I.B., F.W. and A.G. collected the data and drafted the present paper. A.G. designed the qualitative study and carried out the qualitative content analysis of interviews. F.W. carried out the quantitative data analysis. T.V. and P.R. made substantial comments on the content of this manuscript. All authors have read and agreed to the published version of the manuscript.

Funding: The evaluation of the fall prevention program was funded by the foundation GESUND-HEITSFÖRDERUNG SCHWEIZ, grant number 16.113, K40201.

Institutional Review Board Statement: Ethical review and approval were waived for this study as the data collected do not include health-related information about the participants.

Informed Consent Statement: The study participants were informed about the study and had the right to withdraw their participation at any time. They consented to participate by means of a signed form of informed consent.

Data Availability Statement: Requests to access the data can be addressed to ZHAW and Gesundheitsförderung Schweiz.

Acknowledgments: First of all, we are very grateful to all health care providers who took part in our interviews. Second, we would like to thank Tobias Imobersteg and Aro Deparente for their research assistance and Christoph Bauer, Andrea Koppitz, and Silke Neumann for their comments on the interview guideline. Third, we thank Lisa Guggenbühl, Doris Wiegand, and Günter Ackermann from "Gesundheitsförderung Schweiz" for their helpful feedback on an earlier draft of this manuscript. Finally, we would like to thank Andy Biedermann und Flavia Bürgi from Public Health Services, who developed the fall prevention pilot project, for their collaboration.

Conflicts of Interest: The authors declare that they have no competing and conflict of interest.

References

1. Gillespie, L.D.; Robertson, M.C.; Gillespie, W.J.; Sherrington, C.; Gates, S.; Clemson, L.M.; Lamb, S.E. Interventions for Preventing Falls in Older People Living in the Community (Review). *Cochrane Database Syst. Rev.* **2012**, *2012*, CD007146. [CrossRef]
2. Gschwind, Y.J.; Pfenninger, B. *Training Zur Sturzprävention*; Bfu—Beratungsstelle für Unfallverhütung: Bern, Switzerland, 2016.
3. Sattin, R.W. Falls among Older Persons: A Public Health Perspective. *Annu. Rev. Public Health* **1992**, *13*, 489–508. [CrossRef] [PubMed]
4. Chien, M.-H.; Guo, H.-R. Nutritional Status and Falls in Community-Dwelling Older People: A Longitudinal Study of a Population-Based Random Sample. *PLoS ONE* **2014**, *9*, e91044. [CrossRef] [PubMed]
5. Härlein, J.; Halfens, R.J.G.; Dassen, T.; Lahmann, N.A. Falls in Older Hospital Inpatients and the Effect of Cognitive Impairment: A Secondary Analysis of Prevalence Studies. *J. Clin. Nurs.* **2011**, *20*, 175–183. [CrossRef]
6. Muir, S.W.; Gopaul, K.; Montero Odasso, M.M. The Role of Cognitive Impairment in Fall Risk among Older Adults: A Systematic Review and Meta-Analysis. *Age Ageing* **2012**, *41*, 299–308. [CrossRef]
7. Baixinho, C.L.; Madeira, C.; Alves, S.; Henriques, M.A.; Dixe, A. Falls and Preventive Practices among Institutionalized Older People. *Int. J. Environ. Res. Public Health* **2022**, *19*, 7577. [CrossRef]
8. Chen, X.; Van Nguyen, H.; Shen, Q.; Chan, D.K.Y. Characteristics Associated with Recurrent Falls among the Elderly within Aged-Care Wards in a Tertiary Hospital: The Effect of Cognitive Impairment. *Arch. Gerontol. Geriatr.* **2011**, *53*, 2009–2012. [CrossRef]
9. Mirelman, A.; Herman, T.; Brozgol, M.; Dorfman, M.; Sprecher, E.; Schweiger, A.; Giladi, N.; Hausdorff, J.M. Executive Function and Falls in Older Adults: New Findings from a Five-Year Prospective Study Link Fall Risk to Cognition. *PLoS ONE* **2012**, *7*, e40297. [CrossRef]
10. Campbell, A.J.; Borrie, M.J.; Spears, G.F. Risk Factors for Falls in a Community-Based Prospective Study of People 70 Years and Older. *J. Gerontol.* **1989**, *44*, M112–M117. [CrossRef]
11. Oliver, D.; Daly, F.; Martin, F.C.; McMurdo, M.E.T. Risk Factors and Risk Assessment Tools for Falls in Hospital In-Patients: A Systematic Review. *Age Ageing* **2004**, *33*, 122–130. [CrossRef]
12. Müller, C.; Lautenschläger, S.; Voigt-Radloff, S. Potential Analysis for Research on Occupational Therapy-Led Physical Exercise Programmes and Home Environment Adaptation Programmes to Prevent Falls for Elderly People Living at Home. *Int. J. Health Prof.* **2016**, *3*, 85–106. [CrossRef]
13. Sherrington, C.; Lord, S.R.; Herbert, R.D. A Randomized Controlled Trial of Weight-Bearing versus Non-Weight-Bearing Exercise for Improving Physical Ability after Usual Care for Hip Fracture. *Arch. Phys. Med. Rehabil.* **2004**, *85*, 710–716. [CrossRef]
14. Rosie, J.; Taylor, D. Sit-to-Stand as Home Exercise for Mobility-Limited Adults over 80 Years of Age-GrandStand System™ May Keep You Standing? *Age Ageing* **2007**, *36*, 555–562. [CrossRef] [PubMed]
15. Chou, W.C.; Tinetti, M.E.; King, M.B.; Irwin, K.; Fortinsky, R.H. Perceptions of Physicians on the Barriers and Facilitators to Integrating Fall Risk Evaluation and Management into Practice. *J. Gen. Intern. Med.* **2006**, *21*, 117–122. [CrossRef] [PubMed]
16. Loganathan, A.; Ng, C.J.; Tan, M.P.; Low, W.Y. Barriers Faced by Healthcare Professionals When Managing Falls in Older People in Kuala Lumpur, Malaysia: A Qualitative Study. *BMJ Open* **2015**, *5*, e008460. [CrossRef] [PubMed]
17. Gougeon, L.; Johnson, J.; Morse, H. Interprofessional Collaboration in Health Care Teams for the Maintenance of Community-Dwelling Seniors' Health and Well-Being in Canada: A Systematic Review of Trials. *J. Interprofessional Educ. Pract.* **2017**, *7*, 29–37. [CrossRef]
18. Zwarenstein, M.; Reeves, S. Knowledge Translation and Interprofessional Collaboration: Where the Rubber of Evidence-Based Care Hits the Road of Teamwork. *J. Contin. Educ. Health Prof.* **2006**, *26*, 46–54. [CrossRef]
19. Child, S.; Goodwin, V.; Garside, R.; Jones-Hughes, T.; Boddy, K.; Stein, K. Factors Influencing the Implementation of Fall-Prevention Programmes: A Systematic Review and Synthesis of Qualitative Studies. *Implement. Sci.* **2012**, *7*, 1–14. [CrossRef]
20. Baxter, P.; Markle-Reid, M. An Interprofessional Team Approach to Fall Prevention for Older Home Care Clients "at Risk" of Falling: Health Care Providers Share Their Experiences. *Int. J. Integr. Care* **2009**, *9*, 1568–4156. [CrossRef]
21. King, N.; Ross, A. Professional Identities and Interprofessional Relations: Evaluation of Collaborative Community Schemes. *Soc. Work Health Care* **2003**, *38*, 51–72. [CrossRef]
22. Wright, B.A. Behavior Diagnoses by a Multidisciplinary Team. *Geriatr. Nurs.* **1993**, *14*, 30–35. [CrossRef]
23. Légaré, F.; Stacey, D.; Brière, N.; Fraser, K.; Desroches, S.; Dumont, S.; Sales, A.; Puma, C.; Aubé, D. Healthcare Providers' Intentions to Engage in an Interprofessional Approach to Shared Decision-Making in Home Care Programs: A Mixed Methods Study. *J. Interprof. Care* **2013**, *27*, 214–222. [CrossRef] [PubMed]
24. Atwal, A.; Caldwell, K. Do Multidisciplinary Integrated Care Pathways Improve Interprofessional Collaboration? *Scand. J. Caring Sci.* **2002**, *16*, 360–367. [CrossRef] [PubMed]
25. Metzelthin, S.F.; Daniëls, R.; van Rossum, E.; Cox, K.; Habets, H.; de Witte, L.P.; Kempen, G.I.J.M. A Nurse-Led Interdisciplinary Primary Care Approach to Prevent Disability among Community-Dwelling Frail Older People: A Large-Scale Process Evaluation. *Int. J. Nurs. Stud.* **2013**, *50*, 1184–1196. [CrossRef] [PubMed]
26. Van Dongen, J.J.J.; Van Bokhoven, M.A.; Daniëls, R.; Van Der Weijden, T.; Emonts, W.W.G.P.; Beurskens, A. Developing Interprofessional Care Plans in Chronic Care: A Scoping Review. *BMC Fam. Pract.* **2016**, *17*, 137. [CrossRef]
27. Bokhour, B.G. Communication in Interdisciplinary Team Meetings: What Are We Talking About? *J. Interprofessional Care* **2006**, *20*, 349–363. [CrossRef]

28. Molyneux, J. Interprofessional Team Working: What Makes Teams Work Well? *J. Interprofessional Care* **2001**, *15*, 29–35. [CrossRef]
29. Clausen, C.; Strohschein, F.J.; Faremo, S.; Batemans, D.; Posel, N.; Fleiszer, D.M. Developing an Interprofessional Care Plan for an Older Adult Woman with Breast Cancer: From Multiple Voices to a Shared Vision. *Clin. J. Oncol. Nurs.* **2012**, *16*, E18–E26. [CrossRef]
30. Münzer, T.; Gnädinger, M. Erfassung Des Sturzrisikos Und Sturzprävention in Der Hausarztpraxis. *Schweiz Med Forum* **2014**, *14*, 857–861. [CrossRef]
31. Wieber, F.; Baumann, I.; Glässel, A.; Volken, T.; Rüesch, P. *Evaluation Via-Pilotprojekt Sturzprävention. Schlussbericht*; Gesundheitsförderung Schweiz: Bern, Switzerland, 2017.
32. Mays, N.; Pope, C. Assessing Quality in Qualitative Research. *Br. Med. J.* **2000**, *320*, 50–52. [CrossRef]
33. Flick, U. *An Introduction to Qualitative Research*; Sage: Southend Oaks, CA, USA, 2009.
34. Giacomini, M.K.; Cook, D.J. Users' Guides to the Medical Literature: XXIII. Qualitative Research in Health Care A. Are the Results of the Study Valid? *J. Am. Med. Assoc.* **2000**, *284*, 357–362. [CrossRef] [PubMed]
35. Dresing, T.; Pehl, T. *Praxisbuch Interview, Transkription & Analyse. Anleitungen Und Regelsysteme Für Qualitativ Forschende*, 8th ed.; Eigenverlag: Marburg, Germany, 2018.
36. Mayring, P. Qualitative Content Analysis. *Forum Qual. Soc. Res.* **2000**, *1*, 1–10. [CrossRef]
37. Waters, L.; Marrs, S.A.; Tompkins, C.J.; Fix, R.; Finucane, S.; Coogle, C.L.; Grunden, K.; Ihara, E.S.; McIntyre, M.; Parsons, P.; et al. Creating Interprofessional Readiness to Advance Age-Friendly U.S. Healthcare. *Int. J. Environ. Res. Public Health* **2022**, *19*, 5258. [CrossRef] [PubMed]
38. Ostertag, S.; Bosic-Reiniger, J.; Migliaccio, C.; Zins, R. Promoting Older Adult Health with Interprofessional Education through Community Based Health Screening. *Int. J. Environ. Res. Public Health* **2022**, *19*, 6513. [CrossRef]
39. Schmid, F.; Rogan, S.; Glässel, A. A Swiss Health Care Professionals' Perspective on the Meaning of Interprofessional Collaboration in Health Care of People with Ms—A Focus Group Study. *Int. J. Environ. Res. Public Health* **2021**, *18*, 6537. [CrossRef]
40. Nilsen, P.; Timpka, T.; Nordenfelt, L.; Lindqvist, K. Towards Improved Understanding of Injury Prevention Program Sustainability. *Saf. Sci.* **2005**, *43*, 815–833. [CrossRef]
41. Hanson, H.M.; Salmoni, A.W. Stakeholders' Perceptions of Programme Sustainability: Findings from a Community-Based Fall Prevention Programme. *Public Health* **2011**, *125*, 525–532. [CrossRef]
42. Liddle, J.; Lovarini, M.; Clemson, L.; Mackenzie, L.; Tan, A.; Pit, S.W.; Poulos, R.; Tiedemann, A.; Sherrington, C.; Roberts, C.; et al. Making Fall Prevention Routine in Primary Care Practice: Perspectives of Allied Health Professionals. *BMC Health Serv. Res.* **2018**, *18*, 598. [CrossRef]
43. Shahar, E.; Shahar, D.J. On the Causal Structure of Information Bias and Confounding Bias in Randomized Trials. *J. Eval. Clin. Pract.* **2009**, *15*, 1214–1216. [CrossRef]
44. Doidge, J.C.; Harron, K.L. Reflections on Modern Methods: Linkage Error Bias. *Int. J. Epidemiol.* **2019**, *48*, 2050–2060. [CrossRef]
45. Beratungsstelle für Unfallverhütung Statistik Der Nichtberufsunfälle Und Des Sicherheitsniveaus in Der Schweiz. Status. 2019. Available online: https://www.bfu.ch/de/die-bfu/medien/statistik-der-nichtberufsunfaelle-2020 (accessed on 4 August 2022).
46. Rheumaliga. *Abschlussbericht–Wirksamkeit Des Sturzpräventionsprogramms «Sicher Durch Den Alltag» 2016–2020*; Rheumaliga Schweiz: Zurich, Switzerland, 2021.

MDPI
St. Alban-Anlage 66
4052 Basel
Switzerland
Tel. +41 61 683 77 34
Fax +41 61 302 89 18
www.mdpi.com

International Journal of Environmental Research and Public Health Editorial Office
E-mail: ijerph@mdpi.com
www.mdpi.com/journal/ijerph

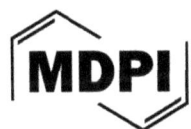

www.ingramcontent.com/pod-product-compliance
Lightning Source LLC
La Vergne TN
LVHW070243100526
838202LV00015B/2169